OFFICE GYNECOLOGY

OFFICE GYNECOLOGY

Second Edition

Morton A. Stenchever, M.D.
Professor and Chairman
Department of Obstetrics and Gynecology
University of Washington School of Medicine
Seattle, Washington

with 176 illustrations

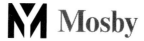 Mosby

St. Louis Baltimore Boston Carlsbad Chicago Naples New York Philadelphia Portland
London Madrid Mexico City Singapore Sydney Tokyo Toronto Wiesbaden

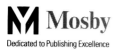

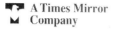

Publisher: Anne S. Patterson
Editor: Susie Baxter
Developmental Editor: Anne Gunter
Project Manager: Linda McKinley
Designer: Liz Young
Production Editor: Paul Stoecklein

Second Edition

Printed in the United States of America

Mosby-Year Book, Inc.
11830 Westline Industrial Drive
St. Louis, Missouri 63146

Library of Congress Cataloging-in-Publication Data

Office gynecology / [edited by] Morton A. Stenchever. – 2nd ed.
    p.   cm.
    Includes bibliographical references and index.
    ISBN 0-8151-8225-2
    1. Gynecology.   I. Stenchever, Morton A.
    [DNLM: 1. Genital Diseases, Female.   WP 140 0324 1996]
  RG101.033   1996
  618.1 – dc20
  DNLM/DLC
  for Library of Congress   96-7317
                                                   CIP

96 97 98 99 00 / 9 8 7 6 5 4 3 2 1

To my wife, *Diane*

Contributors

David M. Barton, M.D., P.A.
Clinical Professor
Department of Obstetrics and Gynecology
University of Washington School of
  Medicine
WAMI Program
Boise, Idaho

Joanna M. Cain, M.D.
Professor and Chair
Department of Obstetrics and Gynecology
Penn State University School of Medicine
Henley, Pennsylvania

Deborah J. Dotters, M.D.
Associate Professor
Division of Gynecologic Oncology
Department of Obstetrics and Gynecology
University of North Carolina School of
  Medicine
Chapel Hill, North Carolina

William Droegemueller, M.D.
Robert A. Ross Distinguished Professor and
  Chairman
Department of Obstetrics and Gynecology
University of North Carolina School of
  Medicine
Chapel Hill, North Carolina

David A. Eschenbach, M.D.
Professor
Department of Obstetrics and Gynecology
University of Washington School of
  Medicine
Seattle, Washington

Gretchen M. Lentz, M.D.
Assistant Professor
Department of Obstetrics and Gynecology
University of Washington School of
  Medicine
Seattle, Washington

Roger E. Moe, M.D.
Professor and Director
Breast Cancer Program
Department of Surgery
University of Washington School of
  Medicine
Seattle, Washington

Kamran S. Moghissi, M.D.
Professor
Department of Obstetrics and Gynecology
Wayne State University School of Medicine
Detroit, Michigan

Donald E. Moore, M.D.
Associate Professor
Department of Obstetrics and Gynecology
University of Washington School of
  Medicine
Seattle, Washington

Susan F. Pokorny, M.D.
Assistant Professor
Department of Obstetrics and Gynecology
  and Pediatrics
Baylor College of Medicine
Houston, Texas

Robert F. Porges, M.D.
Professor and Vice Chairman
Department of Obstetrics and Gynecology
New York University School of Medicine
New York, New York

Barbara J. Roberts
Office Manager
Boise, Idaho

Kirk K. Shy, M.D.
Professor
Department of Obstetrics and Gynecology
University of Washington School of
  Medicine
Seattle, Washington

Richard M. Soderstrom, M.D.
Clinical Professor
Department of Obstetrics and Gynecology
University of Washington School of
  Medicine
Seattle, Washington

Michael R. Soules, M.D.
Professor
Department of Obstetrics and Gynecology
Director
Division of Reproductive Endocrinology
  and Infertility
University of Washington School of
  Medicine
Seattle, Washington

John F. Steege, M.D.
Professor
Department of Obstetrics and Gynecology
University of North Carolina School of
  Medicine
Chapel Hill, North Carolina

Diane H. Stenchever, M.S.W.
Marriage Counselor
Mercer Island, Washington

Morton A. Stenchever, M.D.
Professor and Chairman
Department of Obstetrics and Gynecology
University of Washington School of
  Medicine
Seattle, Washington

Hisham K. Tamimi, M.D.
Professor
Division of Gynecologic Oncology
Department of Obstetrics and Gynecology
University of Washington School of
  Medicine
Seattle, Washington

Jane L. Vollmer
Business Manager
Boise, Idaho

Louis A. Vontver, M.D.
Professor
Department of Obstetrics and Gynecology
University of Washington School of
  Medicine
Seattle, Washington

Pål Wølner-Hanseen, M.D., D.M.S.
Associate Professor
Department of Obstetrics and Gynecology
University of Lund
Lund, Sweden

Paul W. Zarutskie, M.D.
Department of Obstetrics and Gynecology
Mission Hospital
Mission Viejo, California

Preface

A great many changes have taken place in the practice of gynecology during the past few decades. These include changes in patient expectations, technologic advances, and economic and social changes.

Patient expectations and increasing competition among various health-care providers for consumer's business have made it more essential that the office environment be pleasant and the physician and office staff be continuously mindful of the patient's emotional and physical needs. The requirements of insurance carriers and regulatory agencies and the need to seriously address medicolegal considerations make it essential that the office be managed intelligently and efficiently.

Technological advances during the past two decades have been numerous. Essentially, they have made it possible to perform more services for the gynecologic patient in the office, in many instances reducing the need for hospitalizations. Colposcopy and directed biopsy have frequently replaced the need for cone biopsies of the cervix, and endometrial biopsies for endometrial sampling have been demonstrated to be as effective as D & Cs in most cases. Cryocautery, electrocautery procedures (such as LEEP), D & Cs, and, in some instances, hysteroscopy and laparoscopy can be performed in the office setting. Many other procedures can be performed in an outpatient surgery suite, thereby removing the necessity for hospitalization. Many outpatient surgical facilities are built in or near buildings where physicians practice.

In addition, due to social changes that have occurred in the last few decades, physicians must make a greater effort to offer individualized care to each patient within the context of her physical, emotional, and social needs. Physicians and their office staff must become more acquainted with these aspects of patient care in order to take a holistic approach with patients rather than a defined, specialty-oriented one.

This book offers information that not only helps the physician and staff design his/her office appropriately for the modern practice of women's health care, but also provides the most up to date information on each of the subjects that can be adequately dealt with in an office setting. Each contributor is a subject expert in his or her own right. It is my hope that the cumulative effect will be to give the physician information and suggestions to achieve a medically-excellent, environmentally-pleasant, and enjoyable office practice that will benefit the health and well-being of the patient.

Morton A. Stenchever

Contents

PART ONE

OFFICE ORGANIZATION AND GENERAL PATIENT EVALUATION AND CARE

CHAPTER 1

Office Organization

DAVID M. BARTON
BARBARA J. ROBERTS
JANE L. VOLLMER

Good business management is essential to a good medical practice. If the business side of a clinic is neglected and financial difficulties occur, the quality of medical care provided to patients will decline. With a competitive medical practice environment and an increasing number of government regulations, optimal office efficiency is needed.

There are many facets involved in organizing and managing of a medical office. It is virtually impossible to cover all aspects in one chapter. This chapter will acquaint you with the following areas of management:

- Physical organization of an office
- Automated medical office
- Personnel management
- Government regulations
- Business insurance requirements
- Managed health care
- Retirement plans

PHYSICAL ORGANIZATION OF AN OFFICE

How many square feet do I need? What is the approximate cost? Should I own or lease? Where is the best location? What is a well-designed office?

Before these questions can be answered, short-term and long-term goals must be established. Some of the goals could be as follows:

- Number of physicians in the group now
- Number of physicians in the group in 5 to 10 years
- Number of ancillary employees (e.g., nurse practitioner, physician's assistant, ultrasound technician)
- Projected number of patients each physician will see in a day (i.e., style of practice)
- Number of employees required to support the number of physicians and ancillary personnel

The required size of the building varies, depending on specialty. Generally, primary-care physicians require 1000 to 1400 ft^2 per physician.

Parking Space

Several factors determine the size of the parking lot. Some of these factors are local building codes, number of physicians and employees, number of patients seen by each physician per hour, availability of public transportation, and on-time pattern of each physician. As an example, if you are a solo practitioner, with an average of 6 patients per hour and 4 employees, your parking lot should have 10 to 12 spaces: 6 spaces for patients, 4 for employees, 1 for the physician, and 1 for delivery of supplies.

Waiting Room/Reception Area

The reception area (waiting room) is the first area of your office a new patient will see. This area should be aesthetically pleasing to make a good first impression.

The size of the waiting room depends on the projected patient flow of each physician. Each seat in the waiting room requires approximately 12 to 15 ft^2. Durable, fabric-covered seats are more comfortable than vinyl. Reading material should be current, interesting, and varied. A telephone in the waiting room (restricted to local calls only, in a private setting, with a writing space) is a pleasant touch for professional patients.

A television and videocassette recorder (VCR) can also be in the waiting room. If patient education tapes are available for the VCR, it is recommended that an area be screened off and a headset provided for privacy for the patients.

Receptionist's Area

This area should be centrally located in the office complex to permit the receptionist to have visual access to all patients in the waiting room. It is recommended that a "hello and good-bye" area be provided for patients: in other words, one area with one employee to greet patients and another private area with a different employee to collect payments after the patient has completed the visit.

A soundproof window at the front desk has varied opinions. Some space planners recommend this window to enable one employee to accomplish both the hello and good-bye tasks. Others feel that the window separates the receptionist from the patients and decreases the warm, caring attitude a receptionist should project.

The patient's charts should be filed in an open-shelf filing system with covers to pull down at night. The covers provide some protection for patient's charts in case of fire or activation of the sprinkling system. The files should be located for easy access by the receptionist. Adequate space should be provided in front of the filing system to permit good traffic flow and multiple employee use.

The number of telephone lines required depends on patient volume. A peak-hours study should be scheduled periodically with the telephone company to determine whether you are having a busy-signal problem and are subsequently losing calls. An appointment telephone number, bookkeeping and insurance telephone number, and perhaps a medical questions telephone number should be listed in the telephone directory and printed on stationery, statements, appointment cards, new patient brochures, and so on. This will distribute calls to appropriate employees. It is impossible for one person to answer more than three lines and accomplish any other tasks.

Examination Rooms and Procedure Rooms

The number of examination rooms needed should be determined by the number of patient visits per hour. Usually, three examination rooms per physician and a shared procedure room accommodate good patient flow.

The size of the examination rooms depends on the style of practice but should be large enough to be comfortable in when moving around the examination table. As for style of practice, do you always have a nurse accompany you? Will you dictate progress notes in the examination room with the patient present? Will you dictate in your office or at a station in the hallway? Will you use a script or scriber (an employee in the examination room who is writing as the physician discusses the examination with the patient) for progress notes?

Most items needed in the examination room should be within 40 inches of the physician at work. The examination table should be placed diagonally in the room, with the patient facing away from the entry door.

The room should be soundproof. No sinks, electric plugs, or vents should be installed back-to-back between examination rooms. Background music with a volume control in each examination room can also provide privacy. The volume can be decreased before discussion and examination of the patient.

The size of the procedure room is determined by the type of in-office procedures performed; for example, ultrasound, in-office dilation and curettage (D & C), colposcopies, and hysteroscopies. New technology, government regulations, and third-party (insurance company) requirements will increase the types of procedures performed in-office in the future. Plan for room to grow.

Laboratory

The size of the laboratory depends on the kind of tests performed, number of personnel, storage space requirements, and equipment needed. Depending on the amount of equipment needed, plan on providing 145 to 250 ft^2 per technician. The lab should be centrally located in the back office area with easy access from different directions. Toilet facilities with pass-through provisions increase the comfort level of patients.

Consulting Room/Physician's Office

The physician's office should reflect the physician's personality and taste. It should be roomy but not spacious (10×10 ft to 12×15 ft). The physician should be comfortable in this room. A nonclinical surrounding for good physician-patient relationship should be provided.

Nurses' Stations

Nurses' stations should be installed in the back office area. Usually they are insets in the hallways with rotating stools. The stools can be pulled out when in use and returned under the work area when not in use. The station should have adequate writing and storage space and a telephone.

Business Office

The first employee requires 175 ft². Each additional employee requires 75 to 80 ft². How many employees are needed? National surveys indicate that this varies, depending on specialty. An obstetrics and gynecology (ob/gyn) physician generally requires from 3.5 to 4.5 full-time equivalent employees per full-time physician. This number has increased in the last 5 to 10 years because of increased government and insurance companies' regulations. Some space planners recommend that desks be used rather than built-in workstations. Desks can be moved as required with increased patient volume and increased number of employees.

Adequate space and ventilation must be provided for computer equipment.

Hallways

Hallways should be wide enough to permit two people to pass comfortably, preferably 5 feet wide. You must also adhere to local and state building codes.

Conference Room

A conference room (multiple-use area) for staff meetings, medical and business library, employee break area, and so forth enhances the physician's and employee's job satisfaction. The size of this room is determined by the number of physicians and size of the staff.

Summary

One of the most important factors in planning office space is to project growth. This can be accomplished by purchasing enough land to permit growth of the building, constructing the building in such a manner that additional floors can be added later, or purchasing or leasing condominium office space with adjacent vacant space and an option to purchase or lease.

AUTOMATED MEDICAL OFFICE

What are the computer software and hardware needs for a medical office? The following criteria must be established to effectively evaluate the numerous programs available:

- Determine the volume of your practice.
- Select the functions you wish a computer system to perform.
- Calculate the cost.

To assist in determining whether the volume of your practice warrants an automated system, some type of computer functions for the accounts receivable can be cost-effective for a physician seeing as few as 40 patients per week. However, if an office has 300 or fewer monthly transactions, the office may benefit from using a service bureau. A service bureau processes the office's charges and receipts. From these data, the bureau mails the office their accounts receivable status report, statements to mail to patients, insurance claim forms, and various management reports.

If the volume of transactions is greater than 300 per month, an in-house computer (a system that resides and is operated in the office) is warranted. If an in-house computer is the decision, the functions you wish a computer system to perform must be selected. A computer consultant may help you make this evaluation in a more efficient manner.

Some of the functions to consider are as follows:
- Accounts receivable
- Appointment scheduling
- General ledger
- Electronic insurance billing
- Accounts payable
- Payroll
- Medical records
- Research and continuing education

When the desired functions are determined, choose software that can achieve these functions and hardware that can run the chosen software.

Accounts Receivable

The accounts receivable software must be capable of generating monthly patient billing statements, electronic insurance claims, updated patient account status reports, patient recalls, and a wide range of practice and financial analysis reports. The analysis reports can be used in making management decisions. Reports of the number of diagnoses and procedures should also be available.

The program should provide effective password security and backup systems to protect the data. The data should be backed up (duplicated) and stored off-site at frequent, regular intervals. The software should have enough flexibility to support future growth and changes.

An automated recall system can enhance your medical care and provide a subtle marketing technique for an existing patient base. It can provide a way to monitor high-risk patients and at the same time promote preventive medicine.

Appointment Scheduling

One of the advantages of an automated appointment-scheduling system is the accessibility of this information from various locations within the office. A manual system is usually located at one area of the office, thus necessitating a call or trip to this area to obtain scheduling information.

The program should be user-friendly and should require a minimum amount of staff time when scheduling the appointment. The demographics can be updated at the time of the appointment. This program should permit the user to look up the appointment by patient name and provide the date and reason for the visit.

Flexible time slots and the ability to block out time for vacations and holidays, work in appointments, and search for the next available appointment must be accessible.

The day's schedule, the day's charge slips, and the day's collection management status report should automatically be printed.

A predetermined length of appointment should automatically be inserted when the code for the type of or reason for the appointment is keyed.

The program should permit quick new-patient registration, quick cancel and reschedule capability, automatic recall for missed appointments, and automatic cancellation of recall when the appointment is scheduled.

General Ledger, Accounts Payable, Payroll

General ledger, accounts payable, and payroll programs should be user-friendly and integrated (data can be passed from one program to another). This will decrease keying time and errors. Many statistical analysis reports are available from these programs. The program can have safeguards built in to deter fraudulent activity.

Automated Medical Records

As the trend continues toward increased quality assurance, increased regulations, and increased number of malpractice suits, the computerized medical record becomes more feasible. The paper chart has some limitations (e.g., poor accessibility), is often illegible, and is not always properly organized. Computerized medical records allow physicians to do research and quality assurance studies on a daily basis. A cost savings should be achieved by reducing personnel time spent pulling and filing charts.

How are medical progress notes input into the computer? Physicians can dictate progress notes or complete a brief, effectively formatted encounter form that is subsequently keyed in by a clerk. If the physician can type, a terminal can be installed in each examination room. Other data input can go directly into the patient's medical record from the source (laboratory results, letters to referring physicians, etc.).

When the patient is seen, the medical record is retrieved from the terminal in the examination room or a terminal built into the physician's desk. A variety of summary formats and flowcharts should be available to select from the computer menu.

Some ways of overcoming barriers of automated medical charts and human acceptance of computerization of medical records are increased trust in automated systems, involvement of physicians in system design, and increased education on computer capabilities. It is recommended that the computerized medical record be input simultaneously with the paper chart until all physicians and personnel feel comfortable with the system.

Research and Continuing Education

Research capabilities from the data input on each patient should be virtually unlimited. Diagnoses, procedures, ages, and demographic data can be retrieved based on criteria established for the research desired.

Continuing education can be provided by communicating with a variety of databases throughout the world. For example, you can obtain information on medical literature, travel information, and financial data (stocks and bonds); locate new software; and play games.

To communicate outside your office or home, you need a modem. A modem is identified by its transfer rate, the number of bits of information it can send per second. The average modem transfers 1200 to 2400 baud. The modem should be Hayes compatible. The modem is connected to a telephone line. This line can be a dedicated line (used only for computer communications), or a toggle switch can be installed on an existing line for multiple use.

A communications software program is needed to tell your modem what to do. There are a variety of programs available. The program should have a manual that will lead you step by step through installation and use.

Summary

The data entry functions of any program must be easily used by all personnel. The confidentiality and security provisions must include passwords. All data should be backed up on a regular basis. Reliable technical support should be quickly available for all software and hardware. The systems should be flexible, some fields of information should be capable of being customized to meet the special requirements of the practice, and the system should provide room for growth.

The hardware must be installed in a relatively dust-free room with adequate ventilation. A static-free mat should be provided for each terminal. The vendor for the programs must be prepared to train personnel off site and in office. The training should cover the intricacies of the program, familiarity of each component of the hardware, and the mechanics of the printers.

The programs and hardware should be covered by a warranty, with a maintenance contract available at the end of the warranty period.

PERSONNEL MANAGEMENT

Make your office a place where people want to work. Project an attitude that this office is a place where people not only work hard but also play hard. The climate of the office should be positive, congenial, and filled with laughter and project a sense of sincerely caring for each patient and each employee as individuals. An energetic sense of *esprit de corps* should be evident.

A medical clinic with a reputation of providing quality medical care not only has well-qualified, caring physicians, but also employs and retains caring employees. The employees must have effective people skills and the ability to effectively communicate with patients and perceive their needs and expectations. The chemistry of the clinic should project to patients that the physicians and employees work cohesively and effectively as a team.

How are these attitudes maintained with employees?

- Physicians' positive attitudes filter down through the ranks.
- Treating employees with respect encourages loyalty.
- Kindness, fairness, and justice are intangible rewards from the physician and are important to employees.

Manager

An office manager, business manager, or clinic administrator (title varies depending on assigned duties and size of clinic) can be a tremendous asset to the physicians. Some of the typical responsibilities of a manager are as follows:

- Coordinate with an attorney and certified public accountant regarding legal and fiscal matters.
- Maintain personnel policies, job descriptions, and procedure manuals.
- Supervise employees and coordinate duties.
- Conduct office staff training procedures.
- Conduct employees' performance and salary reviews.
- Recruit, interview, and make recommendations for hiring personnel.
- Prepare agendas and coordinate physician and staff meetings.
- Review business insurance policies, and coordinate decisions related to business insurance with the physicians.
- Perform property management tasks.
- Discuss any problems with the physician, and make recommendations for corrective actions.

The manager must have the support and backing of the physicians. The employees must be aware that support and backing are provided, or the manager's effectiveness will be greatly decreased.

Personnel Policies

Regardless of the number of employees, a written personnel policy is mandatory. This policy will be a guide for present and future employees and will decrease conflict regarding employment. The policy should contain information regarding the following:

- Practice goals and objectives
- Normal working hours and overtime pay policy

- Sick leave (i.e., when it starts accumulating, how it accrues, and maximum accrued days)
- Holidays—name the paid holidays
- Vacation—how it accrues, when it can be taken, and carry-forward policy
- Benefits provided (i.e., medical, life, and disability insurance; retirement plans; continuing education; etc.)
- Rules for attendance
- Probationary period—state the period of time
- Performance evaluations and salary reviews—outline when evaluations and reviews will be scheduled
- Termination policy
- Sexual harrassment
- Confidentiality of patients' medical records

It is recommended that personnel policies be reviewed by an attorney to make certain that the policy does not inadvertently create a contractual obligation with employees. The policy should clearly specify that changes can be made at the employer's discretion.

Job Descriptions

A job description must be written for each nonphysician position in the clinic. The job description should contain the following:

- Position title
- Qualifications required for the position
- Duties and responsibilities of the position
- To whom the employee is responsible in performing his or her duties
- Physical requirements and environmental factors in compliance with the Americans with Disabilities Act

Job descriptions are a prerequisite for smooth, ongoing management of personnel. The descriptions should be reviewed and updated on a regular basis.

Salaries and Fringe Benefits

The salaries and fringe benefits provided to employees have a tremendous effect on creating a good work environment and keeping the best personnel from leaving.

Salaries. The salary should clearly relate to the level of responsibility, duties, and qualifications required by the position. Make certain that the salaries paid are comparable to other medical clinics, hospitals, and other job markets in the community.

In establishing salaries, it is important to consider not only the level of responsibility and required qualifications but also the amount of interaction the job requires with patients. As an example, many clinics pay receptionists at the bottom of the clinic's pay scale. Other clinics recognize that receptionists are the first person patients interact with and therefore pay more to attract and retain first-rate people.

Fringe benefits. The benefits offered to employees have become as important to employees as the salaries paid. Job candidates are more aware of the value of fringe benefits, and the benefits package will often be the deciding factor of an excellent candidate accepting employment with the clinic. Some of the benefits most clinics offer are as follows:

- *Paid holidays.* New Year's Day, Memorial Day, Independence Day, Labor Day, Thanksgiving, Christmas, and other days, depending on local customs, are paid holidays.
- *Vacations.* Many management consultants recommend a liberal vacation policy to attract and retain good personnel. This time can vary from 2 weeks after 1 year of employment to 3 to 4 weeks after 5 years. Unused vacation time usually cannot be carried forward from one year to the next, thus encouraging employees to take needed time off. Upon termination, unused vacation is paid on a prorated basis.
- *Sick leave.* Sick leave usually accrues at the rate of ½ to 1 day per month after 6 months of employment. The maximum amount permitted to accrue varies from 10 working days to 30 working days. Some clinics pay employees for unused sick leave at the end of the year to promote good attendance.
- *Medical insurance.* Most clinics have some type of medical insurance. This is one of the most expected and appreciated benefits. Usually, if dependent coverage is desired by employees, the employee pays this portion of the premium.
- *Disability insurance.* Disability insurance can be provided to employees relatively inexpensively and can enhance the benefit package.
- *Uniform allowance.* If employees are required to wear uniforms, a uniform allowance is a common benefit.
- *Life insurance.* Currently a group term life insurance premium is tax deductible if the benefit does not exceed $50,000 (for physicians) and the employees' coverage is prorated by their annual salary. Depending on the clinic's census of physicians and employees, particularly age, this can be an inexpensive benefit.
- *Continuing education.* If the continuing education will enhance the employee's job, it is recommended that time off be granted and the clinic pay for expenses incurred. Usually the clinic's continuing education policy will state the maximum time off permitted and the maximum allowable expenses for a calendar year.
- *Personal time off.* Many clinics (and most large corporations) are including personal time off (PTO) in their benefit package. Usually this is 3 days per calendar year. The days can be taken off for any reason (Christmas shopping, birthdays, etc.).

• *Retirement plans.* The retirement plan is probably the biggest fringe benefit a clinic can offer employees. Usually the physicians wish to have a retirement plan and are required by law to provide this benefit to employees. It is usually necessary to educate the younger employees regarding the value of the plan.

Some employers are offering their employees a "cafeteria," or flexible, benefit plan. This gives the employee a choice of benefits. These plans are authorized under Section 125 of the Internal Revenue Code with numerous rules regulating their use. It is recommended that legal advice be provided if a cafeteria plan is considered.

Make certain that the employees are aware of the dollar value of their combined salary and fringe benefits.

Recruiting and Training

It is expensive to recruit and train new employees. Some personnel turnover is inevitable and is sometimes in the best interest of the practice. Personnel turnover can be kept at a minimum by promoting positive attitudes, providing pleasant working conditions, and offering competitive salaries and fringe benefits.

Recruiting. Recruiting takes time to find the best candidate but will save time later if a less-than-satisfactory employee is hired. If this employee is a poor selection, this will affect other employees' morale and increase personnel turnover, and patients will complain. Pick a candidate with a compatible personality to current employees, one who will fit into the office.

Some recruiting sources are as follows:
• Local medical society
• Local colleges
• Hospital personnel departments
• Advertisements in local newspapers

There are many legal risks in hiring and firing personnel. Physicians and personnel responsible for this task must be cognizant of state and federal labor laws.

The job application form should only ask questions that are job related (i.e., name, address, telephone number, present employment, prior employment history, educational background, and references).

Conduct the interview in a private setting with no distractions for either party. Use the position's job description to compile the questions. The candidate's potential should be considered in addition to qualifications and experience. Show respect to the candidates and make them feel as comfortable as possible. Ask questions that require more than a yes or no answer, make eye contact, and let the candidate do the talking. Give the applicant a time parameter for making a final decision, and stick to that date.

It is usually recommended that the rejected applicants be notified in writing. Thank them for interviewing and mention that their résumé will be kept on file if they so desire. State that the position has been filled, mention only experience and qualifications, and wish them well.

Training. Have the new employee start on a day that is least busy, not a Monday in most clinics. The newcomer should be introduced to the staff, with a short explanation of each staff member's duties, and taken on a tour of the facilities.

An employee familiar with the task should perform the task with the new employee observing. The new employee should be encouraged to ask questions. With the instructor watching, the trainee should perform the task until it is mastered. A written summary of instructions should be given to the new employee for future reference. Someone should be assigned to monitor the performance of the trainee to make certain no bad habits are acquired.

Explain the medical and legal risks to new employees and make certain that they are aware that the physician is medically and legally responsible for all employees' actions. All employees should be tactful and empathetic with patients and fellow employees. Stress confidentiality of all patients' medical records.

Employee cross-training is an advantage to a clinic. Sick leave and vacations are easier to cover. Cross-training familiarizes the employees with the entire operation of the clinic. This reduces conflict among employees because each will appreciate the work of the others. Morale is usually higher with cross-training because the employees experience more variety of duties. It is important to not make any employee feel threatened or to give the impression that workloads will be increased or the number of employees will be cut.

Performance Evaluations

Performance evaluations should be scheduled on a regular basis, usually annually. The annual review should have no surprises for employees. They should be made aware of their performance, good or poor, throughout the year. The evaluation should be realistic, honest, and encouraging to the employee to maintain good performance and improve in needed areas. Recognition for accomplishments and goals for future improvement should be included in the evaluation.

Personnel Records

It is recommended that federal, state, and local laws and regulations be checked to ascertain the length of time personnel records should be kept on file. To provide protection against claims, alleged discrimination, harassment, or inadequate compensation, keep job applications, job descriptions, performance evaluations, documentation of reprimands, and termination notices. Also, keep accident reports on employees, sick and disability records, and group insurance documents.

Summary

Personnel management is not an easy task. The physicians should strive for a positive attitude and treat all employees with respect. A physician is providing a service to patients, and patients have a choice of physicians. The employees assisting the physicians in providing this service should greatly enhance the quality of patient care.

GOVERNMENT REGULATIONS
Occupational Safety and Health Administration

During the past few years, heightened concern for the safety of clinical laboratory workers led the Occupational Safety and Health Administration (OSHA) to specifically address workplace hazards in the clinical laboratory. As a result, OSHA published three Final Rules: *Occupational Exposure to Hazardous Chemicals in Laboratories, Occupational Exposure to Bloodborne Pathogens,* and *Personal Protective Equipment.* The purpose of these rules is to encourage employers and employees to reduce workplace hazards and to implement new or improve existing safety and health programs. A manual should be written addressing specific situations and hazards in your office and kept in an easily accessible place for employees' reference and training along with copies of Material Safety Data Sheets.

Contact your local OSHA office through the U.S. Department of Labor for assistance in developing a manual and organizing your office to comply with their standards.

Clinical Laboratory Improvement Amendments

In 1988, Congress unanimously passed the Clinical Laboratory Improvement Amendments (CLIA), which were designed to provide uniform regulation for laboratory testing regardless of where the tests were performed. There are three levels of certification. The first level is the *waived certification,* which allows any laboratory personnel to perform 10 simple tests (contact your state laboratory for lists). There is no inspection, quality control, or proficiency testing required for this category. The second level is *physician-performed microscopy* (PPM). This level allows the physician and midlevel practitioner to perform 10 additional tests. There is quality control and proficiency testing required for this level but no inspection. The final level is the *certificate of compliance,* which includes all other tests and is subject to all regulations and inspections every 2 years. Each of these categories must be registered with your State Laboratory and Certification

Bureau. Fees are assessed biannually and are calculated according to the level of certification.

Contact your State Laboratory and Certification Bureau for specifics and the latest revisions. As of this writing, three states are exempt from CLIA regulations.

BUSINESS INSURANCE REQUIREMENTS

There are essential insurance coverages necessary to protect physicians and medical clinics against a catastrophic occurrence. Examples of this coverage include the following:
- Professional liability insurance
- Property and equipment insurance
- General liability insurance
- Employee dishonesty insurance
- Workers' compensation insurance
- Fiduciary liability insurance
- Personal disability insurance
- Overhead insurance

Professional Liability Insurance

Professional liability insurance covers charges of alleged negligence or incompetence in performing the practice of medicine. With the increased number of professional liability claims and subsequent escalated settlements, it is imperative that professional liability coverage be purchased and maintained. The amount of coverage needed varies, depending on the physician's specialty and the geographic area in which the physician practices.

Some of the questions to be answered in determining the appropriate policy offered by insurance companies are as follows:
- Can the insurer settle a claim without the physician's knowledge?
- What is the policy's definition of "professional services?"
- Does the policy cover liability for punitive damages?
- Does the policy cover negligent acts of employees?

There are two types of professional liability insurance coverage:
- Claims-made policies
- Occurrence policies

Claims-Made Policies

Claims-made policies cover claims filed or reported while the policy is in force. To continue coverage after the policy has been terminated, a tail policy must be purchased. The cost of the tail policy varies from 110% to 200% (plus) of the premium for the final year of coverage. A modified claims-made policy usually includes a buyout provision; this decreases or eliminates the cost of extended coverage on retirement.

Occurrence Policies

Occurrence policies provide protection for the period of time the policy is in force on claims filed any time in the future. Occurrence policies may not be available and are usually much more expensive than claims-made policies in the early years of coverage.

Multiperil Policies

Many clinics purchase multiperil policies rather than numerous individual policies. Multiperil policies can cover the following:

- *Property and equipment insurance.* Adequate coverage should be purchased for buildings, medical equipment, and administrative equipment. This coverage should be reviewed at least annually and coverage upgraded, depending on increased value of the property.
- *General liability insurance.* Some level of coverage is needed in case an accident or mishap occurs on the premises. As an example, this policy will pay medical and litigation expenses should a patient fall in the office and be injured.
- *Employee dishonesty insurance.* This policy covers embezzlement by an employee. Usually it is necessary to prosecute the employee in order to collect damages.
- *Business interruption insurance.* This provides protection against loss of earnings of a business during the time required to rebuild or repair property damaged or destroyed.

Workers' Compensation Insurance

It is compulsory that workers' compensation insurance be purchased. This insurance covers employees in case of an occupational injury or disease. The benefits include medical expense, loss of pay, and rehabilitation, if necessary.

Fiduciary Liability Insurance or Bond

If a retirement plan is provided, fiduciary coverage is required by law. Currently, the coverage must be at least 10% of the plan's assets. This policy or bond covers the trustees in performing their duties on behalf of the participants of the plan.

Personal Disability Insurance

Personal disability insurance is an important aspect of having an adequate insurance coverage program. In the event of an accident or illness, the policies are designed to replace a portion of the physician's earned income. There are several variables in disability insurance policies:

- *Waiting period.* The waiting period is the period of time between an accident or illness and the date benefits are paid.

- *Percentage.* Percentage of income or maximum amount per month paid as a benefit.
- *Definition of disability.* It is recommended that the definition state that benefits will be paid as long as you are disabled from your own occupation. As an example, if you are a surgeon and sever a hand, if the policy does not state "own occupation," the insurance company will claim that you can perform another occupation (e.g., teach) and you will not have long-term coverage.

Overhead Insurance

If a physician is incapacitated by injury or illness, office expenses continue. Overhead insurance covers expenses such as employees' salaries, rent or lease payments, and utilities. The variances in overhead insurance policies are similar to personal disability insurance.

Summary

It is not financially feasible to insure against every small loss. It is financially feasible to have adequate coverage to avoid a loss that could be devastating. A physician or clinic should have a professional periodically review coverage and exclusions of all policies and make appropriate recommendations. Local professionals can be consulted regarding individual insurance needs.

There are many ramifications and variables associated with insurance policies. This review cannot be deemed to cover all aspects.

MANAGED HEALTH CARE

Shifts in the health care system have created a need to better understand contractual obligations, risks, and responsibilities under managed care to enable physicians to more effectively protect the interests of their patients and their practice.

Particular emphasis is placed on contract analysis, reimbursement issues related to capitation, discounted fee for services, and at-risk arrangements, as well as liability issues related to such programs.

When considering these contracts, it would be advisable to contact the American Medical Association, American Board of Obstetrics and Gynecology, other medical specialty organizations, or your state medical association for more information.

RETIREMENT PLANS

Retirement planning is one of the most important considerations in financial planning. The type of plan a clinic adopts depends primarily on the financial objectives of the physicians, how much the clinic can afford to contribute to the plan, and the ages of the physicians and employees in the clinic. No taxes are paid on the funds contributed to the plan or on the earnings from investments until the funds are distributed to the participants at time of retirement or termination of employment.

Administrative costs will be incurred in adopting and maintaining a plan. Some of these expenses are legal services, accounting services, actuarial services (with some plans), a fiduciary bond, trustees' fees, and investment counseling expense.

The plans can be written with a variety of provisions, providing that they adhere to current Internal Revenue Service rules and regulations. The most common variables in a plan are minimum age, length of service, and vesting period. Usually, the employee can be excluded if under 21 years of age, and the employee has to complete a certain period of employment before the employee is eligible for funding.

Some of the types of plans eligible for adoption are as follows:
• Money purchase pension plans
• Profit-sharing plans
• Defined benefit plans
• 401(k) salary deferral plans

Money Purchase Pension Plans

The money purchase pension plans are funded by a percentage of salary written into the plan document. The percentage can be changed by amending the plan, but it is basically a fixed overhead expense. Some money purchase pension plans are integrated with Social Security to permit additional funding for the higher-paid employees (physicians).

Profit-Sharing Plans

The profit-sharing plans are funded based on the profit of the corporation or entity. This plan provides more flexibility because the plan can be funded from 0% to 15% of compensation.

Defined Benefit Plans

The funding for the defined contribution plans must be calculated by an actuary. The amount of funding depends on the participant's age and goals for annual benefits on retirement. The annual retirement benefit is limited to $90,000, with a cost-of-living adjustment beginning in 1989.

401(k) Salary Deferral Plans

A 401(k) plan gives your employees the opportunity to save additional funds for retirement. Participating employees elect to defer a portion of their compensation to your qualified retirement plan. In doing so, they avoid current income taxes on the deferred amounts and on any plan earnings the amounts generate. No tax will be due until plan benefits are distributed.

401(k) plans are particularly attractive to employees who cannot make deductible Individual Retirement Account contributions or who want to augment their IRA contributions. For 1995, the maximum amount an employee may defer is $9240. You may also make matching contributions on behalf of each participating employee. (The deferral dollar limit is adjusted for inflation each year.)

In addition to the general tax-qualification requirements all plans must meet, 401(k) plans must meet certain other requirements. For instance, all 401(k) salary deferrals made by employees must be completely nonforfeitable. Also, 401(k) plans must meet special nondiscrimination rules.

If your company already has a profit-sharing or other defined contribution plan, a 401(k) option is easy to add. If you are implementing a new qualified plan, the expense and paperwork of adding a 401(k) option along with your plan are minimal.

Summary

Retirement plans are an excellent way of providing funds for retirement and deferring personal income taxes until the funds are distributed. The plans provide a means of financial discipline in preparing for retirement years.

It is mandatory that legal and accounting advice and services be used in establishing and maintaining all retirement plans. Numerous tax acts have been legislated that have changed and updated many rules and regulations pertaining to retirement plans. Professional advice must be provided to keep abreast of current guidelines.

This review is not intended to be all-inclusive in outlining the several types of retirement plans available, the idiosyncrasies of the different plans, or the multiple rules and regulations governing the plans.

BIBLIOGRAPHY

Abbey D, Abbey M: Do you need a computer in your office? *Iowa Med* 9:12, 1985.

Adamson T, Tschann J, Gullion D, et al: Physician communication skills and malpractice claims: a complex relationship, *Health Care Delivery* 356: 360, 1989.

Albert R, Breinhold J: Personnel policies in employee handbooks, *Health Care Law Newsletter* 11:11, 1989.

Allcorn S, Duffield M: Employee training: a path to improved employee performance, *Group Pract J* 7:8, 1988.

Barrett J: Human resource management for solo and small group medical practices, *J Med Pract* 1:239, 1986.

Benjamin C, Baum G: The automated medical record: a practical realization? *Top Health Records Manage* 1:12, 1988.

Bern B, Bern A: What fringe benefits should you give your staff? *Physician Manage* 107:116, 1986.

Birenbaum M: *A guide to OSHA requirements for hospital, independent and physician office laboratories*, ii:1, 1992.

Blide L: Leadership in a computerized health care environment, *Top Health Records Manage* 42:48, 1989.

Bloedorn J: Managing the costs of employment, *J Med Pract Manage* 35:38, 1988.

Blomberg R, Levy E, Anderson A: Assessing the value of employee training, *Health Care Manage Rev* 63:70, 1988.

Bratkovich J, Steele B: Compensation pay for performance boosts productivity, *Personnel J* 78:86, 1989.

Bushhouse F: Your legal risks when hiring and firing, *Physician Manage* 197:201, 1988.

Caldwell A, Sikes J: Do you recall your greatest asset? *Group Pract J* 78:79, 1990.

Caplan C: What belongs in an office manual, *Physician Manage* 219:225, 1987.

Christian W, Troy P: A comparison of methods for orienting new personnel to the human service setting, *J Ment Health Adm* 49:51, 1983.

Conomikes G: *Successful practice management techniques*, Los Angeles, 1988, Conomikes Reports.

Conway S, Messerle J: Searching Medline, *Group Pract J* 26:34, 1990.

Cook J: Training: a five-step program that keeps training on target, *Personnel J* 106:114, 1986.

Cushing M: Criteria for selecting an office system, *Physician Financial News* 7:C4,C6,C13, 1987.

Cushing M: Installing a computer, part I, *Physician Financial News* 19:C1,C2,C9, 1987.

Cushing M: Installing a computer, part II, *Physician Financial News* 1:C3,C4, 1988.

Cushing M: Installing a computer, part III, *Physician Financial News* 5:C3, C6, 1988.

Cushing M: Installing a computer, part IV, *Physician Financial News* 9:C7,C9, 1988.

Daily-Melville C: Design options for small group practices, *Group Pract J* 82:86, 1986.

Doctor's Office 1:3, 1990.

Dodge R, Krakoff I: Clinical data management and analysis using a microcomputer, *Med Pediatr Oncol* 12:20, 1982.

Dresser S: Employee benefits: a la carte, *Assoc Manage* 73:81, 1989.

Feutz S: Legal insights: professional liability insurance, *J Nurs Adm* 5:27, 1989.

FitzGerald R, Howarth B: Employee health benefits plans and federal ERISA law, *Medical Group Management J* 37:9, 1990.

Halcrow: Pay alone won't motivate, *Personnel J* 13:14, 1988.

Helm A: Malpractice liability and your staff, *Physician Manage* 95:102, 1983.

Helpful hiring hints, *Employment Guide* 82:82, 1989.

Henderson C: *The business side of practice*, Chicago, 1989, American Medical Association.

Herndon P: Understanding your office staff compensation, *Internist* 32:33, 1989.

Holstein L: Personnel pitfalls—how to hire and fire without getting sued, *Medical Group Management J* 18:23, 1990.

Johnston T: A training program for medical receptionists, *Med Group Manage* 22:30, 1983.

Kahl K, Casey D: How to evaluate and implement office automation, *Am Med Records Assoc* 20:22, 1984.

Kalogredis V: How to determine the right benefits for your staff, *Physician Manage* 58:62, 1989.

Kaye E: How to reduce stress through office design, *Physician Manage* 84:88, 1985.

Kerfoot K: Nursing management considerations, *Nurs Econ* 42:43, 1988.

Knight C: A changing attitude: the revolution in medical facility design. *Group Pract J* 26:62, 1986.

Kras S, Keschner R, Huber T: *The pension answer book*, ed 4, Greenvale, NY, 1987, Panel.

Liberman A: *Risk and insurance management guide for medical group organizations*, Denver, 1988, Center for Research in Ambulatory Health Care Administration.

Lombardi D: *Handbook of personnel selection and performance evaluation in healthcare*, San Francisco, 1988, Jossey-Bass.

McCord R: Job descriptions: key to an efficient staff, *Physician Manage* 210: 218, 1987.

McCord R: Perfect employees are not born—you train them, *Physician Manage* 53:57, 1988.

Metcalfe D: The computer in general practice, *J Med Eng Technol* 53:55, 1984.

Musselwhite W: Knowledge, pay, and performance, *Training Develop J* 62: 65, 1988.

Peterson H: Computers in medicine, *J Clin Comput* 105:108, 1985.

Planning guide for physician's medical facilities, Chicago, 1979, American Medical Association.

Pollak M: Computer-aided information systems in clinical trials: a physician's perspective, *Comput Programs Biomed* 243:251, 1983.

Practice Personnel Bulletin 3(3):3, 1990.

Practice Personnel Bulletin 3(6):4, 1990.

Rigel S: Is it time for a computer in your practice? Part V. How to evaluate if a computer is appropriate for your practice, *J Dermatol Surg Oncol* 215:216, 1985.

Robinette T: Incentive compensation program works in detailed case study, *Healthc Financ Manage* 36:40, 1983.

Russler D: Exam-room computing, *Group Pract J* 47:51, 1990.

Scroggins C: How to train that new assistant, *Med Econ* 141:153, 1985.

Studney D: Monitoring quality by computer, *Group Pract J* 8:14, 1990.

Sugarman M, Love J: How to set staff salaries, *Physician Manage* 44:50, 1988.

Sweeney D: Ways to get a new employee off to a good start, *Dent Manage* 20:25, 1984.

Tweedy D: *Office space planning and management*, Westport, Conn, 1986, Quorum Books.

Valo C: Managing resources: selecting a patient care information system, *Top Health Records Manage* 64:73, 1988.

Walker C: The use of job evaluation plans in salary administration, *Personnel* 28: 31, 1987.

White W, Hulse C: Guidelines for education and training in your medical group, *Medical Group Management J* 23:51, 1987.

Wirth T, Allcorn S: Managing employee turnover: exit interviews, what can they tell you? *Medical Group Management J* 42:50, 1990.

Wunneburger R: Computerizing a group practice, *Group Pract J* 62:64, 1990.

CHAPTER 2

General Evaluation of the Patient and the Annual Checkup

MORTON A. STENCHEVER

The initial office visit is an extremely important one whether the patient is being seen for an annual checkup or because of a specific complaint. The physician has the opportunity at this time to develop a bond of trust with her on which their future relationship will be built. Confidence will be obtained by displaying to the patient an understanding and nonjudgmental manner in which specific data are collected, sensitive information is shared, feelings and fears are dealt with, and rapport is established. At the first visit a complete history and physical examination should be performed and appropriate laboratory tests ordered. In this way the physician gains knowledge about the problems and needs of the patient and can develop a plan for solutions. At the initial visit the history and physical examination should be a complete one, without corners being cut. The physician should not assume that other physicians are attending to the patient's general medical needs. At subsequent visits specific areas of concern can be addressed, but the patient should be subjected to a complete interval history and a general physical examination at yearly intervals (at least).

This chapter will focus on the ingredients of a general history and physical examination and a discussion of what constitutes normal health maintenance.

DIRECT (NONVERBAL) OBSERVATIONS

It is important to first look at the patient even before speaking. If the physician has the opportunity to observe the patient in the waiting room, this is a good thing to do. The patient may transmit her general demeanor by facial expression and posture. In general, there are five basic impressions that the patient may transmit: happiness, apathy, fear, anger, and sadness.

The happy patient is generally in good personal control and appears self-assured. She transmits a warm, relaxed, responsive impression. Her face is relaxed, generally she smiles, and there is often a sparkle in her eyes. She will greet you with a warm, friendly greeting, and although she may be apprehensive about the first contact, she will generally transmit a sense of good spirits.

Patients with apathy often have a blank facial expression. There is little sparkle in their eyes, and their face may appear masklike. Their lips generally appear thin, and their mouth is noted to be in a neutral position, turning neither up nor down. Their posture is often somewhat slouched, their handshake weak, and their answers to questions short and unemotional. The apathetic patient may suffer from severe emotional distress, or she may be demonstrating a resignation to an imagined or real condition. She may feel overwhelmed by multiple problems.

The frightened patient often shows a tense expression, with her mouth tightly drawn and her eyes darting and narrow. She may be perspiring but may seem to have a dry mouth when she speaks. She often leans forward and demonstrates constant hand activity. Her reactions may be grossly out of proportion to the apparent stimuli.

The angry patient often demonstrates narrowed eyes, furrowed brows, and thin, tight lips. She is often sitting on the edge of her chair and leaning forward as if to pounce. Unlike the defensive pose of the frightened patient, the angry patient radiates aggression. Her voice is often harsh, and she frequently overreacts to questions and answers with short, threatening phrases.

The sad patient often sits in a slouched position and displays large, sad eyes and a turned-down mouth. The eyes are often moist, and there may be tears. This patient is often depressed, and her speech reflects remorse and hopelessness.

By recognizing the patient's demeanor, the physician is often in a position to begin the interview with a question or statement that may demonstrate that he senses the feelings of the patient. Such comments as "You seem tense today" or "You seem sad" or "You seem angry; can you tell me why?" not only demonstrate a sensitivity on the part of the physician, but allow the patient to immediately deal with her underlying concerns.

HISTORY TAKING

Table 2-1 offers a general outline for the taking of a history in an office setting. On the first visit it should be complete, as outlined. On subsequent visits it may be more interval in type and directive, relating to what the physician knows about the patient and to her current complaints.

Chief Complaint

The patient should be encouraged to state in her own words the reason for the visit. Often receptionists ask the patient this when she makes an appointment and, depending on the response, adjust the time of the visit accordingly. Questions such as "What problem brought you to see me?" or "How may I help you?" are good ways to begin. If the receptionist has obtained the reason for the appointment, the physician may refer to that as a start. As the patient tells her story, the physician should not interrupt unless it is to clarify certain points or to offer direction if she digresses. The

TABLE 2-1. Outline for taking a history

Observation—nonverbal	Bleeding problems
Chief complaint	Family history
Gynecologic history	Illnesses and cause of death of first-order
Menstrual history	relatives
Pregnancy history	Congenital malformations, mental retarda-
Infections—vaginal and pelvic	tion, and reproductive wastage
Gynecologic surgical procedures	Occupational and avocational history
Urologic history	Social history
Pelvic pain	Review of systems
Vaginal bleeding	Head
Sexual status	Cardiovascular-respiratory
Contraception history and status	Gastrointestinal
General health problems	Genitourinary
Systemic illnesses	Neuromuscular
Surgical procedures	Psychiatric
Other hospitalizations	Depression
Medications, habits, and allergies	Physical abuse
Medications taken	Sexual abuse
Allergies	Incest
Smoking history	Rape
Alcohol use	
Illicit drug use	

physician should face the patient and maintain direct eye contact. Acknowledgment of important points of the history should be given by either nodding the head or adding a few words. In this way the physician remains involved in the story and demonstrates a sense of caring. When the patient has told the physician her current problem, pertinent open-ended questions should be asked concerning specific points. Although direct questions are worthwhile to establish specific points, it is best to allow the patient to tell her story in her terms and react to open-ended questions. In general, the outline in Table 2-1 is information that should be obtained, but the order in which it is obtained is not necessarily important.

Pertinent Gynecologic History

Several different points make up the gynecologic history. The first involves the menstrual history. The physician should obtain the age of menarche, the duration of each monthly cycle, the number of days of menstrual flow, instances of irregularity of flow, and the dates of the last menstrual period and previous menstrual period. The characteristics of the menstrual flow, including color, amount, and accompanying symptoms such as cramping, sweating, headache, or diarrhea, should be noted. In general, the menstrual cycle ranges between 21 and 40 days and flow lasts 4 to 7 days. Flow is often bright red in color and accompanied by cramping on the day preceding flow and the first day of flow. This is characteristic of an ovulatory cycle, but menstruation that is irregular, dark in color, painless, and either short or extremely long in duration may indicate anovulation. Early cycles in teenagers and later cycles in the premenopausal woman are often anovulatory and may therefore be irregular and different from their usual periods.

Next, the pregnancy history should be obtained. The patient should list each pregnancy that she has experienced, including the year of the pregnancy; duration; type of delivery; size, sex, and current condition of each baby; any complications that may have occurred; and whether or not the infant was breast-fed and if so for how long. Terminations of pregnancies, spontaneous abortions, and ectopic pregnancies should be noted. With these, the time of gestation that they occurred and the circumstances under which they took place should be indicated. Likewise, any unusual pregnancy complication, such as molar pregnancy, should be noted. When serious problems related to pregnancy have occurred, old records should be obtained for appropriate review. Pregnancies that have been complicated by excessive bleeding, chills, fever, infection, toxemia, or other complications should be noted. It is also appropriate to ask the patient about the individuals who fathered each of the pregnancies.

Previous vaginal or pelvic infections should be noted. The patient should be asked to describe the types of infections that she has had in the past, what treatment was received, and any complications that may have occurred. Hospitalizations should be reviewed with respect to cause and outcome.

Every gynecologic surgical procedure that the patient has undergone should be documented. This should include minor operations such as endometrial biopsies; vulvar, vaginal, or cervical biopsies; dilation and curettage; laparoscopic examinations; and any major procedure that the patient has undergone. Dates, types of procedures, diagnoses, significant complications, and lengths of hospitalizations should be noted. Pertinent past records should be obtained.

A urologic history that defines bladder function, incontinence, acute or chronic bladder or kidney infections, and other urologic problems, such as hematuria and passage of urinary stones, should be sought and discussed.

Symptoms relating to pelvic pain or discomfort, dyspareunia, or dysmenorrhea should be discussed. The pain should be described and the presence or absence of a relationship to the menstrual cycle and its association with other events or bleeding noted.

Vaginal bleeding not related to menses should be discussed with respect to its relationship to other events such as coitus or the use of tampons or a contraceptive device.

A sexual history should be taken, including whether the patient is sexually active, the type of relationships that she has, whether she is orgasmic or experiences pain or discomfort with coitus (dyspareunia), and whether she or her partner is experiencing problems of sexual dysfunction. Specific problems should be discussed, and all responses should be dealt with in a nonjudgmental fashion.

Finally, a contraceptive history should be obtained, including all methods used, the length of time that they have been used, and any complications that may have arisen because of their use.

Past General Health

All significant health problems that the patient has experienced during her lifetime should be discussed. These include hospitalizations, operative procedures, and treatment for specific illnesses such as diabetes, hepatitis, tuberculosis, rheumatic fever, and so on. Although many physicians use a history checklist filled out by the patient on the initial visit, a careful physician can often obtain this information as part of the history.

The physician should document all medications taken, the reasons for doing so, and any allergic responses that have been noted.

The patient should be questioned for evidence of bleeding or clotting disorders, including a history of bruisability, bleeding from mucous membranes, or bleeding at the time of minor procedures such as dental extractions.

A smoking history should be elicited, including the amount and length of time that the patient has smoked. She should also be questioned about the use of alcohol; illicit drugs, including marijuana, cocaine, and so on; and the use of prescription drugs, including the type and length of time used. All affirmative answers should be followed by specific questioning concerning the length of use, type of drugs used, and side effects that may have been noted. Alcohol use should be detailed to include the number of drinks per day and any history of binge drinking or previous therapy for alcoholism.

Family History

A detailed family history of all relatives (mother, father, sisters, brothers, children, and grandparents) should be taken and a family tree roughly constructed (Fig. 2-1). All serious illnesses or causes of death for each individual should be noted. A history of congenital malformations, mental retardation, or pregnancy wastage in either the patient or her partner's family should be sought. These questions are particularly important if the patient has suffered reproductive loss problems.

Occupational and Social History

Details about the patient's occupation and that of her partner, including jobs held or performed and any health hazards suffered, should be noted.

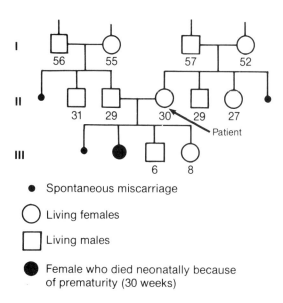

FIGURE 2-1. Family tree of a typical gynecologic patient.

From Stenchever MA: In Herbst AL, Mishell DR, Stenchever MA, et al, editors: *Comprehensive gynecology*, ed 2, St. Louis, 1991, Mosby.

Similarly, hobbies should be discussed in a search for information that may pose health hazards.

A social history should include where and with whom the patient lives, other individuals in the household, areas of the world where the patient and her partner have lived or traveled, and unusual experiences that they may have had.

Review of Systems

A complete review of systems is important and offers the physician an opportunity to discuss several issues that may ordinarily seem to be sensitive. It should include a history of serious headaches, epileptic seizures, dizziness, or fainting spells and, if any of these are found, a discussion of medications that the individual may be taking to combat these symptoms that may affect a future pregnancy.

A complete cardiovascular-respiratory history is important and should include questions about hypertension, heart disease, and chest problems such as asthma, chronic cough, or hemoptysis.

Gastrointestinal symptoms such as a history of functional bowel problems or hepatitis are important to the gynecologist.

Genitourinary problems relating to bladder function, continence, and renal function are important.

Neurologic and neuromuscular impairments should be discussed because they may indicate an underlying generalized condition or may have an effect on future reproduction.

A history of vascular disease, including thrombophlebitis and pulmonary embolism, is important to obtain. If thrombophlebitis or pulmonary embolism has occurred, the history of the circumstances in which it took place should be sought. A relationship to a change in hormonal activities such as pregnancy or birth control pill usage should be noted.

A psychiatric history should be detailed by carefully indicating a history of emotional or mental disease processes, depression, anxiety, or the need for therapy or counseling. The patient should be asked specifically if she has ever been sexually abused in childhood or in her adult life, by a stranger or incestuously, and if she has ever been raped. She should also be asked if she has ever been physically abused or intimidated. If she has, details should be reviewed.

COMPLETE PHYSICAL EXAMINATION

The physician should perform a complete physical examination on every new patient at the first visit and at each annual checkup, especially if he or she is the primary physician caring for the patient. The examination should be viewed as both an opportunity to gain information and to teach the patient information that she should know about herself and her body.

The patient should be completely disrobed and covered by a hospital gown that ensures warmth and modesty. During each step of the examination, she should be encouraged to maintain personal control by being offered options whenever possible. These include whether or not a chaperone should be present and whether or not a drape is used. A chaperone, usually a woman, serves a variety of purposes. She may offer warmth, compassion, and support to the patient during an uncomfortable or potentially embarrassing portion of the examination. She may help the physician carry out procedures and in certain instances offers the physician protection from having his intentions misunderstood by a naive or suspicious patient. Although a chaperone is not absolutely necessary for each visit, one should be available, and the use of such a chaperone should be a circumstance agreed to by the physician and the patient. Local customs vary, and it is important that the physician follow these.

The examination begins with a general evaluation of the patient's appearance. Her weight and blood pressure should be noted, and if postmenopausal, she should be measured for height to document evidence of osteoporosis that occurs because of vertebral compression fractures.

The patient's eyes, ears, nose, throat, and neck should be examined. A funduscopic examination should be performed at least annually to inspect the blood vessels of the retina and to observe the lens for evidence of early cataract formation. The gynecologist should measure intraocular pressures in women over 40 years of age or suggest that this be done by an ophthalmologist. The upper lip and chin should be inspected for the presence of hair follicles, which may indicate androgen activity. The thyroid gland should be palpated for irregularities or increased size (goiter). Specific areas of enlargement, nodularity, hardness, or tenderness should be described because they may indicate thyroid disease. The neck should be palpated for evidence of adenopathy along both the supraclavicular and posterior auricular chains.

The chest should be inspected for symmetry and movement of the diaphragms, percussed for areas of consolidation, and auscultated bilaterally for breath and adventitious sounds. The heart should be examined by palpation for points of maximum impulse, percussed for size, and auscultated for irregularities of rate and evidence of murmurs or other adventitious sounds. The older woman's neck should be auscultated for evidence of vascular bruits. The heart should be auscultated in both the lying and sitting positions.

A careful breast examination should be carried out as described in Chapter 9. During this examination the patient should be taught self-examination of the breasts and encouraged to perform this examination each month.

The abdomen should be examined in the following manner:

1. *Visual inspection.* The abdomen should be inspected for symmetry, scars, protuberances, discoloration of skin, and striations. The hair pattern should be noted. The typical female hair pattern is that of an inverted triangle over the mons pubis. A male pattern involves hair growth between the areas of the mons pubis and the umbilicus in a diamond pattern. A male-type pattern may indicate excessive androgen activity.

2. *Palpation.* The abdomen should be palpated for signs of organomegaly (enlarged organs), particularly the liver, spleen, kidneys, and uterus, and for adnexal masses that may be palpated abdominally. Palpation for fluid waves that may suggest ascites or hematoperitoneum should be carried out. During palpation it is also possible to note the rigidity of the abdomen, which might imply spasm of the rectus muscles secondary to intraabdominal irritation. If the irritation is caused by intraabdominal hemorrhage or infection or by vascular compromise of an organ, the rigidity is often evidence of an acute abdomen. If abdominal tenderness is noted, the physician should seek the phenomenon of rebound, which also signifies intraabdominal irritation. This is elicited by gently pressing the abdomen and then releasing. The release may cause pain under the spot (direct rebound) or in a different portion of the abdomen (referred rebound). The physician should make no sudden or rough movements because such pressure may cause pain even in a normal patient.

3. *Percussion.* Affords the ability to differentiate fluid waves and to outline solid organs and masses.

4. *Auscultation.* The physician should auscultate for bowel sounds. Hypoactive or absent bowel sounds may indicate an ileus caused by peritoneal irritation of the bowel. Hyperactive bowel sounds may indicate intrinsic irritation of the bowel or partial or complete bowel obstruction.

Groins should be palpated for adenopathy and inguinal hernias. The physician should elicit femoral pulses beneath the groin in the femoral triangle, and the two sides should be compared.

Extremities should be examined for evidence of varicose veins, edema, or other lesions. In addition, arterial competency should be judged by palpating pedal pulses on the dorsum of the foot.

Pelvic Examination

A careful pelvic examination should be performed and should include inspection of the introitus, including skin, hair distribution, size of the clitoris, labia majora and minora, urethral opening, perineal body, and anus. Abnormalities should be noted and, where appropriate, evaluated. The introitus should be inspected and the condition of the hymen or its remnants noted. During the inspection of the perineum the presence of lice may be noted.

The speculum examination then follows, and an appropriate Pederson's (narrow) or Graves' speculum is chosen depending on the age of the patient and the patency of the vagina. When the speculum is placed into the vagina, the vaginal epithelium is carefully inspected, and samples may be taken at this point to investigate for infection.

The vaginal epithelium should be inspected and evidence of inflammation or discharge noted and investigated where appropriate with cultures, a saline hanging drop for *Trichomonas,* or a potassium hydroxide (KOH) mount for *Candida.* Odor of the discharge should be noted because a putrid odor may indicate the presence of bacterial vaginosis. This odor can be enhanced when there is doubt by adding a drop of KOH to the discharge on the speculum blade and noting the odor. The KOH aids in the release of the substances that cause the odor (sniff test).

The cervix is inspected for lesions and the condition of the external os (i.e., nulliparous, multiparous, or stellate lacerated) noted. At this point a Papanicolaou smear is generally taken. Although there are many techniques for obtaining a Papanicolaou smear, currently a sweep of the transitional zone (squamocolumnar junction) with a tongue blade or an Ayers' spatula followed by a sampling of the endocervical canal with a cytobrush is an appropriate technique. Figures 2-2 and 2-3 demonstrate this.

After the speculum examination a bimanual examination should be performed by outlining the uterus and the ovaries and describing them in terms of size, shape, position, consistency, and any abnormalities that may be present. A rectovaginal examination follows that will not only help confirm the findings with respect to the uterus and ovaries but will allow the examiner to palpate the rectovaginal septum, the deeper recesses of the cul-de-sac, and the uterosacral ligaments. Scarring and nodularity

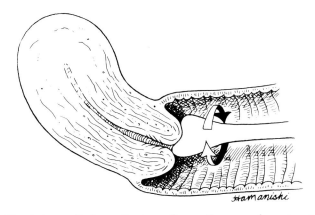

FIGURE 2-2. Obtaining cells from the transformation zone by using Ayers' spatula.

From Stenchever MA: In Herbst AL, Mishell DR, Stenchever MA, et al, editors: *Comprehensive gynecology,* ed 2, St Louis, 1991, Mosby.

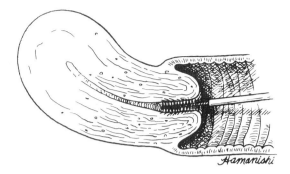

FIGURE 2-3. Obtaining cells from the endocervix by using a cytobrush.

From Stenchever MA: In Herbst AL, Mishell DR, Stenchever MA, et al, editors: *Comprehensive gynecology,* ed 2, St Louis, 1991, Mosby.

in these areas may indicate intraperitoneal pathology, such as endometriosis.

A thorough rectal examination for lesions of the rectum completes the examination. At the time the finger is removed from the rectum, stool present may be checked with guaiac to detect occult blood.

HEALTH MAINTENANCE: THE ANNUAL VISIT

The initial visit and subsequent annual visits allow the physician many opportunities to offer health maintenance advice and to educate the patient with respect to her health needs and understanding of her body. If the visit is an annual visit, an interim health and psychosocial history should be obtained. In addition to documenting health changes or surgical procedures that may have taken place during the year, the woman should be asked general questions regarding her overall well-being. These can include medications or drugs she is now using or whether she has begun to smoke or use alcohol in excess. In addition, she should be asked how she feels, whether she has suffered depression or other emotional distress, whether or not she has been the victim of physical or mental trauma, and whether she has been sexually abused in any way. The conditions of members of her family whose circumstances might affect her well-being should be discussed. In addition, loss and grief situations should be investigated. Several important aspects of the health maintenance visit will now be discussed.

Contraception

The patient's current and past contraceptive history should be noted. If the patient is not using a contraceptive or if her contraceptive is not one that would be expected to be protective, she should be counseled about a method that will work in her situation. Intrauterine devices that have been in place for longer than the period of their known usefulness should be removed and alternative methods suggested. For patients using oral contraceptives, the current health status should be assessed, and the decision of whether to continue with this method should be made. For diaphragm users, replacement of the diaphragm should be done on a 2- to 3-year basis, depending on use. Long-term, nonpermanent contraception, such as the use of a long-acting injectable contraceptive therapy, subdermal implant, or intrauterine device, should be considered. Decisions for sterilization, be it on the male or the female, should be discussed within the social context of the patient's life and her desire or lack of desire for reproduction (see Chapter 3).

Cancer Detection

A good deal of cancer detection can be offered at the annual health maintenance visit. Papanicolaou smears should be performed within the guidelines of the American College of Obstetricians and Gynecologists, which generally suggests an annual Papanicolaou smear for women at risk for cancer of the cervix and one at least every 2 to 3 years for women with two consecutive negative Papanicolaou smears and a low-risk history. The decision of whether or not to perform an annual Papanicolaou smear is generally left to the discretion of the physician and the patient (see Chapter 13). Special instances such as women with a history of intrauterine diethylstilbestrol (DES) exposure should dictate Papanicolaou smears every 6 months, and these should include sampling of the four fornices of the vagina as well as the cervical smear.

Screening for breast cancer has three components: patient self-examination of the breast, annual examination by the physician, and screening mammography. The patient should be taught to do a self-examination of the breast at an early health maintenance visit, preferably during her teens. She should be encouraged to perform this examination monthly after completing her menstrual period and preferably when her breasts are wet. Therefore performing this at the time of a bath or shower is appropriate. All the quadrants of the breast should be carefully palpated. The hand of the side that the breast is being palpated should be placed behind the patient's head so that the pectoralis muscles are flexed and the breast is held firmly beneath the palpating fingers of the opposite hand. After the entire breast is palpated, including the tail that extends into the axilla, the patient should be instructed to palpate the subareola area and to squeeze the nipple for evidence of secretion. Any abnormal lump or secretion should be reported to the physician.

At the annual visit the physician should examine the patient's breasts in a similar fashion in both the lying and sitting positions. Screening mammography should be begun at an early age in women who have a first-degree relative with a history of breast cancer, but a baseline mammogram should be obtained by 35 years of age in all women. American

Cancer Society guidelines should be followed thereafter; these include an annual examination for high-risk patients and examination every 2 to 3 years for others until 50 years of age, at which time annual examinations should be initiated for all women.

Colon cancer, which is common in women, particularly those over 40 years of age, can be screened for in several ways. The first is to perform stool guaiac sampling at least annually and generally on three separate stool specimens. In preparation for this the patient should be instructed to eat a bulky diet high in fiber and to avoid foods that produce peroxide, such as horseradish. Women whose guaiac studies are positive should be referred to a gastroenterologist for flexible sigmoidoscopy and other appropriate evaluation. Whether sigmoidoscopy should be required of all women past 35 years of age is still debated. In those individuals who have a strong family history of colon cancer, this recommendation should be made and studies performed every 3 to 5 years. Because the incidence of carcinoma of the colon increases with age, most authorities advise sigmoidoscopy examinations on women over the age of 65 every 3 to 5 years. A rectal examination should be performed at least annually because a larger number of colon cancers can be reached with the finger in the rectum.

There is no good screening test for ovarian cancer, although 1% of all women are at risk for this disease. Although such assays as Ca-125 may have elevated values in patients with epithelial cancers of the ovary, this test has not been proven to be a good screening test for early cancer. In addition, the use of vaginal ultrasound to detect abnormalities of the ovary has not been demonstrated to be useful as a tool for detecting early ovarian cancer. Nevertheless, physicians should examine the ovaries by palpation at least once a year, and in women with a strong family history of cancer, particularly ovarian cancer, the use of vaginal ultrasound and Ca-125 assays on an annual basis should be considered even though their efficacy has not yet been proven.

The physician may screen for other cancers by carefully interpreting a complete physical examination. Thus abnormalities of the thyroid gland may be investigated, smokers may be screened annually with chest x-rays, urine may be studied for the presence of blood, and so on.

Immunization

The annual health maintenance examination is an excellent opportunity to review the patient's status with respect to immunizations. Table 2-2 reviews some of the immunizations that are available. In general, young women should be assessed for their rubella, measles, and polio immunologic status. All patients should have a tetanus and diphtheria booster shot every 10 years, and women over 60 years of age and women with chronic heart or lung disease should be offered influenza vaccine once a year. It has not been

TABLE 2-2. Immunization recommendations of the American College
of Physicians

Immunization	Administration route	Conditions
Diphtheria-tetanus	IM	Every 10 years
Polio (e-IPV)	SQ	One dose if previously immunized; two additional doses at 4-8 wk and 6-12 mo if never immunized
Measles	SQ	For individuals born after 1957 who have not had measles
Rubella	SQ	For women who are rubella titer negative
Influenza	IM, SQ	Annually in autumn for individuals over 60-65 yr or at high risk
Pneumovax	IM, SQ	Once — usually after 60 yr of age

IM, Intramuscular; *SQ*, subcutaneous.

determined whether pneumonia vaccine (Pneumovax) is effective in preventing pneumonia in older individuals, but because of the failing of the immune system in individuals over 60 years of age, many authorities recommend a one-time-only vaccination for such patients.

Immunizations for specific reasons should be considered. Women who are health care workers and who come in contact with body fluids should be offered hepatitis B vaccination. Women traveling to foreign countries should be given appropriate immunization and disease prophylaxis. Required counseling and immunization can be identified by contacting the Communicable Disease Center in Atlanta, Georgia, or by referring the patient to a travel clinic.

Detection of Other Health Conditions

The annual visit is an excellent time to detect other medical problems, such as developing hypertension, diabetes, arthritis, or other chronic illnesses. The history and physical examination may give direction to the possibility of these conditions occurring, but certain screening laboratory work on an annual basis may be appropriate. A complete blood count, urinalysis, and blood sugar determination should be ordered. Serum lipids to detect a cholesterol problem may be ordered about every 5 years. Other specific laboratory tests should be ordered when the history or physical examination suggests their need. Annual chest x-ray and electrocardiogram (ECG) are not necessary unless the patient gives a history suggesting that they would be helpful. Annual chest x-ray for heavy smokers, as an example, is probably warranted. Women at high risk for human immunodeficiency virus (HIV) infection should be offered screening for their condition. These include intravenous drug users and women associated with at-risk men.

When specific problems are detected or suspected, referrals to the appropriate specialist should be considered.

Weight Control

The annual visit is an excellent time for the physician to counsel the patient regarding weight control. Although there is wide latitude of what is acceptable from a health standpoint, patients who are 15% or more under ideal weight probably have an eating disorder such as anorexia nervosa or bulimia, and those who are more than 20% over ideal weight probably suffer from some form of obesity. Table 2-3 is a Metropolitan Life table of desired weights for women. The physician may use these to determine whether or not a patient falls into the desired range. If she does not, a careful dietary history should be taken to get some idea of the types of foods she eats and the number of calories she consumes daily. Having the patient record everything she eats for a 3-day period will give the physician an opportunity to make this determination. If her weight is low, she should carefully be evaluated for the possibility of anorexia nervosa or bulimia. These data should be coupled with her exercise history to determine whether she takes in enough calories to compensate for the amount of activity she ordinarily experiences.

TABLE 2-3.   Height and weight table for women*

Height		Weight (lb)		
Feet	Inches	Small frame	Medium frame	Large frame
4	10	102-111	109-121	118-131
4	11	103-113	111-123	120-134
5	0	104-115	113-126	122-137
5	1	106-118	115-129	125-140
5	2	108-121	118-132	128-143
5	3	111-124	121-135	131-147
5	4	114-127	124-138	134-151
5	5	117-130	127-141	137-155
5	6	120-133	130-144	140-159
5	7	123-136	133-147	143-163
5	8	126-139	136-150	146-167
5	9	129-142	139-153	149-170
5	10	132-145	142-156	152-173
5	11	135-148	145-159	155-176
6	0	138-151	148-162	158-179

*Weights at ages 25 to 29 years based on the lowest mortality. Weights is in pounds according to frame (in indoor clothing weighing 3 lb, shoes with 1 in. heels).
From *1983 Metropolitan Height and Weight Tables*, Metropolitan Life Insurance Company, Health and Safety Division.

If the patient's weight is 20% or more above her ideal, the dietary history can be helpful both in determining the types and quantities of foods she eats and also in helping reeducate her to a lower caloric diet, generally one that is lower in fat content. In general, patients who have a weight of 20% to 40% above ideal are said to be mildly obese and probably do not have any increased health risks. Loss of weight by these individuals is usually considered for cosmetic reasons. Individuals who have weights of 40% to 100% in excess of their ideal weight are said to be moderately obese and should, for health reasons, be placed on a reducing diet generally with the support of a lay group such as Weight Watchers, TOPS (Taking Off Pounds Sensibly), or some commercial group such as NutriSystem. The goal of such groups is to change the patient's eating habits to a diet that is low in fat and calories. Individuals whose weight is in excess of 100% above ideal weight require medical management and are at medical risk. They should be referred to individuals who specialize in the care of such obese patients.

At times knowledge of the serum lipids is a helpful management tool in getting patients to go on a reducing diet. Often in a mildly or moderately obese individual, a weight loss of 10 to 20 lb will reduce cholesterol as much as 50 to 75 mg. The desire of patients to reduce their serum cholesterol may be strong enough to influence them to change their dietary habits. Individuals with cholesterol values in excess of 300 mg/dl should be investigated for the possibility of hypothyroidism, diabetes, or familial hyperlipidemias.

Grief and Loss

Grief and loss are common human experiences and may occur in women of any age. The loss of a child, spouse, close relative, or friend can precipitate an acute grief reaction. But similar reactions may occur in an individual experiencing spontaneous abortion or the loss of a body part or organ, when faced with the realization of infertility and childlessness, because of the loss of a job, or because of a change in a relationship, such as separation or divorce. Other losses, such as the loss of a pet, may also stimulate an acute grief reaction.

Lindemann describes the acute grief syndrome as one that has both psychologic and somatic components. The syndrome includes complaints of tightness in the throat and chest, a choking sensation, a feeling of shortness of breath, and frequent sighing. There is often an empty feeling in the abdomen, muscle weakness, and the feeling of tension and mental pain. The symptoms may come in waves lasting from minutes to an hour and may become dreaded by the sufferer. In severe bereavement situations, disorders of the sensorium involving a sense of unreality, a tendency to place emotional distance between themselves and other people, and a preoccupation with imagery of the deceased may occur. In bereavement the bereaved may assume the mannerisms of the deceased person and even attempt to perform the work of the lost loved one. In such situations as the death of the mother, the bereaved daughter may see the mother's face when she looks at herself in the mirror and may assume her mother's mannerisms of speech and gestures. The bereaved individual may believe that the deceased person is nearby and can communicate. Grieving is almost always associated with guilt that may involve the events of the loss or the tasks left unfinished before the loss occurred. Often an individual who is grieving will feel a lack of warmth and may demonstrate hostility toward others. A normal grief period is variable depending on what is being grieved, but when loss of life is involved, it generally lasts from 6 to 18 months. Generally it ends when the individual appropriately experiences the pain and suffering and places the memory of the deceased person in the proper place within the bereaved individual's life, thereby establishing new relationships and new life directions. At times, when the loss of a spouse is suffered by an older individual, the grieving period may be extended and may even last the rest of the individual's life. This is probably due, in part, to the inability of the older individual to adequately replace the lost spouse with other relationships or experiences.

Certain abnormal grief reactions have been noted by Lindemann. The first of these is the delayed reaction, which essentially involves the postponement of grieving. This is often seen when an automobile accident occurs in which one individual is killed and another is left seriously injured. The injured person may postpone grief until such time as the injuries are healed. Thus the occurrence of grief may seem to be at an inappropriate time and in an inappropriate manner out of context with the current life situation.

A second variation of abnormal grief is the distorted reaction. In this situation the bereaved person takes on the characteristics of the deceased without evidence of a sense of loss. This may include the symptoms the lost person experienced before death.

A third abnormal reaction is the development of psychosomatic symptoms such as ulcerative colitis, rheumatoid arthritis, and asthma.

Other types of pathologic grief reactions include severe alterations of relationships with friends and relatives, inappropriate hostility toward others, behavior patterns resembling psychoses, a long-term, continuing inability to make decisions or to take initiative, and the performance of activities that are both socially and economically destructive.

Finally, a condition known as agitated depression may occur in which the bereaved individual develops tension, agitation, insomnia, feelings of worthlessness, and fantasies of a need for punishment. Suicide is a prominent danger in such situations. Individuals suffering from agitated depression generally have a past history of depression, and this problem usually occurs in individuals who have been intimately associated with the lost individual, such as mothers who have lost young children.

Patients who have experienced loss should be evaluated for the grief reaction and for abnormal variance. When these are discovered, appropriate counseling and referral should be offered. When a patient reports the immediate loss of a loved one, it is appropriate for the physician to review the grief reaction that the patient can anticipate and to warn her about making sudden decisions that may be physically and economically detrimental to her best interests.

General Considerations

The annual health maintenance visit is an opportunity to instruct the patient in general good health habits and to consider safety issues. Patients should be encouraged to get 7 to 8 hours of sleep per night. This is particularly important for older women. A modest exercise program should be encouraged to improve cardiovascular efficiency. This may be a weight-bearing type of exercise, such as walking, jogging, or aerobic dancing, or a non–weight-bearing exercise, such as swimming or cycling. Older women who are at risk for falls and associated injuries, should be encouraged to participate in exercises that improve flexibility and balance. If the patient participates in such activities as cycling, horseback riding, or motorcycle riding, she should be urged to wear a helmet. She should be cautioned not to participate in sports or other exercise activities that are beyond her capability.

The patient should be asked whether there are firearms in the home. If there are, caution concerning their use and safety measures associated with their use should be stressed. She should be encouraged to wear seat belts when riding in a motor vehicle. Hearing problems should be discussed, and situations that hinder hearing in at-risk circumstances, such as jogging on a busy thoroughfare while listening to a Walkman, should be discussed. She should be informed about the importance of appropriate footwear for activities she may undertake. This is particularly important for older women, who are at risk for falls. Skin exposure to ultraviolet radiation should be discussed and proper precautions to avoid overexposure noted.

Patients should be asked about depression and possible suicidal ideation. Destructive habits, such as the use of tobacco, alcohol, or drugs, should be noted and remedial suggestions given.

It is important for the physician to use the annual visit as an opportunity to do many things to help promote the general health and well-being of the patient. In so doing, mortality and morbidity may be postponed and the patient given the opportunity to enjoy an excellent quality of life for as long as possible.

42   *Office Gynecology*

BIBLIOGRAPHY

American College of Obstetricians and Gynecologists: *Cervical cytology: evaluation and management of abnormalities*, Washington, DC, 1984, ACOG Technical Bulletin No 81.

American College of Obstetricians and Gynecologists: *The Obstetricians and Gynecologists and Primary Preventive Health Care*, Washington, DC, 1993, ACOG Task Force on Primary and Preventive Care.

Byyne RL: Establishing guidelines for preventive medicine, *Contemp Obstet Gynecol* 31:43, 1988.

Casper RC, Eckert ED, Halmi KA, et al: Bulimia: its incidence and clinical importance in patients with anorexia nervosa, *Br J Psych* 27:1030, 1980.

Frank E, Anderson C, Rubinstein D: Frequency of sexual dysfunction in normal couples, *N Engl J Med* 299:111, 1978.

Hammond DC: Screening for sexual dysfunction, *Clin Obstet Gynecol* 27:732, 1984.

Johnson WG, Schlundt DG: Eating disorders: assessment and treatment, *Clin Obstet Gynecol* 28:598, 1985.

Kalucy RC, Crisp AH, Lacy JH, et al: Prevalence and prognosis of anorexia nervosa, *Aust N Z J Psychiatry* 11:251, 1977.

Kendell RE, Hall DJ, Harley A, et al: The epidemiology of anorexia nervosa, *Psychol Med* 2:200, 1973.

Kline NS: *From sad to glad*, New York, 1974, GP Putnam's Sons.

Leppert PC, Pahlka BS: Grieving characteristics after spontaneous abortion: a management approach, *Obstet Gynecol* 64:119, 1984.

Lindemann E: Symptomatology and management of acute grief, *Am J Psychiatry* 101:141, 1944.

Lundin T: Long term outcome of bereavement, *Br J Psychiatry* 145:424, 1984.

Papanicolaou GN, Trout HF: *Diagnosis of uterine cancer by vaginal smears*, New York, 1943, The Commonwealth Fund.

Quackenbush J: The death of a pet: how it can affect owners, *Vet Clin North Am* 15:395, 1985.

Shy K, Chu J, Mandelson M, et al: Papanicolaou smear screening interval and risk of cervical cancer, *Obstet Gynecol* 74:838, 1989.

Stenchever MA: History and examination of the patient. In Droegemueller W, Herbst AL, Mishell DR, et al, editors: *Comprehensive gynecology*, ed 2, St Louis, 1991, Mosby.

Stunkard AJ: Current status of treatment for obesity in adults. In Stukard AJ, Stellar E, editors: *Eating and its disorders*, New York, 1984, Raven Press.

Taylor PT, Andersen WA, Barber SR, et al: The screening Papanicolaou smear: contribution of the endocervical brush, *Obstet Gynecol* 70:734, 1987.

The health consequences of smoking, Washington, DC, 1973, US Department of Health, Education and Welfare.

Warren NP: Anorexia nervosa and the related eating disorders, *Clin Obstet Gynecol* 28:588, 1985.

CHAPTER **3**

Contraception

KIRK K. SHY

Data on the sexual and reproductive behavior of women in the 1988 National Survey of Family Growth indicate a few significant changes when compared with 1982. The proportion of never-married women currently in a sexual relationship increased for *all* age categories, and the proportion of nonmarried cohabiting women increased from 1 in 20 to 1 in 10. Thirty-four percent of women 18 to 19 years old had multiple partners in the previous 1-year period. This indicates the increasing necessity for contraceptive methods that also provide protection against sexually transmitted disease (STD).

Between 1982 and 1987, condom and oral contraceptive use increased significantly among sexually active women. The increase in condom use was greatest (to 16%) for unmarried women. This emphasizes the mounting concern about STD and the increasing proportion of women with favorable opinions about oral contraception and condoms. Oral contraceptives and condoms are the dominant contraceptive methods among U.S. women (Table 3-1).

After an increase in sexual activity among adolescents during the 1980s, between 1990 and 1993 the proportion of high school students who reported being sexually experienced remained stable. Furthermore, during 1991 and 1992, in most states, live birth and gonorrhea rates declined among 15- to 19-year-old males and females. This was associated with an increased use of condoms in this age group. This may be attributed to human immunodeficiency virus (HIV) education and prevention programs for youth. The

TABLE 3-1. Estimated number and percent distribution of contraceptive methods among sexually active U.S. women (15-44)*

Contraceptive method	Number (millions)	Percent of sexually active women
Sterilization	13.8	33
Female	8.1	19
Male	5.7	14
Pill	13.2	32
Condom	6.9	17
Intrauterine device	1.1	3
Diaphragm	1.7	4
Foam	0.6	1
Suppository	0.6	1
Sponge	1.1	3
Periodic abstinence	1.7	4
Withdrawal	2.3	6
Douche	0.6	1
Total contraceptors†	38.0	92
Noncontraceptors	3.3	8

*1987 Ortho Bill Control Study. Data are from Forrest DJ, Fordyce RR: *Fam Plann Perspect* 20:112, 1988.
†Numbers and percentages do not add up because some women used more than one method.

direction of these changes is encouraging, but the contraceptive challenges remain. Pregnancy rates among U.S. teenagers are greater than for any other developed country. At least 1 in 5 sexually active teenagers and poor women do not use contraception.

EFFECTIVENESS

"How effective is it?" is probably the most common question from patients considering a new contraceptive method. This question is best answered with data specific to a particular couple's circumstances. Unfortunately, a data-based answer is not possible. Instead, we must rely on summary data and clinical opinion.

Table 3-2 depicts the failure rates for various forms of contraception in a study of over 17,000 married women observed for an average of 9.5 years. These extensive data from the Oxford/Family Planning Association are valuable because generally data from other studies are based on either smaller samples or interview-based surveys. The particular data in this table are a reference point for contraceptive counseling. However, it must be emphasized that contraceptive failure rates from this table vary widely according to many factors, including duration of use, age (Fig. 3-1), education, and income. As any of these four factors increase, failure rates fall.

TABLE 3-2. Observed failure rates for different methods of contraception*

Method	Failure rate (per 100 woman-years)
Oral Contraceptive	
Combination	
> 50 μg estrogen	0.32
50 μg estrogen	0.16
< 50 μg estrogen	0.27
Progestin-only	1.2
Diaphragm	1.9
Condom	3.6
Intrauterine device	
Lippe's Loop D	1.3
Copper-TCu-380A	<0.8
Copper-7	1.5
Rhythm	15.5
Withdrawal	6.7
Spermicides	11.9
Sterilization	
Female	0.13
Male	0.02

*Data are from married women 25 years or more followed for an average of 9.5 years at British family planning clinics (from Vessey M, Lawless M, Yates D: *Lancet* 1:841, 1982), except for data concerning the Copper-TCu-380A (from Trussell J, Hatcher RA, Cates W, et al: *Stud Fam Plann* 21:51, 1990).

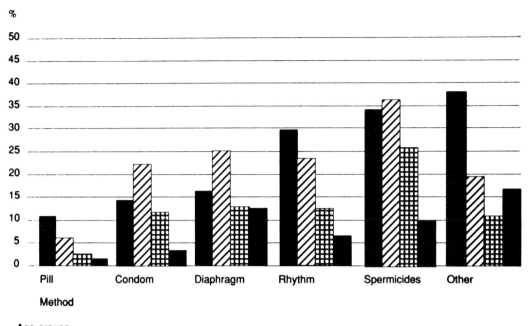

%

Age-groups

■ <20   ▨ 20–24   ⊞ 25–34   ■ 35–44

FIGURE 3-1.   Percentage of women experiencing contraceptive failure during the first 12 months of use, by age and method, standardized by race and marital status.

From Jones EF, Forrest JD: Fam Plann Perspect 21:103, 1989.

Furthermore, reporting of contraceptive failure rates is unavoidably troubled by ambiguity and bias:

1. Method failure rates reported in the literature typically are calculated incorrectly. This occurs because women who would not become pregnant even without contraception (e.g., because of infertility or chance) are included (erroneously) in the denominator. Thus reported method failure rates are generally too low.

2. Less effective contraceptive methods are commonly chosen by couples with a lower inherent likelihood of pregnancy either because of a low frequency of intercourse or because of suspected subfecundity. Thus pregnancy risk for less effective contraceptive methods may be under-estimated.

3. Contraceptive failure rates are not standardized for the characteristics of populations that tend to choose different classes of contraceptive methods. Nonwhite and poor patients tend to choose barrier contraception. Because unwanted pregnancy is more common in this population (regardless of contraceptive method), unwanted pregnancy rates with barrier methods are biased upward; correspondingly, pregnancy rates with oral contraceptives are biased downward.

4. Unwanted pregnancies that result in abortion are typically underreported in large surveys of contraceptive failure. Proper counting of these pregnancies results in an increase in failure rates for all contraceptive methods. Underreporting of abortion is greatest among patients relying on condoms and spermicides.

5. Many studies use an outdated methodology known as the Pearl index (failure per 100 woman-years of exposure). Misleadingly low failure rates occur because couples drop out of the analysis when they experience trouble with the method, and couples tend to continue (and contribute a nonrepresentative large number of years) when the method has been particularly successful for them. Life-table methods are superior to the Pearl index.

6. There is no reliable method to adjust for frequency of intercourse in comparing pregnancy rates across contraception methods.

Fundamentally, low reported contraceptive failure rates do not protect women from unwanted pregnancy; consistent, properly applied contraceptive methods do. In counseling patients, factors such as perceived safety, convenience, and cost are often more important in preventing an unwanted pregnancy than the theoretic contraceptive effectiveness of a method.

FERTILITY AWARENESS AND NATURAL FAMILY PLANNING

Fertility awareness methods are based on daily recording and charting of physiologic changes during the normal menstrual cycle. Charting permits identification of fertile days on which intercourse without contraception has a high likelihood of pregnancy. Charting along with other methods of contraception during the fertile period is called *fertility awareness*. Charting along with abstinence during the fertile days to avoid pregnancy is called *natural family planning*. This includes the rhythm (or calendar) method, basal body temperature (BBT) charting and the symptothermal method, and cervical mucus charting. The phrase "natural family planning" must be considered somewhat of a misnomer. Avoiding intercourse when pregnancy is most likely to occur can hardly be considered natural. Conversely, other, more medically oriented contraceptive techniques are not "unnatural."

Fertility awareness and natural family planning are based on three underlying assumptions:

1. The ovum is capable of fertilization for only approximately 24 hours after ovulation.

2. Sperm maintain their fertilizing ability for only about 48 hours after intercourse.

3. Ovulation usually occurs 12 to 16 days before the onset of menses.

Assumptions 1 and 2 are difficult to validate directly, and contemporary evidence suggests that fertile intervals for both ovum and sperm are considerably longer than these assumptions suggest. Cycle length varies to a greater or lesser degree in most women. These difficulties result in higher pregnancy rates with natural family planning than with medical methods of contraception.

Pregnancy rates with natural family planning are loosely related to specific techniques. Highest pregnancy rates occur when the calendar method is used alone. The World Health Organization reported a multi-center contraceptive study of the ovulation (Billings) method that is based on women's examination of their cervical mucus. The overall reported pregnancy rate was 19.6 pregnancies per 100 woman-years. Most pregnancies were associated with a couple's conscious departure from the rules. Across natural family planning methods, pregnancy rates are probably lowest with the BBT method and intercourse confined to the postovulatory phase.

Calendar Method

The calendar method and other natural family planning techniques rely on precise definitions of menstrual cycle day number and a series of rules that specify safe and unsafe (fertile) days for intercourse. The first day of menstrual bleeding (or even light spotting) is by definition the first numbered day of the menstrual cycle. Cycle length must be counted for eight cycles before beginning use of this method. With this information fertile days can be predicted at the onset of a menstrual period. The first fertile menstrual cycle day number is calculated by subtracting 18 from the length of the shortest cycle (during the preceding 8 months). The last fertile menstrual cycle day number is calculated by subtracting 11 from the length of the longest cycle.

Thus for a constant 24-day cycle length, the first fertile (unsafe) day number is 6, and the last fertile (unsafe) day number is 13. For a woman with cycle length varying from 26 to 29 days, the first fertile (unsafe) day number is 8, and the last fertile (unsafe) day number is 18.

Basal Body Temperature Method

The basal body temperature (BBT) method is used to identify the postovulatory period during which conception is unlikely. This is a retrospective determination. Based on evaluation of temperature charts from the three preceding menstrual periods, the onset of the postovulatory interval in the present cycle is estimated. Because the day of ovulation is best determined by retrospective evaluation of the BBT chart, use of the current BBT chart provides only limited information for the current cycle.

Ovulation is suggested in a BBT chart by a sharp rise of 0.4 to 0.6°F between two successive days, a subsequent sustained temperature plateau for several days, and a temperature dip, or nadir, preceding the initial sharp temperature rise. Classically these temperature changes result in a biphasic BBT curve (Figure 3-2). Evaluation of temperatures is simplified by charting. Temperature elevation results from thermogenic properties of progesterone from the corpus luteum after ovulation. Actual temperatures have little importance. Variability in day-to-day temperatures is normal, producing irregularity in the shape of the curve. Variability is increased by sleep disturbance, intercurrent illness, and other factors.

For reliable information, temperature should be taken daily before rising from bed. Satisfactory results can be obtained with ordinary oral, glass thermometers. Measurement and recording are simplified with electronic digital thermometers.

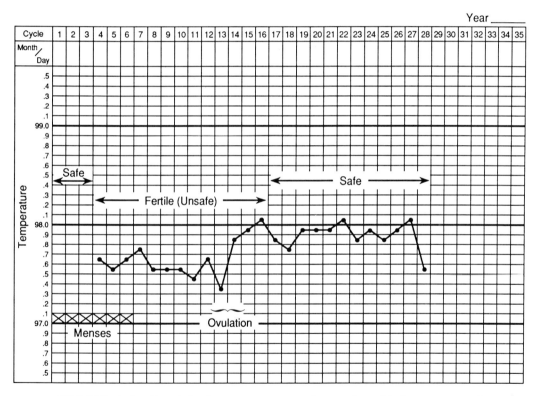

FIGURE 3-2. Basal body temperature chart of a 28-day menstrual cycle. Retrospective evaluation indicates that ovulation probably occurred in conjunction with a temperature dip on day 13 or the subsequent temperature elevation on day 14. Usual cycle day number of ovulation should be based on the three preceding cycles. Because of chance variability from cycle to cycle in the day of ovulation, intercourse as early as day 4 of the menstrual cycle could result in a pregnancy. Thus "unsafe" (fertile) days begin 4 days after the onset of menstruation and continue until 3 days of successive temperature elevation. Note that although menstruation continues on days 4 to 6, these are unsafe (fertile) days nonetheless.

Avoiding intercourse throughout the preovulatory phase of the cycle is the approach least likely to fail and result in pregnancy. However, intercourse during the first 3 days of menses may be permitted. Because of chance variability from cycle to cycle in the day of ovulation and because sperm can probably survive for 72 hours, intercourse as early as day 4 of the menstrual cycle could result in a pregnancy. Thus intercourse should be avoided on day 4 of the menstrual cycle (the fourth day of menstruation) until 4 days after ovulation determined on the basis of the preceding three to four BBT charts. For women with menstrual periods longer than 3 days, alternative contraception is necessary during the latter days of menstruation.

Most women do not ovulate every cycle, and this is reflected in BBT charts. Absence of ovulation in a particular cycle is indicated by absence of a temperature rise or persistence of the temperature elevation for 10 days or less. Use of BBT curves as a measure of ovulation has been validated with luteinizing hormone and progesterone measurement together with serial ultrasound measurements of follicular development.

Cervical Mucus Charting

Cervical mucus charting for contraception is also known as the ovulation method and as the Billings method, after its developer. The method is based on sequential cervical mucus changes produced by alterations in estrogen and progesterone secretion during the menstrual cycle. Women's recognition of these changes allows for the prediction of ovulation and observance of sexual abstinence for contraception.

Amount, viscosity, color, and spinnbarkeit ("stretchiness" between spread fingers) are characteristics that aid in the prediction of ovulation (Table 3-3). Menstrual bleeding precedes an interval of a few "dry days" with little or no vaginal secretions. This is followed by the onset of "mucus symptoms" and "cloudy, sticky" secretions. At ovulation, cervical mucus increases substantially and is associated with the stretchy characteristic termed *spinnbarkeit*. At this time, cervical mucus typically can be stretched 2 to 4 inches between two fingers. After ovulation, the quantity of cervical mucus diminishes, and it loses its spinnbarkeit, becoming progressively thicker and more cloudy and opaque.

Women are instructed to wipe the vulva with toilet paper before and after micturition and make note of secretions present. In addition, a finger should be inserted into the vagina and the degree of wetness determined. An attempt should also be made with the finger to collect any cervical mucus present.

For this method to be effective, intercourse should be avoided at the onset of any vaginal moisture or cervical mucus. Abstinence should continue until the evening of the fourth day after the peak day of maximal mucus secretion

TABLE 3-3. Cervical mucus characteristics according to mucus type and time of cycle

Mucus type and time of cycle	Amount	Viscosity	Color	Spinnbarkeit (in.)
DRY DAYS				
Postmenstruation	Moderate	Thick	Cloudy, yellow, or white	<1
ONSET OF MUCUS SYMPTOMS AND CLOUDY OR STICKY SECRETION				
Nearing ovulation	Increasing	Somewhat thick to thin	Mixed cloudy and clear	1-1½
PEAK SYMPTOMS				
Ovulation	Maximum	Thin and slippery	Clear	6-8
Postovulation (about 3 days)	Decreasing	Thin	Mixed cloudy and clear	4-6
TACKY MUCUS				
Nearing menstruation	Minimal	Thick	Cloudy	<1-1½

associated with ovulation. Intercourse can then resume throughout the postovulatory phase until menstruation.

Avoiding intercourse during the entire preovulatory interval from the onset of menstruation until the fourth peak day enhances the contraceptive effectiveness of cervical mucus charting. Women with short cycles may exhibit the first mucus symptoms during menstruation, when these symptoms are difficult to detect. Although mucus symptoms typically precede ovulation by 3 days or more, outliers of sperm viability (i.e., greater than 3 days) or short preovulatory mucus symptoms (less than 3 days) permit conception. Finally, semen in the vagina may interfere with detection of the true onset of peak symptoms. For the same reason, this contraceptive method loses effectiveness in the presence of vaginal infections and after douching.

Summary

Although failure rates with these methods are substantially greater than with other medical methods of contraception, failure rates are a fraction of the rates for couples without any form of contraception. However, it must be understood that a certain percent of the contraceptive effectiveness of these methods is attributable to fewer acts of sexual intercourse, and not its timing alone. Women with irregular menstrual cycles (typically older or younger patients) are not good candidates. Combining natural family planning methods (e.g., basal body temperature and cervical mucus charting) improves their overall effectiveness. When uncertain, addition of barrier methods is recommended. Use of condoms is the only method that does not interfere with cervical mucus charting. Because natural methods are the least studied contraceptive method, their side effects have been only superficially investigated. Poorly substantiated concerns have been raised about increased birth defects in contraceptive failures after natural family planning.

ORAL CONTRACEPTIVES

Almost all oral contraceptives (OCs) are *combination pills* that contain an estrogen and a progestin. The progestin alone is probably sufficient to provide satisfactory contraception for most women. Addition of estrogen and cyclic administration with a 7-day pill-free interval controls the menstrual cycle and makes it predictable. All low-dose combination OCs (35 μg or less) now contain the estrogen ethinyl estradiol. Formerly mestranol was used with little difference in effects. Contemporary OCs contain one of several progestins (ethynodiol diacetate, norethindrone, norethindrone acetate, norgestrel, or norethynodrel), including two new ones (desogestrel and norgestimate).

Mechanism of Action

Estrogen has at least four effects that prevent conception. Ovulation is inhibited. In the pituitary, an alteration occurs in sensitivity to gonadotropin-releasing hormone (GnRH); in the brain, steroids exert a direct effect on GnRH pulse generation. For agents with 50 μg or less estrogen, ovulation occurs in 2% to 5% of cases, thus the importance of other estrogenic and progestational effects, particularly inhibition of implantation, accelerated ovum transport, and promotion of luteolysis (premature degeneration of the corpus luteum).

Although progesterone normally prepares the endometrium for implantation of the conceptus, progestins have several contraceptive effects. In the presence of progestins, *hostile cervical mucus* develops that is scanty, cellular, and exhibits decreased ferning and spinnbarkeit. Capacitation is inhibited. Ovulation may be inhibited by progestins in the same manner that estrogens interfere with ovulation.

Classes of Oral Contraceptives

Since the 1960s, most clinical research has been directed to decreasing the steroid dosage in an effort to reduce steroid-related side effects and complications. As a result, a variety of classes of OCs have been developed: combination, sequential, minipills, and triphasic.

Monophasic combination oral contraceptives dominate the OC marketplace in the United States (Fig. 3-3). All contain a synthetic estrogen and progestin in a fixed ratio. These pills are administered for 21 days with a 7-day hiatus during which menstruation usually occurs. To increase compliance, some brands of combination pills are packaged with seven additional inert pills to complete a 28-day pill package cycle. During the past two decades, the estrogen dosage of many combined oral contraceptives has been reduced; these new preparations are termed *low-dose* combined OCs, and they should not be confused with minipills, which are discussed below.

Sequential OCs are no longer manufactured in the United States because of their association with endometrial cancer. (Endometrial cancer was

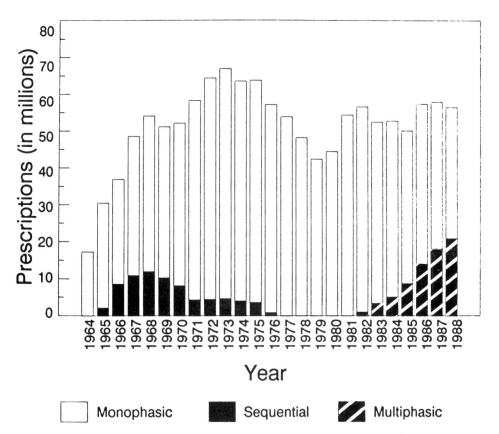

FIGURE 3-3. Number of retail oral contraceptive prescriptions by formulation type, 1964 to 1988, United States.

From Gerstman BB, Gross TP, Kennedy DL, et al: Am J Public Health 81:90, 1991.

probably related to the high estrogen dosage in certain of the sequential pills, such as Oracon, and not the sequential dosing pattern. Thus low-estrogen sequentials available in Europe have not been associated with endometrial cancer.) With sequentials, estrogens are administered daily for 21 days, and progestins are added only for the last 7 days. Again a 7-day hiatus with menstruation completes the 28-day cycle.

Minipills have been available in the United States since 1973; however, they occupy only a small proportion of the market. No estrogens are contained in minipills. Instead they contain only the progestins that are available in the combination preparations, but in minipills the progestin dosage is considerably less (35% that of low-dose combination pills). Minipills must be taken every day. As a result menses are commonly irregular.

Triphasic OCs have three different estrogen-progestin ratios during the contraceptive pill cycle, more closely approximating the cyclic hormonal changes that occur in the normal menstrual cycle. This dosing scheme permits a modest reduction in progestin dosage.

Risks and Side Effects of Hormonal Contraception

Four specific diseases of the circulatory system are associated with OCs: venous thromboembolism, ischemic heart disease (including myocardial infarction), cerebrovascular disease and stroke, and hypertension. The pathogenesis and risk factors for each of these conditions vary, but the results of major cohort studies (British Royal College Study, Oxford/Family Planning Association Study, and The Walnut Creek Study) show more clearly than ever that the increased risk of death caused by these conditions and OCs is concentrated among women over 35, especially women who smoke. These vascular diseases and their respective risk factors for women using OC are listed in Table 3-4.

Oral contraceptives increase venous thromboembolic disease overtly and subclinically as measured by ^{125}I-fibrinogen uptake and plasma fibrinogen chromatography. British studies indicated that overt superficial or deep thromboembolic disease directly attributable to OCs (principally ≥ 50 μg estrogen) occurs annually in approximately 2 of 1000 OC users. Subclinical thrombosis is much more frequent. This risk of venous thromboembolic disease begins during the first month of use and thereafter remains relatively constant. After discontinuation, this risk resolves entirely within 1 month. Venous thromboembolic disease is the leading cause of death directly related to OCs. For all OC users, the number of cases of venous thromboembolism per 10,000 woman-years of use is approximately 11, compared with 3 cases for nonusers. Risk increases directly with age and smoking. During the postoperative period, the attributable risk of deep vein thrombosis or pulmonary embolism associated with oral contraceptives is high: 30 cases per 10,000 women per year.

TABLE 3-4. Circulatory system disease and use of oral contraceptives: summary of cohort and case-control studies of white women in the United Kingdom and the United States

Disease	Relative risk	Duration of use	Estrogen	Progestin	Past use	Other risk factors
			Dose			
Venous thrombo-embolic disease	2-4	No	Yes	No?	No	ABO blood type, smoking?, age
Ischemic heart disease	2-6	Yes?	Yes	Yes?	?	Age, smoking, hypertension, high choles-terol level, dia-betes
Stroke, throm-botic	9	?	?	?	?	Hypertension
Stroke, hemor-rhagic	1.5-4	Yes?	No?	Yes	Yes?	Smoking, hyper-tension, race
Hypertension	1-3	Yes?	?	Yes	No	Age, race

From Kols MA, Rinehart W, Piotrow PT, et al: *Popul Rep A* 6:190, 1982.

These venous thrombotic effects are similar to the changes seen late in pregnancy, and they are related primarily to the estrogenic component of combination OCs. Venous thromboembolic disease in OC users is mediated by two factors: accelerated intravenous coagulation and impaired fibrino-lytic activity. Accelerated intravenous coagulation results from estrogen's action to reduce antithrombin III activity. Normally, antithrombin III inactivates factor X and thrombin. Blunting of the process leads to greater thrombin and fibrin production (Fig. 3-4). OCs containing 75 to 150 μg of mestranol or ethinyl estradiol decrease antithrombin III activity to a greater extent than OCs containing 50 μg or less. Antithrombin III activity is not altered when progesterone is given in the absence of estrogens. The impaired fibrinolytic activity caused by OCs results from their action to reduce plasminogen activator concentration (Fig. 3-5). Normally, the fibrinolytic capacity of the blood derives from the conversion of circulating plasminogen to plasmin, an enzyme that degrades fibrin and fibrinogen. Production of plasmin is facilitated by plasminogen activator.

In addition to increasing the risk of venous thromboembolic disease, OCs increase the risks of myocardial infarction, thrombotic stroke, and hemorrhagic stroke (Table 3-4). These are also the effects of aging on the vasculature. Nonetheless, the Food and Drug Administration (FDA) has instructed manufacturers to revise labeling for OC products to reflect

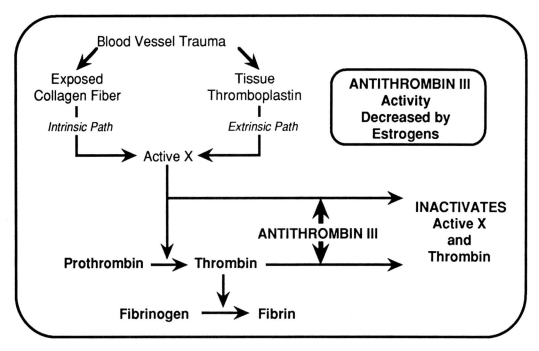

FIGURE 3-4. Estrogens affect the clotting cascade by decreasing antithrombin III activity. (Normally, through a series of steps, antithrombin III slows fibrin formation.)

current scientific opinion that the benefits of OC for healthy nonsmoking women over 40 may outweigh the possible risks. The risks of stroke and myocardial infarction are related to both estrogen and progestin dosages. For myocardial infarction among OC users, the major factors, besides age, that influence risk are cigarette smoking, history of preeclampsia or hypertension, type II hyperlipoproteinemia, and diabetes mellitus. For thrombotic stroke the only factor is hypertension, and for hemorrhagic stroke only cigarette smoking, hypertension, and black race. In the same way that age multiplies the thromboembolic risks of OCs, epidemiologic data indicate that these additional factors multiply the risks of myocardial infarction and stroke with OCs.

This background information suggests that the pathogenesis of myocardial infarction and stroke attributable to OCs has two components: factors related to duration of use and factors not related to duration of use (Table 3-5). Accelerated platelet aggregation and fibrin deposition, as well as decreased antithrombin III activity and decreased plasminogen-activator concentration in the vascular endothelium, all result from OCs and contribute to myocardial infarction and strokes. These metabolic changes are *not* related to duration of use. Autopsies of women who die with myocardial infarction while on oral contraceptives reveal that the infarc-

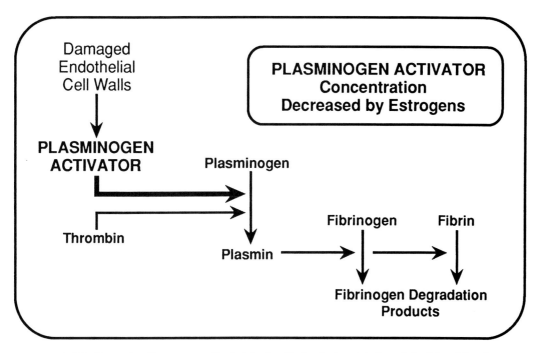

FIGURE 3-5. Estrogens diminish the fibrinolytic activity of the blood by decreasing the concentration of plasminogen activator. (Normally, plasminogen activator facilitates fibrinogen and fibrin degradation.)

TABLE 3-5. Pathogenesis of myocardial infarction and stroke related to oral contraception

---

FACTORS UNRELATED TO DURATION OF USE

Platelet aggregation
Fibrin deposition
Antithrombin III activity

FACTORS RELATED TO DURATION OF USE

Blood pressure
Glucose tolerance
High-density lipoprotein cholesterol

---

tions usually have thrombotic rather than atheromatous origin. These acute thrombotic effects of current use are largely related to estrogen content.

The pathogenesis of myocardial infarction and stroke related to duration of OC use has not been systematically investigated. However, the most likely source of the increased risk is accelerated atherogenesis. Oral contraceptives have been observed to have effects on each of the three major factors believed to influence the occurrence of atherosclerotic cardiovascular disease: blood pressure, glucose tolerance, and serum high-density lipoproteins (HDL). Although OCs elevate blood pressure in most women, on the average this elevation is small (1 to 2 mm Hg diastolic, 5 mm Hg systolic). Nonetheless, this leads to a threefold to sixfold increase in the rate of overt hypertension. The decreased glucose tolerance appears to be associated with both the estrogen and progestin components of OCs. The progestogenic component of many oral contraceptives decreases HDLs, whereas they are increased by the estrogen component. On the other hand, low-density lipoproteins (LDL) are increased by estrogens and are decreased by progestins. Thus the net effect of a particular oral contraceptive on lipoprotein cholesterol depends on the specific estrogen progestin composition. High LDL and low HDL cholesterol concentrations are associated with increased risk of coronary heart disease.

Epidemiologic studies have found an association between progestin dose and cardiovascular disease, hypertension, coronary artery disease, stroke, myocardial infarction, and death from these entities Other works such as the Framingham studies suggest that these adverse cardiovascular events are caused by alterations in lipoprotein metabolism.

Of the two most common contraceptive progestins, norgestrel and norethindrone, on a weight basis norgestrel is considerably more potent. This potency difference concerns not only progestational effects but also androgenic and antiestrogenic side effects of progestins. These nonprogestational side effects are responsible for the reduction in HDL with combination oral contraceptives.

Understandably, considerable effort has been devoted to minimize the adverse lipoprotein changes (particularly reduction in HDL cholesterol) associated with oral contraceptives. Notably, among the combination pills with norgestrel there has been an emphasis on products with lower progestin dosage. Thus total milligrams of norgestrel for a cycle of Lo-Ovral are 6.3, versus 1.925 mg of norgestrel for the newer product Triphasil.

It should be emphasized that after stopping OCs, excess cardiovascular risk ceases almost immediately. This conclusion is based on the Nurses' Health Study, in which over 100,000 women were studied, many for 10 years or more.

Other metabolic effects of OCs are less significant. Included are higher peripheral blood glucose levels and a compensatory increase in serum insulin. This may result from decreased insulin receptors and insulin binding induced by progestins. Expression of gallbladder disease may be accelerated in women who are already susceptible to this disease. Endocrine function test results from the thyroid and adrenal are altered. In part, these changes result from increased serum binding globulins for these hormones. Endocrine function test results should be considered with this in mind. Test alterations induced by OCs are of no clinical significance and return to normal soon after OCs are discontinued.

Norgestimate and Desogestrel

Norgestimate and desogestrel are two new progestins in OCs available in the United States. Like their predecessors, these new progestins are 19-nortestosterones. Both norgestimate and desogestrel are derived from norgestrel. The half-life of norgestimate is 45 to 71 hours, and it and its metabolites are biologically active. These features prolong the activity of norgestimate in vivo, and in theory they may improve contraceptive efficacy (if a pill is missed) and reduce breakthrough bleeding. Desogestrel is rapidly metabolized in a first pass through the liver and bowel mucosa. Consequently, the parent compound (desogestrel) is inactive; only its metabolite (3-ketodesogestrel) has biologic activity. These new progestins have less androgenic activity than the progestins contained in other OCs. As a result, the lipid profile of women using norgestimate-containing OCs is favorable. For women using desogestrel-containing OCs, the lipid profile is neutral or positive. Although this is desirable, whether changes in lipid metabolism result in further reduction in OC-related mortality is uncertain. Mortality is already exceedingly low.

Androgen-related side effects, such as acne and hirsutism, may be less for OCs with these new progestins. However, few randomized trials comparing the new progestin OCs with the established pills have been completed. Several lines of evidence suggest fewer androgenic side effects:

1. Androgen receptor binding affinity of norgestimate and 3-keto-desogestrel (the active metabolite of desogestrel) is less than levonorgestrel (Fig. 3-6).

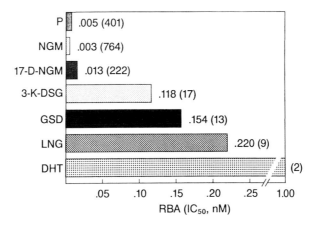

FIGURE 3-6. Relative binding affinities (RBAs) to androgen receptors in rat prostate. *P*, progesterone; *17-D-NGM*, 17-deacetyl norgestimate; *DHT*, dihydrotestosterone; *GSD*, gestodene; *3-K-DSG*, 3-ketodesogestrel; *LNG*, levonorgestrel; *NGM*, norgestimate.

From Darney PD: *Am J Med* 98(1A) 104S, 1995.

2. Sex hormone–binding globulin concentrations increase more with desogestrel and norgestimate than with other progestins. Sex hormone–binding globulins are inversely related to a compound's androgenicity.

3. Free serum testosterone concentrations are less among women with OCs containing desogestrel and norgestimate. In turn, clinical studies have shown that the number of women with acne or hirsutism (either preexisting or newly emergent) is reduced in women who use OCs with the new progestins. Weight gain has many determinants, and it is uncertain whether the new progestins have an effect on it.

Oral Contraceptives and Cancer

Oral contraceptives protect against ovarian cancer, and because in the United States and Europe the annual incidence of ovarian cancer is 10 to 20 cases per 100,000 women of all ages (accounting for 6% of all female cancer deaths), a beneficial effect of OCs is highly significant. Oral contraceptive use produces this protective effect to essentially the same degree as pregnancy. Twelve months of combined OC use has about the same effect in reducing ovarian cancer as a live birth. Reduction in ovarian cancer risk is not related to timing of use. Protection remains for as long as 10 years after use ceases and appears to be greatest with longer durations of use. The mechanism by which OCs protect against ovarian cancer may be related to inhibition of ovulation. With each ovulation, minor trauma occurs to the surface epithelium of the ovary, and as a consequence of ovulation the epithelium is exposed to estrogen-rich follicular fluid. Results in the United States suggest that OC use averts about 1700 cases of ovarian cancer each year in women 20 to 54 years of age.

Evidence links combination OCs with a reduced risk of endometrial cancer. This is significant because the protective effect is large and the annual rate of endometrial cancer in developing countries is high, 10 to 25 cases per 100,000 women of all ages. The protective effect increases with duration of use and is greatest in nulliparous women who otherwise are at greater risk for endometrial cancer. Estrogens promote endometrial growth that may eventually lead to cancer, whereas progestin opposes this effect. Thus OC formulations with high progestin content may offer the most protection against endometrial cancer. Researchers at the U.S. Centers for Disease Control estimate that OC use in the United States prevents about 2000 cases of endometrial cancer each year.

The relationship between OCs and breast cancer is more controversial. Studies on the relationship between breast cancer and OCs have largely been restricted to premenopausal development of cancer, in part because few OC users have passed menopause. There are fundamental reasons to be suspicious about a causal relationship. Number of years of regular menstrual cycles is directly related to breast cancer risk. Among women before their first full-term pregnancy, proliferation of breast epithelium is significantly greater among OC users. Although most studies have not shown a relationship, more recent studies of OCs and breast cancer have reported an increased risk in one subgroup or another. Subgroups at increased risk are not consistent across studies, and it is possible that the observed high-risk groups are simply a statistical artifact related to the large number of comparisons. Women with long-term use, particularly before the first full-term pregnancy, are the subgroup most consistently identified at risk for breast cancer in the OC studies that found this association. The Cancer and Steroid Hormone Study funded by the National Institutes of Child Health and Human Development is the largest U.S. study, and no convincing link with breast cancer was demonstrated. Undoubtedly, considerably more research will be necessary to clarify this matter. In 1989 the Fertility and Maternal Health Advisory Committee to the FDA concluded that the evidence linking OCs and breast cancer was too inconclusive to warrant changes in current practice patterns or drug labeling. This authoritative viewpoint can serve as a point of reference in counseling patients.

The association of OCs with other cancers is either uncertain or of limited clinical significance because of their rare occurrence. Long-term OC users increase by several times their risks of liver cancer and hepatocellular adenoma. Given the extremely rare nature of these tumors, this finding has limited significance. Studies evaluating the relationship between OC use and cervical cancer are inconclusive. Because of differences in sexual practices between OC users and nonusers, and because sexual practices are tied directly to the development of cervical cancer, it is difficult to isolate the independent effects of OCs. This matter is further confused because nonusers of OCs commonly use barrier methods of contraception, which are protective against cervical cancer. Finally, the U.S. Walnut Creek Cohort Study reported that OC users were at increased risk of malignant melanoma. This was not confirmed in two other large British cohort studies, and a valid association appears doubtful.

Health Benefits of Oral Contraceptives

In addition to protection against ovarian and endometrial carcinoma, OCs have several additional health benefits. Risk of ectopic pregnancy is all but eliminated because anovulation results from the pill. Iron-deficiency anemia is reduced because of decreased menstrual flow with the OCs. Dysmenorrhea is relieved because OCs inhibit prostaglandin production, the direct cause of menstrual pain. Benign breast disease is diminished in OC users. This effect appears related to progestin dosage. As progestin dosage is reduced in modern OCs, much of the protection from benign breast disease may be lost. Functional ovarian cysts (corpus luteum and follicular cysts) are reduced because of anovulation with OCs. Recent case reports linking ovarian cysts to triphasic OC formulations have not been substantiated.

Contraindications to Women with Combined Oral Contraceptives

Keep in mind the *absolute contraindications*. Most are obvious considering the risks discussed previously:
1. Thromboembolic disease or history thereof
2. Cerebrovascular accident or history thereof
3. Coronary artery or ischemic heart disease or history thereof
4. Impaired liver function (active)
5. Hepatic adenoma, cancer, or history thereof
6. Breast cancer or history thereof
7. Estrogen-dependent neoplasia or history thereof
8. Pregnancy
9. Previous cholestasis during pregnancy

There are several other strong relative contraindications to OCs. In each case, the medical risks of an unwanted pregnancy must be considered. This should be done in the context of the feasibility of alternative contraception and the patient's view regarding elective abortion. Strong relative complications include vascular or migraine headaches (particularly if they begin after beginning OCs). Risk of stroke may be higher in this group. Hypertension and its attendant morbidity may be increased with OCs. Long-leg casts or other forced immobility may increase risk of deep vein thrombophlebitis. Another obvious relative contraindication is heavy smoking at ages 35 years or more because of the synergistic effects of these factors and OCs for cardiovascular disease. Consideration should be given to other conditions in organ systems affected by combined OCs, including diabetes (glucose tolerance altered by progestins), or necessary for metabolism of contraceptive steroids, such as active gall bladder disease. (The liver is necessary for conjugation and excretion of contraceptive steroids.)

Initial Selection and Starting Combination Oral Contraceptives

Triphasic OCs offer the theoretic advantage of lower complication rates because of lower steroid dosage. However, compared with monophasic OCs, the dosage reduction is small, and reduced complications with triphasics have yet to be demonstrated. The contraceptive benefits observed with monophasic OCs may be diminished at lower triphasic steroid dosages. Further, prescribing flexibility is diminished with triphasic OCs. Thus the benefit for triphasic over monophasic OCs is small.

The initial selection should have a daily dosage of 35 μg of estrogen. Lower dosages have higher rates of troublesome endometrial bleeding, which may affect continuation rates. Progestin dosage should be 1 mg or less norethindrone or 0.125 mg or less norgestrel. There is little evidence that higher progestin dosages provide either greater effectiveness or cycle control. The development of new progestins (norgestimate and desogestrel) offers the theoretic advantage of fewer androgenic side effects. These formulations are probably best when the treatment objective extends beyond contraception to reduction of hirsutism or acne. For a patient with contraceptive failure at 35 μg estrogen or less, 50-μg pills should be considered. Otherwise, the increased cardiovascular risk is not warranted. Estrogen dosages greater than 50 μg are not indicated for contraception.

There are several options for beginning OC use:

1. Now (only if absence of pregnancy can be ensured); will provide the earliest possible onset of contraception and may be associated with a relatively long interval of unpredictable bleeding
2. Five days after the onset of the next normal menstrual period
3. On the first day of the next menstrual period
4. On the first Sunday after the onset of the next normal menstrual period (will generally result in menstruation-free weekends)

With the last three options, effective contraception begins with the first pill. For new pill users, condoms or other backup methods of contraception should be discussed, considering the large number of women who stop using OCs soon after beginning. Condoms are also indicated for all couples not in a mutually monogamous relationship.

Management of Oral Contraception and Common Side Effects

Patients should have a 3-month visit after beginning OCs. This ensures early recognition of a significant elevation in blood pressure soon after beginning OCs. At this time, compliance with pill-taking instructions should be verified. Patients without risk factors for complications of OC may be followed annually. Special laboratory studies of lipoprotein cholesterol and glucose tolerance are necessary only for the same indications as in other women who do not use OC.

The following common side effects of oral contraception may mandate a change in OC:

1. Intermenstrual bleeding
   - Exclude causes other than OCs, such as pelvic inflammatory disease, cervicitis, or pregnancy-related conditions (e.g., ectopic pregnancy).
   - If initiation of OCs is recent and the bleeding is not excessive, encourage the patient to continue with the present medication because bleeding problems generally resolve spontaneously within 3 months.
   - Pills should be taken at precisely the same time daily.
   - Consider the influence of intercurrent illness or other drugs (e.g., antibiotics, which may interfere with the enterohepatic circulation of contraceptive steroids) on OC absorption or metabolism.

- Consider change from norethindrone products to norgestimate or desogen products, which may have better cycle control.
- If these measures are not successful, consider an OC with 50 μg of estrogen.

2. Nausea
   - Rule out intercurrent disease or early pregnancy.
   - Advise that this problem usually decreases or resolves completely within 3 to 4 months.
   - If vomiting occurs, patients should take an additional pill from an extra pill package designated for use only in this circumstance.
   - Consider changing to a combination pill with only 20 μg of estrogen, which should decrease nausea significantly, or to a progestin-only pill, which is unlikely to cause nausea.

3. Amenorrhea
   - Exclude pregnancy.
   - Light or scanty menstruation is the rule with OCs. Amenorrhea is not rare, and its presence has no bearing on contraceptive effectiveness, health risks, or resumption of fertility after stopping OC. Many women find amenorrhea an unanticipated benefit of OCs.
   - If the patient is concerned, consider changing to an OC with a higher estrogen dosage.

4. Breast tenderness
   - Exclude pregnancy and localized breast disease.
   - Change in breast size is common for women using OCs.
   - Determine if the problem is worsened by jogging or other exercise.
   - Supportive bras can reduce discomfort.
   - Change to an OC with less estrogen, progestin, or less of both.

5. Weight gain
   - Although uncommon, weight gain may be a direct result of OCs.
   - Cyclic weight gain related to fluid retention generally begins during the first cycles of OC use. Increased fat deposition in the breasts, hips, and thighs is not uncommon after a few months of use. These types of weight gain may respond to lower estrogen dosage.
   - Long-term insidious weight gain may result from the androgenicity of contraceptive progestins. Conventional dieting and exercise may be helpful, but it may be necessary to discontinue OCs.

6. Skin changes
   - Oral contraceptives typically improve acne or complaints of oily skin. This is most evident for OCs with the new progestins of low androgenicity, such as norgestimate and desogen.
   - Other skin changes, such as chloasma (facial pigmentation that is common during pregnancy), telangiectasia, or unexplained hair loss, may be the direct result of OCs. Because these skin

changes may be permanent, consideration should be given to stopping OCs.

7. Chlamydial cervicitis
   • Chlamydial infections are more common in OC users. This may be related to the larger ectropion (endocervical columnar epithelium exposed on the surface near the cervical os) induced by OCs. An increase in chlamydial pelvic inflammatory disease (PID) has not been observed, and some researchers suggest that OCs diminish risk of PID. Except in mutually monogamous relationships, OC users should use condoms as protection from sexually transmitted disease.

Oral Contraceptive (Combination Pill) Effectiveness

Typical failure rates during the first year of use are 3%. The lowest expected failure rates are 0.1%.

Progestin-Only Oral Contraceptives: The Minipill

The minipill differs substantially from combination OC's:
1. Only progestins and no estrogens are used.
2. Dosage of progestin is less with the minipill than with low-dose combination OCs (e.g., norethindrone: 1 mg daily for Ortho-Novum 1/35 versus 0.35 mg daily for Micronor; norgestrel: 0.075 mg daily for Ovrette versus 0.05 to 0.125 mg daily for Triphasil).
3. An active contraceptive tablet must be taken daily without a 7-day contraceptive pill hiatus.

Because of lower steroid dosage, contraceptive effectiveness and risks are both somewhat lower with the minipill than with combination pills. A Pearl index of about 2 has been reported for both Micronor and Ovrette. Ovulation is not completely suppressed in all minipill users. Women with regular or frequent menses while using the minipill may be ovulating and at greater pregnancy risk. Lower medical risks have been deduced based on lower steroid dosages in the minipill. However, use of the minipill is so uncommon that supportive data are lacking. The minipill then has substantial theoretic benefit for women with risk factors for adverse cardiovascular events. One specific group is heavy smokers over the age of 35 years. Nursing mothers are another group for whom the minipill may be particularly effective. Progestins do not suppress lactation, but estrogens in combination pills do. Studies indicate that both contraceptive estrogens and progestins are detectable in breast milk. Adverse effects have not been demonstrated in infants.

Particular side effects and risks of the minipill include irregular menses and an increased proportion of ectopic pregnancy for contraceptive failures. Ectopic pregnancy results from the action of progesterone to reduce tubal motility.

LONG-ACTING HORMONAL CONTRACEPTION

Long-acting hormonal contraception invites considerable interest among patients and family planners. Interruptions at the time of intercourse such as putting on a condom are eliminated. Daily necessity to remember a pill is unnecessary. "User failures" are decreased, and total failures approach rates with sterilization. Until recently, only a single long-acting contraceptive was available, the injectable Depo-Provera (depot medroxyprogesterone acetate). Its acceptance in the United States has been limited by controversy concerning potential carcinogenesis. However, it has considerable acceptance worldwide, and with patient consent it is often used in the United States. In 1991 the subdermal implant Norplant (levonorgestrel in a Silastic capsule) became available. Concerns about carcinogenesis have not been raised.

Depo-Provera

Depo-Provera is medroxyprogesterone acetate in oil for intramuscular depot administration and long-term release. To ensure that a woman is not pregnant at the time of administration, injections are best given within 5 to 7 days of the last menstrual period. This method of administration minimizes irregular menstrual bleeding. Standard dosage is 150 mg intramuscularly every 3 months. (Contraceptive effectiveness may extend to 4 months.) Care must be taken to shake the vial thoroughly to suspend all the microcrystalline sediment. The oil vehicle is viscous and unless heated may be difficult to draw into the syringe. Injections are generally into the hip. However, in obese women an intramuscular site in the hip may be difficult to obtain with a standard needle. Inadvertent administration into the subcutaneous fat may result in eratic absorption of the drug, and the deltoid may be a preferable site in obese women. For proper absorption, the injection site should not be massaged.

Failure rates for all users are well under 1%. It is uncertain whether failure rates are related to body weight. Mechanisms of action are the same as for OCs.

Menstrual disturbance and its management. Menstrual disturbance, initially metrorrhagia and later amenorrhea, will occur for most women who use Depo-Provera (Fig. 3-7). At 1 year approximately 50% of women are amenorrheic, increasing to 75% at 4 years. Heavy, health-threatening bleeding is rare; in fact, iron stores and hematocrit typically increase. Prophylactic treatment with oral estrogen to prevent abnormal bleeding has not been successful, and oral estrogen treatment reduces the benefits of Depo-Provera. For moderate or prolonged bleeding 25 μg of estradiol three times daily may be effective. If this is unsuccessful or if the initial complaint is heavy bleeding, a cycle of combined OCs can be used. It can be repeated

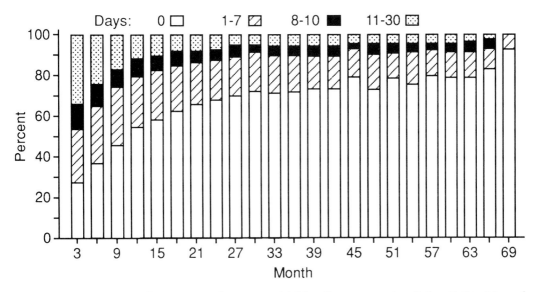

FIGURE 3-7. Percentage of women with bleeding or spotting 0, 1 to 7, 8 to 10, and 11 to 30 days per 30-day cycle while receiving depot medroxyprogesterone acetate (Depo-Provera) every 3 months.

From Schwallie PC, Assenzo JR: *Fertil Steril* 24:331, 1973.

one time if bleeding continues. For continued bleeding dilation and curettage (D&C) should be considered.

Weight change and cardiovascular effects. Most women gain weight while using Depo-Provera. Weight gain averages 1 to 5 kg during the first year of use, and increases may continue throughout its use. The weight gain is from increased fat and not fluid retention.

Because Depo-Provera is not an estrogen, there is little reason to be concerned about estrogenic cardiovascular risks with Depo-Provera. Furthermore, studies of the coagulation and fibrinolytic systems have not demonstrated changes with Depo-Provera regardless of dose. There are no case studies to support an association between Depo-Provera and thrombophlebitis; however, follow-up studies have not been large enough to demonstrate this effect.

Whether Depo-Provera has a significant effect on lipoprotein metabolism is uncertain. Similarly, effects on glucose metabolism are mixed.

The cancer question. Most human studies of Depo-Provera and cancer have had too few patients to detect small or modest increases. These studies have typically followed women from a single clinic or program for 1 to 5 years. This study design is inefficient for detecting associations with rare or relatively uncommon diseases such as cancer. The case-control method (cancer cases and disease-free controls compared on use of the drug [exposure]) is considerably more efficient for studies of Depo-Provera and cancer. A relatively large, hospital-based case-control study from the World Health Organization was largely reassuring for breast cancer and cervical cancer.

The cancer concern related to Depo-Provera stems from studies of rats, dogs (beagles), and monkeys. In these species, both benign and malignant tumors were more common in the animals receiving Depo-Provera than in the nontreated controls. However, these comparisons are flawed because in rats Depo-Provera has strong estrogenic effects, producing an increase in prolactin, which induces breast nodules and malignancy. On the other hand, in women Depo-Provera has no estrogenic effect and does not increase prolactin. Several researchers have concluded that in dogs any progestin given at high enough dosage for a long enough period of time will result in breast tumors. Breast tumor development after Depo-Provera administration to beagles appears to be mediated by growth hormone, which is not elevated with this drug in humans. In monkeys, only breast nodules were detected (at 1 to 10 times the equivalent human dose of Depo-Provera); no malignancy occurred.

Recently, case-control studies from Costa Rica (performed by the U.S. Centers for Disease Control) and New Zealand reported an inconsistent risk of breast cancer with Depo-Provera. In the Costa Rica study, breast cancer risk was increased 2.6 times among all Depo-Provera users. There was no dose-response effect demonstrated, and risk was the same regardless of duration of use. Even duration of use less than 1 year was associated with a 2.3-fold increase in risk, a finding with limited biologic plausibility. In the New Zealand study, overall an increased risk was not observed. However, for women 25 to 34 years of age the risk of breast cancer was 2 times greater in the Depo-Provera group. This risk increased further for women who had used the drug for 6 years or more. Data for these recent studies are from interviews and subject to recall bias. The World Health Organization collaborative study did not demonstrate a significantly increased risk for breast cancer among women using Depo-Provera.

Reproductive effects. On average, former Depo-Provera users require as long as 9 months longer to conceive than women who discontinue barrier contraception or the intrauterine device (Fig. 3-8). At 2 years, pregnancy rates are the same. No evidence suggests that fertility is permanently altered by Depo-Provera. By 6 months after discontinuation, menses will return to 50% of women. Long-term users conceive as rapidly as women who have had only a few injections, suggesting that there is no cumulative effect.

It is unlikely that Depo-Provera has a significant teratologic effect. Ovulation will not occur until drug levels are almost undetectable, with little potential for teratogenesis. Studies suggesting the potential for limb reduction after intrauterine exposure to Depo-Provera have largely been dispelled on the basis of recall bias and nonreproducibility. High doses have

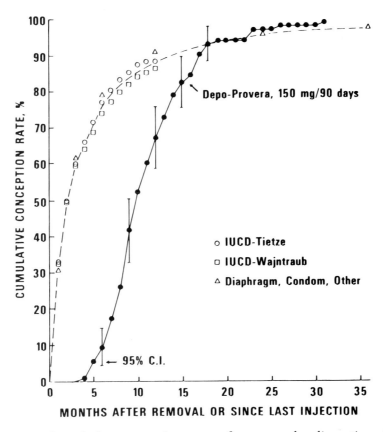

FIGURE 3-8. Cumulative conception rates of women who discontinued Depo-Provera and other methods to become pregnant.

From Schwallie PC, Assenzo JR: *Contraception* 10:181, 1974.

been associated with masculinization of the female fetus. Considering the rare occurrence of pregnancy with Depo-Provera and the unlikely occurrence of significant congenital birth defect regardless of the cause, it is unlikely that the issue of teratogenicity can ever be completely settled. Nonetheless, the likelihood that this will occur is remote at best.

Depo-Provera does not interfere with lactation, and this is a significant benefit compared with oral contraceptives, which contain estrogens that suppress milk production. Milk constituents, protein, fat, and lactose, are unaffected. Studies following children to 10 years after exposure to Depo-Provera in breast milk found no difference in growth or in physical or mental development.

Norplant

Norplant is a long-acting subdermal contraceptive implant of the progestin levonorgestrel. The implants are distributed as a system kit containing a set

of 6 Silastic (dimethylsiloxane/methylvinylsiloxane copolymer) capsules
each with 36 mg of crystalline levonorgestrel. The capsules are 2.4 mm
in diameter and 34 mm long with sealed ends. The new aspect of this
product is long-term (5 year), highly effective hormonal contraception at
drug levels lower than all current oral contraceptive pills. Norplant's
mode of action is the same as for oral contraceptive pills. Local levonorgestrel absorption from Norplant bypasses the liver, avoiding the first-
pass effect. Initial levonorgestrel levels of 0.50 µg/ml fall to approximately
0.35 µg/ml by 9 months and remain at this level until removal of the
implants at 5 years. Levels are less in obese women. In these women
adipose tissue about the implant may slow absorption, dilutional effects
may be greater, or steroid metabolism may be faster. Since Norplant
became available in 1991, it has been used extensively (estimated 891,000
implants between February 1991 and December 1993). Norplant has been
effective, with high continuation rates among well-selected and motivated
teenagers.

Effectiveness. Pregnancy rates from U.S. studies with Norplant have
been higher than rates from international studies. Worldwide pregnancy
rates (Pearl index) at 1, 2, 3, 4, and 5 years of use were 0.2%, 0.2%, 0.9%,
0.5% and 1.1% respectively, versus U.S. pregnancy rates of 0.0%, 2.1%,
3.1%, 0.0%, and 0.0%. Higher U.S. pregnancy rates have been attributed to
greater body weight in U.S. study subjects and to the increased density of
the Silastic tubing used in the Norplant produced for the United States.
(Increased tubing density results in lower serum levonorgestrel levels and
presumably higher likelihood of ovulation.) Currently, commercial Norplant for the United States is being manufactured with the low-density
Silastic. Pregnancy rates are greatest for women weighing 70 kg or more
at insertion (Table 3-6). Note that for the less dense tubing even for women
weighing 70 kg or more, the pregnancy rate is only 2.4% over 5 years. This

TABLE 3-6. Norplant capsules: gross cumulative pregnancy rates at 5 years of use,
by weight and density of tubing

| | | Cumulative pregnancy rates | | |
| | | | Tubing density | |
Weight (kg) at insertion	N	All types	Less	More
<50	532	0.2	0.0	0.3
50-59	1041	3.5	2.0	4.3
60-69	585	3.5	1.5	4.5
>70	309	7.6	2.4	9.3
Total	2469	3.5	1.6	4.9

From Sivin I: *Stud Fam Plann* 19:81, 1988.

is lower than for any other reversible contraceptive. Capsules in place for 6 or more years have unacceptably high pregnancy rates.

Twenty percent of pregnancies in Norplant users are ectopic. Thus this diagnosis must be considered in any pregnant Norplant patient, particularly if she has risk factors. However, to put this into proper perspective, worldwide the ectopic pregnancy rate with Norplant has been 0.28 per 1000 woman-years of use. In the United States during 1985, for all women 15 to 44 years of age the ectopic pregnancy rate was 1.5 per 1000 woman-years. Norplant, then, can be expected to decrease the overall risk of ectopic pregnancy.

Advantages. Norplant's advantages are obvious: highly effective contraception, little need for patient motivation or compliance, and rapid reversibility. As a progestin-only contraceptive, side effects and risks of estrogens are avoided.

Disadvantages. Norplant has two principal disadvantages: disruption of menstrual bleeding patterns and difficult removal. Irregular cycles are the most common reason for discontinuing Norplant.

After 6 months of use, approximately 70% of users have irregular cycles, and 20% to 25% have regular cycles. The remaining 5% to 8% of women have amenorrhea as long as Norplant is in place (Fig. 3-9). After first-year attrition for menstrual and other complaints, approximately 40% of continuing users have menstrual irregularity.

Norplant users with regular bleeding patterns are at greater risk of pregnancy. In a study (sponsored by the Population Council at the University of Southern California) over 5 years of use 17.4% of women with regular cycles became pregnant, versus a 4.4% pregnancy rate among women with irregular cycles and no pregnancies among women with amenorrhea. Women with regular menstrual cycles on Norplant may ovulate regularly, explaining the greater pregnancy rate in this group. However, these findings require confirmation in other studies because the Silastic tubing in the Norplant used in this U.S. study was more dense (and associated with lower serum levonorgestrel levels) than the Silastic tubing presently manufactured.

Removal requires considerably more time and skill than insertion. Fibrous capsules develop around the Norplant capsules, becoming thicker with time, and this is the major technical problem. Among experienced practitioners, removal averaged 25 minutes with a range of 12 to 60 minutes. If (as directed) insertion was immediately subdermal, and not deeper into subcutaneous fat, removal is substantially easier. Pain at removal is not excessive and is largely eliminated with placement of a local anesthetic. If continuing contraception is desired after removal of the capsules, new capsules can be inserted through the same incision into a different part of the arm.

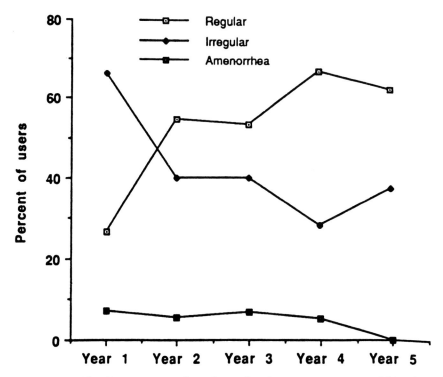

FIGURE 3-9. Bleeding patterns based on the dominant pattern of bleeding for each year of implant use. (Discontinuation among Norplant users with irregular bleeding during the first year of use was an important reason for a lower percentage of users with irregular bleeding in years 2 to 5.)

From Shoupe D, Mishell DR, Bopp BL, et al: *Obstet Gynecol* 77:256, 1991.

Side effects and metabolic considerations. Infection at the insertion site and spontaneous expulsion are less than 1%. This is significant because most Norplant data have been collected outside the United States, where sanitation standards may have been lower.

Next to menstrual problems, headache is the most common side effect and was responsible for 19% of Norplant terminations. Weight gain, mastalgia, galactorrhea, mood changes, and acne may also be associated with Norplant.

Studies of Norplant's effect on serum lipoprotein and carbohydrate metabolism do not demonstrate consistent evidence of any adverse effect. In spite of abnormal menses, hemoglobin levels generally increase.

In 1995, the Food and Drug Administration (FDA) reported on serious adverse events in Norplant users during the first 3 years of FDA approval. This report was positive. There were few hospitalizations among an estimated 891,000 insertions. The largest category was 24 hospitalizations for infection. Other potential complications such as stroke occurred less frequently than would have been predicted based on the age distribution of the Norplant users.

Indications, contraindications, and insertion. Norplant is indicated for sexually active women who desire long-term contraception. Included are women who

1. Desire spacing of future pregnancies
2. Desire a highly effective, long-term method of contraception
3. Have experienced serious or minor estrogen-related side effects using oral contraceptives
4. Have difficulty remembering to take birth control pills every day, have contraindications or difficulty using IUDs, or desire a non-coitus-related method of contraception
5. Have completed their childbearing but do not desire permanent sterilization
6. Have a history of anemia with heavy menstrual bleeding
7. Are considering sterilization but are not yet ready to undergo surgery*

Contraindications include active thrombophlebitis or thromboembolic disease, undiagnosed genital bleeding, acute liver disease, benign or undiagnosed liver tumors, and known or suspected breast cancer.

Insertion can be performed at any time in the menstrual cycle. Pregnancy should always be ruled out. Many practitioners choose to insert Norplant within 2 days of menstruation. Because levonorgestrel levels are highest within 24 hours of insertion, when inserted during menstruation (or at any time to a woman using OC), contraception is immediate.

Insertion is through a 2-mm preanesthetized incision in the inner skin of the upper arm. This site was chosen because it has little trauma, making migration of the implants less likely. The implants are placed just beneath the skin in a fan distribution with all the ends nearly touching to facilitate removal from a single incision. Insertion itself is through a specially designed trochar sleeve. The process itself is largely painless, requiring 5 to 10 minutes. To reduce bruising after the insertions, a pressure bandage should be applied to the incision for 24 hours.

Reproductive effects. Forty-eight hours after removing Norplant, levonorgestrel can no longer be detected in the serum. Most women begin to menstruate regularly within 30 days. Pregnancy rates are comparable to women attempting pregnancy without prior hormonal contraception. Data are limited, but there is little to suggest a teratogenic effect or a change in the subsequent risk of ectopic pregnancy.

POSTCOITAL CONTRACEPTION

Postcoital contraception is an emergency method designed to prevent pregnancy after an unprotected intercourse or a contraceptive accident. Two methods are available: hormonal (the so-called morning after pill) and

*Darney PD, Klaisle CM, Tanner S, et al: Sustained-release contraceptives, *Curr Prob Obstet Gynecol Fert* 13:87, 1990.

intrauterine device (IUD) insertion. Conception rates may be as high as 30% after intercourse on the 2 days preceding ovulation. The success of postcoital contraception, without regard to cycle day, is greater than 97%.

Presently, the oral contraceptive Ovral (0.5 mg norgestrel and 50 μg ethinyl estradiol) is the most commonly used agent for postcoital contraception. Two tablets are administered initially, followed after 12 hours by two additional tablets. If vomiting occurs, an additional dose should be administered with an antiemetic. Use should begin within 72 hours of intercourse, although effectiveness (albeit reduced) may remain at longer intervals after intercourse. Before initiating postcoital contraception, preexisting unrecognized pregnancy should be excluded. Any other recent unprotected intercourse should be considered along with the estimated day of the menstrual cycle and the likelihood of ovulation.

Insertion of a postcoital IUD will effectively prevent pregnancy, and insertion can be as long as 5 days after intercourse. Although studied for only copper-containing IUDs, other IUDs are probably equally effective. The IUD can remain in place and provide continuing contraception. Postcoital IUDs are contraindicated for women at risk of pelvic inflammatory disease (in the presence of mucopurulent cervicitis, multiple recent sexual partners, etc.). Postcoital contraception is frequently used for victims of sexual assault. Proper evaluation for STDs is a necessity, and uncertainty regarding STDs should preclude an IUD for rape victims.

All patients should be seen at 2 weeks after treatment. At this time, contraceptive failures can be detected. Culture for STD should be repeated, and the patient's future contraception methods should be discussed.

INTRAUTERINE CONTRACEPTIVE DEVICE

The IUD has been associated with considerable controversy and change during the past 15 years. The controversy concerns the Dalkon Shield IUD and its association with spontaneous septic abortion and PID. The changes concern a loss from the marketplace of all the former standard IUDs and their replacement with the TCu-380A (ParaGard), a highly successful IUD with 10 years of effectiveness.

Infections caused by the Dalkon Shield resulted from bacteria entering the endometrial cavity on a string extending from the vagina through the cervix to the IUD and the endometrial cavity. The string is necessary for removal of the IUD. Unlike other IUDs, the Dalkon Shield's string was braided, and this permitted bacteria to be "wicked" in the string and carried into the endometrial cavity. All modern IUDs have had strings, but they are monofilaments that do not "wick".

Unfortunately, in the absence of substantial supporting studies, most cases of PID that occurred in association with other IUD designs were assumed to have been caused by the IUD, in the same way that the Dalkon Shield caused PID. Consequently, IUD manufacturers were subjected to considerable PID-related litigation. Although ruled overwhelmingly for the defendants, IUD manufacturers, the costs of litigation became so onerous that almost all manufacture and distribution of IUDs ceased in the United States.

In 1987 GynoPharma (a U.S. company specializing in gynecologic and contraceptive products) received a license from the Population Council, developers of the TCu-380A, to sell this IUD in the United States. The TCu-380A (Paragard) is now the principal IUD in the United States. It has major advantages over older IUDs in contraceptive effectiveness (which rivals the effectiveness of OCs) and contraceptive lifetime, which is 10 years.

Modern History of the Intrauterine Device

The first modern IUDs were made of polyethylene, a biologically inert plastic. The Lippe's Loop was internationally distributed in the 1960s and became the most used nonmedicated IUD.

In the late 1960s copper was added to polyethylene IUDs, substantially increasing their effectiveness. Because the copper IUDs were significantly smaller than their polyethylene predecessors, a reduction in side effects accompanied their high effectiveness. (In the 1970s a progesterone-impregnated IUD, the Progestasert, was developed.) The initial copper IUDs—the copper 7 and the copper T—had a surface area of 200 mm^2 copper. The copper was in the form of a wire only 0.2 mm thick. Extended use caused this wire to fragment. Thus it was necessary to change these IUDs every few years.

Second- and third-generation copper IUDs incorporate changes that diminish fragmentation of the copper wire and increase duration of effectiveness (Table 3-7). Wire thickness was increased to 0.3 or 0.4 mm, and solid copper collars or sleeves were added. The Paragard T380A has an exposed copper surface area of 380 mm^2. The polyethylene portion of the IUD is imbedded with barium sulfate to render it radiopaque. Its increased copper surface area further increases contraceptive effectiveness.

Mechanism of Action

The mechanism of action for IUDs is not precisely understood. Recent evidence suggests that the IUD exerts its action before the ovum reaches the uterus. In a study from the Dominican Republic, ova were recovered from tubal flushes (a research technique) soon after ovulation in 39% of IUD users compared with 56% of noncontraceptors. Further, eggs with a microscopic appearance of fertilization were recovered from 50% of noncontraceptors who had intercourse during the fertile period. In contrast under the same circumstances for IUD users, no fertilized eggs were found

TABLE 3-7. Annual pregnancy rates with long-term intrauterine device use

Device	Annual Pearl index			
	1 yr	4 yr	5 yr	6 yr
FIRST GENERATION				
Copper T 200	3.1	1.1	–	–
Copper 7	2.6	1.0	–	–
SECOND GENERATION				
Multiload Cu 250	0.6	0.6	0.8	–
Nova-T	0.8	0.5	0.5	–
THIRD GENERATION				
CuT-380A	0.5	0.6	0.3	0.3
Multiload Cu 375	0.4	0.6	0.4	0.4

From Newton J, Tacchi D: *Lancet* 1:1322, 1990.

in the fallopian tubes and no ova were found in the endometrial cavity. The authors concluded that the principal mode of action of IUDs is *not* to disrupt the implantation site of a fertilized ovum.

Intrauterine devices incite an intense endometrial foreign body response characterized by infiltration with white blood cells, production of prostaglandins, and elaboration of proteolytic enzymes. These changes inhibit sperm transport and survival, making fertilization difficult or impossible. Copper also interferes with the normal activity of carbonic anhydrase and possibly alkaline phosphatase, the enzymes necessary for fertilization. This occurs because of copper's competition with zinc, a heavy metal necessary for enzymatic action. Progesterone-medicated IUDs also produce an atrophic endometrium that is not receptive to fertilized ova.

Effectiveness

The reported failure rates for the TCu-380A (0.5 to 0.8 pregnancies per 100 woman-years) are considerably lower than failure rates reported with the Lippe's Loop or the first-generation copper devices (Table 3-7). Obviously, failure rates vary by age and parity status, limiting direct comparison with oral contraceptives. Nonetheless, it is apparent that IUDs provide effective contraception with little absolute difference in pregnancy rates between the TCu-380A and oral contraceptives.

Management of pregnancy with an IUD. If a pregnancy occurs with an IUD, the location of the pregnancy (and IUD) should be verified with pelvic ultrasound. A significant proportion of such pregnancies are ectopic. If the IUD string is visible through the cervix (particularly if the string is normal in length and not shortened, which would indicate that the IUD has been drawn up into the uterus), removal of the IUD by simple traction on the string will enhance the likelihood that the pregnancy will continue to term. Often this process is technically simple because a common cause of pregnancy is partial extrusion of the IUD from the uterus into the cervix, where the IUD has little effect. Removal of the IUD may interrupt as many as 25% of concomitant pregnancies. When an IUD is left in place during pregnancy, the likelihood of spontaneous abortion increases to 50%.

Left in place throughout pregnancy, IUDs may result in sepsis and maternal death. The gravity of this association must be expressed clearly to the patient. This may be particularly problematic in cases where the IUD string is not visible and removal of the IUD will probably interrupt the pregnancy. Even in the absence of recognized sepsis prematurity is increased when a failed IUD is left in place. If the IUD has perforated the uterus to an extrauterine position clearly outside the endometrial cavity, sepsis and prematurity are probably less likely.

Intrauterine devices and ectopic pregnancy. The incidence of ectopic pregnancy is not increased with the TCu-380A. Available data suggest the reverse – a reduction in the incidence of ectopic pregnancy compared with women who do not use contraception. (An exception to this rule is the progesterone-medicated IUD, which increases the incidence of ectopic pregnancy. This may be related to progesterone's action to reduce fallopian tubal motility and later ovum transport through the tube to the uterus.) However, because the incidence of intrauterine pregnancy is low in women who use IUDs, the ratio of ectopic to intrauterine pregnancy is increased. In women with IUDs, as many as 10% of pregnancies are ectopic. If pregnancy is suspected, patients with IUDs should be advised to notify their physician immediately to exclude ectopic pregnancy.

Intrauterine Device and Pelvic Inflammatory Disease

Since withdrawal from the marketplace of the Dalkon Shield and many of its immediate successors, there is widespread recognition that the IUD is a cause of pelvic inflammatory disease (PID) in some women. Because bacteria are wicked along the Dalkon Shield's string into the endometrial cavity, PID commonly occurred with the Dalkon Shield much later after insertion. On the other hand, the principal cause of PID with other IUDs is bacteria that enter the endometrial cavity during the insertion process. Under these circumstances, PID typically occurs within 3 months of insertion. A recent publication suggests that levonorgestrel (progestin)-medicated IUDs are less likely to be associated with PID than copper medicated IUDs. This finding is attributed to thicker, less penetrable cervical mucus as well as less endometrial bleeding due to the progestin effects.

There is little doubt that PID related to the IUD can have serious consequences. A Seattle study indicated that women with primary tubal infertility (presumably stemming from PID) were 11 times more likely to have used the Dalkon Shield IUD than other women who conceived. Note that in this study the copper IUDs contributed little to the risk of tubal infertility (Table 3-8).

In general, duration of use is not thought to influence risk of PID. However, risk of severe PID may be greater in long-term users, particularly PID related to actinomyces.

Insertion and Removal

Contraindications to insertion. Candidate selection is crucial to minimize infection and other side effects associated with IUDs. Candidates should be in a mutually monogamous relationship at little risk of STDs and not immunosuppressed (not receiving steroid therapy, not positive for HIV, etc.). Additional relative contraindications include history of PID or ectopic pregnancy. Worsening anemia or dysmenorrhea may occur if an IUD is inserted. Menorrhagia may complicate IUD use in women with uterine fibroids. Placement of an IUD in a patient with valvular heart disease may increase her risk of bacterial endocarditis. Women with histories of vasovagal reactions or fainting may have this problem during IUD placement.

Insertion procedures. Insertion need not be timed to a particular phase of the menstrual cycle. Insertion during menses reduces the risk of an unrecognized pregnancy; however, the cervix is fully dilated at menses and midcycle, facilitating insertion at these times. Infection and expulsion are greater for insertions at menses.

Emphasis should be given to several matters in the written insertion instructions that accompany the IUD package. Careful bimanual examination should be performed to determine uterine position. (Nonrecognition of a retroverted uterus is the leading cause of IUD perforation.) Vaginal secretions should be cleansed from the cervical os with an antiseptic

TABLE 3-8. Intrauterine device (IUD) and relative risk of pelvic inflammatory disease (PID) and primary tubal infertility, according to type of IUD

IUD	Relative risk of PID	Relative risk of primary tubal infertility	
		IUD ever used	**IUD only used**
Any IUD	—	2.6	—
Dalkon Shield	8.3	6.8	11.3
Progestasert	2.2	—	—
Copper IUD	1.9	1.9	1.3
Lippe's Loop	1.2		
Saf-T-Coil	1.3	3.2	4.4

Data from Lee NC, Rubin GL, Ory HW, et al: *Obstet Gynecol* 62:1, 1983; and Daling JR, Weiss NS, Metch BJ, et al: *N Engl J Med* 312:937, 1985.

solution. A paracervical block can be placed if a difficult insertion is anticipated, for example, in a nullipara or young patient. In the absence of a paracervical block, a small amount of local anesthetic in the anterior cervical lip before grasping with a tenaculum reduces pain and increases patient confidence. Sounding the uterus determines the length of the uterus, an aid to correct IUD placement, and sounding facilitates directed passage of the IUD and its inserter through the internal cervical os. Particular attention should be given to the written instructions for the withdrawal technique for insertion of an IUD. Incorrect attempts to push the IUD into place with the insertion rod increase greatly the risk of uterine perforation during insertion.

Removal of the IUD. In most circumstances, IUD removal is technically simple, fast, and without undue patient distress. Removal is likely to be more difficult if the IUD has been in place for an extended period. In this circumstance, the string may be fragile, and the IUD may have become imbedded in the endometrium. Obviously, inability to see the IUD string extending through the cervical os indicates a difficult removal.

For every removal, traction on the IUD string should be *gentle*. If the uterus is sharply retroflexed or anteflexed, using a tenaculum to straighten the cervical-uterine canal reduces the amount of traction required.

If a difficult removal is anticipated, the process can be facilitated with mechanical cervical dilation. This can be accomplished with a paracervical block and conventional dilators or with a laminaria. If the IUD string breaks, removal can still be accomplished with short-jawed alligator forceps. Such an instrument has been designed specially for IUD removal. Bronchoscopy forceps have a longer handle but also function effectively for this purpose.

If IUD strings are not visible and removal is planned, strings can usually be retrieved from the cervix with a narrow forceps. If not, it is generally possible to use a uterine sound to "palpate" the endometrial cavity and locate the IUD. If the IUD is not palpated in this way, determination of its intrauterine or extrauterine position should be completed with diagnostic ultrasound.

Side Effects and Complications

As with other contraceptive methods, IUDs can cause annoying side effects and some serious complications. In spite of this, continuation rates for IUDs (Table 3-9) are as high as with any other reversible method of contraception. Removal for side effects is greatest in the first and second years of use and slightly greater among nulliparas. In general, if there is concern that the IUD is causing a troublesome side effect or promoting a potentially serious complication, the best course is removal of the IUD and use of a different contraceptive method.

TABLE 3-9. Net cummulative rates per 100 CuT-380A acceptors by year and parity*

	1 year		2 years		3 years		4 years		5 years		6 years	
	Parous	All	Parous	All	Parous	All	Parous	All	Parous	All	Parous	All
Pregnancy	0.5	0.6	0.8	0.9	1.1	1.4	1.2	1.6	1.5	1.9	1.5	1.9
Expulsion	5.2	5.7	7.0	8.0	8.1	9.3	9.3	10.4	9.6	10.6	9.6	10.6
Bleeding/pain	9.5	11.8	17.3	20.3	23.2	28.7	25.8	28.1	29.2	30.8	31.6	32.2
Other medical	1.6	2.5	3.1	4.4	4.1	5.8	5.4	7.2	8.8	7.3	8.8	7.6
Continuation	79.9	77.0	64.8	60.7	64.6	49.6	47.9	43.2	43.4	39.1	41.0	37.0
Number completed	1082	3196	1347	2973	936	1182	788	941	606	686	445	445

Data from GynoPharma Inc: Prescribing information, ParaGard T380A Intrauterine Copper Contraceptive.
*Rates were calculated by combining the experience on a weighted basis from both The Population Council (PC, 3536 acceptors) and World Health Organization (WHO, 1396 acceptors) trials. Of the women completing 1, 2, 3, and 4 years of use, 64%, 51%, 25%, and 16%, respectively, were from the PC study. The rates in years 5 and 6 are derived from the WHO trials.

Bleeding and pain are the most common reasons for IUD removal. Approximately 10% of TCu-380A IUDs are removed for this reason during the first year of use. If menses are considered to be heavy or excessive and the patient wants to continue the IUD, hematocrit should be measured. Excess bleeding can be a sign of indolent pelvic infection.

Uterine perforation is rare. Within 3 months of pregnancy, the uterus has not regained its nonpregnant tone, increasing the likelihood of perforation. In large clinical trials, the ratio of perforation to insertion is 1.2:1000. Copper-containing IUDs in the peritoneal cavity should be removed as soon as possible because copper induces an intense inflammatory response, which may rapidly result in adherence to the omentum or bowel.

Expulsion of the IUD occurs in 5% to 6% of TCu-380A users, most often during the first 3 months after insertion. This problem is more common in young or nulliparous women. Partial expulsion may result in pregnancy. Women should be taught to feel their IUD string after menses. Lengthening of the string is evidence for partial expulsion of the IUD into the cervix. Clinicians should record string length in the medical record after insertion.

CONDOMS

More condoms, more consistently is now the major public health directive for contraception and prevention of STDs. This, of course, is in response to the acquired immunodeficiency syndrome (AIDS) epidemic. Unlike most other developed nations, widespread approval of condoms is a relatively new phenomenon in the United States. In fact, their sale for contraception was outlawed by Congress in 1873. In certain states, it was a criminal offense for one person to inform another that using a condom might prevent pregnancy. Similar laws remained in effect in some localities until 1975. Today, use of condoms to prevent transmission of STDs – especially AIDS – has become more important than pregnancy prevention.

Male Condom

Most male condoms have fundamentally the same shape and thickness. They are manufactured by relatively few factories (50) worldwide. All are made from Latex tapped from rubber trees. Chemicals are added to promote polymerization and hence elasticity. Each condom is formed by a dripping process using glass molds.

The contraceptive effectiveness of condoms depends on the likelihood of breakage and slippage. *Consumer Reports* indicates that approximately 1 in 140 condoms break during vaginal intercourse. The FDA's role is to ensure that standards for the manufacture of condoms are maintained. The government's tolerance for failure is 1.5%. Each condom is checked for holes by testing electrical resistance across the condom. Inflation and tensile strength testing are done on lot samples. A recent study by *Consumer*

Reports showed that high standards were met for most brands of condoms sold in the United States. Natural membrane, or "skin," condoms (made from lamb cecum) typically withstand more than 10 times the pressure of latex condoms. Nonoxynol-9 (a surfactant that disrupts sperm's cell wall) has been applied to the inner and outer surface of certain brands of condoms. However, contraceptive foam should also be added if breakage occurs. To reduce slippage of the condom during intercourse, one brand (Mentor) is sold with an applicator and an adhesive to hold the condom in position on the penis. Slippage is also reduced by holding the rim of the condom firmly on the penis during removal soon after ejaculation.

Bacteria are unable to penetrate either latex or skin condoms. Latex condoms also prevent transmission of viruses, but hepatitis B virus (42 nm) has been demonstrated to pass through natural membrane condoms. Therefore latex condoms should be used whenever sexually transmitted disease is an issue.

Condoms are available with several features to enhance acceptance:
1. Lubricants—"dry" silicon-based lubricants are most common; wet-lubricated condoms use a water-based surgical jelly.
2. Spermicide—concentrations vary from 1% to 12%; if irritation is a problem, a lower concentration should be used.
3. Texture-ribbing or stippling around the shaft.
4. Contour—some are contoured for a more snug fit, others are tapered or flared.
5. Color—a wide color range is available.

Certain features and precautions should be observed for all condoms. They should have a reservoir tip. Condoms with signs of deterioration should not be used. Oil-based lubricants weaken latex considerably, and mineral oil, baby oil, vegetable oil, petroleum jelly, cold creams, and hand lotions containing such oils should all be avoided. Lubricants safe for condoms are water based. They include K-Y Lubricating Jelly and Today Personal Lubricant. Although foam increases the effectiveness of condoms, the principal contraceptive effect is from the condom itself. Couples should not decide against barrier methods because too much effort (foam *and* condoms) is involved. Properly used condoms alone are effective contraception.

Female Condom (Reality)

The Reality female condom was approved by the FDA in 1992. It is the first barrier contraceptive for women that offers limited protection against STDs. This is important because women are up to 17 times more likely to get an HIV infection from an HIV-positive male than are men from an HIV-positive woman.

The female condom is a thin (0.5 mm) polyurethane sheath that is 7.8 cm

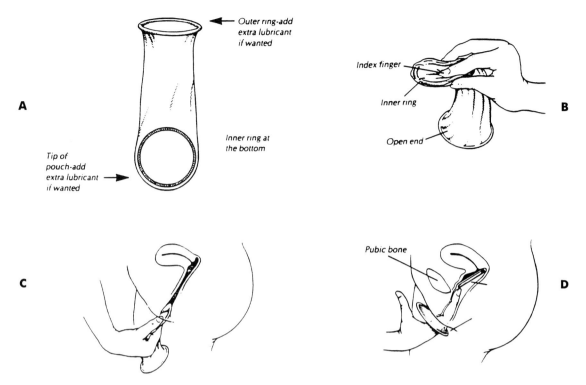

FIGURE 3-10. Reality female condom. **A,** Inner and outer rings are polyurethane, as is the sheath. **B,** In preparation: 1. Hold pouch with open end hanging down. While holding the outside of the pouch, squeeze the inner ring with thumb and middle finger. 2. Place index finger between the thumb and middle finger while squeezing the inner ring. **C,** For insertion: 1. While squeezing the condom, spread the vulvar lips with the other hand. 2. Insert the "squeezed" Reality condom. **D,** Final positioning: 1. Push the inner ring and pouch the rest of the way into the vagina with the index finger. 2. The inner ring should be past the pubic bone.

in diameter and 17 cm in length (Fig. 3-10). The sheath has two polyurethane rings: an inner ring at the closed end of the sheath that lies inside the vagina and a larger ring that remains outside the vagina. The inner ring serves as an insertion mechanism and an internal anchor. The condom is prelubricated with silicone-based lubricant, and additional lubricant is provided. The condom can be inserted up to 8 hours before intercourse.

Data on pregnancy protection with the female condom are sparse. The manufacturer indicates an annual pregnancy rate of 26% estimated by doubling the 6-month pregnancy rate. Because of the urgency to provide STD protection controlled by women, the female condom received an expedited FDA review. Further studies are needed to clarify contraceptive effectiveness.

Information on the acceptability of the female condom is also limited.

One small study from a New York City hospital indicated high levels of acceptability particularly related to feelings of protection and confidence engendered by the device. Least-liked features were difficulties with insertion and removal. A majority of women and over 40% of their partners preferred the female condom compared with the male condom. Again, the device is new and little studied. More data are needed to determine where the female condom fits into the contraceptive armamentarium.

VAGINAL SPERMICIDES AND OTHER BARRIER CONTRACEPTION

Spermicidal preparations consist of two components: an inert base (foam, jelly, or cream) and a spermicidal chemical (nonoxynol-9 or octoxinol-9). Spermicides can be used alone without a barrier and are administered as foam, jellies, creams, and suppositories. Used alone, failure rates are considerably higher than for spermicides used with diaphragm, cervical cap, or condoms (see Table 3-1).

Diaphragm

Diaphragms are dome-shaped rubber caps with a flexible rim. Before intercourse, the diaphragm is inserted into the vagina with the posterior rim resting in the posterior vaginal fornix and the anterior rim fitting snugly behind the pubic synthesis. Contraceptive jelly in the dome covers the cervix, blocking passage of sperm. As with the condom, the diaphragm confers some protection against sexually transmitted infections.

Two types of diaphragm are commonly used: flat spring rim, a thin rim with gentle spring strength; and arching spring rim, a sturdy rim with considerable strength (Fig. 3-11). In general, sturdier rims are helpful for women with pelvic relaxation, and gentle spring strength is sufficient for women with more vulvar tone. An additional advantage for diaphragms with sturdy rims is their tendency to "pop" into place, requiring less manipulation for proper positioning.

Diaphragms have certain noncontraceptive risks and benefits. Urinary track infections are more common. Some women are sensitive to the contraceptive jelly. These problems can be reduced by choosing a diaphragm with a less rigid rim or by choosing a different contraceptive jelly. Noncontraceptive benefits include reduced risk of sexually transmitted disease and reduced risk of cervical cancer.

The goal for fitting a diaphragm is to fit the largest size that remains comfortable for the patient. Tight fit usually decreases substantially after relaxation and during sexual arousal. The most serious problem in diaphragm fitting is the incorrect choice of a size that is too small.

Diaphragm users should be instructed to do the following:
1. Use contraceptive jelly or cream before each intercourse.
2. After intercourse, leave the diaphragm in place for at least 6 to 8 hours.

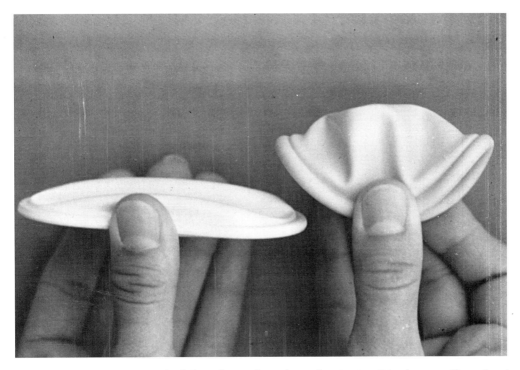

FIGURE 3-11. On the left is the Ortho-White Flat Spring Diaphragm. Note that it bends in only two planes. This rim is less noticeable to some users. On the right is the All-Flex Arching Spring Diaphragm. It bends in three places. The sturdy spring facilitates proper placement of the diaphragm.

3. If intercourse will occur more than once within the 6-hour period during which the diaphragm must be left in place, insert a vaginal spermicide for each intercourse.
4. To minimize the small risk of toxic shock syndrome, wash hands carefully before inserting the diaphragm, do not wear the diaphragm for more than 24 consecutive hours, do not use during a menstrual period, do not use for 12 weeks after delivery, and wash the diaphragm after each use.
5. Inspect the diaphragm for holes before each use.
6. Keep the diaphragm away from petroleum products, which cause the diaphragm to deteriorate.

Cervical Cap

The cervical cap is a cup-shaped device that fits over the cervix and is held in place (at least partially) by suction between its firm flexible rim and the surface of the cervix (Fig. 3-12). The device received FDA approval in May 1988 after an initiative spearheaded by the National Women's Health Network. Presently there is only a single manufacturer (Lamberts Ltd.,

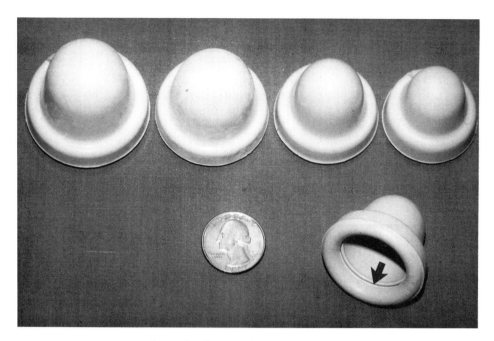

FIGURE 3-12. Pictured are the five available sizes (22, 25, 28, and 31 mm inside diameter) of the Prentif Cavity-Rim Cervical Cap. Arrow indicates the hollow rim that creates suction to hold this cap on the cervix. (Quarter indicates relative size.)

Luton, England) for cervical caps distributed in the United States. The name of its cap is the Prentif Cavity-Rim Cervical Cap. Like the diaphragm, it must be used with a contraceptive jelly.

Principal benefits of the cervical cap are longer periods of effectiveness and decreased messiness. The amount of time the cap can be left on the cervix for contraception is controversial. The FDA advises 48 hours or less. The National Women's Health Network extends the effective period to 72 hours.

A principal disadvantage for the cap is difficulty in fitting. Practitioners are required to complete a certified training program. Only four sizes of the cap are manufactured, and this limits the proportion of women who can be properly fitted. Before fitting, the cervix should be inspected with a speculum. A round cervix is easiest to fit, and a midplane or mildly retroverted uterus is best. Asymmetric cervical length is problematic. The cap itself should cover at least 75% of the cervix, and gaps between the cap and the cervix should be 2 mm or less. Checks should indicate a seal of the cap on the cervix, and the cap should remain in place despite firm pressure from the examining hand. As many as 25% of women have a cervix that is incompatible with the cervical cap (Fig. 3-13).

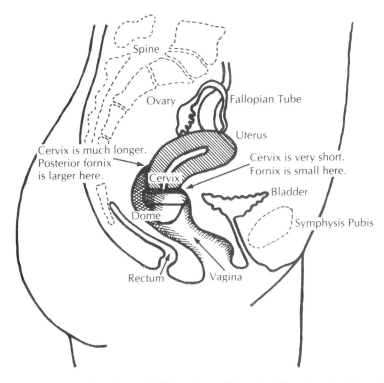

FIGURE 3-13. Example of poorly fitting Prentif Cavity-Rim Cervical Cap. Here the intravaginal cervix is assymmetric, with a short anterior course and a much longer posterior course. This makes the cap fitting unstable.

From Brokaw AK, Baker NN, Haney SL: *Nurse Pract* 13:;49, 1988.

In a randomized clinical trial comparing the cap with the diaphragm, pregnancy rates, although high, were the same – 16% for each year of use. Abnormal Papanicolaou smears occurred in 4% of cap users compared with 1.7% of diaphragm users. Cap users had more complaints of vaginal odor and dislodgement. Diaphragm users complained more about interrupted sex and messiness.

STERILIZATION AND ABORTION

Fundamental to effective sterilization counseling is respect for patient autonomy. A gynecologist's position makes it difficult to weigh the relative emotional costs of sterilization regret versus costs of regret induced by an unwanted pregnancy after the decision for no further children. Doctors may feel more responsible for sterilization regret because they had an active role in the surgical procedure. However, for some patients the predicament of an unwanted pregnancy is worse.

Because tubal reanastomosis is frequently ineffective, the permanence of tubal sterilization must be emphasized. Couples with unstable marriages should consider postponing sterilization until the status of the marriage is clarified. If federal funds will be used for the sterilization procedure, patients must (except in certain emergencies) wait 30 days after signing the consent document.

For couples, consider that vasectomy is an excellent alternative to female tubal sterilization. Couples should be counseled that vasectomy is more effective, safer, and less expensive.

The principal method for female sterilization in the United States is laproscopic electrocautery—either bipolar or unipolar. Laproscopic placement of clips or Silastic rings is also common. Minilaparotomy with partial tubal resection is just as effective and requires less technolgy than laproscopic methods. Failure rates are the same: less than 1% during the first year. Transcervical methods are experimental, and hysterectomy for sterilization alone is not justified. Long-term complications have not been proven except for ectopic pregnancy, which is more common among pregnancies conceived after tubal sterilization. As many as 50% of pregnancies after sterilization by electrocautery are ectopic.

Elective termination of pregnancy is best performed in an office seting, where complication rates have been demonstrated to be lowest and unnecessary charges are eliminated. Because the overwhelmng majority of elective abortions are in the first trimester, the vacum curettage method is most common. The technique has been imroved by introduction of a flexible suction cannula that minimizes patient distress by reducing the need for mechanical dilation. Clarifiation of the role of adjunctive techniques (*Laminaria* or synthetic osmotic dilators) and prophylactic antibiotics has made the procedure technially simpler and has reduced infectious complications. In the near future, medical methods may replace surgical methods for termination of pregnancies at 7 menstrual weeks or less. Unfortunately, in spite of improving technology, fewer practitioners today are performing abortions, which increasingly are available only in large urban centers.

Counselors for patients planning or considering an elective termination of pregnancy must give accurate information about the procedure, provide adequate time for ventilation about feelings, and permit the expression of grief. Misconceptions about the safety of abortion or future fertility are commonplace. A helpful reference for women is the fact that abortion (regardless of gestational age) is safer than term delivery. Fertility is not altered by elective abortion. All patients (including women with prior elective abortions) have an element of grief when a pregnancy is lost. Expectation of this grief by the counselor will speed its expression and the recovery of the patient.

BIBLIOGRAPHY

Albertson BD, Zinaman MJ: The prediction of ovulation and monitoring of the fertile period, *Adv Contracept* 3:263, 1987.

Alvarez F, Branche V, Fernandez E, et al: New insights on the mode of action of intrauterine devices in women, *Fertil Steril* 49:768, 1988.

American College of Obstetricians and Gynecologists: The intrauterine device, *Am Coll Obstet Gynecol Techn Bull* 104:1, 1987.

American College of Obstetricians and Gynecologists: Oral contraception, *Am Coll Obstet Gynecol Techn Bull* 106:1, 1987.

American Health Consultants: New Advantage 24 contraceptive gel claims 24-hour effectiveness, *Contraceptive Technology Update* 45, April 1995.

Archer DF: Management of bleeding in women using subdermal implants, *Contemp Ob Gyn* 11:1-5, 1995.

Beilenson PL, Miola ES, Farmer M: Politics and practice: introducing Norplant into a school-based health center in Baltimore, *Am J Public Health* 85:309, 1995.

Bernstein GS, Clark VA, Coulson AH, et al: *Use effectiveness of cervical caps*, Final Report to NICHD, Contract No. 1-HD-1-2804, 1986.

Billings EL, Billings JJ, Brown JB, et al: Symptoms and hormonal changes accompanying ovulation, *Lancet* 1:282, 1972.

Billings JJ: *Natural family planning: the ovulation method*, ed 2, Collegetown, Minn, 1973, Liturgical Press.

Bottiger LE, Boman G, Eklund G, et al: Oral contraceptives and thromboembolic disease: effects of lowering estrogen content, *Lancet* 1:1097, 1980.

Bradley DD, Wingerd J, Petitti DB, et al: Serum high-density-lipoprotein cholesterol in women using oral contraceptives, estrogens, and progestins, *N Engl J Med* 299:17, 1978.

Brinton LA, Vessey MP, Flavel R, et al: Risk factors for benign breast disease, *Am J Epidemiol* 113:203, 1981.

Brokaw AK, Baker NN, Haney SL: Fitting the cervical cap, *Nurse Pract* 13:49, 1988.

The Cancer and Steroid Hormone Study of the Centers for Disease Control and the National Institutes of Child Health and Human Development: Oral-contraceptive use and the risk of breast cancer, *N Engl J Med* 315:405, 1986.

The Cancer and Steroid Hormone Study of the Centers for Disease Control and the National Institutes of Child Health and Human Development: The reduction in risk of ovarian cancer associated with oral contraceptive use, *N Engl J Med* 316:650, 1987.

Casagrande JT, Louie EW, Pike MC, et al: "Incessant ovulation" and ovarian cancer, *Lancet* 2:170, 1979.

Cates W, Stewart FH, Tussell J: Commentary: the quest for women's prophylactic methods, hope vs science, *Am J Public Health* 82:1479, 1992.

Centers for Disease Control: Adolescent health: state of the nation—pregnancy, sexually transmitted diseases, and related risk behaviors among US adolescents, Atlanta, 1995, US Department of Health and Human Services, Public Health Service, DSHS publication no. (CDC) 099-4630.

The cervical cap, *Med Letter* 30:93, 1988.

Chapdelaine A, Desmarasis JL, Derman RJ: Clinical evidence of the minimal androgenic activity of norgestimate, *Int J Fertil* 34:347, 1989.

Church CA, Rinehart W: Counseling clients about the pill, *Popul Rep A* 8:1, 1990.

Connell EB: The female condom—a new contraceptive option, *Contemp Ob Gyn* 39:20, 1994.

Consumers' Union: How reliable are condoms? *Consumer Report* 1:1-6, 1995.

Daling JR, Weiss NS, Metch BJ, et al: Primary tubal infertility in relation to the use of an intrauterine device, *N Engl J Med* 312:937, 1985.

Darney PD: The androgenicity of progestins, *Am J Med* 98(1A):1045, 1995.

Darney PD, Klaisle CM, Tanner S, et al: Sustained-release contraceptives, *Curr Probl Obstet Gynecol Fertil* 13:87, 1990.

Farley TM, Rosenberg MJ, Rowe PJ, et al: Intrauterine devices and pelvic inflammatory disease: an international perspective, *Lancet* 339:785, 1992.

Fihn SK, Latham RH, Roberts P, et al: Association between diaphragm use and urinary tract infection, *JAMA* 254: 240, 1985.

Filshie M, Guillebaud J: *Contraception science and practice*, London, 1989, Butterworths.

Flynn AM, Lynch SS: Cervical mucous and identification of the fertile phase of the menstrual cycle, *Br J Obstet Gynaecol* 83:656, 1976.

Foreman H, Stadel BV, Schlesselman S: Intrauterine device usage and fetal loss, *Obstet Gynecol* 58:669, 1981.

Forrest JD, Fordyce RR: U.S. women's contraceptive attitudes and practice: how have they changed in the 1980's? *Fam Plann Perspect* 20:112, 1988.

Forrest JD, Singh S: The sexual and reproductive behavior of American women, 1982-1988, *Fam Plann Perspect* 22:206, 1990.

Gerofi JP, Spencer B: Condoms. In Corson SL, Dermano RJ, Tyrer LB, editors: *Fertility control*, ed 2, London, Ont, 1994, Goldin.

Gerstman BB, Gross TP, Kennedy DL, et al: Trends in the content and use of oral contraceptives in the United States, *Am J Public Health* 81:90, 1991.

Gevers-Leuven JA, Dersjant-Roorda MC, Helmerhorst FM, et al: Effects of oral contraceptives on liver metabolism, *Am J Obstet Gynecol* 163:1410, 1990.

Godsland IF, Crook D, Simpson R, et al: The effects of different formulations of oral contraceptive agents on lipid and carbohydrate metabolism, *N Engl J Med* 323:1375, 1990.

Gollub EL, Stein Z, El-Sadr W: Short-term acceptability of the female condom among staff and patients at a New York City hospital, *Fam Plann Perspect* 27:155, 1995.

Grady WR, Hirsch MB, Keen N, et al: Contraceptive failure and continuation among married women in the United States: estimates from the 1982 National Survey of Family Growth, *Fam Plann Perspect* 18:200, 1986.

Gregersen E, Benete G: The female condom: a pilot study of the acceptability of a new female barrier method, *Acta Obstet Gynecol Scand* 69:73, 1990.

Grimes DA, Hughes JM: Use of multiphasic oral contraceptives and hospitalizations of women with functional ovarian cysts in the United States, *Obstet Gynecol* 73:1037, 1989.

Grimes DA, Mishell DR: Congenital limb reduction deformaties and oral contraceptives, *Am J Obstet Gynecol* 158: 439, 1988.

Grou F, Rodrigues I: The morning-after pill—how long after? *Am J Obstet Gynecol* 171:1529, 1994.

Hatcher RA, Stewart F, Trussell J, et al: *Contraceptive technology*, New York, 1990, Irvington.

Henshaw SK, Van Vort J: Abortion services in the United States, 1987 and 1988, *Fam Plann Perspect* 20:288, 1990.

Jones EF, Forrest JD: Contraceptive failure in the United States: revised estimates from the 1982 National Survey of Family Growth, *Fam Plann Perspect* 21:103, 1989.

Klaus H, Goebel JM, Muraski B, et al: Use-effectiveness and client satisfaction in six centers teaching the Billings ovulation method, *Contraception* 19: 613, 1979.

Kolbe LJ, Kann L, Collins JL: Overview of the Youth Risk Surveillance System, *Public Health Rep* 108(suppl 1):2, 1993.

Kols MA, Rinehart W, Piotrow PT, et al: Oral contraceptives in the 1980s, *Popul Rep A* 6:190, 1982.

Lee NC, Rosero-Bixby L, Oberle MW, et al: A case-control study of breast cancer and hormonal contraception in Costa Rica, *J Natl Cancer Inst* 79:1247, 1987.

Lee NC, Rubin GL, Borucki R: The intrauterine device and pelvic inflammatory disease revisited: new results from the Women's Health Study, *Obstet Gynecol* 72:1, 1988.

Lee NC, Rubin GL, Ory HW, et al: Type of intrauterine device and risk of pelvic inflammatory disease, *Obstet Gynecol* 62:1, 1983.

Liang AP, Levenson AG, Layde PM, et al: Risk of breast, uterine corpus, and ovarian cancer in women receiving medroxyprogesterone injections, *JAMA* 249:2909, 1983.

Lippes J, Malik, Tatum HJ: The postcoital copper T, *Adv Planned Parenth* 11:24, 1976.

Liskin L, Pile JM, Quillin WF: Vasectomy—safe and simple, *Popul Rep D* 4:61, 1983.

Liskin L, Rinehart W, Blackburn R, et al: Minilaporatory and laporascopy: safe, effective and widely used, *Popul Rep C* 9:125, 1985.

Liskin LS, Quillin WF: Long-acting progestins—promise and prospects, *Popul Rep K* 11:17, 1983.

Louv WC, Austin H, Perlman J, et al: Oral contraceptive use and risk of chlamydial and gonococcal infections, *Am J Obstet Gynecol* 160:396, 1989.

Lytle CD, Carney PG, Vohra S, et al: Virus leakage through natural membrane condoms, *Sex Transm Dis* 17:58, 1990.

Marshall J: Cervical-mucous and basal body-temperature method of regulating births, *Lancet* 2:282, 1976.

Mastroianni L: Rhythm: systematized chance-taking, *Fam Plann Perspect* 6:209, 1974.

McCarthy JJ, Rockette HE: Prediction of ovulation with basal body temperature, *J Reprod Med* 31:742, 1986.

Meade TW, Greenberg G, Thompson SG: Progestogens and cardiovascular reactions associated with oral contraceptives and a comparison of the safety of 50- and 30-μg oestrogen preparations. *Br Med J* 1:1157, 1980.

Mishell DR, Kletzky OA, Brenner PF, et al: The effect of contraceptive steroids on hypothalamic-pituitary function, *Am J Obstet Gynecol* 128:60, 1977.

Moghissi KS: Cervical mucous changes and ovulation prediction and detection, *J Reprod Med* 31:748, 1986.

Neuberger J, Forman D, Doll R, et al: Oral contraceptives and hepatocellular carcinoma, *Br Med J* 292:1355, 1986.

Newton J, Tacchi D: Long-term use of copper intrauterine devices, *Lancet* 1:1322, 1990.

Notelovitz M, Feldman EB, Gillespy M, et al: Lipid and lipoprotein changes in women taking low-dose, triphasic oral contraceptives: a controlled, comparative, 12-month clinical trial, *Am J Obstet Gynecol* 160:1269, 1989.

Olsson H: Oral contraceptives and breast cancer—a review, *Acta Oncologica* 28:849, 1989.

Oral contraceptive use in older women, *FDA Drug Bull* 20:1, 1990.

Ory HW, Forrest JD, Lincoln R: *Making choices: evaluating health risks and benefits of birth control methods*, New York, 1983, The Alan Guttmacher Institute.

Paul C, Skegg DC, Spears GF: Depot medroxyprogesterone (Depo-Provera) and risk of breast cancer, *Br Med J* 299:759, 1989.

Porter JB, Hunter JR, Danielson DA, et al: Oral contraceptives and nonfatal vascular disease—recent experience, *Obstet Gynecol* 59:299, 1982.

Postcoital contraception, *Lancet* 1:855, 1983.

Ramcharan S, Pellegrin FA, Ray R, et al: *The Walnut Creek Contraceptive Drug Study: a prospective study of the side effects of oral contraceptives*, vol 3, *An interim report—a comparison of disease occurrence leading to hospitalization or death in users and nonusers of oral contraceptives*, Bethesda, Md, US Department of Health and Human Services, National Institute of Child Health and Human Behavior, Center for Population Research Monographs, NIH Publication No. 81-564, 1981.

Rebar RW, Zeserson K: Characteristics of the new progestogens in combination oral contraceptives, *Contraception* 44:1, 1991.

Richard BW, Lasagna LL: Drug regulation in the United States and the United Kingdom: the Depo-Provera story, *Ann Intern Med* 106:886, 1987.

Rosenberg MJ, Gollub EL: Commentary: methods women can use that may prevent sexually transmitted disease, including HIV, *Am J Public Health* 82:1473, 1992.

Rosenfield A, Maine D, Rochat R, et al: The Food and Drug Administration and medroxyprogesterone acetate, *JAMA* 249:2922, 1983.

Royal College of General Practitioners: *Oral contraceptives and health: an interim report from the Oral Contraceptive Study of the Royal College of General Practitioners*, New York, 1974, Pitman.

Schwallie PC, Assenzo JR: Contraceptive use-efficacy study utilizing medroxyprogesterone acetate administered as an intramuscular injection once every 90 days, *Fertil Steril* 24:331, 1973.

Schwallie PC, Assenzo JR: The effect of depo-medroxyprogesterone acetate on pituitary and ovarian function, and the return of fertility following its discontinuation: a review, *Contraception* 10:181, 1974.

Shoupe D, Mishell DR: Subdermal implant system for long-term contraception, *Am J Obstet Gynecol* 160:1286, 1989.

Shoupe D, Mishell DR, Bopp BL, et al: The significance of bleeding patterns in Norplant implant users, *Obstet Gynecol* 77:256, 1991.

Si S, Jun-kang C, Pei-juan Y, et al: A cross-over study of three oral contraceptives containing ethinyloestradiol and either desogestrel or levonorgestrel, *Contraception* 45:523, 1992.

Sivin I: International experience with Norplant and Norplant-2 contraceptives, *Stud Fam Plann* 19:81, 1988.

Sivin I, Tatum HJ: Four years of experience with the TCu-380A intrauterine contraceptive device, *Fertil Steril* 36:159, 1981.

Spellacy WN, Kabra PS, Buhi WC, et al: Pituitary and ovarian responsiveness to a graded gonadotropin releasing factor stimulation test in women using a low-estrogen or regular type of oral contraceptive, *Am J Obstet Gynecol* 137:109, 1980.

Stadel BV: Oral contraceptives and cardiovascular disease, *N Engl J Med* 305:612,672, 1981.

Stadel BV, Lai S: Oral contraceptives and premenopausal breast cancer in nulliparous women, *Contraception* 38:287, 1988.

Stampfer MJ, Willett WC, Colditz GA, et al: A prospective study of past use of oral contraceptive agents and risk of cardiovascular diseases, *N Engl J Med* 319:1313, 1988.

Toivonen J, Luukkainen T, Allonen H: Protective effect of intrauterine release of levonorgestrel on pelvic infection: three years' experience of levonorgestrel- and copper-releasing intrauterine devices, *Obstet Gynecol* 77:261, 1991.

Treiman K, Liskin L: IUDs — new look, *Popul Rep B* 16:1, 1988.

Trussell J, Grummer-Straun L: Contraceptive failure of the ovulation method of periodic abstinence, *Fam Plann Perspect* 22:65, 1990.

Trussell J, Hatcher RA, Cates W, et al: Contraceptive failure in the United States: an update, *Stud Fam Plann* 21:51, 1990.

UK National Case-Control Study Group: Oral contraceptive use and breast cancer risk in young women, *Lancet* 1:973, 1989.

Vessey MP, Lawless A, McPherson K, et al: Fertility after stopping use of intrauterine contraceptive device, *Lancet* 1:106, 1983.

Vessey M, Lawless M, Yeates D: Efficacy of different contraceptive methods, *Lancet* 1:841, 1982.

Vessey MP, McPherson K, Johnson B: Mortality among women participating in the Oxford/Family Planning Association Contraceptive Study, *Lancet* 2:731, 1977.

Vessey MP, Yeates D, Flavel R, et al: Pelvic inflammatory disease and the intrauterine device: findings in a large cohort study, *Br Med J* 282:855, 1981.

Wahl P, Walden C, Knopp R: Effect of estrogen/progestin potency on lipid/lipoprotein cholesterol, *N Engl J Med* 308:862, 1983.

Washington AE, Gore S, Schacter J, et al: Oral contraceptives, *Chlamydia trachomatis* infection, and pelvic inflammatory disease, *JAMA* 253:2246, 1985.

Weiss NS, Sayvetz TA: Incidence of endometrial cancer in relation to the use of oral contraceptives, *N Engl J Med* 302:551, 1980.

Wharton C, Blackburn R: Low-dose pills, *Popul Rep A* 7:1, 1988.

What role do lipid levels play in managing OC patients? *Contracept Technol Update* 8:29, 1987.

WHO Collaborative Study of Neoplasia and Steroid Contraceptives: Breast cancer, cervical cancer, and depot medroxyprogesterone acetate, *Lancet* 2:1207, 1984.

WHO Collaborative Study of Neoplasia and Steroid Contraceptives: Breast cancer and Depo-medroxyprogesterone acetate (DMPA): a multinational study, *Lancet* 338(8771):833, 1991.

Wingrave SJ, Kay CR: Oral contraceptives and gallbladder disease, *Lancet* 2:957, 1982.

World Health Organization: A prospective multicentre trial of the ovulation method of natural family planning. II. The effectiveness phase, *Fertil Steril* 36:591, 1981.

World Health Organization: Injectible hormonal contraceptives: technical and safety aspects, Geneva, 1982, WHO Offset Publication No. 65.

Wynn V, Adams PW, Godsland I, et al: Comparison of effects of different combined oral contraceptive formulations on carbohydrate and lipid metabolism, *Lancet* 1:1045, 1979.

Wysowski DK, Green L: Serious adverse events in Norplant users reported to the Food and Drug Administration's MedWatch Spontaneous Reporting System, *Obstet Gynecol* 85:538, 1995.

Yuzpe A, Smith P, Rademaker A: A multicenter clinical investigation employing ethinyl estradiol combined with *dl*-norgestrel as a postcoital contraceptive agent, *Fertil Steril* 37:508, 1982.

CHAPTER 4

Psychosocial Problems: Detection and Management

DIANE H. STENCHEVER

SELF-ESTEEM
SEXUAL ABUSE
RAPE
  Medical Care
  Medicolegal Concerns
  Psychologic Support
DOMESTIC VIOLENCE AND
  ABUSE

SEXUAL RESPONSE AND
  DYSFUNCTION
  Inhibited Sexual Desire
  Vaginismus
  Orgasmic Dysfunction
  Dyspareunia

The individual is the product of her experiences. Early in life as her personality develops, so does she develop a vision of herself. Positive experiences and nurturing forces tend to build a strong self-esteem; however, attacks against her mental and physical well-being will distort her self-image and may influence the choices that she makes later in life as well as her overall personal development.

Every individual faces change and loss throughout her lifetime. These tend to multiply with age. They may include losses in career and social opportunities, physical losses such as body parts, and the loss of friends or loved ones through separation, death, or divorce. Later in life, the loss of physical or mental abilities either by illness or accident may occur. Often loss activates a grieving process. The ability to grieve and come to terms with loss effectively may determine how future life experiences will be handled. The inability to resolve grief appropriately may leave the individual unable to deal with new life choices effectively. This may lead to poor choices, and the individual may focus on the grief-provoking effect and see all other events in a relationship relative to that effect. The consequences may be poorly developed relationships, lost opportunities, and the selection of a less productive choice when presented with several alternatives.

A knowledgeable and sensitive gynecologist caring for women who have particular life crises and changes can help them understand the impact of the problems they face and the consequences of the choices they will make. It is possible to provide or refer the patient to specific counseling to help her through these critical life events as they occur. Because counseling patients may not be the major role of the gynecologist in a particular situation, it is appropriate for physicians to develop a list of individual counselors and agencies to which the patient can be referred. A responsibility of the physician is to be familiar with the specific resources available in order to make an appropriate referral when such is indicated.

This chapter will discuss some of the major psychologic and social problems that can arise during a woman's lifetime and offer suggestions on how the physician can be helpful.

SELF-ESTEEM

Because self-esteem begins to develop in early childhood, the gynecologist often aids the development of the young woman's self-esteem through his or her patient, the mother. Young women who are just beginning their child-rearing responsibilities can be encouraged to continuously reinforce the child's self-worth as an individual by verbal and nonverbal means such as touching the child, talking to the child in gentle ways, offering positive praise for the child's actions, and as the child becomes older setting limits that are socially acceptable within the framework of the family. They should be encouraged to limit punishment to reinforcement of the needs for the limits set. Intimidation, verbal abuse, and physical abuse should be avoided. Physicians may be helpful in offering advice or reading material and discussing specific issues directly with the young mother or her partner. In some instances, the parents may be referred for parenting classes. Positive reinforcement of the child's self-worth mixed with warmth and love tends to build self-esteem. Negative statements and actions tend to tear it down. Because children have nothing with which to compare, if the message from the parents and other significant individuals in their life is negative, they will tend to believe the message to be true and develop a negative self-esteem for life. When this is the case, physicians and other counselors treating the patient in future life situations may need to begin by building self-esteem before other progress can be made.

SEXUAL ABUSE

Physical or sexual abuse can have serious consequences, particularly if experienced in childhood. If such conditions are noted, they should be dealt with energetically because they will have long-standing influences on the child. The physician must communicate to the child that she is a victim and in no way responsible for what has happened. Contrary statements may have a lasting effect on the child's developing self-esteem. Many children seen after the event may show little in the way of symptoms or affect but should still be considered to be traumatized and counseled fully.

Incest must be placed within the context of sexual abuse of the child. Incest in general is defined as sexual intimacy with or without coitus involving a close family member. The act may include fondling, exposure, or penetration of an orifice by the phallus. Although it is difficult to estimate the incidence of incest, it has been estimated that at least 10% of all childhood abuse cases involve sexual abuse and that perhaps 350,000 or more children per year are sexually abused in the United States. A number of studies have estimated as many as 15% to 25% of all adult women and 12% of all men have experienced incest at some time during their life, most often in childhood.

Childhood sexual abuse is usually separated into those events in which the child is victimized by a stranger and those by a family member. In general, sexual abuse by a stranger is a single occurrence and is almost always reported to the police. The child will generally clearly define what happened, and the act may take the form of a variety of sexual activities often involving enticement, coercion, or physical force. Under such circumstances, the child must be interviewed carefully and allowed to tell what happened, and the police or protective services should be notified. The child should be evaluated as a rape victim and be offered appropriate prophylaxis against infection and referral to a mental health care or rape crisis center for continuing counseling and therapy. The molester should be apprehended if possible and removed from the child's environment. Most communities have sexual abuse crisis intervention centers, and they are equipped to handle childhood sexual abuse. In each case the child should be carefully told that he or she was a victim of a wrongful act and in no way was he or she to blame. Any statement that implies the child might in some way have enticed the perpetrator to perform the act is inappropriate and may have a prolonged and lasting detrimental effect on the child.

The welfare of the molested child's siblings must be considered as well. Another aspect of child sexual abuse is the effect the act has on the parents. Often they feel helplessness and anger because they failed to protect their child. They may feel that the child is twice brutalized, first by the act and then by the legal system, which may cause the child to repeat trauma through a court situation and may lead to the release of the perpetrator or a mild sentence. In the case of either of these possibilities the family may feel frustration because the crime is not properly punished.

Perhaps as many as 80% of childhood sexual assaults are perpetrated by a parent, guardian, other family member, or maternal significant other. Although different states define incest differently with respect to whether coitus takes place, to the child the assault will have serious implications. Incest occurs in all social groups, including cultures where it is a stated taboo.

Incest victims may exhibit anger directed both inwardly and toward society, the child's mother, and men in general. Anger toward the mother may be made worse by a sense that she was not protective in this situation. Children who have been victimized by incest often feel guilty during adolescence. Many may be afraid to withdraw from the incestuous relationship because they fear that doing so would destroy the family and the security it provides. Such victims may feel humiliated and develop a weak self-image. They may then have difficulty developing an appropriate relationship with members of the opposite sex. They may make poor choices with respect to interpersonal relationships in the future and frequently choose a chaotic relationship after they leave home. Some children demonstrate normal psychologic development when evaluated in the future, but most exhibit guilt, anger, behavior problems, unexplained physical complaints, lying, stealing, school failure, running away, and sleep disturbances. Young teenagers demonstrating some of these findings could certainly be questioned by the gynecologist about the possibility of an incestuous relationship. Appropriate questions (e.g., "Were you physically or sexually abused or raped as a child or adolescent?") should be asked as part of a routine history. Affirmative answers to these direct questions should be followed up with detailed but discreet questioning with respect to the circumstances involved. The physician should be nonjudgmental and should try to decide on the appropriate counseling for the patient at the particular time she is being seen.

Incest victims as adults frequently choose partners with inadequate personalities who may be capable of physical and sexual violence. This may be their unconscious desire to find familiar relationships. They may, however, be impeded by their poor self-image from developing stronger and more positive relationships.

RAPE

Rape is defined as any act of sexual intimacy without mutual consent that is performed by one person on another by force, by threat of force, or by the inability of the victim to give appropriate consent.

Rape is a common act. A 1987 report from the U.S. Department of Justice placed the annual incidence of sexual assault in females at 73 per 100,000. This accounted for about 6% of all violent crimes but probably represents only a fraction of those rapes that were actually committed. Victims may be reluctant to report rapes to authorities because of embarrassment, fear of retribution, guilt feelings, or simply because they do not understand their rights. Individuals in permanent relationships may feel that the disclosure of a rape may lead to the destruction of their relationship.

Society has many misconceptions about a rape victim, especially if the victim is a female. There is a feeling that an individual may encourage the rape by behavior or dress, and there is a misconception that no one is raped unless they wish to be, often reflecting basic promiscuity in the individual. Sexual assault victims are accused of seduction of innocent men or of lying about the assault in order to make trouble for someone else.

Rape is reported in individuals of all ages, races, and socioeconomic groups. The very young, very old, and mentally or physically handicapped are particularly susceptible. The perpetrator may be a stranger but often is someone known to the individual.

There are variations of sexual assault that must be noted. First is sexual assault in marriage, which is forced coitus or related sexual acts in a marital relationship without the consent of the partner. This often occurs in conjunction with physical abuse. The second is "date rape." In this situation the woman may voluntarily participate in sexual play but coitus is performed, often forcibly, without her consent. Often, date rape is not reported because the victim may believe she contributed to the act by participating in foreplay. However, long-term, serious damage to self-esteem often occurs.

Most states criminalize sexual intercourse with females under a specific age. This is generally referred to as statutory rape. Consent of the female is irrelevant in this situation because the statute defines that she is incapable of consenting.

The rape causes the victim to lose control over his or her life during the actual event, and this often leads to anxiety and fear. If the attack is life-threatening, shock associated with physical and psychologic symptoms may occur. Burgess and Holmstrom identified two phases of the rape/ trauma syndrome. The immediate, or acute, phase lasts from hours to days and may be associated with paralysis of the individual's usual coping mechanisms. The victim may appear to be exhibiting emotions from complete loss of control to a well-controlled behavior pattern. The reaction depends on a number of factors, including the relationship of the victim to the attacker, whether force was used, and the length of time the victim was held against her will. The physical complaints may be associated with specific injuries that occurred during the rape or general complaints of soreness, eating problems, headaches, and sleep disturbances. Behavior problems include fear, mood swings, irritability, guilt, anger, depression, and difficulty in concentrating. The victim may experience flashbacks to the attack. If the patient is seen during this particular period of time, it is the physician's responsibility to assess the specific medical problems and offer a program of emotional support and reassurance.

The second phase of the rape/trauma syndrome involves long-term adjustment and has been called the reorganization phase. Flashbacks and nightmares may continue, and phobias may develop. These phobias may be directed against members of the opposite sex, the sex act itself, or nonrelated circumstances such as fears of crowds or other situations. The victim may, during this period of time, institute a number of lifestyle changes, including job, residence, friends, and significant others. If the victim has contracted a sexually transmitted disease or a pregnancy, resolution of this phase may last from months to years and generally involves an attempt on the part of the victim to regain control over her life. Often the rape leads to divorce or to separation from permanent relationships. Although marriages get into difficulty after rape, counseling is rarely sought, and this leads to at least one half of the relationships being destroyed. This occurs because the severe emotional trauma often changes both the victim and her partner because they do not grieve properly for the event and deal with their fears of the significance of the event. Part of the problem is that they fear that the event may be repeated at some other time. Partners will experience these tragedies differently, and the way in which they deal with these differences may drive the couple apart. If the victim is a female, she often develops anxiety over the event while her partner develops anger because men are socialized to be protectors and are helpless in a rape situation. It is often noted that this anger is turned against the victim and leads to a sense of blame because she may not have protected herself from the situation or fought to repel it. The victim may wish to talk about the experience and deal with it in verbal fashion; the tendency for the partner is often to try to forget it and move on.

When the physician realizes that the patient is experiencing or contemplating a major lifestyle change during the postrape period, it is appropriate to point out the reasons why this is happening and to help the victim obtain counseling.

The physician has many responsibilities in the care of a rape victim. This section will be limited to discussing the care of a female who has been raped. In this situation, the physician's responsibility is divided into three categories: medical, legal, and supportive.

Medical Care

It is important to obtain informed consent before the examination is begun and specimens are collected. In addition to fulfilling legal requirements, obtaining informed consent also helps the victim participate in regaining control of her body and her situation. The physician should consider having a third party, preferably a female, present. This should reduce any feelings of vulnerability the victim may experience and can help reassure the victim and provide emotional support.

The medical responsibility of the physician is to first treat injuries and perform tests to prevent and to treat infections and pregnancies. In one sexual assault center between 12% and 40% of victims who were sexually assaulted had acute injuries. Most were minor and required simple repair, but 1% required hospitalization and major operative repair. The victim, however, almost always perceives the experience as life-threatening because in many cases it is. Injuries often occur when the victim is restrained or physically coerced into the physical act. Thus the physician should seek signs of injury such as bruises, abrasions, and lacerations about the neck, back, buttocks, and extremities. If a knife is used as the coercion tactic, small cuts may be found in several areas of the body. Erythema, lacerations, and edema of the vulva or rectum can be present because these areas were manipulated with the hands or penis. These are particularly common findings in children or virginal victims but may occur in any woman and should be looked for. Lacerations of the hymen or vagina are common in the very young and the elderly. Lacerations around the urethra, the rectum, and at times the vaginal vault that perforate into the abdominal cavity may be noted. Bite marks may be found in any of these regions. At times foreign objects are inserted into the vagina, urethra, or rectum and may be found. With oral penetration, injuries may be noted in the mouth and pharynx.

Infection is a major concern, although the risk of contracting an infection is similar to that seen in the general population. In a recent Seattle study, rape victims were found to have, at the time of the rape, a higher incidence of sexually transmitted infections than the control population, and it was felt that many of these women had these infections before the rape. Infections may occur in the vagina, pharynx, and rectum. A specific history of the attack should help the physician in seeking sources. Cultures should be performed for *Neisseria gonorrhoeae* and *Chlamydia trachomatis*. Investigation for syphilis by using either darkfield studies or serology at the time the victim is seen and at a follow-up visit is indicated. Although the victim is also at risk for infections from herpesvirus, hepatitis B virus, cytomegalovirus, human immunodeficiency virus, and other sexually transmitted diseases, in most cases those screening tests cannot be performed at the time the victim is seen in the acute stage. These should be reserved for follow-up visits when indicated.

Cervical mucus should be cultured for *N. gonorrhoeae* and *C. trachomatis*. In addition, cultures of the rectum and oral pharynx are indicated if the history suggests that they would be positive. A wet mount for *Trichomonas vaginalis* and a potassium hydroxide mount for *Candida albicans* can be useful.

At follow-up the patient should once again be investigated for signs and symptoms of sexually transmitted disease and appropriate repeat cultures and serologies obtained.

Prophylactic antibiotics are useful in the management of the acute rape victim. An appropriate prophylaxis for gonorrhea and *Chlamydia* should be given (i.e., ceftriaxone, 250 mg intramuscularly [single dose] and doxycycline, 100 mg orally twice daily for 7 days). In patients who are pregnant, erythromycin may be substituted for tetracycline.

The patient's menstrual history, birth control regimen, and known pregnancy status should be assessed. If the patient is at risk for pregnancy at the time of assault, an appropriate morning-after prophylaxis can be offered. One that is appropriate is two combined oral contraceptive pills such as Ortho-Novum 1/35 or Ovral given immediately and repeated in 12 hours. The chance of pregnancy is often minimal but has been estimated to be between 2% and 4% of victims having a single unprotected coitus. The risk is higher, of course, if the patient is midcycle.

Medicolegal Concerns

Medicolegal aspects should be the next concern of the physician caring for an acute rape victim. To be meaningful, materials should be collected shortly after the assault takes place. The victim should be encouraged to come immediately to a rape crisis center or physician's office where she can be evaluated before bathing, urinating, defecating, washing out her mouth, changing clothes, or cleaning her fingernails. In general, evidence for coitus is present in the vagina for as long as 48 hours after the attack. In other orifices the evidence may last only up to 6 hours. The patient's history and physical examination are important to document her condition at the time she is seen. As much data as possible should be included in such a report. Documentation of the use of force, evidence for sexual contact, and the obtaining of materials that may help identify the offender are paramount concerns. To document that force was used a physician should carefully describe every injury noted and illustrate with either drawings or photographs. Detail is important because injuries suffered by sexual assault victims are often seen in common patterns.

Documentation of sexual contact begins with a history that should include when the patient last had intercourse before the attack. If sperm or semen is found in the vagina or cervix of the victim, it must not be confused with substances present from a consenting sexual act before the attack. Secretions from the vagina or rectum should be investigated to seek motile sperm and the presence of acid phosphatase. Nonmotile sperm may be present as well if the attack occurred 12 to 20 hours previously. Motile sperm may last as long as 2 to 3 days in the endocervix. It is often difficult to ascertain whether ejaculation occurred in the mouth because residual seminal fluid is rapidly destroyed by bacteria and salivary enzymes. Some of the fluid may be found staining the skin or clothing several hours after an attack, and this should be sought. Because acid phosphatase is an enzyme found in high concentration in seminal fluid, substances removed for analysis should be tested for this enzyme. In general motile sperm are present in the vagina for up to 8 hours, in the pharynx for up to 6 hours, and in the cervix for up to 5 days. Nonmotile sperm may occur in the vagina from 7 to 9 days, for an unknown period of time in the pharynx, for 20 to 24 hours in the rectum, and for up to 17 days in the cervix. Acid phosphatase may be present for up to 48 hours in the vagina and similarly in the cervix but is often minimally detectable in the pharynx or rectum. The acid phosphatase may be present in the cervix similar in time to the vagina.

In addition to documenting that intercourse has taken place, it is important to try to identify the perpetrator. All clothing immediately associated with the area of assault should be collected, labeled, and submitted to the authorities. Smears of the vaginal secretions or a Papanicolaou smear should be made to permanently document the presence of sperm. Vaginal secretions for acid phosphatase reaction should be collected by wet or dry swab and refrigerated until the pathologist can process them. Pubic hair combings should be obtained to attempt to identify the pubic hair of the assaulter. Saliva should be collected from the victim to ascertain whether she secretes an antigen that could differentiate her from substances obtained from the perpetrator. Fingernail scrapings should be obtained for skin or blood if the victim scratched the perpetrator. This may allow for DNA testing, which is available in most areas and acceptable in many courts of law. All materials collected should be labeled and turned over to legal authorities or a pathologist, depending on the system in effect. Receipts should be obtained, and this should be documented in the patient's chart.

Psychologic Support

When the physical needs of the patient have been met and the physician has carefully documented the information concerning the rape, he or she should then discuss with the victim the degree of injury suffered, the probability of infection or pregnancy, and a general course that the victim might expect to follow with respect to these. Follow-up appointments to aid prevention of infection and pregnancy should be carried out and appropriate medications prescribed. The physician should allow the victim to discuss her anxieties and should correct her misconceptions. The physician should reassure her insofar as possible that her well-being will be restored. Health personnel trained to handle rape trauma victims and to facilitate counseling should be notified and introduced to the victim at that time if possible, and follow-up appointments should be made. She should not be released until specific plans are made and she understands what these are. A follow-up visit should take place between 1 and 4 weeks later to reevaluate the patient's medical, infectious disease, pregnancy, and psychologic status. An assessment should then be made for the degree of follow-up counseling that will be necessary, and the need should be identified to the patient and plans agreed to. At every step of the way the victim must be made to realize that she is a victim and holds no blame. In every situation she should be allowed to discuss her feelings and her current concepts of her problems. Even though the patient may appear to be in excellent emotional control, the physician must not be misled and must still treat her with the full resources available to a rape victim. Even the best-adjusted patient will experience the stages of the rape/trauma syndrome and must be helped through each stage as much as possible. It is important that health care workers at no time make any comments suggesting that the patient was anything but a victim. Women in this situation are sensitive to any accusations and insinuations that they are in any way responsible. In fact they may actually believe that in some way they may have been. Health care workers should make every effort to avoid giving this impression.

DOMESTIC VIOLENCE AND ABUSE

Abuse may be defined as aggressive behavior including acts of a sexual or physical nature, verbal belittling, or intimidation. The acts may be premeditated, as when one individual wishes to gain control over another, or spontaneous, occurring out of response to anger or frustration. *Domestic violence* and *spouse abuse* are terms that refer to violence that occurs between partners who are in an ongoing relationship regardless of whether they are married. In addition to physical abuse it may include passive neglect, emotional or mental anguish, financial exploitation, denial of care, and in some cases self-inflicted abuse to create guilt. Verbal abuse, threats of violence, throwing an object at someone, pushing, slapping, kicking, hitting, beating up, threatening with a weapon, and using a weapon are all degrees of abuse. Intimidation is generally a part of the syndrome.

In 1985 the Surgeon General of the United States sponsored a workshop on violence and public health in an effort to focus attention on this and similar problems. Although it is difficult to estimate the actual occurrence of domestic violence in the United States, it is thought to be as high as 2 million cases annually. The Federal Bureau of Investigation (FBI) has estimated that perhaps only 1 in 60 cases of domestic violence are actually reported. Perhaps as many as 50% of all relationships are associated with violent acts at one time or another. As many as 25% of women treated for injuries in emergency room settings are victims of spousal abuse, but only 3% are recognized as such. Additionally, 85% of women who are mothers of child abuse victims are themselves abused. Current studies document that women in the United States are more likely to be injured, raped, or killed by a current or former male partner than by all other types of assailants combined. In a 1984 study by the U.S. Department of Justice, Bureau of Justice Statistics, 57% of 450,000 cases of family violence committed by spouses or ex-spouses demonstrated that the wife was the victim in 93% of the cases. In one quarter of these cases, at least three similar incidents had been reported within the previous 6 months. Similar findings were reported by the FBI in 1990. Recently, the American Medical Association published guidelines on domestic violence. It reported that 47% of husbands who beat their wives do so three or more times per year. Of women who have ever been married, 14% reported having been raped by their current or former husband. Rape is a significant form of abuse in 54% of violent marriages. Furthermore, it has been estimated that between one-third and one-half of female homicide victims are murdered by their male partners, whereas only 12% of male homicide victims are killed by their spouses.

Walker states that in her experience and the experience of others, batterers and their victims move easily between suicidal and homicidal intent. Suicide threats in a relationship on the part of the batterer or the victim may be a warning that a homicide may actually occur. Victims often feel that they have no other choice in life. Counseling can help identify other choices.

The battered-wife syndrome has been defined as a symptom complex occurring as a result of violence in which a woman has at any time received deliberate, severe, and repeated (more than three times) physical abuse from her husband with the minimal injury of severe bruising. Such women often give a history of having been beaten as a child, raised in a single-parent household, married as a teenager, and impregnated before marriage. They often appear in medical facilities with a variety of somatic complaints, including headache, insomnia, choking sensation, hyperventilation, gastrointestinal symptoms, and chest, pelvic, and back pain. They are often noncompliant with the physician's advice and recommendations. They appear shy, frightened, embarrassed, evasive, anxious, or passive, and they often cry. The batterer may accompany the woman and stay close to the examination room to monitor what is said. Often the patient's explanation does not fit her injuries, and she frequently gives a history of multiple emergency room visits for trauma and other causes and often has a history of a prescription of tranquilizers. Physicians, when confronting such individuals, should ask direct questions about whether she is being physically abused, especially when there is evidence for injury. Direct questions are necessary because most victims will not readily admit to physical violence out of shame, guilt, or fear. Questions such as "Have you ever been physically injured by anyone recently or in the past?" and "Has anyone at home injured you or attempted to hurt you?" are appropriate.

Physical examination should lead the physician to look for evidence for injury such as bruises, healed burns, fresh burns, or other signs of trauma. Sunglasses should be removed to seek eye injuries. Because domestic violence victims often suffer from posttraumatic stress syndrome, individuals who seem to fall into this category should be investigated for the possibility of a history of domestic violence.

Often there is a cycle of battering that begins with a tension-building phase followed by a gradual increase in tension until specific acts of violence occur. The battering itself may be associated with heavy alcohol or drug consumption on the part of the batterer so that this is blamed for the event. However, it may be merely the excuse that leads to the event. After the battering the batterer may apologize profusely and ask for forgiveness. He often showers the victim with gifts and promises never to repeat the act. He may show remorse. However, within a short time the cycle begins again, and eventually beatings become more frequent and the remorse stage shorter or nonexistent.

As with other victim-associated acts, several myths exist about battered women. These include a thought that such women are always from a lower socioeconomic group, that they enjoy the abuse (or they would take the children and leave), that they probably provoke the beating, and that any woman who is serious about solving her problem could have the batterer arrested and put in jail. In addition, it is thought that if the battered woman remarries she will choose another violent man. Battering occurs in women of all social groups, and women often remain in the relationship for complex and multiple reasons often involved with the loss of control over self, fear, and economic necessity. The cycle of violence occurs regardless of what the victim does, and many women who leave such a relationship remain single or remarry men who are nonviolent.

Although most states have laws to control domestic violence, this has not effectively deterred the acts of domestic violence in the United States. In fact there is evidence that the incidence is mounting steadily. Often the crime is a misdemeanor, jail time may be overnight or not at all, and the perpetrator may be sentenced to anger management classes that may or may not be enforced. Because many of the batterers will not admit that they have a problem and do not wish to be in such classes, little benefit may be obtained. In fact, when husbands are jailed, wives have been known to provide bail so that the husband does not miss work and deprive the family of financial benefits.

Family counseling and intervention can be extremely dangerous because it often raises issues that exacerbate the violence and increase the risk of serious harm to the woman and her children. Individual violence elimination counseling teaches nonviolent methods of problem solving and should be completed before any family therapy is attempted.

Physicians should help patients develop alternatives for a life outside a violent marriage or, if the patient is not willing to leave the marriage, should help her construct an exit plan that can be put into effect if another violent experience should occur. The plan includes preparation of a bag packed with clothing changes for herself and her children, cash, checkbook, savings account books, and identification papers such as birth certificates, social security cards, and voter registration cards. This bag should be kept in a safe place with either a friend or a relative. Financial records, including mortgage papers, rent receipts, and automobile titles, may also be set aside for the patient's use. She should practice exactly how she will leave the house and where she would go as she would in a fire drill. In addition, physicians should learn about community resources for battered women and their children and make appropriate referrals so that the woman may obtain counseling for herself, her children, and the batterer should she decide to stay in the relationship. In most communities such shelters are overburdened; in at least one major city it has been estimated that half of the homeless women are victims of domestic violence.

The American College of Obstetricians and Gynecologists (ACOG) has prepared a patient education pamphlet, *The Abused Woman*, that can be placed in physicians' offices and made available to women in this predicament. Women have been known to pick up such a pamphlet and use it as a resource information document even when they are unwilling to speak about it to the physician.

Another form of domestic violence is that of violence directed to the elderly family member. Abuse of the elderly has been estimated to occur in as many as 2 million people in the United States per year. Indeed, it has been estimated that perhaps 1 in every 10 elderly individuals living in a family situation is a victim of abuse. It may be more difficult to identify such situations because the elderly tend to be more isolated and are reluctant to report such abuse because this may remove them from the family situation. Often the personality of the caregiver is the determinant of whether abuse will occur to the elderly rather than the stress and circumstances of the caring condition.

Characteristically, the abused person is one beyond the age of 75 years, frequently with physical impairment, usually white, widowed, and living with relatives. Often the person abusing her is a young adult within the family; however, it may also be a caregiver or a spouse. The diagnosis is difficult but can be made when the details of the injury do not match the injury itself. Similarities between elder abuse and child abuse are therefore apparent, and the physician should approach the elder individual who may seem to have been abused in the same way he or she would approach a potential child abuse victim.

After identification of the problem, treatment and counseling must be directed both to the individual and to the family members involved. This should be done in the same fashion as domestic violence problems are handled in other situations.

All 50 states and the District of Columbia have passed legislation protecting the elderly from domestic violence and neglect. Forty-two states have mandatory reporting laws.

SEXUAL RESPONSE AND DYSFUNCTION

Although sexual gratification is a major human experience, it is also an extremely personal one, and what constitutes sexual satisfaction varies from one individual to another. As with so many human experiences that involve emotion, variations occur in any individual from time to time and depend on a number of factors, including but not limited to state of health, fatigue, state of emotional well-being, the presence of stressful stimuli, the influence of alcohol or drugs (including illicit and prescription items), and the condition and input of the partner. Masters and Johnson concluded after evaluating the sexual cycles of 700 subjects under laboratory conditions that a sexual cycle does exist and includes an excitement or seduction phase that is initiated by either external or internal stimuli and that seems to be under the influence of the parasympathetic arm of the autonomic nervous system. During the excitement phase several physiologic responses such as deep breathing, increased heart rate, increased blood pressure, and a feeling of total body warmth in conjunction with erotic feelings are noted. There is an increase in sexual tension during this phase, accompanied by generalized vasocongestion as manifested by breast engorgement; the development of macular-papillary erythematous rashes on the breast, chest, and abdomen (the sexual flush); and engorgement of the labia majora and labia minora. The clitoris generally swells, becomes erect, and is pressed tightly against the clitoral hood. A transudate lubricant generally occurs in the vagina, and the Bartholin's glands may secrete small amounts of liquid. With the deep breathing the uterus may tent up into the pelvis, and a myotonic effect, including nipple erection, is noted. Because these responses primarily result from parasympathetic stimulation, individuals who are taking medications that interfere with the parasympathetic receptors may experience difficulty in obtaining adequate levels of excitation.

The excitation phase is followed by the plateau stage, which is associated with an increased amount of vasocongestion throughout the body and engorgement of the breasts, labia, and lower third of the vagina. Engorgement of the lower aspect of the vagina may cause a decrease in diameter of the vagina by as much as 50%, increasing the friction of the vagina against the penis. The clitoris during this stage is tightly retracted against the pubic symphysis, and the vagina is noted to be lengthened and dilated in its upper two thirds.

The plateau stage is followed by orgasm, at which point the sexual tension that has been built up in the entire body is released. A myotonic response involving all of the muscle systems of the body occurs, and individuals may experience carpal spasm and extremely rarely grand mal seizures. The sphincter muscles of the vagina and anus contract. The uterus often contracts in a rhythmic fashion, but the intensity varies from woman to woman. The orgasmic phase is influenced by the sympathetic nervous system, and individuals taking medications that interfere with sympathetic receptors may be unable to achieve orgasm. Most careful questioning of the patient with respect to her sexual response gives some insight into whether a problem may exist in the excitement stage or the orgasmic stage and offer a clue as to the potential cause.

After orgasm, resolution (the last stage of the sexual cycle) occurs. During this stage the woman returns to her preexcitement level. Although prolonged refractory periods are noted in the male, this has not been the case in women. Therefore new cycles may be stimulated shortly after orgasm. The resolution period is generally accompanied by a feeling of personal satisfaction and well-being.

Although several lay publications have suggested that the cervix is important in sexual response because the cervix seems to have a rich nerve supply, no scientific data support this theory. Sexual gratification and orgasmic behavior seem to be associated with receptors in the clitoris, mons pubis, labia, and possibly pressure receptors in the pelvis. It is important to understand this and to use this information in counseling women who are about to undergo pelvic surgical procedures.

After menopause vaginal epithelium may undergo atrophy, vaginal pH changes, and there is a decrease in the quantity of vaginal secretions and a decrease in general circulation to the vagina and the uterus. In addition, relaxation of pelvic support structures may occur, and a cystocele, rectocele, or prolapse of the uterus may be noted. These factors may decrease a woman's ability to enjoy coitus, but most of these can be reversed by replacement estrogen therapy. Because postmenopausal women generally are married to men of their own age group and because general health conditions and medications may influence the husband's sexual response as well as the woman's, it is important for a physician to discuss sexual matters with the patient by asking such questions as ''Are you currently sexually active?'' ''Is coitus enjoyable?'' ''Are you able to appreciate arousal as you have in the past?'' and ''Are you orgasmic?'' Negative answers should be investigated both from the standpoint of the woman's desire and ability and those of her partner. Often the sympathetic physician can uncover sexual dysfunction within a couple and direct help and counseling toward the individual in need.

As many as 50% of marriages will at one time or another experience problems of sexual dysfunction. In couples who undergo marriage counseling the percentages are generally higher. Although sexual dysfunction does not necessarily detract from a happy marriage, the physician should try to assess whether the couple desires to overcome sexual dysfunction.

Sexual dysfunction may occur because of a previous negative sexual experience or may be secondary to an emotional or physical illness. It may be related to a specific current problem within the marriage or to factors that have occurred in the past, perhaps unrelated to the marriage. Drugs and alcohol often play a role. A small amount of alcohol may decrease inhibitions and improve sexual response, but increased amounts of alcohol act as a depressant and generally decrease the individual's ability to become sexually aroused or to become vaginally lubricated. Narcotics and sedative-type drugs also depress sexual responsiveness, and drugs that affect the autonomic nervous system can have a profound effect on arousal and orgasm.

Inhibited Sexual Desire

The most common sexual dysfunction is inhibited sexual desire. Couples are often incompatible with respect to individual libidinal drive. The starting point in therapy is to discuss what each individual expects and requires. If lack of sexual arousal is due to past experience or problems in the present relationship, this is best approached by resolving those conflicts through a counseling program. At times the problem is simply that the couple does not give a high enough priority to their sexual relationship because of other responsibilities. They should be encouraged to change their priorities and make time available for sufficient foreplay and arousal at a time when they are not totally fatigued. If drug or alcohol abuse is a contributing factor, this problem should be dealt with. If prescription drugs are involved, attempts should be made to change therapeutic approaches.

Vaginismus

A second problem leading to sexual dysfunction is vaginismus. In vaginismus there is an involuntary spasm of the vaginal, introital, and levator ani muscles. Penetration is either painful or impossible, and when coitus is attempted, the patient generally experiences pain, which increases the degree of spasm in the muscles. Thus not only does the patient experience pain but also the fear of pain as coitus or pelvic examination is contemplated. She may have difficulty inserting a tampon or vaginal medications, and when the levator spasm is continuous and strong, she may begin to experience chronic pelvic pain. In some cases, vaginismus is primary; that is, the patient has never experienced successful coitus. In such instances, the problem is generally based on poor early sexual education, sexual abuse, or aversion to sexuality in general. Thus the individual has a form of conversion hysteria. It is not uncommon to find that the problem first occurred because of a lack of appropriate learning about sex secondary to cultural or familial teaching, such as sex is evil, painful, or undesirable. Secondary vaginismus often occurs after the individual has had an unpleasant sexual experience such as a rape or has experienced an injury in the vaginal area that has led to a painful coital experience. Once the pattern of pain has been established, the cycle of vaginismus may be seen.

The physician should examine the patient carefully to ascertain whether any physical reason for the vaginismus exists (e.g., scarring after a surgical procedure or acute vaginitis). If such is the case, the condition should be treated medically. If the problem is one of poor learning or understanding about sexual matters, the physician should attempt to reeducate the patient in an appropriate fashion. Often a woman suffering from primary vaginismus believes that there is an obstruction to coitus of a physical nature, and she should be reassured that this is not the case. She then may be taught desensitizing techniques such as sitting in a warm bathtub under circumstances that are completely controlled by her and allowing her to digitally dilate her vagina by gentle pressure against the levator muscles by using first one, then two, and perhaps three fingers. This activity can then be transferred to her partner, and after adequate relaxation of the levator muscles is obtained, coitus can be attempted. The patient should be instructed not to have coitus until this point is reached; thus she may enjoy arousal and sex play without the fear that coitus will follow. In some cases vaginal dilators can be used instead of the fingers to demonstrate to the patient that there is indeed room for the penis. Desensitization and relief of vaginismus is generally a relatively simple procedure that takes a short period of time.

Orgasmic Dysfunction

A third dysfunction, orgasmic dysfunction, is common. As many as 10% to 15% of all women state that they have never experienced orgasms with any form of sexual stimulation, and perhaps another 25% state that they have had difficulty reaching an orgasm on specific occasions. Some women are orgasmic secondary to masturbation or oral sex but not with penile intercourse. A careful history differentiates these individuals. If the patient has never experienced orgasm, she may be taught masturbatory techniques. Once she has achieved an orgasm, transference to coitus may occur. She should communicate to her partner those activities that prepare her for and allow her to have an orgasm. These should be added to the coital experience. They may include digital stimulation of the mons and vulva by the partner before and during coitus and in some cases the use of a vibrator during coitus. It is important that couples discuss their individual needs with each other and practice methods that allow them both to fully enjoy the experience.

Dyspareunia

The final sexual dysfunction is dyspareunia. It often has an organic basis. The physician, by careful history and physical examination, should attempt to understand the reason for the dyspareunia and find means to correct it. Often dyspareunia occurs at the point of insertion of the penis, and levator spasm may be the cause. Vaginal spasm for whatever reason may be discovered. This can be treated as noted previously. If the dyspareunia occurs with deeper penetration, the problem may be centered in the urinary tract, such as urethritis, cystitis, or trigonitis, or it may happen because of some vaginal problem such as poor healing of a vaginal laceration or episiotomy. Deeper in the pelvis, pelvic inflammatory disease or endometriosis may be the cause. If no cause can be found, the patient should be approached in much the same way as a woman suffering from vaginismus. Reeducation and change of coital position can be suggested and may be helpful.

The key to managing sexual dysfunction in an office practice is a careful history with specific and direct questions relating to the patient's coital experience, a sympathetic, nonjudgmental approach to the patient's responses, and an attempt to direct therapy at the specific complaint. In every case the individual must be treated as a member of a couple with the needs and problems of the partner taken into consideration. Several health care workers have an interest in sexual counseling, and the busy physician may wish to avail himself or herself of these services. Often sexual dysfunction is a result of other marital problems, and referral to a marriage counselor may be appropriate.

BIBLIOGRAPHY

American College of Obstetricians and Gynecologists: *The abused woman*, Patient Education Pamphlet APO83, Washington, DC, 1989, ACOG.

American College of Obstetricians and Gynecologists: *Sexual assault*, Technical Bulletin No 172, Washington, DC, 1992, ACOG.

American College of Obstetricians and Gynecologists: *Domestic Violence*, Technical Bulletin No 209, Washington, DC, 1995, ACOG.

American Medical Association: *Domestic and treatment guidelines on domestic violence*, Chicago, 1992, American Medical Association.

American Medical Association Council on Scientific Affairs: Violence against women: relevance for medical practitioners, *JAMA* 267:3184, 1992.

Bachmann GA, Moeller TP, Benett J: Childhood sexual abuse and the consequences in adult women, *Obstet Gynecol* 71:631, 1988.

Batten DA: Incest: a review of the literature, *Med Sci Law* 23:245, 1983.

Behrman S: Hostility to kith and kin, *Br Med J* 2:538, 1975.

Bergman B, Brismar B: A five year follow-up study of 117 battered women, *Am J Public Health* 81:1486, 1991.

Briere J, Runtz M: Symptomatology associated with childhood sexual victimization in a non-clinical adult sample, *Clin Abuse Neglect* 12:51, 1988.

Browne A, Williams KR: Gender, intimacy, and lethal violence: trends from 1976-1987, *Gender in Society,* 7:78, 1993.

Bowden ML, Grant ST, Vogel B, et al: The elderly, disabled, and handicapped adult burned through abuse and neglect, *Burns Incl Therm Inj* 14:447, 1988.

Browning DH, Boatman B: Incest: children at risk, *Am J Psychiatry* 134:69, 1977.

Burgess AW, Holmstrom LL: *Rape: victims at crisis,* Bowie, Md, 1974, Robert J Brady.

Campbell JC, Poland ML, Waller JB, Ager J: Correlates of battering during pregnancies, *Res Nurs Health* 15:219, 1992.

Carrington L, Heimbach DM, Marvin JA: Risk management in children with burn injuries, *J Burn Care Rehab* 9:75, 1988.

Centers for Disease Control and Prevention: Physical violence during the 12 months preceding child birth. Alaska, Maine, Oklahoma, and West Virginia 1990-1991, *MMWR CDC Surveill Summ* 43:132, 1994.

Davis LD: Beliefs of service providers about abused women and abusing men, *Soc Work* 29:2, 1984.

Dickstein LJ: Spouse abuse and other domestic violence, *Psychiatr Clin North Am* 11:611, 1988.

Ehrlich P, Anetzberger G: Survey of state public health departments on procedures for reporting elder abuse, *Public Health Rep* 106:151, 1991.

Elbow M: Theoretical considerations of violent marriages, *Soc Casework* 58:515, 1977.

Frank E, Anderson C, Rubinstein D: Frequency of sexual dysfunction in "normal" couples, *N Engl J Med* 299:111, 1978.

Frazer M: Domestic violence: a medicolegal review, *J Forensic Sci* 31:1409, 1986.

Gayford JJ: Battered wives: research on battered wives, *R Soc Health J* 95:288, 1975.

Gelles RJ: Violence in the family: a review of research in the seventies, *J Marriage Fam* 42:873, 1980.

Gentry CE: Incestuous abuse of children: the need for an objective view, *Child Welfare* 58:355, 1978.

Giordano NH, Giordano JA: Elder abuse: a review of the literature, *Soc Work* 29:232, 1984.

Glaser JB, Jammerschlag MR, McCormack WM: Epidemiology of sexually transmitted diseases in rape victims, *Rev Infect Dis* 11:246, 1989.

Goldberg WG, Tomlanovich MC: Domestic violence victims in emergency departments: new findings, *JAMA* 251:3259, 1984.

Green BL: *A clinical approach to marital problems,* Springfield, Ill, 1970, Charles C Thomas.

Hamburger LK, Saunders DG, Hovey M: Prevalence of domestic violence in community practice and rate of physician injury, *Fam Med* 24:283, 1992.

Hammond DC: Screening for sexual dysfunction, *Clin Obstet Gynecol* 27:732, 1984.

Hilberman E: Overview: the "wife-beater's wife" reconsidered, *Am J Psychiatry* 137:1336, 1980.

Hilberman E, Monson K: Sixty battered women, *Victimatology* 2:460, 1977.

Jenny C, Hooton TM, Bowers A, et al: Sexually transmitted diseases in victims of rape, *N Engl J Med* 322:713, 1990.

Jones J, Dorgherty J, Schelble D, et al: Emergency department protocol for the diagnosis and evaluation of geriatric abuse, *Ann Emerg Med* 17:1006, 1988.

Jones JG: Sexual abuse of children, *Am J Dis Child* 136:142, 1982.

Kaplan HS: *The new sex therapy,* New York, 1974, Brunner/Mazel.

Khan M, Sexton M: Sexual abuse of young children, *Clin Pediatr (Phila)* 22:369, 1983.

Klaus PA, Rand MR: *Family violence,* Washington, DC, 1984, US Department of Justice, Bureau of Justice Statistics.

LaFerla JJ: Inhibited sexual desire and orgasmic dysfunction in women, *Clin Obstet Gynecol* 27:738, 1984.

Lamont J: Vaginismus, *Am J Obstet Gynecol* 131:632, 1978.

Masters WH, Johnson VE: *Human sexual inadequacy,* Boston, 1970, Little, Brown.

Masters WH, Johnson VE: *Human sexual response,* Boston, 1966, Little, Brown.

Mercy JA, Saltzman LE: Fatal violence among spouses in the United States 1976-1985, *Am J Public Health* 79:595, 1989.

Morgan SM: *Conjugal terrorism: a psychological and community treatment model of wife abuse,* Palo Alto, Calif, 1982, R&E Research Associates.

Mowbray CA: Shedding light on elder abuse, *J Gerontol Nurs* 15:20, 1989.

Nadelson CC, Notman MT, Zackson H, et al: Followup study of rape victims, *Am J Psychiatry* 139:1267, 1982.

Parker B, Schumacher DN: The battered wife syndrome and violence in the nuclear family of origin: a controlled pilot study, *Am J Public Health* 67:760, 1977.

Pedrick-Cornell C, Gelles RJ: Elderly abuse: the status of current knowledge, *Fam Relat* 31:457, 1982.

Pillemer K, Finkelhov D: Causes of elder abuse: caregiver stress versus problem relatives, *Am J Orthopsychiatry* 59:179, 1989.

Pillemer K, Suitor JJ: Violence and violent feelings: what causes them among family care givers? *J Gerontol* 47:S165, 1992.

Rounsaville B, Weissman MM: Battered woman: a medical problem requiring detection, *Int J Psychiatr Med* 8:191, 1977.

Sager CJ: Sexual dysfunction in marital discord. In Kaplan HS, editor: *The new sex therapy,* New York, 1974, Brunner/Mazel.

Sarafino EP: An estimate of nation wide incidence of sexual offenses against children, *Child Welfare* 58:127, 1979.

Select Committee on Aging: *Domestic violence against the elderly.* Hearings before the Subcommittee on Human Services. House of Representatives, April 21, 1980. Washington, DC, 1980, US Government Printing Office.

Sgroi SM: Sexual molestation of children: the last frontier of child abuse, *Child Today* 4:18, 1975.

Steege JR: Dyspareunia in vaginismus, *Clin Obstet Gynecol* 27:750, 1984.

US Department of Health and Human Services: *Surgeon General's Workshop on Violence in Public Health: report,* DHHS Publication No HRS-D-MC 86-1, Washington, DC, 1986, Public Health Service, Health Resources and Service Administration.

US Department of Justice: *Uniform crime reports for the United States, 1987,* Publication No 14, Washington, DC, 1987, US Government Printing Office.

Viken RM: Family violence: aids to recognition, *Postgrad Med* 71:115, 1982.

Walker LE: *The battered woman syndrome,* New York, 1984, Springer.

CHAPTER 5

Pediatric Gynecology

SUSAN F. POKORNY

This chapter considers gynecologic conditions that the gynecologist is likely to encounter in children from infancy until the prepubertal period. Congenital anomalies and neoplasia will not be covered.

Psychosocial factors are heavily entwined with biobehavioral variations of gynecologic conditions seen in children and young adolescents. These factors make the historical detail of any given gynecologic condition suspect and mandate that a thorough, age-appropriate genital examination be performed before any therapeutic intervention.

The history is usually obtained from individuals who do not use or who misapply anatomically correct terms or who use colloquialisms. Furthermore the caregiver will express or ignore concerns which are not the same as those of the child. Some of the more frequent remarks include "She keeps pulling at herself" and "She says it hurts down there." Many parents treat these complaints casually and explain to the child that if she is going to touch herself "down there" she should do it in the bedroom, or she might feel better if she took a warm bath. At the other extreme, some caregivers overreact to the aforementioned symptoms and report that they think the child has some type of perversion or has been sexually abused. The main thing the clinician must remember is that once the child's caregiver has decided that something *might* be wrong with the child's genitalia, the situation has taken on the proportions of a medical emergency, and accompanying psychosocial issues must be addressed. The parent should be asked directly what it is about the child's symptoms that concerns him or her the most; if allowed to express these concerns, the parent is then more receptive to reassurances and therapeutic interventions.

EXAMINATION

The goal of any examination is to obtain the maximum amount of information about the patient's physical status. At the same time, education specific to the patient's cognitive and physiologic stage of development should be given. Prepubertal girls can always be taught proper toilet hygiene techniques and about the propriety of reporting sexually abusive activities. Peripubertal girls need the same information but can also be taught menstrual hygiene techniques and the physical dangers of premature sexual intercourse. Postpubertal girls should receive contraceptive and preconception counseling information.

Over 90% of childhood gynecologic conditions can be diagnosed by a detailed visual inspection of the external genitalia without the use of instruments. Compliance, which is crucial to the performance of an adequate genital examination, can be gained by reassuring the patient that she has control over the examination and that discomfort will be avoided. Compliance can be augmented by explaining the type and usefulness of the information that can be obtained from the examination and by actively involving the patient in the examination process. These premises are true for a 2-year-old or a 20-year-old patient.

Positioning of the patient is just as important for gynecologic examinations of children as it is for adults. The examiner should be seated, with the child in the supine position and her feet in stirrups or in the examiner's lap. A good light source is mandatory. The head of the child should be elevated for direct eye contact and constant communication between the patient and examiner.

Getting the child to assume this position can sometimes be trying. Engaging the child in the visual examination by using a handheld mirror is helpful. While she sits on the examination table, the patient can be shown that she can see her shoes by looking in the mirror. The mirror can be repositioned to show her how she will be able to see her "girl parts." It is helpful to position and to demonstrate the "mirror trick" to the extremely anxious patient while she is fully clothed. Once the child is reassured and understands what needs to be done, she will comply with instructions about removing clothing so that the examination can proceed.

For the small, prepubertal child who shows anxiety when she sees the examiner or when the parent attempts to place her on the examination table, allow the child to remain on the parent's lap for the examination. Elevate the head of the gynecology table so that the parent is in a slightly reclined sitting position with the feet in the stirrups (yes, even fathers can do this!). The child is then positioned with her legs straddled across the parent's thighs. The parent can hold the handheld mirror so that both the patient and parent can see the genital area. This is an excellent position because the parent's arms enwrap and reassure the child and the child's elevated position aids the examination.

Once the child is positioned for the examination, some means of magnifying the tissue is necessary because frequently minute detail is helpful to the diagnosis and because the external genital structures of children are small. A handheld magnifying glass or a colposcope can be used.

To adequately visualize the small structures of the vestibule, fingers placed bilaterally on the labia majora and slightly posterior to the vaginal orifice can spread the tissues laterally and posteriorly. If the vestibule is deep or the aforementioned attempt is unsatisfactory, the examiner should gently grasp the labia majora in the same area as the two fingers were placed but now using two hands, and gently spread the tissues laterally and posteriorly as before while pulling toward the examiner. While this is being done, the child needs reassurance and should be instructed to take deep breaths. This invariably allows the vestibular tissues to fan out and give the examiner a good, albeit brief, view of the hymen, vaginal opening, and other vestibular structures.

Placing the child in the knee-chest position is more anxiety provoking but should be attempted. This position adds to the hymen evaluation (Figs. 5-1 and 5-2) and allows better visualization of the vaginal canal. If there is minimal discharge or inflammation, if the child can relax, and if one has a well-focused intense light, frequently the vagina will balloon open and the cervix can be seen at the apex.

Instruments are rarely needed for the genital examination of prepubertal females. The atrophic mucosa is sensitive to touch and can be easily torn by inflexible instruments. Even cotton swabs used to obtain secretions are abrasive and painful. Vaginal secretions for a wet mount, cultures, and forensic material can be obtained in a nontraumatic manner by employing a catheter-in-a-catheter technique. With aseptic technique, the proximal 4 inches of butterfly intravenous tubing is passed into the distal 4 inches of a soft number 12 bladder catheter. A 1-cc tuberculin syringe with 0.5 to

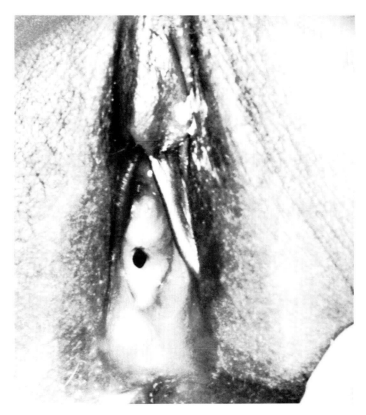

FIGURE 5-1. Normal external genitalia of a prepubertal female in the supine position when using the lateral-spread technique.

1.0 cc of aspirating fluid is attached to the hub of the butterfly tubing (Fig. 5-3). The outer bladder catheter keeps the vaginal walls from sucking against the inner catheter so that a large amount of the aspirating fluid can be flushed in and out of the upper portion of the vagina several times before it is aspirated back into the syringe and the catheters removed from the vagina. This technique provides enough material for a wet mount, a Gram stain, forensic studies, and multiple cultures.

If the vaginal canal and cervix must be examined, a small-diameter endoscope with irrigating properties is the ideal instrument. The irrigating capacity of these instruments allows debris to be flushed away. After the vagina is lavaged, one gently squeezes the vulvar tissues around the scope, and the irrigating fluid (bladder irrigant in most cases) will expand the vaginal canal so that the entire canal and the cervix can be seen (Fig. 5-4). Speculums, even nasal speculums, cannot be opened sufficiently to see all aspects to the prepubertal vagina without damaging the hymen. The otoscope and the Cameron-Myers vaginoscope will not damage the hymen but have such small portals that they are inefficient.

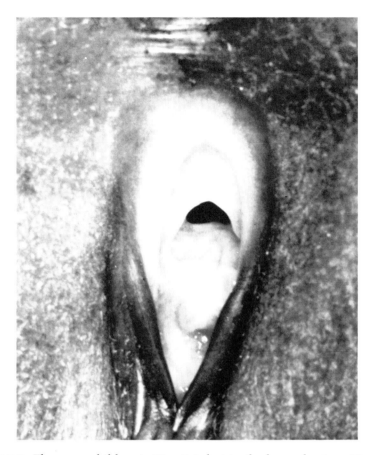

FIGURE 5-2. The same child as in Fig. 5-1, but in the knee-chest position.

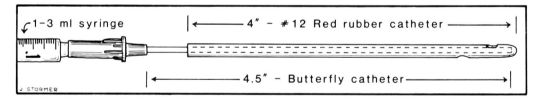

FIGURE 5-3. Catheter-in-catheter aspirator used to obtain secretions from the prepubertal vagina.

From Pokorny SF, Stormer J: *Am J Obstet Gynecol* 156:581, 1987.

Vaginoscopy can be successfully performed in the office on a cooperative child if a small amount of topical anesthetic cream or ointment is placed on the vulva and a flexible endoscope is used. For office vaginoscopy, the child should be positioned semireclined on the gynecology examination table with her buttocks over the dip tray basin, which is used to catch the irrigation fluid.

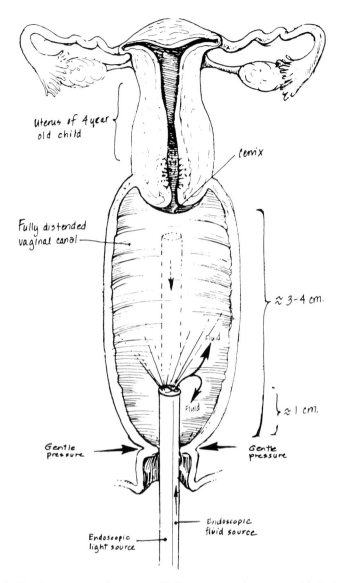

FIGURE 5-4. Vaginoscopy using a small-diameter endoscope with irrigating fluid. The latter lavages debris from the vagina and expands the vaginal canal for good inspection of the cervix and vagina.

From Pokorny SF: In Stoval T, Mann W, editors: *Textbook of gynecologic surgery,* New York, Churchill Livingstone, 1996.

HORMONAL STATUS AND ANATOMY

Before examining the child for anatomic landmarks, minute variations, and lesions, the clinician must have a concept of the appropriate hormonal status of a child's tissue. The neonatal term infant has been excessively stimulated with maternal hormones; small breast buds, thickened vulvar mucosa, mucoid leukorrhea, and low levels of gonadotropins are the consequence. Immediately after birth, with the loss of maternal estrogens, not infrequently there is a small withdrawal menstrual bleed from the neonatal endocervix and endometrium. This marks the end of maternal estrogen stimulation, but not the end of the estrogen effect. The neonatal vulvar mucosa does not immediately become atrophic; in fact, the vulvar tissues remain well estrogenized for several years. This affords the diapered neonate and infant protection from severe irritative vulvitis caused by urine and feces but does make them more susceptible to *Monilia* vulvitis. When the child reaches the age of toilet training, most estrogen effect on the vulva is gone, and it becomes atrophic (Fig. 5-5). The tables are now turned, and the child is no longer susceptible to *Monilia* vulvitis, but she will develop a significant vulvitis from fecal contamination.

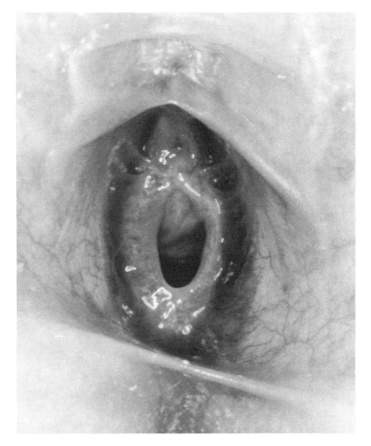

FIGURE 5-5. Vulva of a 3-year-old. Note the denseness of capillaries on the vestibular sulcus (erythema of atrophic mucosa can be confused with inflammation). Also note the bands and crepts of the minor vestibular glands in the periurethral sulcus.

From Pokorny SF: *Curr Probl Obstet Gynecol Fertil* 13:202, 1990.

The estrogen effect is apparent in the thickened vulvar mucosa of the neonate and creates a moist white-pink appearance; capillaries cannot be seen with magnification. These same findings in a 3-year-old to 7-year-old child would be distinctly abnormal (Fig. 5-6). As this child enters puberty one again sees estrogen's effect on the vulva.

It is important for the clinician to differentiate between abnormal erythema caused by inflammation and normal erythema caused by atrophic changes. From 3 years on to the prepubertal years of 9 to 11 years of age, road map capillary beds should be visible, especially with magnification, on the atrophic vulvar mucosa of the unestrogenized child. This capillary density is greatest in the sulcus of the vestibule. Inflammation of the tissue causes a more generalized redness and an edematous thickening of the tissue that obscures the capillary beds so easily seen on the atrophic mucosa.

The most obvious landmark on the perineum of the prepubertal female (Fig. 5-7) is the clitoris, which has extreme variability in size and in the amount of surrounding subcutaneous fat; no extensive endocrine or karyotypic evaluation is warranted unless the diameter of the glans clitoris is 0.5 cm or greater.

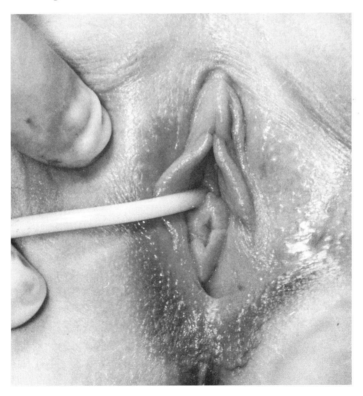

FIGURE 5-6. Vulva of a 3-year-old with an estrogen-producing ovarian cyst and premature thelarche.

From Pokorny SF: *Curr Probl Obstet Gynecol Fertil* 13:202, 1990.

The labia minora are the next most prominent structures to be identified. They form the lateral anterior margins of the vestibule and course medially toward the midline under the clitoral complex. The mucosa of the vulva is demarcated by the clitoris superiorly, the labia minora anteriolaterally, Hart's line posteriolaterally, and the midline posterior forchette; this mucosal, as opposed to skin-covered, area is the vestibule. The urethral and vaginal orifices are centered in the vestibule midline. The sulcus between the vaginal orifice and the posterior forchette, the fossa navicularis, can be

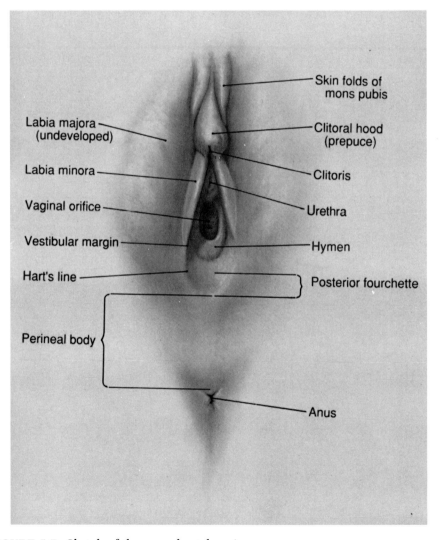

FIGURE 5-7. Sketch of the prepubertal perineum.

From Pokorny SF: In Heger A, Emans SJ, editors: *Evaluation of the sexually abused child*, New York, 1992, Oxford University Press.

deep and form a considerable pocket, or it can be shallow and almost nonexistent.

It is important for the clinician to be anatomically meticulous about describing and locating individual variations and lesions of the vulva of the prepubertal child, who may not be able to concisely describe what has happened to her or localize the symptom she is experiencing. Asking the child to point to or touch with her own finger the site where she hurts, itches, or was touched helps clarify some of these issues.

HYMEN

The hymen is a collar of fibroelastic tissue that surrounds the mouth of the vagina. How this collar is configured varies from child to child (Fig. 5-8). It is noteworthy that the posterior or crescent hymen has no hymenal tissue in the suburethral area. Not infrequently, the annular or circumferential hymen will have a cleft in its collar clockwise somewhere between 10 and 2 o'clock if one is looking at a child in the supine position, with 12 o'clock being toward the urethra and 6 o'clock toward the anus.

The vaginal orifice diameter can be greatly influenced by this hymenal configuration and by the height of this hymenal collar. It is also influenced by the degree of perineal muscular relaxation that the child has at the time the diameter measurements are taken and by the position of the child (see Figs. 5-1 and 5-2).

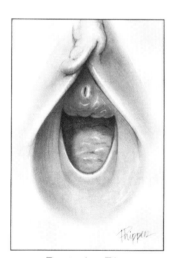

Posterior Rim

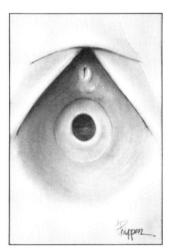

Circumferential
Smooth Rim

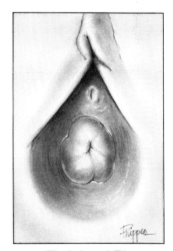

Fimbriated Rim

FIGURE 5-8. Various hymen configurations.

From Pokorny SF: *Am J Obstet Gynecol* 157:950, 1987.

The majority of hymens have a smooth, free, thin margin with no irregularities, mounds, or indentations. When such variations are noted, however, it is imperative that they be described in anatomically descriptive terms, *not* action descriptive terms such as *ruptured*, *marital*, or *virginal*. The greatest hymen contour variability occurs in the suburethral area from 9 o'clock clockwise around to 3 o'clock; occasionally one will see symmetric scallops, flaps, or wings of tissue of the same color and thickness as the remainder of the hymen in this area. The scallops that grace the free margins of the fimbriated hymen are uniform in their arrangement. In evaluating these scalloped hymen contours, it is important to document the integrity of the hymenal collar and to confirm that the scallop indentations do not represent breaks that extend through the collar of tissue down to the vaginal wall (Fig. 5-9).

Hymenal tags of the newborn are small exophytic mucosal lesions of small dimensions, 1 mm by 3 mm, and the majority resolve. Occasionally one will persist, and in the older child these tags are typically isolated,

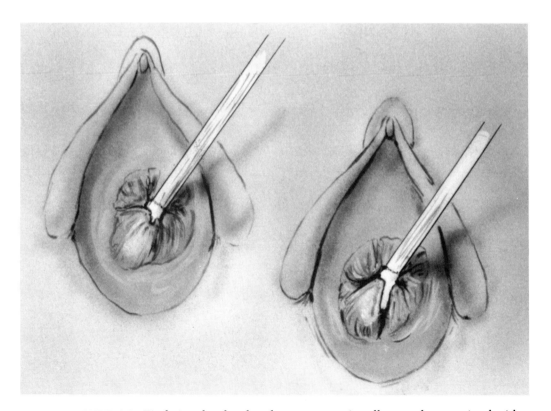

FIGURE 5-9. Fimbriated redundant hymens occasionally must be examined with a small probe or swab to determine whether an indentation extends to the base of the hymen collar. A tear at the 6 o'clock position is illustrated.

From Pokorny SF: *Curr Probl Obstet Gynecol Fertil* 13:202, 1990.

asymmetric mounds of tissue; their thickness and color resemble the hymen. Occasionally, they outgrow their blood supply, become more polypoid, and create an inflammatory and occasionally bloody discharge. When these latter alterations occur, it is difficult to distinguish them from a pedunculated friable condyloma acuminata or other neoplasm; excisional biopsy is warranted.

An isolated mound of tissue on the hymen rim at 6 o'clock can represent the remnant of a septated hymen that broke loose from its suburethral attachment (Fig. 5-10). Most other bumps on the hymen margin, other than those mentioned previously, are believed to be acquired. Biopsy material of erythematous, thickened hymenal bumps has proved many of these bumps to be inflammatory (Fig. 5-11) or histologically suggestive of condylomata acuminata. It is unclear whether inflammation alone can cause an isolated hymenal bump to form or whether a traumatic event must precede its formation.

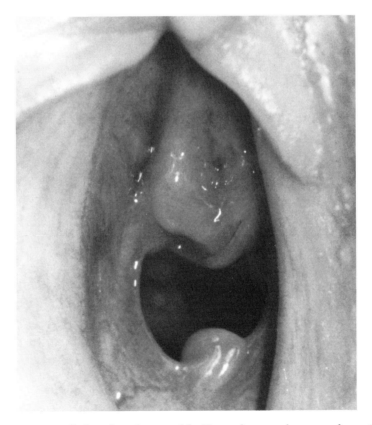

FIGURE 5-10. Vestibule of a 5-year-old. Note the patulous urethra. A biopsy specimen of a mound of tissue on the hymen margin at the 6 o'clock position is fibroelastic tissue compatible with a hymenal septal remnant.

From Pokorny SF: *Curr Probl Obstet Gynecol Fertil* 13:202, 1990.

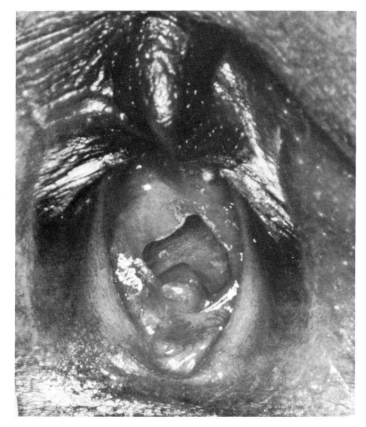

FIGURE 5-11. Vulva of a 4-year-old child. A biopsy of the mound of erythematous tissue at the 6 o'clock position on the hymen rim revealed chronic inflammation.

From Pokorny SF: *Curr Probl Obstet Gynecol Fertil* 13:202, 1990.

It has been proposed that symmetric bumps of the hymen represent retractions of a traumatic hymen laceration at 6 o'clock (Figs. 5-12 and 5-13). Certainly interpretation of bumps and breaks on the hymen is controversial, but in the author's reported series of 265 prepubertal hymens, bumps and breaks were three times more likely to be associated with sexual abuse than with other pediatric gynecologic conditions, including perineal injuries from falls.

Besides the previously mentioned hymenal configurations and alterations, from 3% to 4% of females have a significant congenital hymenal variation such as an imperforate, microperforate, or septated hymen. Although described in the literature, the cribriform hymen seems exceedingly rare, if it exists at all. In the prepubertal child, an anteriorly placed microperforate hymen is frequently mistaken for an imperforate hymen (Fig. 5-14). If one probes with a soft catheter immediately posterior to the urethra, the small hymenal perforation may be demonstrated. This needs no

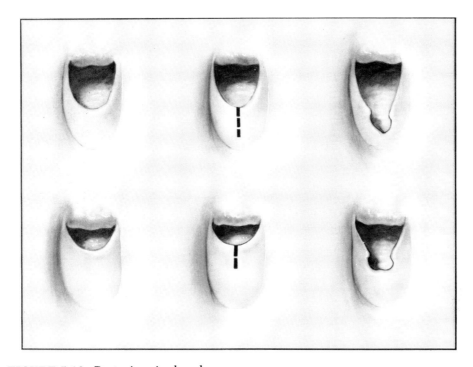

FIGURE 5-12. Posterior rim breaks.

From Pokorny SF, Kozinetz CA: *Adolesc Pediatr Gynecol* 1:99, 1988.

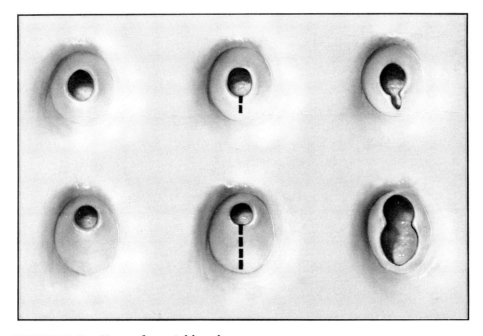

FIGURE 5-13. Circumferential breaks.

From Pokorny SF, Kozinetz CA: *Adolesc Pediatr Gynecol* 1:99, 1988.

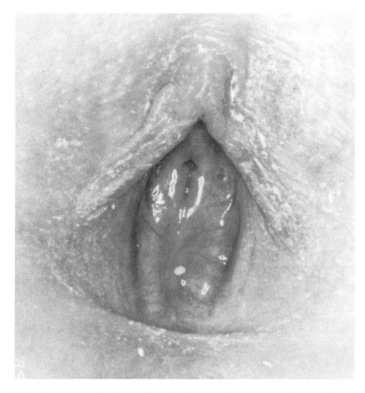

FIGURE 5-14. A seemingly imperforate hymen in a prepubertal female. A small probe is passed into the vagina via a microperforate opening in the suburethral area.

From Pokorny SF, Pokorny WJ: In Ashcraft KW, Holder TM, editors: *Pediatric surgery*, ed 2, Philadelphia, 1991, Saunders.

surgical intervention because drainage is not impeded, and under estrogen stimulation at the time of puberty, this introitus frequently enlarges. The concept that children with microperforate hymens have more problems with vulvovaginitis because of poor drainage has never been scientifically proved. On the contrary, the hymenal barrier might act as a protection to the atrophic mucosa of the vagina.

When an imperforate hymen is detected at birth because of a small hydrocolpos that does not extend above the pelvic brim, the hymenotomy can be performed in the nursery. The infant is stabilized in the dorsal lithotomy position by assistants, local anesthetic applied, a cruciform incision made in the bulging membrane, and the redundant margins excised. Because of the extremely well estrogenized mucosa of the neonate, hemostasis is rarely a problem and can usually be managed by silver-nitrate cauterization.

Periurethral cysts in the neonate are frequently confused with a small hydromucocolpos and bulging imperforate hymen (Fig. 5-15). If one carefully probes in the suburethral area, the anteriorly placed vaginal

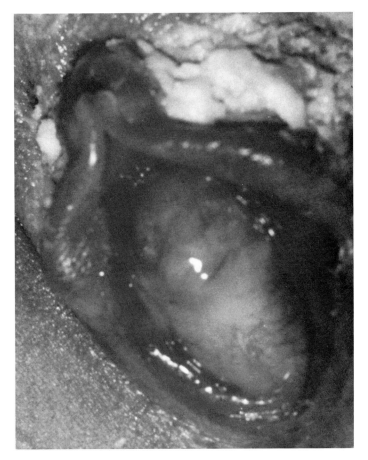

FIGURE 5-15. A periurethral cyst in the newborn that gives the appearance of an imperforate hymen and small hydromucocolpos.

From Pokorny SF, Pokorny WJ: In Ashcraft KW, Holder TM, editors: *Pediatric surgery,* ed 2, Philadelphia, 1991, Saunders.

introitus will be found. The probe or feeding tube can then be glided posteriorly past the cyst and into the vagina, thus proving the patency of the latter. The hymen may be stretched thinly over the 2-cm to 3-cm yellowish suburethral cyst (Fig. 5-16). These cysts spontaneously resolve over the first month or so of life and do not require excision or drainage unless they become infected or symptomatic.

The most common, distinctly aberrant hymenal variation is the *septated hymen*, in which a bridge of tissue vertically separates two distinct vaginal orifices. It is important to distinguish a septated hymen from a longitudinally duplicated vagina; the former has no association with upper-tract müllerian duplication anomalies, whereas the latter does. This distinction can be easily made by placing a probe or catheter through one orifice and out the other in the case of the septated hymen (Fig. 5-17).

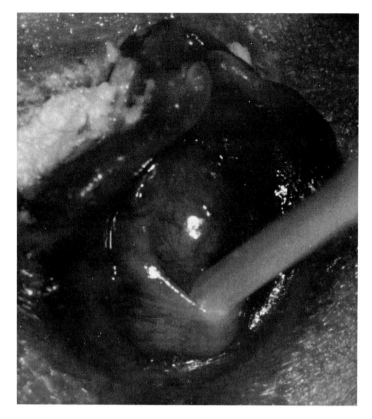

FIGURE 5-16. The same case as in Fig. 5-13 illustrates that the hymen was stretched thinly over the yellowish periurethral cyst, which spontaneously resolved over several months.

From Pokorny SF, Pokorny WJ: In Ashcraft KW, Holder TM, editors: *Pediatric surgery,* ed 2, Philadelphia, 1991, Saunders.

Occasionally one examines a child who seems to have no hymenal tissue at all; if any can be visualized, it is only in irregularly placed nubbins of tissue surrounding the mouth of the vagina (Fig. 5-18). All children are born with a hymen, and falls and severe blows to the adjacent perineal or vulvar tissues do not result in these findings. In adult patients hymenal caruncles occur after the stretch trauma of vaginal childbirth. By the same token, hymenal remnants or caruncles are evidence of significant stretch trauma to the prepubertal child's vaginal introitus and are the most consistent residual physical findings of severe childhood sexual abuse involving vaginal penetration. As such, hymenal caruncles in the prepubertal child should not be ignored by the clinician and should be reported to the proper authorities for investigation of sexual abuse.

VULVOVAGINITIS

By far, vulvovaginitis is the most common entity for which a child is brought to the gynecologist. Vulvovaginitis should be conceptualized as two distinct

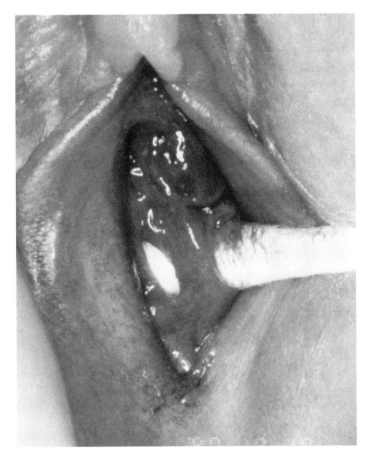

FIGURE 5-17. Septated hymen with a probe that confirms that this is not a müllerian duplication.

entities: vulvitis, in which the inflammation is confined predominantly to the external genitalia; and vaginitis, in which the inflammation comes predominantly from the vagina. These two entities, in children, have distinctly different etiologies and different clinical presentations, both of which depend on the estrogen status of the child.

By conceptualizing vulvitis and vaginitis as distinct pathophysiologic processes, one can more easily identify the etiologic process and intervene therapeutically. Clearly a severe vulvitis can and will spill over and cause an inflammatory discharge or reaction in the vagina. By the same token, constant chapping of the vulva from vaginal discharge will ultimately cause a vulvitis, no matter how fastidious the child or caregiver is in hygiene practices.

A historical recounting of when and how the first manifestations of the problem occurred helps distinguish the two entities. The child with a history of vulvitis typically offers complaints of pain, pruritus, or dysuria, usually accompanied by erythematous tissue changes. The child with vaginitis

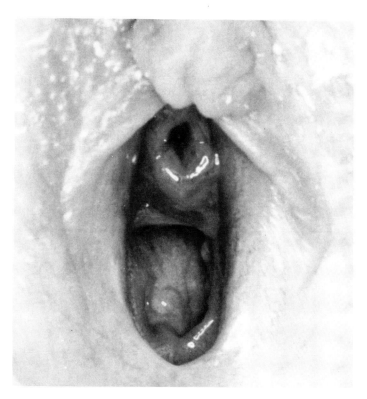

FIGURE 5-18. Remnants-only hymen of a 7½-year-old. The perpetrator confessed to multiple episodes of penile-vaginal penetration several years earlier.

From Pokorny S: In Kaufman R, Fredrich EG, Gardner HL, editors: *Benign diseases of the vulva and vagina*, Chicago, 1989, Year Book Medical.

frequently denies a problem. Discharge is a variable and minor manifestation of vulvitis, but it is a more persistent and major manifestation of vaginitis. Physical manifestations of vulvitis are always ultimately visible on the external genitalia, although etiologies are more frequently elusive. With vaginitis proper cultures or vaginoscopy are necessary for diagnosis, and typically a specific etiology will be found. Although rarely associated with serious morbidity, caregivers of a child with vulvitis, which can be a chronic condition, are more demanding of a therapeutic intervention. By comparison, vaginitis is more frequently associated with serious morbidity, but caregivers are more likely to ignore its manifestations.

Vulvitis

Vulvitis implies that the predominant pathophysiologic process is on the skin or mucosal surface of the vulva. The symptoms are distressing to the child and her caregiver, who will place pressure on the clinician for a quick solution. Because of the more superficial nature of this entity, the clinician should ultimately if not initially be able to see physical signs of the pathophysiologic process on the external genitalia and direct therapeutic interventions toward them.

Erythema is the most common sign of vulvitis. In the estrogenized diapered infant, the most common microbial etiology is *Monilia* candidiasis. This is easily identified by its fiery red edematous mucosal and skin reaction, cheesy white discharge, and positive KOH findings. The most common cause of vulvitis in infants, however, is actually a chemical dermatitis that usually spares the mucosal surface of the vulva and is caused by feces or urine irritation. Therapy is use of antifungals for the former and removal of the irritant and symptomatic treatment for the latter.

When the child moves into the toilet-training period, the estrogen effect on the vulvar mucosa wanes. At about the time the child's toilet habits become less supervised and the mucosa becomes atrophic, the child's vulva becomes more easily inflamed by exogenous irritants such as fecal contamination, caustic soaps (perfumed soaps and bubble baths), pinworms, and sexual abuse.

The clinician is dependent on the child's caregiver to investigate what possible irritants are in the child's environment. Many times the irritant is something that was used on or by the child at an earlier age (e.g., antifungal creams or bubble bath), and it must now be explained to the caregiver why and how the child's body has converted these old standbys into irritants. In this same light, genital manipulations for sexually abusive purposes or for genital hygiene, which were tolerated by the child at an earlier age, become intolerable and symptomatic in the older, less estrogenized, and now verbal child. For example, an occasional caregiver will use a cotton swab to wipe the vaginal canal of an infant in much the same way as they would clean the child's ear canal. The atrophic mucosa of the older child will react to vigorous scrubbing and wiping in an inflammatory and symptomatic manner. Not only does atrophic mucosa react differently, but it also looks different from that of an infant (see Fig. 5-5). Some parents who compulsively cared for an infant with recurrent *Candida* must be educated about the erythema of the atrophic mucosa in their older child.

Recurrent use of oral antibiotics in a child can lead to a supercolonization and ultimately overgrowth of *Candida* in the older unestrogenized child. More commonly, when one sees a florid *Candida* vulvitis in the older child, one should consider the possibility of an underlying skin disorder. A follow-up examination after a course of an antifungal agent is occasionally necessary before the underlying skin disorder can be appreciated. Conversely, the vesicular-like appearance of the satellite lesions of *Monilia* frequently persist after the confluent erythematous florid stage of a *Monilia* vulvitis has resolved. These satellite lesions can be confused with herpes simplex lesions.

Enterobius vermicularis is the most common microbe to cause a vulvitis in the older child and can be easily treated with mebendazole, 100 mg (Vermox). Many clinicians advocate attempts to spot the small, 2-mm- to 3-mm-long, threadlike white worms by nocturnal searches of the child's perineum or by adhesive tape samples of the perirectal area in attempts to detect the *Enterobius* eggs before treatment. In areas of the south where these parasites are indigenous, the diagnosis can be made by a history of perirectal pruritus or an erythematous perirectal halo that spreads anteriorly over the vulva. In addition to mebendazole, the caregiver should be educated regarding shortening family members' fingernails to decrease the possibility of anal-to-oral recontamination. Also, all bedding, underwear, and bedclothes should be washed in hot water on the day of treatment.

Most vulvitis in the older unestrogenized child can be resolved with minimal pharmacologic intervention if the irritant can be removed. The most common irritants are perfumed or harsh soaps, fecal contamination secondary to poor hygiene habits, and unusual hygiene or abusive sexual practices by the child's caregiver. Diagnosing sexual or inappropriate caregiver manipulations of the genital area that cause a traumatic vulvitis is difficult. Because of threats of harm to themselves or loved ones, the abused child will probably deny abuse. Occasionally a child will reveal unusual genital hygiene practices if the clinician requests that they "play like" or show or tell how they clean themselves after using the toilet. Some caregivers are so defensive about this matter that it helps to instruct the child that she should be the only one who is allowed to cleanse herself or apply creams to the vulva.

The first line of treatment of inflamed vulvar tissue is symptomatic. Tub or sitz baths, with or without an antibacterial soap, are the first step. Following these baths, which should occur several times a day to decrease fecal contamination and urine irritation, the inflamed tissue should be dried with a hair dryer or by leaving it exposed to air; caution should be taken not to burn the child with hot settings. It is dramatic just how frequently and how rapidly these measures resolve much of the inflammation. The hardest part of the treatment is convincing the child's caregiver that there is not a simple pharmacologic cure.

In cases of severe vulvitis from *Monilia*, before attempts at applying an antifungal cream, symptomatic measures might need to be applied for 24 to 48 hours. Many creams are painful when applied to the acutely and severely inflamed tissues. Before application of any cream to the vulva, the child and caregiver must be forewarned to do a small test application at the time the bath water is drawn and available. If the cream stings or burns the child, she can quickly return to the bath to wash it off and wait 24 more hours before trying to use it again. It is rare that a vulvitis will be so severe as to require oral antibiotics for an associated cellulitis. A child with a recurrent and apparent vulvitis with minimal or no discharge and no inflammatory cells in a vaginal wash does not require an examination under anesthesia even if the etiology remains elusive. The family and child must accept the chronic nature of the disorder and learn to symptomatically treat it.

Vaginitis

Vaginitis is almost never a problem in the diapered, estrogenized child. The most commonly noted vaginal drainage in an infant occurs in the first week or so of life when a mucoid, frequently blood-streaked discharge is noted on the child's genital area. This represents a sloughing of genital cells, predominantly endocervical and endometrial, following the withdrawal of maternal hormonal stimulation of the child's reproductive system. A congenital anomaly such as a rectovaginal fistula must be sought if an estrogenized infant has a persistent copious purulent vaginal discharge.

Vaginitis is not as common or as symptomatic as vulvitis in the older unestrogenized child. Many well-meaning mothers change their child's underwear and bathe her before the first office visit (similar to an adult woman douching before an office visit for vaginal discharge). To avoid this, it helps to instruct the child not to take a bath on the day of the evaluation and to bring with her the previous 3-day collection of unwashed underwear. This is an important step because it is difficult to quantify the amount of discharge the parent is describing. Certainly, when one sees copious or blood-stained discharge no matter how long the history, one is much more aggressive about establishing an etiology. On the other hand, if only small yellow streaks are seen on the child's panties and there is no history of larger or bloody stains, the evaluation can proceed more leisurely. As has been stated, the findings on the external genitalia can be minimal to nonexistent, depending on how long the drainage has occurred and how fastidious the child and caregiver are with genital hygiene. Some children change their underwear three to five times a day with frequent bathing and have almost no evidence of vulvar chapping (vulvitis) from the vaginitis. Other children have a telltale line of hyperpigmentation or crusting on the most dependent portion of the labia majora, which indicates prolonged chapping from the moisture of the discharge. Occasionally the skin reacts with a significant hyperkeratosis along the most dependent aspect of the labia majora (Fig. 5-19).

Once the clinician is convinced that there is a significant discharge, the next step is to sample the upper vaginal secretions for a wet mount and appropriate cultures. This can be done by the vaginal aspiration described earlier in this chapter. If the wet mount demonstrates only parabasal

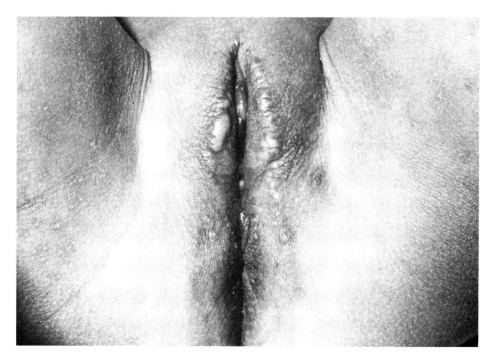

FIGURE 5-19. Hyperkeratosis along the dependent aspect of the labia majora secondary to chronic drainage and chapping from a vaginal foreign object.

epithelial cells with no other signs of inflammation, such as white blood cells (WBCs) or bacteria, one must assume that the discharge was from a minor vulvitis that has spontaneously resolved.

Once a positive (inflammatory) wet mount has been obtained, diagnostic procedures must move forward to find an etiology. The first step is to culture the vaginal wash material. Appropriate cultures should be started for not only sexually transmitted diseases such as gonorrhea and *Chlamydia* infection but also for anaerobic and aerobic organisms. The laboratory should be instructed to do colony counts and identify all organisms identified; otherwise one will get the feedback of "normal vaginal flora," which implies the usual mixture of skin and enteric organisms found in the adult female's vagina. This is not what is wanted. When one requests that all organisms be identified with accompanying colony counts, invariably one finds a specific overgrowth of a specific organism. The specific treatment of such organisms by an oral antibiotic clears the discharge almost overnight. If one does not have a laboratory that does specific cultures, and there are multiple WBCs and bacteria in the vaginal wet mount, an empiric trial of a broad-spectrum antibiotic is warranted. *Shigella* and *Salmonella* vaginitis can cause a particularly bloody discharge, but so can an excessive overgrowth of many enteric organisms. The one organism that is extremely difficult to eradicate is group B streptococcus, particularly in children, who tend to be carriers of this organism in their oropharynx. These children can be symptomatically helped by frequent tub or sitz baths with a liquid antibacterial soap that they slosh into their genital area; this will decrease the bacterial load and thereby their symptom of yellowish vaginal discharge. Although many studies have been performed on the vaginal microflora of the child, few of these studies differentiate between children with estrogen-primed vaginas (i.e., the infant and the young peripubertal female and the unestrogenized child). Furthermore, these studies are difficult to perform on a broad spectrum of both symptomatic and asymptomatic children.

Foreign Objects

Once efforts have been made to identify and treat a specific vaginal organism and the vaginal drainage persists or immediately recurs after treatment, the child's vagina must be explored to rule out neoplasm and a foreign object. When performing vaginoscopy one should also consider the possibility of anomalous drainage from a congenital malformation such as a rudimentary uterine horn or an ectopic ureter.

Occasionally a child uses crayons or facial blush to make streaks or stains on her panties because of the secondary gains she obtains from this behavior. These fictitious discharges are another reason the clinician should attempt to see the discharge for which the child is being evaluated.

The most commonly found vaginal foreign object is toilet paper wads. Frequently these can be seen in the lower portion of the vagina as greyish white objects. If toilet paper is a consideration, efforts should be taken to lavage the vagina. This is accomplished in much the same way that office vaginoscopy is described earlier in this chapter. After anesthetizing the vulva with a topical anesthetic, the child should be positioned with her buttocks on the edge of the gynecology table over the drip basin and a lubricated bladder catheter placed into her vagina; a dilute bactericidal soap solution can be used for the lavage. It is not uncommon for these children to return months later with a recurrent problem. Because of this, at the time of their initial treatment, efforts should be made to understand their toilet hygiene practices and to encourage modification. Occasionally it is necessary to switch them from toilet paper to other types of genital hygiene products.

Certainly if vaginal cultures do not identify a specific treatable organism and if efforts to lavage the child's vagina offer no solution or resolution to a bloody or copious foul-smelling discharge, vaginoscopy, usually under anesthesia, must be performed to rule out a foreign object. It is dramatic to find radiopaque objects on roentgenograms, but this is an unnecessary step; most plastic and rubber toys and small objects go undetected by preoperative studies. On rare occasion, a foreign object can be milked from the vagina at the time a rectal examination is performed. In the majority of cases, the child must be anesthetized for removal of the foreign object, particularly if it has existed for some time, because foreign objects have a tendency to become embedded in the vaginal wall. Care must be taken to avoid damaging adjacent organs, specifically the bowel and bladder, while removing the object.

COMMON PREPUBERTAL LESIONS
Urethral Prolapse

The appearance of a prolapsed urethra depends on the accompanying degree of inflammation, edema, and necrosis. In its milder state, it looks like a cherry-red donut or a prolapsed cervix; in the extreme situation, the urethral meatus is obscured and the prolapse looks like a fungating neoplastic mass that can be 2 to 3 cm in diameter. Many children are totally asymptomatic except for some bloody vulvar discharge. Occasionally the child has urinary tract symptoms such as dysuria and, in rare situations, urinary retention.

The etiology of urethral prolapse is connected to the hypoestrogenic state of the latency and childhood years. The majority of cases resolve with topical estrogen cream applied to the vulva after a sitz bath once or twice daily for up to 2 weeks. If the child shows signs of absorbing too much estrogen (as manifested by complaints of breast tenderness, formation of breast buds, or hyperpigmentation of the vulva), the dose or duration of treatment can be lessened. The estrogen effect continues to be exerted for a few weeks after discontinuation of use of the estrogen cream (Figs. 5-20 and 5-21).

With this treatment, the prolapse usually completely resolves. In some children there remains a somewhat patulous but uninflamed collar of periurethral tissue. If the child remains asymptomatic, no other treatment is necessary. Occasionally a child remains bothered because the protuberant, patulous urethral tissue extends out of the vestibule and keeps the vulva moist and chapped by secretions. In these instances, surgical excision of the remaining prolapse seems warranted. This excision is performed under general anesthesia. A Foley catheter is placed in the bladder and the prolapse excised at its base. With 4-0 or 5-0 polyglactin 910 (Vicryl) or chromic suture, the urethral mucosa is approximated to the periurethral vestibular mucosa. This is a highly vascular lesion; hemostasis is aided by excising the entire lesion and by close spacing of sutures. The catheter can be removed and the child discharged home from the day surgery area with instructions to continue sitz baths and the topical estrogen cream for 1 week. Surgical excision might be offered initially to the child who has such a severe prolapse that she has significant urinary symptoms.

Condylomata Acuminata (Venereal Warts)

As condylomata acuminata become more prevalent in the adult population, they are seen more frequently in children. Caused by the papilloma virus,

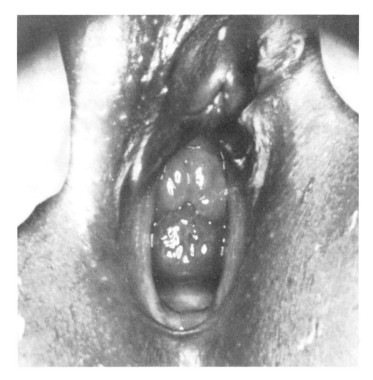

FIGURE 5-20. Large urethral prolapse before estrogen treatment. Note the attenuated thin hymen.

these lesions do not have their typical warty appearance when they occur on the unestrogenized prepubertal vulva. In this situation they are frequently flesh colored with small red punctuations (Fig. 5-22) that represent the tips of capillaries coursing through each papule. A small uninflamed condyloma can easily be overlooked by the unwary examiner. On the other hand, if large, these lesions can become inflamed, erythematous, and friable and require excisional biopsy to differentiate them from other neoplasm of the external genitalia. Guidelines for management must remain flexible. Currently it seems prudent to symptomatically manage condylomata acuminata that occur before 2 years of age, even if they occasionally bleed, because many spontaneously resolve. In the older unestrogenized child, the condylomata produce an inflammatory discharge that chaps the vulva and causes pain and pruritus. Furthermore, the further the child is from the possibility of maternal transmission via passage through the birth canal, the more likely it is that the child acquired the condylomata by sexual transmission. These factors increase the need for excisional biopsy of the condylomata in the older child for strain typing because of epidemiologic and medicolegal reasons. At the same time the child is anesthetized for the excisional biopsy, ablative procedures can be applied to the remainder of the condylomata. There is some concern that

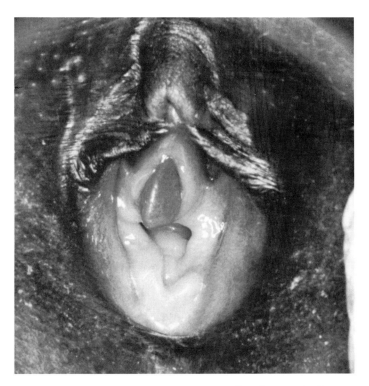

FIGURE 5-21. Same patient as in Fig. 5-20, 3 weeks after topical estrogen cream. Note that a small asymptomatic fragment of prolapse remains at the urethral orifice. Also note the estrogen effect on the hymen, which is more pronounced with a disruption in its integrity at 4 o'clock.

cystoscopy can carry the papillomavirus into the bladder; by the same token the need to perform vaginoscopy or proctoscopy to rule out asymptomatic vaginal and anal condylomata in children should be carefully examined. If typing of the condylomata is not needed for medicolegal reasons and the condylomata are small and asymptomatic in the older child, ablation of the lesions under anesthesia may not be warranted.

Labial/Vulvar Agglutination

The unestrogenized vulvar tissues of the young female have an unusual tendency to agglutinate. This occurrence is believed to be caused by low estrogen levels and by vulvitis. Most cases are asymptomatic and are brought to the attention of the physician because of anatomic concerns. When followed over the course of a year, over 80% spontaneously resolve. The child might develop symptoms of urethritis and vulvitis caused by pooling of urine behind the agglutinated tissue.

Severe cases of agglutination (Fig. 5-23) are occasionally confused with an imperforate hymen or ambiguous genitalia caused by androgen excess.

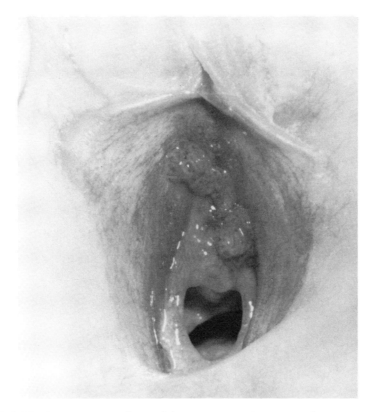

FIGURE 5-22. Appearance of condylomata acuminata on the unestrogenized prepubertal vestibule. The small red punctuations are typical and represent capillaries just below the surface, which makes these lesions extremely friable.

In the former situation, one should always be able to find a normal urethral orifice on the floor of the vestibule; an imperforate hymen is seen in the same plane as the urethral orifice. Ambiguous genitalia arc prcscnt from birth, and agglutination is an acquired lesion. If ambiguous genitalia result from early embryologic androgen excess, as in congenital adrenal hyperplasia, the labia minora become incorporated into the anterior sheath of the phallus. In severe labial and vulvar agglutination, one can always find a line of demarcation between the clitoral hood (prepuce) and the labia minora that course to the midline under the clitoris.

Agglutination can be treated with local application of estrogen cream in the same manner as for urethral prolapse. One should anticipate seeing resolution of the agglutination within a month of treatment. It is common for agglutination to recur, especially if underlying vulvar irritants remain in the child's environs.

Families need much reassuring over this lesion, and patience is important. Surgery is rarely necessary and should be reserved for long-standing agglutination in which the child has developed the equivalent

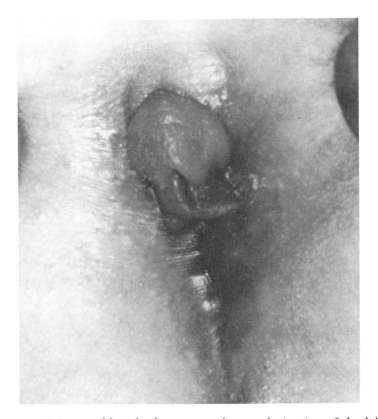

FIGURE 5-23. A 3-year-old with almost complete agglutination of the labial and vulvar tissues. This child was toilet trained and had no symptoms. Note the line of demarcation between the clitoral hood and the labia minora, which helps distinguish this from an intersex problem.

From Pokorny SF, Pokorny WJ: In Ashcraft KW, Holder TM, editors: *Pediatric surgery,* ed 2, Philadelphia, 1991, Saunders.

of a skin bridge over the vulva. Occasionally surgery is necessary when the child has such urinary symptoms that bladder catheterization is necessary and the urethra cannot be visualized. The agglutinated tissues should never be forcefully separated because the psychosocial and physical trauma to the child is real and the raw surfaces more readily reagglutinate.

GENITAL TRAUMA AND SEXUAL ABUSE OF THE PREPUBERTAL CHILD

Genital injuries engender anxiety in patient and caregiver. For psychosocial reasons, this anxiety is greatest when the patient is a young female child and trauma is possibly secondary to sexual abuse. Concern about this latter social malady has mandated that more and more children be brought to the doctor's office or emergency center for a genital examination. Sometimes this concern about abuse is not directly expressed and the patient is brought for a vague complaint on the pretense of concern about a minor problem or

TABLE 5-1. Examinations of sexual assault survivors: psychosocial guidelines

1. Health care providers are the only professionals who are socially sanctioned to perform genital examinations.
2. In a court of law, someone must examine and report the findings from the site of the crime (i.e., the genital area).
3. Physicians must realize that they should not attempt to become the "judge and jury" for alleged cases of sexual assault and abuse.
4. Physicians who perform genital examinations on sexual assault survivors are requested to obtain medicolegal evidence from the site of the crime. This should be done atraumatically, both physically and psychologically.
5. Medicolegal evidence consists of debris found on the survivor's body that will substantiate her story (e.g., grass particles, sperm, hair, cloth fibers). Rape kits used by many communities have clear instructions that outline the ways and means of obtaining this medicolegal evidence. Obviously if considerable time has passed since the alleged episode, a rape kit is not necessary.
6. Other important medicolegal evidence consists of documented physical changes on the survivor's body that would indicate that he or she had been traumatized or sexually exposed. Documenting a sexually transmitted disease or certain types of genital trauma in a young child falls into this category.
7. In-depth interviews are not encouraged in the anxiety-laden atmosphere of an emergency center when an acute genital injury is involved. Verbatim recordings of the survivor's statement of events surrounding the injury should be made. Questions, if necessary, should be carefully phrased in an open-ended manner. Care must be taken to not place words or ideas into the mind of the young survivor; leading questions can hurt future efforts to prosecute.

injury. Not uncommonly, resources to investigate alleged sexual abuse are mobilized because of the genital site of the injury in spite of the child giving a concise history of how the injury occurred. Just as frequently, if the parent directly expresses concern about sexual abuse, the physician's anxiety about "getting involved" is so great that the child is not uncommonly shuffled from one doctor to another.

For the inexperienced, guidelines for developing a perspective or frame of mind to approach these cases are outlined in Table 5-1. These guidelines are meant to simplify a complex and changing social situation so that the physician can concentrate on doing no harm and alleviating suffering in the young patient.

Accidental injuries are usually the result of a fall. The most serious injuries of this nature are impalement injuries. Straddle injuries are painful but are rarely serious if not associated with an expanding hematoma. The clinician must realize that the atrophic mucosa of the unestrogenized female's vulva will bleed out of proportion to the seriousness of the wound. By contrast, penetrating impalement and rape injuries in a young girl may not be as hemorrhagic externally, but serious life-threatening associated injury to adjacent viscera and major vessels may have occurred.

Initial steps toward management must be to ascertain the cause of the injury. It is worth getting a good description of the object the patient supposedly fell onto and the height from which she fell. If impalement is unlikely, a conservative approach with appropriate observation in the emergency center can be initiated. Bleeding frequently stops by keeping the child quiet and by placing the child in a supine position with a pressure dressing against her perineum. If injury to adjacent organs is suspected or hemostasis cannot be obtained, no matter how minor the wound, management must proceed to an examination under anesthesia. Cleansing and debridement of the wound is necessary whether anesthesia is used or not. Sutures, which should only be placed in a child under anesthesia, may be necessary for hemostasis and to approximate deep wounds. They are unnecessary and will pull out if used on the surface of anything other than direct midline perineal body wounds.

The clinician must realize that many sexually abused children have no physical signs of the abuse, even if seen within 24 hours of the abuse. Attempts at forced traumatic vaginal penetration are rare; this usually occurs in the case of stranger rape, and in these situations the child will give an explicit history.

Young children are not cognitively aware of their anatomy; therefore many young females give a history of vaginal penetration because they perceive the pressure of an adult finger or phallus against their vestibule as vaginal penetration. Some children are gradually and chronically dilated and therefore escape significant vaginal or perineal lacerations with phallic vaginal penetration. Erythema, ecchymoses, and abrasions are usually seen in these latter situations if the child is examined within hours of the sexual abuse. If seen days after the abuse, these chronically abused survivors maintain the hymenal alterations described earlier in this chapter as hymenal caruncles.

HORMONAL ALTERATIONS

Tanner has described physical characteristics of the breast and pubic hair that indicate progressive advancement of physiologic maturity. The clinician must be aware of the sequence and the tempo through which normal maturation proceeds so that investigations can be initiated when the peripubertal girl manifests an alternate course or when the young female begins to develop (breasts before the age of 8 and menses before 10 years old).

The least-mature Tanner stage is stage 1; the most mature, stage 5. A distinctive stage for breast development is Tanner stage 4. At this point the areola forms a separate mound from the remainder of the breast tissue contour. Breast stages 3 and 5 have similar contours, with the areola conforming to the curve of the general breast tissue. One cannot differentiate late stage 3 from early stage 5 unless one has sequentially examined the patient and noted that she has progressed through Tanner stage 4, which not all girls do. Breast stage 2 is a breast bud that is firm and frequently tender, and stage 1 has no palpable breast tissue, and the areola remains small and unpigmented.

The distinctive pubic hair stage is stage 3, when mature, coarse, curly pubic hair courses over the mons pubis. Stage 2 has the same hair type, but it is localized only along the labia majora. Stage 4 pubic hair has a triangular pattern, and stage 5 extends to the thighs. Stage 1 has no mature coarse hair at all.

The most common hormonal entity in perpubertal children that is brought to the attention of the gynecologist is premature, unilateral or bilateral thelarche in a child less than 8 years of age. Without evidence of a growth spurt or signs of estrogen stimulation (see Fig. 5-6) on the vulvar tissues, the child should be reevaluated in 3 months. The small breasts, Tanner stage 2 or 3, usually resolve. End-organ sensitivity to low estrogen levels is an explanation for these cases.

If the premature thelarche recurs, progresses, or is associated with a growth spurt or vulvar estrogenization, evaluation for precocious puberty must begin. Estradiol levels, thyroid function studies, imaging of the central nervous system (CNS) and the ovaries, and a bone age should be obtained. Gonadotropin-releasing hormone stimulation tests are useful to differentiate true (CNS-driven ovarian stimulation) precocious puberty from pseudoprecocious puberty (changes secondary to an endogenous or exogenous estrogen source). A long-bone survey is necessary to detect the polycystic fibrotic changes of the McCune-Albright syndrome and should be obtained in a child with precocious puberty and café au lait spots.

A child will not have isolated premature menarche without some degree of estrogenization of the vulvar tissues. A maturation index is a rough quantitative means for following disease progression or therapeutic effectiveness, but it is not necessary to confirm that the lower genital tract is responding to estrogen because one can see the tissue changes or can find navicular exfoliated cells with small nuclei on a wet mount.

Isolated premature pubarche is not uncommon but is not brought to the attention of the physician as frequently as premature thelarche. It rarely is the herald to precocious puberty, but a search for androgen-producing tumors must be sought in progressive and excessive cases.

BIBLIOGRAPHY

Altchek A: Pediatric vulvovaginitis, *J Reprod Med* 29:359, 1984.

Chadwick DL, Berkowitz CD, Kerns DL, et al: *Color atlas of child sexual abuse,* Chicago, 1990, Year Book Medical.

Cowell CA: The gynecologic examination of infants, children, and young adolescents, *Pediatr Clin North Am* 28:247, 1981.

Emans SJ, Woods ER, Flagg NT, et al: Genital findings in sexually abused symptomatic and asymptomatic girls, *Pediatrics* 79:778, 1987.

Emans SJH, Goldstein DP: *Pediatric and adolescent gynecology,* ed 3, Boston, 1990, Little, Brown.

Hammerschlag MR, Alpert S, Rosner I, et al: Microbiology of the vagina in children: normal and potentially pathogenic organisms, *Pediatrics* 62:57, 1978.

Herman-Giddens ME, Berson NL: Harmful genital care practices in children, *JAMA* 261:577, 1989.

Huffman JW: *The gynecology of childhood and adolescence,* ed 2, Philadelphia, 1981, Saunders.

Jenny C, Kuhns MLD, Arakawa F: Hymens in newborn female infants, *Pediatrics* 80:399, 1987.

Jenny C, Sutherland SE, Sandahl BB: Developmental approach to preventing the sexual abuse of children, *Pediatrics* 78:1034, 1986.

Mercer LJ, Mueller CM, Hajj SN: Medical treatment of urethral prolapse in the premenarchal female, *Adolesc Pediatr Gynecol* 1:181, 1988.

Mor N, Merlob P, Reisner SH: Types of hymen in the newborn infant, *Eur J Obstet Gynecol Reprod Biol* 22:225, 1986.

Paradise JE, Campos JM, Friedman HM, et al: Vulvovaginitis in premenar

cheal girls: clinical features and diagnostic evaluation, *Pediatrics* 70:193, 1982.

Pokorny S: Pediatric vulvovaginitis. In Kaufman R, Fredrich EG, Gardner HL, editors: *Benign diseases of the vulva and vagina,* Chicago, 1989, Year Book Medical.

Pokorny SF: Configuration of the prepubertal hymen, *Am J Obstet Gynecol* 157:950, 1987.

Pokorny SF: Child abuse and infections, *Obstet Gynecol Clin North Am* 16:401, 1989.

Pokorny SF: Physical examination of the reproductive systems of female children and adolescents, *Curr Probl Obstet Gynecol Fertil* 13:202, 1990.

Pokorny SF: Anatomical terms of female external genitalia. In Heger A, Emans SJ, editors: *Evaluation of the sexually abused child,* New York, 1992, Oxford University Press.

Pokorny SF: Vaginoscopy. In Stoval T, Mann W, editors: *Textbook of gynecologic surgery,* Churchill Livingstone, New York, 1996.

Pokorny SF, Kozinetz CA: Configuration and other anatomic details of the prepubertal hymen, *Adolesc Pediatr Gynecol* 1:97, 1988.

Pokorny SF, Pokorny WJ: Pediatric gynecology. In Ashkraft KW, Holder TM, editors: *Pediatric surgery,* ed 2, Philadelphia, 1991, Saunders.

Pokorny SF, Pokorny WJ, Kramer W: Acute genital injury in the prepubertal female, *Am J Obstet Gynecol* 166:1461, 1992.

Pokorny SF, Stormer J: Atraumatic removal of secretions from the prepubertal vagina, *Am J Obstet Gynecol* 156:581, 1987.

Yordan EE, Yordan RA: The hymen and Tanner staging of the breast, *Adolesc Pediatr Gynecol* 5:76, 1992.

CHAPTER 6

Management of Menopause

DONALD E. MOORE

Data in the last decade support a return to the philosophy of "estrogen forever" for postmenopausal women, something that was popular in the 1960s and early 1970s. The benefits of estrogen replacement therapy (ERT) to the cardiovascular and skeletal systems outweigh the risk to the endometrium. On the other hand, the effect of breast cancer on the risk-benefit ratio is unclear. Significant improvement in vasomotor stability

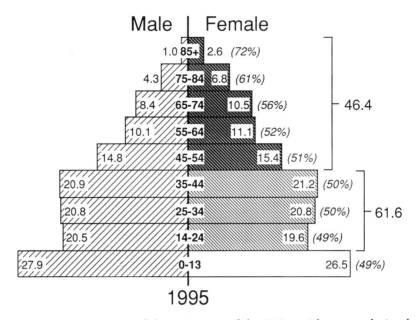

FIGURE 6-1. Age structure of the estimates of the U.S. resident population by age and sex, July 1, 1995 (in millions) (U.S. Bureau of the Census) (total males = 128,685,000; total females = 134,749,000). Percentages and bracketed numbers refer to the population in the respective group who are female.

is well documented. Data on improved sexual functioning are emerging. The dosage for conjugated equine estrogens (CEE) is well established for the prevention of osteoporosis but only assumed for the cardiovascular system. The use, dosage, and effects of progestins (including progesterone), estradiol patches, and nonsteroidal therapies are developing.

In the United States today, there are approximately 35.5 million women who are 50 years of age or older; this is about 28% of all women (U.S. Bureau of the Census, 1995). In the near future, the population will continue to age and live longer so that this ratio will also increase. Notice in Fig. 6-1 that roughly 50% of the population is female until the age of 50 years, when the percentage of the population that is female increases. In fact, 56% of the population 50 years of age and older are women.

Phases of life related to menopause are illustrated in Fig. 6-2. Menopause is defined as the date of the last spontaneous menstrual period. The perimenopausal period is the 1 to 2 years before and after menopause; the climacteric period is the time during which the symptoms related to menopause occur.

ENDOCRINOLOGY, PHYSIOLOGY, AND CAUSES OF OVARIAN FAILURE

Fertility remains relatively stable until about the age of 37 years in women and then begins to fall rapidly. Although the reason for this decline is

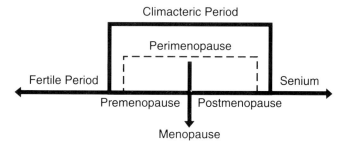

FIGURE 6-2. The climacteric period.

Redrawn from Jaszmann LJB: In Campbell S, editor: *The management of the menopause and post-menopause years*, Baltimore, 1976, University Park Press.

unclear, the explanation probably lies somewhere in our better understanding the influence of the decline in the number of oocytes in the ovaries with age. Women at birth have approximately 1 million primordial follicles. This number declines to about 450,000 at puberty, 20,000 at 38 years, and 0 or very few after menopause (Fig. 6-3). This decline of about 1000 per month before puberty, 1000 to 2000 per month before 35 years of age, and 100 to 400 per month after 35 years of age seems to be due to natural atresia and is not greatly influenced by ovulation, birth control pills, or pregnancy (Fig. 6-3). Most women continue to have normal-length cycles and continue to ovulate right up to near the last menstrual cycle, although 40% develop oligomenorrhea and anovulation during the last 2 years. The spontaneous abortion rate increases in women over 40 years to 25% to 50%. Furthermore, the rate of chromosomal abnormalities in the unfertilized oocytes of women undergoing in vitro fertilization (IVF) after the age of 35 years is higher than in those 35 or younger (47% vs. 25%) ($P < .05$).

There are some changes in the way the ovaries and the body produce androgens and estrogens before and after menopause. Although the metabolic clearance rates (MCRs) do not differ for androstenedione, testosterone, estrone, and estradiol before and after menopause, the serum levels of these four hormones decrease after menopause, as ovarian production decreases. The levels of androstenedione are about half, and testosterone levels are about 80% of those of premenopausal women (Fig. 6-4). The postmenopausal serum levels of estrone are about one third and estradiol one ninth that of the levels in premenopausal women. Estrone and estradiol also do not cycle or fluctuate as they do in premenopausal women. After oophorectomy in a postmenopausal woman, serum levels of estrone and estradiol do not change, but those of androstenedione and testosterone decrease (Fig. 6-4).

A study by Longcope, Hunter, and Franz in 42 postmenopausal women undergoing hysterectomy found a major ovarian arteriovenous gradient for testosterone in about 50% of women and for estradiol in fewer than 20%.

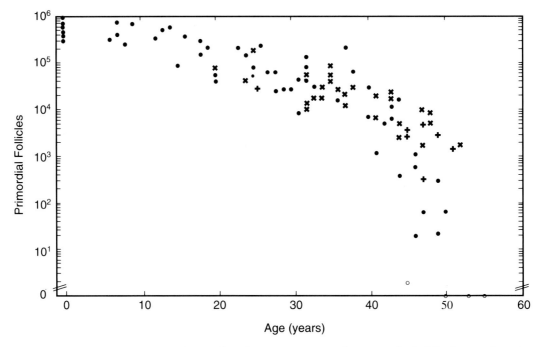

FIGURE 6-3. The relationship between age and primordial follicle number is compared by using data from four studies. +, Stillborns and girls or premenopausal women with regular menses; •, perimenopausal women; ○, postmenopausal women.

Redrawn from Richardson SJ, Nelson JF: *Ann N Y Acad Sci* 592:13, 1990.

For androstenedione, dehydroepiandrosterone, and estrone the gradients did not signify important ovarian secretion. There is no evidence for secretion of dihydrotestosterone, estrone sulfate, or dehydroepiandrosterone (DHEA) sulfate. After menopause much of the estrone arises from the aromatization of androstenedione in body fat; the amount of aromatization of androstenedione to estrone and testosterone to estradiol more than doubles in postmenopausal women and relates directly to the amount of body fat. Follicle-stimulating hormone (FSH) and luteinizing hormone (LH) levels rise steadily during the first 12 months after menopause and then either level off or decrease.

The most common cause of ovarian failure is natural menopause at the average age of 51 years (with a range of 40 to 58) (Fig. 6-5). Before 40 years of age "natural" ovarian failure is considered "premature." Other women are born without functioning ovaries (Turner's syndrome and gonadal dysgenesis). Both irradiation and chemotherapy for the treatment of breast cancer, leukemia, or other cancers can cause ovarian failure. Surgical castration causes menopause in about 30% of U.S. women. After the age of

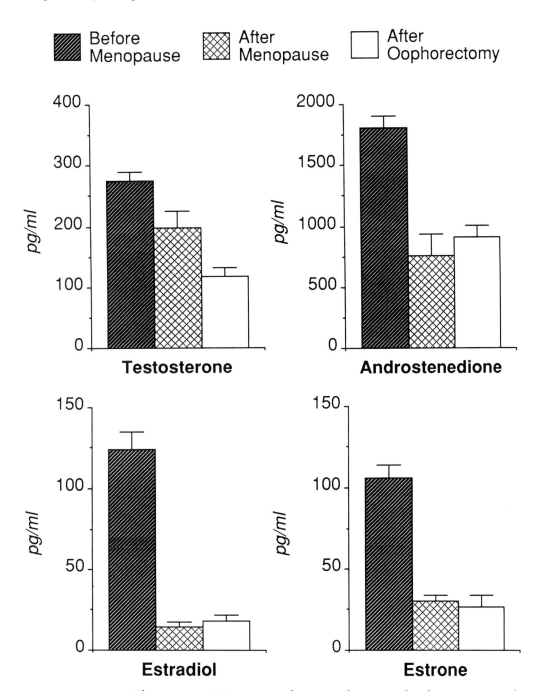

FIGURE 6-4. The mean ± S.E. serum androgen and estrogen levels in women with endometrial cancer before menopause ($n = 5$) and after menopause ($n = 16$) and 6 to 8 weeks after oophorectomy ($n = 16$). These levels were not significantly different from those without endometrial cancer.

Modified from Judd HL: *Clin Obstet Gynecol* 19:775, 1976.

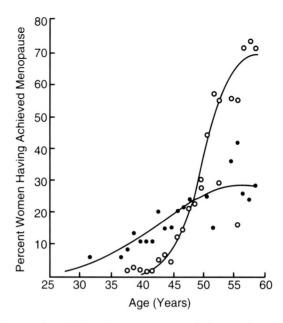

FIGURE 6-5. Observed and fitted percentages of the study respondents having achieved operative (●) or natural (○) menopause as a function of age.

Redrawn from Krailo MD, Pike MC: *Am J Epidemiol* 117:356, 1983.

45 it is often customary to remove the ovaries at the time of hysterectomy in an attempt to reduce the small risk of future ovarian cancer. Rarely are the ovaries so diseased by infection, tumor, or endometriosis that removal of both is required.

Surgical versus Natural Menopause

Approximately 1 in 50,000 women over the age of 40 years develop ovarian cancer each year. However, there is some question whether bilateral oophorectomy will protect a woman from developing ovarian cancer because a similar cancer of the peritoneal surfaces can develop despite bilateral oophorectomy. Furthermore, surgical extirpation of both ovaries before menopause increases the risks of cardiovascular disease and osteoporosis. The benefits of ovarian conservation before menopause probably outweigh the risks of ovarian cancer in the general population, unless, perhaps, estrogen therapy compliance were perfect. The benefits of ovarian conservation after menopause are unknown, but the ovary does continue to produce testosterone after menopause.

SYMPTOMS AND SIGNS OF OVARIAN FAILURE
Physiology and Treatment of Hot Flashes

Seventy-five percent of women report vasomotor symptoms at menopause. These symptoms are severe in about 15%. The prevalence of vasomotor symptoms tapers to 25% 5 years after menopause and 15% 16 years after menopause. Some women in their seventies and eighties still report hot flashes. Women with surgically induced menopause tend to have a higher prevalence and severity of hot flashes.

Cultural differences may affect the reporting of hot flashes. Postmenopausal women from Western societies report far more frequent hot flashes than their counterparts in Japan and Indonesia or Mayan women in Yucatan, Mexico.

Usually hot flashes occur spontaneously, but stress, emotions, external heat, a confining space, caffeine, or alcohol may trigger hot flashes. External temperature can modulate hot flashes; there is a significant reduction in both the frequency and intensity of hot flashes during the daytime and in a cool as compared with a warm room.

A hot flash is commonly 1 to 5 minutes in duration but occasionally ranges from seconds to 15 minutes or more. Hot flashes are described as waves of heat, drenching sweats, anxiety, and palpitations. Women report a sense of impending hot flash before the flash actually starts. The heart rate and skin blood flow increase, particularly in the hands and fingers. There is a rapid drop in skin resistance and an increase in skin conductance. The finger temperature rises 1 to 7°C, and sweating commences. As a result of the vasodilation and sweating there is heat loss and a drop in internal temperature of 0.1 to 0.9°C. Shivering may occur and facilitate the return of body temperature to normal. Vasoconstriction may do the same. The temperature of the toes also increases concomitantly with the finger temperature.

There is an apparent resetting of the body's thermostat or temperature set point in the hypothalamus that the body perceives as a need to eliminate heat. The resultant response in the skin apparently results in the objective and symptomatic changes.

Some women develop insomnia from the vasomotor symptoms. The lack of sleep compounded by an age-related decrease in rapid eye movement (REM) sleep can lead to depression, irritability, a loss of the sense of worth, and memory loss. However, as a group, postmenopausal women do not experience more depression than premenopausal women do.

Even men, after orchiectomy, can experience vasomotor symptoms.

Serum levels of estrogens are lower in postmenopausal women with hot flashes than in those with no hot flashes.

Women with gonadal dysgenesis do not experience hot flashes until they are exposed and then withdrawn from estrogen treatment.

During a hot flash there is an episodic release of LH and gonadotropin-releasing hormone (GnRH)) (Fig. 6-6). However, LH and GnRH are thought only to be secondary responses to a neurotransmitter from higher centers in the brain. Epinephrine has been shown to increase while norepinephrine decreases during hot flashes. There is also some increase in β-endorphin, β-lipotropin, and adrenocorticotropic hormone (ACTH) concentrations during hot flashes. Cortisol, DHEA, and androstenedione levels also increase.

Clinical risk factors for vasomotor symptoms include an ectomorphic body structure; a strong family history of osteoporosis; a calcium intake less than recommended; inactivity, cigarette smoking, and alcohol abuse; and early hypoestrogenicity caused genetically, by early or surgical menopause, by hypothalamic pituitary failure, by excessive exercise, or by certain hormonal excesses such as glucocorticoid excess or thyrotoxicosis.

Because hot flashes are the consequence of ovarian failure, estrogen is the standard against which all other treatments must be compared. Several double-blind crossover, placebo-controlled studies have demonstrated the efficacy of estrogen over placebo in treating hot flashes. A prototype of this study was performed by Coope in a general practice in 1976. A double-blind crossover study of 30 menopausal women was performed by using CEE versus placebo. For the first 3 months the two groups were randomly allocated to either CEE therapy or placebo. The conjugated estrogen (Premarin)-treated group ingested 1.25 mg daily 21 out of 28 days with a 7-day gap between each course. The placebo group was given lactose tablets identical in taste and appearance to Premarin. After 3 months each group

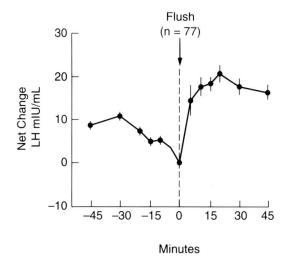

FIGURE 6-6. Mean (± SEM) serum LH concentration during 77 flush episodes expressed as a net change in milli-international units per milliliter from the onset of the flush at 0 on the *x*-axis. This graph incorporates 5-minute sampling from 20 minutes before to 20 minutes after each flush episode. It can be seen that the flush onset is coincident with a rise in serum LH levels.

Redrawn from Casper R, Yen SSC: In Yen SSC, Jaffee RD, editors: *Reproductive endocrinology, physiology, pathophysiology, and clinical management,* ed 3, Philadelphia, 1991, Saunders, p. 394.

crossed over to the opposite medication. The group initiated with estrogen had a 90% decrease in the average number of hot flashes per week; the placebo group had a 50% reduction (Fig. 6-7). After crossing over from placebo to Premarin therapy the initial placebo group had a sharp further reduction in hot flashes while taking Premarin. In contrast, the initial estrogen group, after switching to placebo, had a return of their hot flashes to baseline.

Melis, Gambacciani, Cagnacci, and others randomized patients to placebo versus the dopamine antagonist veralipride, 100 mg per day for 30 days. There was a significant reduction in vasomotor symptoms, an increase in plasma prolactin, and a decrease in plasma LH but no change in LH

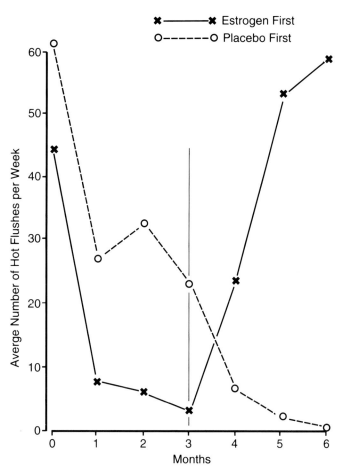

FIGURE 6-7. Prevalence of hot flushes in 30 postmenopausal women randomly assigned to either placebo or CEE treatment for 3 months and then crossed over to the opposite medication for an additional 3 months in a double-blind clinical trial.

Redrawn from Coope J: In Campbell S, editor: *The management of the menopause and post-menopausal years*, Baltimore, 1976, University Park Press.

pulsatility in the patients ingesting veralipride. After infusion of the opioid antagonist naloxone in the patients receiving veralipride therapy LH levels increased, suggesting involvement of the opioid system.

One of the treatments, that of clonidine, does not decrease the number of objective signs of hot flashes but does decrease the perception of hot flashes.

A double-blind, crossover, placebo-controlled study using transdermal estradiol showed an increased efficacy with estradiol (Estraderm) over placebo for hot flashes. Medroxyprogesterone acetate and lofexidine also reduce the incidence of hot flashes.

Genitourinary Atrophy

Those genitourinary tissues that are embryonically estrogen dependent remain so for life. After estrogen withdrawal, these tissues atrophy. The thick stratified squamous epithelium of the vaginal mucosa of the reproductive-aged woman regresses to a thickness of two to three cells in the estrogen-deprived postmenopausal woman. Vaginal dryness, atrophy, and dyspareunia can result and lead to atrophic vaginitis or sexual dysfunction.

The same happens to the urethral mucosa, with a consequent 30% reduction in urethral closure pressure. The trigone of the bladder attenuates because of atrophy; urinary urgency and frequency result. The supportive tissues of the pelvic organs weaken and result in a loss of support to the base of the bladder and urethra. The urethrovesical junction may prolapse, thereby removing itself from the abdominal cavity. The vulva, cervix, and uterus decrease in size. The cervix may become flush with the back of the vagina. These changes increase the likelihood of urinary incontinence and inadequate control of urination.

The symptoms of dyspareunia and urinary incontinence must be explored routinely, aggressively, and empathetically with the patient by the physician. Otherwise, the problems may not be identified because many women feel embarrassed by them.

Most of these changes can be treated by ERT. With ERT the vaginal mucosa thickens, the pH of the vagina decreases, and there is a decrease in vaginal dryness. Estrogen therapy can be delivered either vaginally or orally with the same efficacy. A dosage of 0.3 mg of CEE daily, oral or vaginal, produces a satisfactory therapeutic result in most women with vaginal mucosal atrophy; 0.1 to 0.2 mg of estradiol in a vaginal cream is also effective.

Similarly, ERT has a beneficial effect on the estrogen-dependent tissues of the urinary tract. The urethral mucosa thickens, and the proximal portion of the urethra becomes less prolapsed and returns to the abdominal cavity. Upon return of the proximal part of the urethra to the abdomen the pelvic diaphragm becomes more effective in preventing the loss of urine with coughing, sneezing, or any other Valsalva maneuver. Furthermore, once the proximal portion of the urethra becomes more of an abdominal organ, the intraabdominal pressure is transmitted equally to both the bladder and the urethra. Therefore a postmenopausal woman with urinary incontinence and other urinary tract symptoms may benefit from a trial of ERT; approximately 50% show improvement.

Skin

The skin after menopause is thought to undergo some degree of atrophy and loss of collagen. In hypoestrogenic animals the epidermis undergoes atrophy, the number of capillaries decreases, and collagen fibers fragment. In women, skin collagen content declines in relation to menopausal age but not chronologic age. Skin thickness tends to decrease at the rate of about 1.2% per year and collagen at the rate of 2.1% per year in early menopause. Estrogen therapy helps the skin of these women look healthier. Estrogen decreases the fragmentation in the dermis of estrogen-deficient women and increases the capillaries. The skin thickens, and the skin collagen and water content increase. Brincat and Studd compared a group of postmenopausal women with and without ERT and found that the ERT group had more collagen in their skin than the untreated group. ERT seems to effect a return of skin thickness and collagen even in late postmenopause and acts prophylactically in early postmenopause. Brincat et al. suggest that the behavior of the connective tissue element in skin may reflect similar changes in the organic matrix in bone.

Sexual Function

Both males and females show a decreasing total sexual outlet with aging, according to Kinsey, Pomeroy, Martin, and Gebhard. Total sexual outlet in single women is about once every 2 weeks and does not change with age (Fig. 6-8). The total sexual outlet per week in married females is approximately two per week in women in their twenties, which gradually decreases to once every other week in the sixties, and follows a pattern of male activity (Fig. 6-9). The decreasing frequency of sexual intercourse and orgasm in marriage may be more a result of the aging of the husband rather than a change in sexual capacity in the female.

After menopause five basic sexual changes may occur: diminished sexual response, dyspareunia from vulvar and vaginal atrophy, decreased sexual activity, decline in sexual desire, and a dysfunctional male partner. Furthermore, age-related chronic illnesses such as hypertension, diabetes, and cancer may affect the ability and desire to perform. The anxiety associated with these states may compromise vaginal blood flow. Intact ovaries through the production of androgens may play a role in arousal,

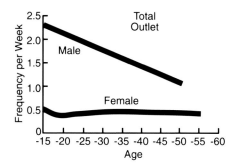

FIGURE 6-8. Comparison of aging and sexual outlet patterns among single females and males.

Redrawn from Kinsey AC, Pomeroy WB, Martin CE, Gebhard PH: *Sexual behavior in the human female*, Philadelphia, 1953, Saunders.

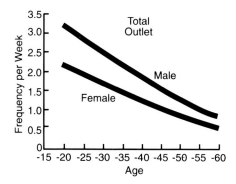

FIGURE 6-9. Comparison of aging and sexual outlet patterns among married females and males.

Redrawn from Kinsey AC, Pomeroy WB, Martin CE, Gebhard PH: *Sexual behavior in the human female*, Philadelphia, 1953, Saunders.

desire, fantasy, and sexual gratification, and their removal might diminish these. Despite these physiologic changes, the most important factor in vaginal health is continued sexual activity and the presence of a functioning desired male.

Masters and Johnson found a reduced rapidity and intensity of physiologic response in postmenopausal women. None of the women past the age of 60 years demonstrated the superficial, vasocongestive skin response or skin flush. In those who did develop the skin flush under the age of 60 years, the flush was limited to the epigastrium, anterior portion of the chest, neck, face, and forehead. General muscle tension elevation and response to sexual stimuli decreased. Irritation of the urethra and bladder occurred with some regularity, particularly in those postmenopausal women who did not lubricate well. There was a greater frequency of a sensation of urinary urgency shortly after coitus, sometimes lasting in some individuals 2 to 3 days after extended coitus. The commonly noted orgasmic-phase rectal contractions seen in younger women occurred infrequently in postmenopausal women. The clitoral response to sexual stimulation was similar to that seen in younger women. The flattening, separation, and elevation of the labia majora that are seen in younger women tended to disappear in postmenopausal women. The thickening seen in the labia minora of younger women during advanced excitement-phase levels of sexual response that extend the vaginal barrel by approximately 1 cm tended to decrease or even disappear in the older women. Bartholin's gland secretion and vaginal lubrication decreased and, although present in the age groups up to 70 years, was not demonstrated in the 71-year-old to 80-year-old age group. The walls of the vagina were tissue paper thin and were a light pinkish color. The vagina became shorter in length and narrower in transcervical width and lost some of its expansive ability. The few women in Masters and Johnson's study group who did maintain sexual activity on a regular basis experienced vaginal lubrication similar to that expected in a premenopausal woman. Orgasmic platform contractions recurred less frequently than in younger women except in the women who continued to maintain regular coitus. Masters and Johnson conclude that despite the reduction in all four phases of the sexual cycle with advancing years the postmenopausal woman is fully capable of sexual performance at orgasmic response levels, particularly if she continues regular sexual activity.

Sarrel reported the results of a study of 50 couples who had a problem with sex after menopause. Twenty-two percent reported problems with the woman only, 18% in the man only, and 60% in both partners. In these latter couples difficulty occurred when the women began to experience dyspareunia, anorgasmia, or both.

Sarrel and Whitehead interviewed 178 postmenopausal women. Thirteen percent reported no sexual difficulties. Some of these women were taking ERT. Of the remaining 154 women, 45% reported a loss of sexual desire, and 10% experienced sexual aversion. Twenty-seven percent reported dyspareunia and vaginal dryness. Twenty-one percent had vaginismus by medical examination. Thirty-six percent reported excitement-phase disorders, including touch sensation impairment (they did not want to be touched), loss of clitoral sensation, vaginal dryness, and urinary incontinence. In the women with dyspareunia and vaginal dryness in the second study, 79% responded favorably to ERT. The nonresponders were found to have vaginismus. Twenty-seven percent reported becoming nonorgasmic at menopause.

Many of these problems can be treated adequately by the gynecologist, the internist, or the family physician and may not need a sex therapist. For example, Sarrel studied a subgroup of the 38 men of the 50 couples described previously who reported problems with erection. The problem was corrected in 28 (74%) of these men when the women were given hormonal replacement therapy. No other sex therapy was required for these 28 men.

Sarrel reports marked improvement in sexual function after ERT. Clitoral sensitivity increased significantly, and women who were nonorgasmic experienced a return of orgasmic capacity and an increase in the level of sexual desire. None of these women was given androgens. Certainly as a first attempt ERT is warranted. If the response is unsatisfactory and serum levels of estradiol are low, consider an increase in the dose before referral to a sex therapist. The appropriate dose of estrogen and the effect of progestins on sexual function after menopause and in the perimenopausal state are not yet well determined.

According to Sarrel the increase in the vibration threshold needed to attain orgasm seen in postmenopausal women decreases to the premenopausal level when ERT is given. The decreased blood flow to the vagina after menopause also returns to normal after the administration of CEE. The same findings were seen with blood flow to the vulva with estradiol. This positive effect was reversed with 10 mg of medroxyprogesterone when added to estradiol in the vulvar study.

CARDIOVASCULAR DISEASE

Stampfer, Colditz, and Willett note that the leading cause of death in women in the United States is coronary artery disease, as it is in men. Bush points out that in the United States in 1986 cardiovascular disease accounted for nearly 53% of all deaths in women over 50 years of age as compared with 4% of deaths caused by breast cancer, 18% caused by other forms of cancer, and 2% resulting from accidents and suicides (National Center for Health Statistics) (Fig. 6-10).

The risk of cardiovascular disease increases greatly with age, although in every age group the rate is higher in men. The mortality rate for cardiovascular disease for women seems to lag behind men by about 5 to 10 years. Although within any age group more men than women die per 100,000 relative population (Fig. 6-11), the total number of women who die of cardiovascular disease is greater than the total number of men, because women tend to live longer than men and therefore as a group are older. For example, in 1986 in the United States, 337,024 women as compared with 333,348 men died of ischemic heart disease or cerebral vascular disease.

Bush observed that there is no sharp increase in mortality in the years after menopause. A possible explanation may be the subtle reduction of estrogen production by the ovaries beginning at about 35 years of age and continuing as a slow process for 10 to 15 or more years. Menopause per se does not seem to affect this increasing rate. Age and cigarette smoking, on

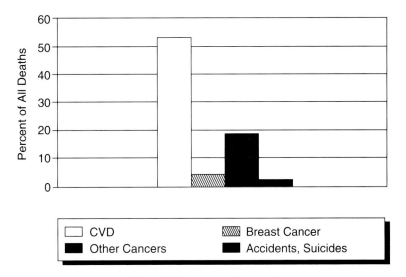

FIGURE 6-10. Percentage of deaths from specific conditions among women over 50 years of age (United States, 1986).

Redrawn from Bush TL: *Ann N Y Acad Sci* 592:263, 1990.

the other hand, are powerful confounding factors; for example, between the ages of 47 and 52 years there is a 100% increase in the rate of coronary artery disease mortality. Likewise, smokers tend to have both an early menopause and a greater risk for coronary artery disease. Studies that do not control for age and smoking may draw misleading conclusions. For example, in the Nurses' Health Study cohort in which the relationship between natural menopause and nonfatal myocardial infarction was studied, the relative risk (RR) associated with natural menopause was 1.7 (95% confidence interval [CI] 1.1 to 2.8); however, after controlling for smoking and age by using 1-year age groups and smoking the RR was 1.0 (95% CI, 0.8 to 1.3).

In contrast to natural menopause, surgical menopause has a profound and immediate effect on cardiovascular disease. The RR of calcification of the abdominal aorta was found to be 5.5 after surgical menopause (95% CI, 1.9 to 15.8). Again in the Nurses' Health Study the RR of coronary heart disease among women with bilateral oophorectomy after adjusting for age and smoking was 2.2 (95% CI, 1.2 to 4.2). Under the age of 35 years, women who underwent bilateral oophorectomy had seven times the risk of cardiovascular disease when compared with premenopausal women. This increased risk was not seen in women receiving ERT (RR of 0.9; 95% CI, 0.6 to 1.6).

Despite the failure to demonstrate a negative effect of natural menopause on coronary artery disease, the use of estrogen therapy seems to have a beneficial effect. The Lipid Research Clinics Program Follow-up Study followed a cohort of 2270 white women for an average of 8.5 years. Of the women not using estrogen, 2.6% died from cardiovascular disease as compared with 1% of the estrogen users. The estimated protective effect in estrogen users was 0.37 (95% confidence limits [CL], 0.16 to 0.88) and was still demonstrated after exclusion of all women who had cardiovascular disease at the initiation of therapy. About half of the protective effect of estrogen was mediated through increased high-density lipoprotein (HDL) levels. Unfortunately, this study did not separate those women with natural from those with surgical menopause.

In 1994 Grodstein and Stampfer performed a metaanalysis of all the epidemiologic studies to date. They found an overall RR for coronary artery disease of 0.65 (95% CI, 0.60 to 0.70) for women who had ever taken ERT and 0.49 (95% CI, 0.43 to 0.56) for women currently taking ERT. In 1991 Stampfer and co-workers reported the largest study to date, the Nurses' Health Study. The RR was 0.56 (95% CI, 0.40 to 0.80) for current users and 0.83 (95% CI, 0.65 to 1.05) for past users. This protective effect did not seem to be related to duration of use and was independent of age.

The cardiovascular response to estrogen may be trimodal, with hypoestrogenicity being detrimental, low physiologic doses being beneficial,

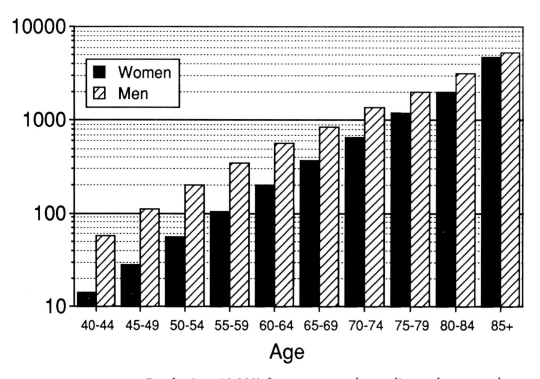

FIGURE 6-11. Deaths (per 10,000) from coronary heart disease by age and sex (United States, 1986).

Redrawn from Bush TL: *Ann N Y Acad Sci* 592:263, 1990.

and high doses detrimental. The Framingham double-blind, placebo-controlled trial in men with a previous myocardial infarction found no therapeutic efficacy in preventing mortality, a higher incidence of nonfatal pulmonary embolism and thrombophlebitis, and a higher incidence of nonfatal myocardial infarction with dosages of CEEs of 2.5 mg and 5.0 mg. Likewise, the higher potency of the estrogen component in birth control pills may be responsible for the adverse effects on the cardiovascular system. As the dosages of estrogen (and progestins) have decreased in oral contraceptives over the last three decades, so have the adverse effects.

Because cardiovascular disease is such a major cause of mortality in women in their postmenopausal years, the theoretical cumulative net number of lives saved by using estrogen for 25 years has been estimated by Lobo to be about 5561 per 100,000 users aged 50 to 75 years (Table 6-1) despite the adverse effects on the gallbladder, endometrium, and breast. This is the equivalent of a 41% reduction in overall mortality in users versus nonusers. The beneficial effect on the cardiovascular system is an estrogenic one.

The calculations performed in Table 6-1 are dependent on the values assigned to the relative risks for breast cancer and cardiovascular disease. For example, if the relative risk of death from breast cancer associated with ERT were 2.0 instead of 1.1 and the relative risk for coronary artery disease were reduced to 1.0, the number of osteoporotic-related deaths saved by the use of ERT would be too few to overcome the increased mortality from breast cancer (Table 6-1). These manipulations of the assumptions of Table 6-1 illustrate the importance of the cardiovascular protective effect of ERT.

These relationships might have clinical importance. For example, in a woman low at risk for cardiovascular disease and osteoporosis, the net effect of ERT might be detrimental, and she probably should not take ERT for more than a short time, particularly if at risk for breast cancer. For

TABLE 6-1. Estimated changes in mortality induced by daily estrogen replacement therapy (0.625 mg) in women aged 50 to 75 years

Condition	Risk	Cumulative change in mortality/100,000
Osteoporotic fractures	0.4	−563
Gallbladder disease	1.5	+2
Endometrial cancer	2.0	+63*
Breast cancer	1.1	+187
Ischemia heart disease	0.5	−5250
Net change		−5561
Net change (%)		−41

Originally adapted from Henderson BE, Ross RH, Paganini-Hill A, Mack TM: *Am J Obstet Gynecol* 154:1181, 1986; and Lobo RA: *Ann N Y Acad Sci* 592:286, 1990.
*Case fatality rate estimate at 0.05.

example, Sullivan, Zwagg, Hughes, and associates identified a group of women with normal coronary arteries on arteriography. These women had a high survival rate the next 10 years, and ERT had no measureable impact.

Whether the addition of a progestin to ERT might reduce this protective effect is still under study. In most studies to date so few of the estrogen users were taking progestogens (1% in the Lipid Research Clinics Program Follow-up Study) that no conclusions can yet be drawn about the effects of progestins on the cardiovascular system. The effect of progestins on HDL cholesterol and the cardiovascular system may be dose and potency dependent. For example, the progestins levonorgestrel (250 μg) and medroxyprogesterone acetate (10 mg) in a study by Ottosson et al. had detrimental effects on HDL cholesterol, and micronized progesterone (200 mg) had no effect. Until the effect on the cardiovascular system becomes clarified, a recommended strategy is to provide as small a dosage of progestin as possible that still protects the endometrium.

Lipoproteins change at menopause. Both total cholesterol and low-density lipoprotein (LDL) cholesterol increase after menopause. There is no major change in HDL cholesterol. In men, for every 1% increase in total cholesterol there is a 2% increase in the risk of myocardial infarction, and for every 11% reduction in LDL cholesterol there is a 19% reduction in coronary artery disease risk. In women a 10-mg/dl increase in HDL cholesterol is associated with a 40% to 50% decrease in cardiovascular risk.

Low-density lipoprotein and intermediate-density lipoprotein (IDL) cholesterol are the major deleterious cholesterol moities. They consist of a phospholipid outer core soluble in blood and an internal core densely packed with cholesterol esters. Oxidizing forms of LDL cholesterol can also contribute to intimal injury, and they appear to bind permanently and lead to extremely atherogenic characteristics. HDL collects cholesterol and transports it back to the liver for degradation and reformation of other lipoproteins. The most active form is HDL_2. In the liver, hepatic lipase destroys HDL cholesterol. Estrogen degrades hepatic lipase.

Estrogens and progestins have other effects than just on the lipoproteins. The research of Adams, Kaplan, Manuck, et al. in monkeys suggests that contraceptive estrogens (equivalent to Ovral and Demulen) may have a direct beneficial effect on blood vessels that may negate or confuse the interpretation of lipoprotein changes in response to the combination pill. In these studies in monkeys, ethinyl estradiol combined with a progestin protected the coronary arteries from the negative effects of a moderately atherogenic diet and from the progestinic lowering of HDL cholesterol when compared with untreated controls. Estrogen seemed to protect the intima of the vessels directly, offsetting the detrimental lipoprotein effects of the progestin. One must keep in mind, however, that estrogen in high doses has an adverse effect on the coagulation system, increasing the risk for thrombosis in the peripheral vessels and in the coronary arteries.

Estrogens other than those in the large epidemiologic studies (mainly CEE or Premarin) also seem to have beneficial effects. For example, in a randomized, double-blind, placebo-controlled, crossover study by Walsh, Sacks, and Schiff of micronized estradiol, transdermal estradiol, and placebo, oral estrogens increased hepatic catabolism of LDL cholesterol, which in turn lowered the plasma LDL concentration.

Paganini-Hill, Ross, and Henderson demonstrated a 50% reduction in the death rate from stroke in estrogen users as compared with nonusers. A similar protective effect of estradiol, CEE, and oral contraceptives was seen on all types of stroke and on acute stroke in a population-based cohort study in Sweden. Blood pressure is not increased in ERT users.

Not all studies have demonstrated a beneficial effect of ERT on the cardiovascular system. In a large epidemiologic study of 603 white females aged 45 to 69 years, Thompson, Meade, and Greenberg from Middlesex, United Kingdom, found no major cardiovascular risk or benefit associated with ERT. Although the gross relative risk was slightly elevated, when the data were analyzed with other cardiovascular risk factors taken into account, the relative risk was reduced. The dosages and types of estrogens differed from those used in the United States.

Sitruk-Ware and de Palacios pointed out a possible explanation for the discordant findings related to ERT and the cardiovascular system. They found in a review of ERT that the risk in women of cardiovascular disease either remained unchanged or increased in users as compared with nonusers in epidemiologic studies published before 1980. Since 1980 a protective effect has been demonstrated, simultaneous with the greater use of lower, natural dosages of estrogen.

OSTEOPOROSIS

Most women in their eighties and nineties are affected by osteoporosis. About 50% of those affected sustain some form of osteoporotic fracture, and one-sixth of those with fractures of the hip die of complications. Twenty-five percent of white women over 60 years of age have spinal compression fractures caused by osteoporosis. The financial toll of osteoporotic fractures is estimated to be $7.5 billion per year in the United States. The classic fractures of osteoporosis are vertebral, hip, surgical neck of the humerus, the ribs, the pelvis, and Colles' fracture of the radius.

Both men and women lose bone with aging (osteopenia). In women, bone loss begins slowly at about the age of 35 years and accelerates at menopause. Immediately after menopause the rate of bone loss is approximately 5% per year for spinal trabecular bone and 1% to 2% for cortical bone. Although the rate of loss tends to slow down within a few years, by the age of 80 white women experience a 50% reduction in bone mass, resulting in osteoporosis and consequent fractures.

The rate of fracture of the distal portion of the forearm and ankle increases soon after menopause and levels off at about the age of 65 years. The rate of fracture of the hip, which contains both cortical and cancellous bone, increases exponentiaily throughout life. The incidence of vertebral fractures follows an intermediate pattern that increases soon after menopause and continues to increase gradually with age. Although men also have a gradually increasing incidence of bone fractures with age, the rate is much less than in women after menopause without estrogen.

Osteoporosis results from reduced bone density and the resultant architectural changes; after bone density decreases below a certain threshold, fractures begin to occur. Maximum adult bone mass is genetically determined, driven, and sustained by threshold amounts of dietary calcium and is attained by adolescence or early adulthood. The amount of bone mass at menopause and the rate of loss after menopause determine the risk of osteoporosis and fracture. Women of Afro-Caribbean origin have greater bone density than do white or Asian women and, despite similar rates of bone loss after menopause, run a much lower risk of osteoporosis and fracture. In a cross-sectional study of the bone density in black and white, healthy, nonobese women aged 24 to 65 years, Lucky, Meier, Mandeli, and colleagues found higher bone density in blacks than in whites at both lumbar spine and radius and at all ages. The cross-sectional rate of decline of vertebral bone density was similar between races; however, radial density increased 3.8% per decade in premenopausal blacks under 46 years of age, and it declined 3.2% per decade ($P < .09$) in premenopausal whites. These findings suggest that attainment of higher peak bone mass and delayed onset of bone loss contribute to the lower incidence of osteoporotic fractures in black women.

Women who consume two or more alcoholic drinks per day and women who smoke have significantly lower bone density than nondrinkers do. The effect of cigarette smoking is seen predominantly in the spine. Whereas alcohol intake and cigarette smoking may lower bone mass, excessive exercise or calcium supplementation above daily requirements does not increase bone density beyond the genetic limit. The goal is to maintain bone density at the genetic limit.

The primary influence on bone density loss seems to be the duration of hypoestrogenicity and not chronologic age. Urinary hydroxyproline/ creatinine but not serum osteocalcin or urinary calcium/creatinine secretion is a significant predictor of bone mineral density at the lumbar spine and the femoral neck, independent of age. These data are consistent with the hypothesis that age-related bone loss after menopause occurs in the presence of initially increased (but subsequently decreasing) bone turnover with maintenance of a relative excess of bone resorption.

Estrogen Replacement Therapy and Bone Loss

To date, estrogen has shown the greatest efficacy in preventing postmenopausal osteoporosis. In the late 1970s and early 1980s, several prospective studies demonstrated that both mestranol and CEE prevented bone loss in menopausal women when compared with placebo (Fig. 6-12). A typical study was published in 1981; Christiansen, Christensen, and Transbol treated postmenopausal women for 24 months with either placebo or a combination of estrogen and progestin. At 24 months subjects switched to either placebo or the combination of estrogen and progestin. Note in Fig. 6-9 that the placebo group continued to lose bone mineral as measured by photon absorptiometry (^{125}I) on the distal part of the forearms. The combination group had a gradual increase in bone mineral, and this began to decrease after switching over to placebo. The placebo group when switched over to combination estrogen and progestin began to regain some of their bone mineral or at least did not continue to lose bone mineral. Many of these studies focused on corticol bone; similar findings were seen in spinal and trabecular bone.

Although Hillard, Whitcroft, Marsh, and associates also found in 1994 that the majority of subjects who took either transdermal or oral HRT for

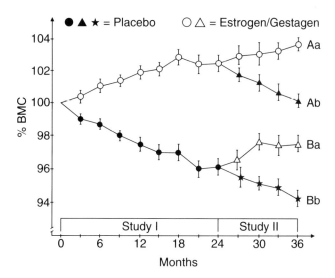

FIGURE 6-12. Bone mineral content as a function of time and treatment in women who had passed through natural menopause 6 months to 3 years before. The estrogen was a combination of estradiol, 4 mg, and estriol, 2 mg, and norethindrone acetate 1 mg or placebo.

Redrawn from Christensen C, Christensen MS, Transbol IB: *Lancet* 2:459, 1981.

3 years had increased bone density in both the lumbar spine and femoral neck, 12% of women lost a significant amount of bone from the femoral neck despite adequate compliance. They suggest that women taking ERT primarily for hip fracture prevention consider a follow-up bone density measurement to establish the efficacy of treatment.

Osteoporosis results in fractures. Again, in the late 1970s several case-control studies demonstrated a protective odds ratio if estrogens were started within 5 years of menopause. Weiss, Ure, Ballard, and others interviewed 327 women with fractures of the hip or lower portion of the forearm. A random sample of 567 women served as controls. A relative protective effect against fractures was seen in women who had used ERT for more than 5 years (RR ~ 0.4 to 0.5; CI, 0.3 to 0.6). More recent studies concur.

Most of the subjects in these studies were using CEEs, which in the United States has been and still is Premarin. The minimum effective dose of CEEs or Premarin is thought to be 0.625 mg daily when the end point of mineral bone content is used. The daily addition of 1500 mg of calcium seems to improve the efficacy of 0.3 mg of Premarin. The addition of progestins to ERT seems to be beneficial. There is even some evidence that progestins alone may prevent bone loss by a different mechanism, perhaps by stimulating bone formation.

Calcium

Impaired calcium metabolism is most prominent after the age of 70 years and appears to be caused by decreased cutaneous synthesis and intestinal absorption of vitamin D or decreased tissue responsiveness to its active metabolites. Its effects are aggravated by the relatively low dietary calcium intake and decreased sun exposure by most elderly persons. For example, in an upper-middle-class white community in Rancho Bernardo, California, the median intake of calcium in women aged 50 to 79 years was less than 800 mg a day in 426 of 531, or 80% (Fig. 6-13). This leads to mild but sustained secondary hyperparathyroidism and increased bone turnover.

Osteoporotic women have decreased calcium absorption and decreased serum 1,25-dihydroxyvitamin D and are usually in negative calcium balance. Estrogen therapy improves calcium balance in postmenopausal women by increasing serum, 1,25-dihydroxyvitamin D levels. This effect appears to be mediated indirectly through stimulation of renal 1α-hydroxylase by increased serum immunoreactive parathyroid hormone (PTH).

Stevenson, Whitehead, Padwick, and colleagues found no correlation between current dietary calcium intake in postmenopausal women and either total-body calcium or bone density (Fig. 6-14). In fact, calcium intake above 200 to 400 mg per day was of no apparent benefit to postmenopausal

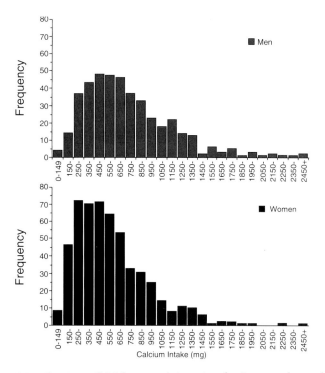

FIGURE 6-13. Distribution of 24-hour calcium intake in men *(upper)* and women *(lower)* aged 50 to 79 years at baseline.

Redrawn from Holbrook TL, Barrett-Connor E, Wingard DL: *Lancet* 2:1046, 1988.

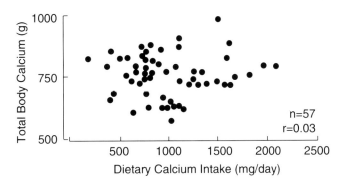

FIGURE 6-14. Relationship of dietary calcium intake and total-body calcium in healthy postmenopausal women.

Redrawn from Stevenson JC: *Obstet Gynecol* 75(suppl):36, 1990.

cortical and trabecular bone. About 10% of women take in even less than this minimum standard of 200 mg per day of calcium. In contrast, Holbrook, Barrett-Connor, and Wingard found a strong correlation between dietary intake of calcium and fracture of the hip in 531 women aged 50 to 79 years, even after adjustment for cigarette smoking, alcohol intake, exercise, and obesity. Perhaps some clarification of these divergent findings is provided by the work of Dawson-Hughes, Dallal, Krall, and others. In a placebo-controlled study of calcium supplementation they found that women who had undergone menopause 5 or fewer years earlier did not show any effect on bone loss in their spines with supplementation of calcium. Among the women who had been postmenopausal for 6 years or more and who were given placebo, bone loss was less rapid in the group with higher dietary calcium intake. In those with lower dietary calcium intake (less than 400 mg per day), calcium supplementation was more effective than placebo at the femoral neck, radius, and spine. Those women ingesting more than 400 mg of calcium per day and who had been postmenopausal for 6 years or more and received supplemental calcium maintained bone density at the hip and radius but lost bone from the spine. They concluded that postmenopausal women who are at least 6 years postmenopausal and whose dietary intake of calcium is less than 400 mg per day can significantly reduce bone loss by increasing their calcium intake to 500 mg of calcium per day or more. In other groups of postmenopausal women calcium supplementation may have either no effect or little effect.

A 1994 study by Aloai, Vaswani, Yeh, and associates showed elemental calcium supplementation (1700 g per day) more effective than placebo but less effective than the combination of ERT and calcium.

A follow-up study of 957 men and women aged 50 to 79 years found that the age-adjusted risk of hip fracture was inversely associated with dietary calcium (RR, 0.6 per 198 mg per 1000 kcal). This strongly supports the hypothesis that sufficient dietary calcium intake protects against hip fracture.

Exercise

If stress is applied to a bone, it will become denser. Krolner, Toft, Nielsen, and Tondevold carried out an 8-month exercise program in 16 healthy women aged 50 to 73 years with previous Colles' fractures. The bone mineral content in their lumbar vertebrae was superior to that in the lumbar vertebrae of 15 healthy nonexercising control subjects. Stevenson and Stevenson, Lees, Devenport, et al. found that postmenopausal women who engage in regular weight-bearing exercise have greater femoral neck and proximal femur bone density than do inactive women (Fig. 6-15). Simkin, Ayalon, and Leichter found an increase in bone density in the distal portion of the radius of 14 postmenopausal women after 5 months of arm exercises (performed three times a week) when compared with a control group of nonexercising women. These same findings were noted in male and female swimmers in the vertebral bone mineral content and in the femoral neck. In contrast, Rockwell, Sorensen, Baker, and others found a 4% decrease in lumbar spine bone density in weight-training premenopausal women as

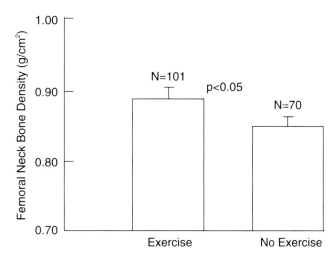

FIGURE 6-15. Femoral neck bone density in postmenopausal women who did versus those who did not take regular weight-bearing exercise.

Redrawn from Stevenson JC: *Obstet Gynecol* 75(suppl):36, 1990.

compared with sedentary women. The beneficial effects of exercise on bone density may not be enough to overcome the effect of estrogen deficiency.

A retirement community study in 1995 out of Rancho Bernardo by Greendale, Barrett-Connor, Edelstein, and associates found that a protective effect of current and lifelong exercise on hip bone mineral density, but not on osteoporotic fracture. They conclude that the risk of osteoporotic fracture was unaltered by exercise.

Therapy after Osteoporosis Has Developed

Once osteoporosis has occurred, apparently efficacious treatments include ERT, disodium etidronate (a bisphosphonate), and stanozolol (an anabolic steroid).

CANCER
Endometrial Cancer

Multiple studies starting in the mid-1970s suggested a fivefold to sevenfold increase in the risk of endometrial cancer associated with unopposed estrogen therapy. A metaanalysis of 30 studies by Grady, Gebretsadik, Kerlikowske, and colleagues and another by Herrinton and Weiss showed that interrupting the estrogen for 5 to 7 days per month did not reduce the increased risk and that the increased risk persisted for several years after discontinuation of the estrogen. Using data from the Cancer and Steroid Hormone Study, Rubin, Peterson, Lee, and associates found an elevated risk of endometrial cancer 6 or more years after discontinuation of unopposed ERT.

The risk of endometrial cancer increases with increasing dose and duration of use of unopposed estrogen replacement therapy (Fig. 6-16).

Despite the increased risk of endometrial cancer in women who use unopposed estrogen, the excessive number of cases that develop seems to be of lower severity. For example, in a study by Chu, Schweid, and Weiss women on ERT who subsequently developed endometrial cancer had a longer life expectancy than women who had not taken ERT.

The increased risk is eliminated with the addition of a progestin. Using endometrial hyperplasia as a guide to therapeutic effects, Whitehead and Fraser, as well as Whitehead, Hillard, and Crook have recommended at least 12 to 13 days per month of a progestin. The substantial protective effect that the addition of a progestin has on endometrial cancer must be weighed against any potential but as yet unclarified adverse effect the progestin may have on the cardiovascular system and breast cancer.

In general, most authors do not recommend routine endometrial biopsies in asymptomatic postmenopausal women who are not using ERT because the background incidence of endometrial cancer is estimated at 1 per 1000 per year. Because the risk increases fourfold to sevenfold in unopposed estrogen therapy (70 per 1000 in 10 years), yearly endometrial biopsies might be considered in a woman taking an estrogen without a progestin or in any woman receiving ERT with an abnormal bleeding

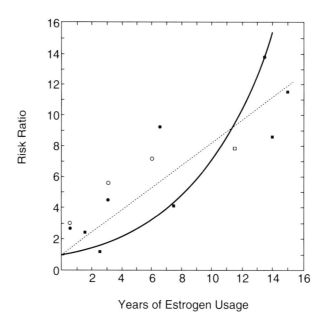

FIGURE 6-16. Dose response between the risk ratio for endometrial cancer and the length of estrogen usage: linear fit *(gray line)* versus exponential fit *(solid line.)*

Redrawn from Cramer DW, Knapp RC: *Obstet Gynecol* 54:521, 1979.

pattern. It is disturbing, however, that the presence or absence of bleeding does not correlate well with endometrial histology.

Colon Cancer

A recent study by Calle, Miracle-McMahill, Thun, and Heath published in 1995 found a decreased risk of colon cancer in women who had been taking ERT. Use of ERT was associated with an RR of 0.71 (95% CI, 0.61 to 0.83); in current users the RR was 0.55 (95% CI, 0.40 to 0.76). There was a significant trend of decreasing risk with increasing years of use among all users.

Ovarian Cancer

A recent study from Atlanta found an increased risk of ovarian cancer, both in current and former users who had used ERT for 6 or more years. The RR was 1.72 (95% CI, 1.01 to 2.90) for current users and 1.48 (95% CI, 0.99 to 2.22) for former users relative to those who had never used ERT.

Breast Cancer

In contrast to cardiovascular disease the incidence of breast cancer begins to decline around the age of menopause. This suggests a detrimental effect of ovarian hormonal production on breast cancer. Furthermore, late menopause is associated with an increased breast cancer risk, early menopause reduces the risk of cancer, and bilateral oophorectomy is associated with an even greater reduction in risk.

Because endogenous estrogens seem to increase the risk for breast cancer it has been assumed for decades that exogenous estrogens would increase the risk as well. Over 30 studies have looked at the relationship between ERT and breast cancer, including seven prospective cohort studies. These epidemiologic studies have been reviewed in at least five meta-analyses; three concluded that there is an increased risk, and two reported no increased risk. For example, Colditz, Egan, and Stampfer reported in 1993 a 23% increased risk in postmenopausal women who had used HRT at least 10 years (RR 1.23, 95% CI, 1.08 to 1.40). No increased risk was seen in former users.

Dupont, Page, Rogers, and Parl in 1989 reported no increased risk in women who ingested lower doses of CEE. Sillero-Arenas, Delgado-Rodriguez, Radiguez-Canteras, et al. in 1992 reported a 63% increased risk in current users who had gone through a natural menopause. Steinberg, Thacker, Smith, et al. in 1991 reported an increased risk of 30% after 15 years of estrogen use (RR 1.3, CI, 1.2 to 1.6), although the increase was mostly in women using estradiol. A family history of breast cancer doubled the risk.

Two recent studies in 1995 illustrate the inconsistencies in the data. Colditz, Hankinson, Hunter, et al. analyzed the Nurses' Health Study and found an increased risk of breast cancer among older women (ages 60 to 64) with 5 or more years of ERT use (RR 1.71, 95% CI, 1.34 to 2.18). In contrast, Stanford, Weiss, Voigt, et al. in a case-control study in Seattle found no increase in risk.

The addition of a progestin to the estrogen replacement therapy seems to have no impact on the risk for breast cancer. Colditz, Egan, and Stampfer found no significant change in the RR in women who ingested both an estrogen and progestin, and Stanford, Weiss, Voigt, et al. continued to find no increased risk.

In the United States physicians primarily prescribe oral conjugated equine estrogens; in Europe they primarily prescribe estradiol. For example, Bergkvist, Adami, Persson, et al. in Sweden found in a prospective study of 23,244 women that the risk of breast cancer reached 1.7 after 9 years of use (95% CI, 1.1 to 2.7) in women who were taking estradiol as compared with the population at large. The increased risk associated with the use of estradiol reached significance, but with the use of conjugated estrogens it did not; however, only a few women were using CEE. The total risk of breast cancer was highest among the women who took ERT combined with a progestin.

ESTROGEN, PROGESTIN, AND OTHER PHARMACEUTICAL PREPARATIONS

Premarin (CEE) in daily dosages of 0.625 mg meets most of the goals of ERT. However, it does have two unique problems: it consists of multiple types of estrogens, and its metabolism is slow. For example, equilin, one of 30 or so estrogens found in Premarin, is still measurable in serum 13 weeks after ingestion. Furthermore, an occasional woman does not absorb CEE well orally, and a few women have troublesome side effects. Because Premarin has been the major source of estrogen therapy in the United States since the 1940s, most epidemiologic studies that require large populations to identify small changes in uncommon events can say much about Premarin and little about other preparations. However, many other preparations and modes of delivery of estrogens are available and effective. The following is a select discussion of some of the other options.

Continuous Estrogen/Progestin Therapy

Udoff, Langenberg, and Adashi in 1995 reviewed 42 studies that reported the use of a continuous daily regimen of an estrogen and a progestin given to postmenopausal women with intact uteri. They found compliance rates of approximately 80%, amenorrhea in at least 75% after the first 6 months of use, reasonable endometrial protection (endometrial hyperplasia less than 1%), and a favorable impact on lipoproteins.

Magos, Brincat, Studd, et al. used a combination of oral CEE (0.625 mg/day) and norethindrone acetate (NET/AC) (0.35 mg/day). Sixty-five percent were immediately amenorrheic and stayed so on continued therapy. To achieve amenorrhea the NET/AC dosage had to be increased to as high as 1.4 mg per day in a few patients. The endometrium was atrophic or hypoplastic after 6 months of therapy.

Use of a Progestin Every Third Month

A few investigators have tried postmenopausal women on ERT with a progestin given for 2 weeks every 3 months. Although the trials have been limited to 1 or 2 years, they show promise. The endometrium becomes secretory. According to Hirvonen, Salmi, Puolakka, et al. endometrial hyperplasia was prevented, but the 3-month regimen was not able to reverse preexisting hyperplasia. This regimen may require regular assessment of the endometrium.

Estradiol

Estradiol, the naturally occurring and most potent estrogen in the human female, can be given orally, vaginally, transdermally, or intramuscularly. Oral preparations of estradiol are micronized and provided in 1-, 2-, or 4-mg (1000 to 4000 µg) tablets. One or two milligrams are usually enough to treat the vasomotor symptoms of most women; however, sometimes as much as 4 mg of estradiol must be used orally per day. Approximately 90% of the estradiol is converted by the gastrointestinal tract and liver to estrone and estrone sulfate, and only 10% of the unconjugated estrogens in the serum remains as estradiol. This is in contrast to the other modes of delivery in which the serum levels of estradiol are the dominate form of the absorbed unconjugated estrogens.

Vaginal estradiol is provided as a cream in a calibrated applicator. One gram of preparation contains 100 µg of estradiol (one tenth the oral dose) and usually results in peak blood levels of 100 pg/ml of estradiol 2 to 12 hours after insertion. About 100 to 200 µg of vaginal estradiol is usually effective in controlling vasomotor symptoms; a woman can titrate her dosage to her symptoms by adjusting her nightly dose. Vaginal estradiol and transdermal estradiol are particularly effective in women who do not respond well to oral CEEs.

Transdermal Estradiol

Estradiol transdermal patches are supplied in two different dosages. Estraderm 0.05 has a contact surface of 10 cm^2 and contains 4 mg of estradiol. The 0.05 (50 µg) refers to the number of milligrams of estradiol delivered per day to the skin surface. The second dosage is Estraderm 0.1

(100 μg), which has a 20-cm² contact surface, contains 8 mg of estradiol, and delivers 0.1 mg, or 100 μg, of estradiol to the skin per day. One or two patches are used at one time and are changed twice a week. Mild skin irritation occurs in about 30% of patients.

A patch-releasing progesterone is presently impractical because of the need for a large size to deliver enough progesterone to be effective.

Nonnatural progestins have greater potency than progesterone and require a smaller patch size. Norethindrone acetate is an example. By delivering norethindrone acetate in combination with estradiol transdermally, Whitehead, Hillard, and Crook observed a lower required dosage of norethindrone acetate to suppress the endometrium and no reduction of the estrogen-induced beneficial effect on lipoproteins.

Pang, Lozano, Cedars, et al. conclude that serum estradiol levels were significantly lower in postmenopausal women using the estradiol patch with cyclic medroxyprogesterone acetate than in women using the estradiol patch alone. They hypothesized an increased metabolic clearance of estradiol as a result of the induction of hepatic enzymes by the progestin.

The effect of transdermal estradiol and progestins on the vertebrae in a controlled study in postmenopausal women was found by dual-photon absorptiometry to prevent a decrease in bone density for at least 2 years. Women were given a transdermal estradiol patch twice weekly 3 weeks a month. The delivery rate was 50 μg per day. Oral micronized progesterone, 200 mg a day, dydrogesterone, 20 mg a day, or promegestone, 250 μg a day, was administered the last 10 days of the estradiol cycle. After 2 months the estrogen dosage was increased, decreased, or maintained depending on the clinical results and serum levels of estradiol. This transdermal estradiol dosage is considerably lower than the usual oral dosage (1000 to 4000 μg/day) yet was sufficient to provide effective relief of climacteric symptoms. The control group received no medication, not even calcium supplementation. Similar positive effects on the vertebrae and proximal portion of the femur were seen by Stevenson, Cust, Canger, et al. with the estradiol patch for 18 months.

Stanczyk, Shoupe, Nunez, et al. found that both the subdermal pellet and transdermal patch increased HDL cholesterol levels significantly at 6 months of therapy. The total cholesterol/HDL ratio decreased significantly as well.

Injectable Estradiols

Estradiol valerate and estradiol cypionate are injectable estradiols and are given once a month. For example, 1 mg of estradiol valerate can be given intramuscularly once a month. The serum levels of estradiol are initially elevated, rapidly fall over the course of 2 weeks, and taper off by 4 weeks. Other methods, because of their more steady serum levels, are preferable.

Progestins

To offset the effect of the increased risk for endometrial cancer, the progestin should be given for at least 12 to 13 days per month. It is at that time that the increased incidence of hyperplasia is reduced close to zero. Administering 2.5 mg of medroxyprogesterone acetate for 6 or 7 days per month is not enough to completely prevent the hyperplasia associated with 0.625 mg Premarin, although it greatly reduces it.

Regular monthly bleeding is the major side effect of the progestins. Other side effects include breast tenderness, bloating, edema, abdominal cramps, anxiety, irritability, depression, and a premenstrual tension–like syndrome. About 5% of patients cannot take progestins at all. The C-19 nortestosterone derivatives, norgestrel, norethindrone, and norethindrone acetate, tend to be androgenic and associated with acne and greasy skin and hair. The C-21 derivative medroxyprogesterone acetate is associated with depression and anxiety.

Oral micronized progesterone at 100 mg combined with estradiol and given 21 or 25 days out of the month has been found effective and well tolerated in a multicenter study of postmenopausal women in France in 1994. The endometrium was found to be well protected during the 6-month trial. Over 90% of the women became amenorrheic.

Transdermal norethindrone acetate in preliminary trials shows some promise. To reduce the side effects, reduce the dosage or use an alternate progestin.

The incidence of withdrawal bleeding with each cycle of unopposed estrogen regimens is approximately 25%. When progestins are added, about 85% of women have regular monthly withdrawal bleeding.

The effects of progestins on lipoproteins relate to potency and dosage. In a study of 58 postmenopausal women taking 2 mg of estradiol valerate daily, the women received a 10-day sequential addition of levonorgestrel, medroxyprogesterone acetate, or micronized progesterone. Low-dose natural progesterone has no major effect on HDL_2 cholesterol, whereas levonorgestrel, medroxyprogesterone acetate, and norethindrone acetate all had a detrimental effect on HDL_2 cholesterol.

Androgens

The ovaries continue to produce androgens after menopause. Therefore there probably would be no benefit to add androgens to ERTs for women with intact ovaries. In women with both ovaries removed, the efficacy, safety, and dosage of androgens have not been determined. Sherwin, Gelfand, and Brender have found androgens to enhance the intensity of sexual desire and arousal and the frequency of sexual fantasies but not sexual activity per se in oophorectomized women. The measurement of serum levels of testosterone may be helpful as well. If androgen therapy is to be used, natural testosterone would be preferable, particularly if titrated to a level not only of improved symptomatology but also to physiologic blood levels of testosterone. Just as there may be detrimental effects on the cardiovascular system with high dosages of estrogen, so too might there be disadvantages with supraphysiologic quantities of androgens.

Calcium Supplements

Retail sales of calcium supplements totaled more than $177 million in 1987. There are some 40 different calcium supplements. There appears to be no difference in the amount of calcium absorbed from the various calcium salts in the commercial supplements, milk, and calcium-fortified orange juice. Therefore the main basis for comparison is cost. According to Hegarty and Stewart, the cost per year of the various sources of calcium that would provide 800 mg of calcium per day ranged, in January 1988 in Houston, from $11 to $412. Milk, which has other benefits as well, was $175 to $266 per year.

Other Therapeutic Approaches

Tamoxifen has been shown to be effective in a pilot trial of tamoxifen versus placebo. Powles observed a reduction in LDL cholesterol and apolipoprotein B with tamoxifen. There is some evidence that postmenopausal bone loss may be reduced by tamoxifen and that tamoxifen is estrogenic rather than antiestrogenic on the female genital tract.

Transdermal Clonidine

A randomized, prospective, double-blind, placebo-controlled study of transdermal clonidine demonstrated a highly significant reduction in the number of hot flashes, few side effects, and no significant effect on blood pressure.

BIBLIOGRAPHY

Adami HO, Persson I: Hormone replacement and breast cancer, *JAMA* 272: 178, 1995.

Adams MR, Kaplan JR, Manuck SB, et al: Inhibition of coronary artery atherosclerosis by 17-beta estradiol in ovariectomized monkeys: lack of an effect of added progesterone, *Arteriosclerosis* 10: 1051, 1990.

Aitken JM, Hart DM, Lindsay R: Oestrogen replacement therapy for prevention of osteoporosis after oophorectomy, *Br Med J* 3:515, 1973.

Aloai J, Vaswani A, Yeh J, et al: Calcium supplementation with and without hormone replacement therapy to prevent postmenopausal bone loss, *Ann Intern Med* 120:97, 1994.

Beggs VE, Calhoun KS, Wolchik SA: Sexual anxiety and female sexual arousal: a comparison of arousal during sexual anxiety stimuli and sexual pleasure stimuli, *Arch Sex Behav* 16: 311, 1987.

Berg G, Gottqall T, Hammar M, Lindgren R: Climacteric symptoms among women aged 60-62 in Linkoping, Sweden, in 1986, *Maturitas* 10:193, 1988.

Bergkvist L, Adami HO, Persson I, et al: The risk of breast cancer after estrogen and estrogen-progestin replacement, *N Engl J Med* 321:293, 1989.

Bergman A, Brenner PF: Alterations in the urogenital system. In Mishell DR Jr, editor: *Menopause: physiology and pharmacology*, Chicago, 1987, Year Book Medical.

Bergman A, Brenner PF: Beneficial effects of pharmacologic agents: genitourinary. In Mishell DR Jr, editor: *Menopause: physiology and pharmacology*, Chicago, 1987, Year Book Medical.

Boccardo F, Bruzzi P, Rubagotti A, et al: Estrogen-like action of tamoxifen on vaginal epithelium in breast cancer patients, *Oncology* 38:281, 1981.

Bortnichak EA, Freeman DH Jr, Ostfield AM, et al: The association between cholesterol cholelithiasis and coronary heart disease in Framingham, Massachusetts, *Am J Epidemiol* 121:19, 1985.

Brincat M, Studd J: Skin and the menopause. In Mishell DR Jr, editor: *Menopause: physiology and pharmacology*, Chicago, 1987, Year Book Medical.

Bullock JL, Massey FM, Gambrell RD Jr: Use of medroxyprogesterone acetate to prevent menopausal symptoms, *Obstet Gynecol* 46:165, 1975.

Bush TL: The epidemiology of cardiovascular disease in postmenopausal women, *Ann N Y Acad Sci* 592:263, 1990.

Bush TL, Barrett-Connor E, Cowan LD, et al: Cardiovascular mortality and noncontraceptive use of estrogen in women: results from the Lipid Research Clinics Program Follow-up Study, *Circulation* 75:1102, 1987.

Callantine MR, Martin PL, Bolding OT, et al: Micronized 17β-estradiol for oral estrogen therapy in menopausal women, *Obstet Gynecol* 46:37, 1975.

Calle E, Miracle-McMahill H, Thun M, Heath C Jr: Estrogen replacement therapy and risk of fatal colon cancer in a prospective cohort of postmenopausal women, *J Natl Cancer Inst* 87:517, 1995.

Cann CE, Genant HK, Ettinger B, Gordan GS: Spinal mineral loss in oophorectomized women: determination by quantitative computed tomography, *JAMA* 244:2056, 1980.

Casper R, Yen SSC: The menopause and perimenopausal period. In Yen SSC, Jaffee RD, editors: *Reproductive endocrinology, physiology, pathophysiology, and clinical management*, ed 2, Philadelphia, 1986, Saunders.

Christiansen C, Christensen MS, Transbol I: Bone mass in postmenopausal women after withdrawal of oestrogen/gestagen replacement therapy, *Lancet* 2:459, 1981.

Christiansen C, Riis BJ: 17β-Estradiol and continuous norethisterone: a unique treatment for established osteoporosis in elderly women, *J Clin Endocrinol Metab* 71:836, 1990.

Chu J, Schweid AI, Weiss NS: Survival among women with endometrial cancer: a comparison of estrogen users and nonusers, *Am J Obstet Gynecol* 143:569, 1982.

Cohn SH, Abesamis C, Yasumura S, et al: Comparative skeletal mass and radial bone content in black and white women, *Metabolism* 26:171, 1977.

Colditz GA, Egan KM, Stampfer MJ: Hormone replacement therapy and risk of breast cancer: results from epidemiologic studies, *Am J Obstet Gynecol* 168:1473, 1993.

Colditz GA, Hankinson SE, Hunter DJ, et al: The use of estrogens and progestins and the risk of breast cancer in postmenopausal women, *N Engl J Med* 332:1589, 1995.

Colditz GA, Willett WC, Stampfer MJ, et al: Menopause and the risk of coronary heart disease in women, *N Engl J Med* 316:1105, 1987.

Coope J: Double-blind cross-over study of estrogen replacement therapy. In Campbell S, editor: *The management of the menopause and post-menopausal years*, Baltimore, 1976, University Park Press.

Coronary Drug Project Research Group: Project TCD: initial findings leading to modifications of its research protocol, *JAMA* 214:1303, 1970.

Coronary Drug Project Research Group: Project TCD: findings leading to discontinuation of the 2.5 mg/day estrogen group, *JAMA* 226:652, 1973.

Cramer DW, Knapp R. Review of epidemiologic studies of endometrial cancer and exogenous estrogen, *Obstet Gynecol* 54:521, 1979.

Damewood MD, Grochow LB. Prospects for fertility after chemotherapy or radiation for neoplastic disease, *Fertil Steril* 45:443, 1986.

Dawson-Hughes B, Dallal GE, Krall EA, et al: A controlled trial of the effect of calcium supplementation on bone density in post menopausal women, *N Engl J Med* 323:878, 1990.

Dewhurst CJ: Frequency and severity of menopausal symptoms. In Campbell S, editor: *The management of the menopause and post-menopausal years*, Baltimore, 1976, University Park Press.

Dupont WD, Page DL, Rogers LW, Parl FF: Influence of exogenous estrogens, proliferative breast disease, and other variables on breast cancer risk, *Cancer* 63:948, 1989.

Erlik Y, Meldrum DR, Judd HL: Estrogen levels in postmenopausal women with hot flashes, *Obstet Gynecol* 59:403, 1982.

Ettinger B, Cann C, Genant HK: Menopausal bone loss: effects of conjugated oestrogen and/or high calcium diet, *Maturitas* 6:108, 1984.

Falkeborn M, Persson I, Terent A, et al: Hormone replacement therapy and the risk of stroke, *Arch Intern Med* 153:1201, 1993.

Federation C, Schwartz D, Mayaux MJ: Female fecundity as a function of age: results of artificial insemination in 2193 nulliparous women with azoospermic husbands, *N Engl J Med* 306:404, 1982.

Gallagher JC, Riggs BL, DeLuca HF: Effect of estrogen on calcium absorption and serum vitamin D metabolites in postmenopausal osteoporosis, *J Clin Endocrinol Metab* 51:1359, 1980.

Gillet J, Andre G, Faguer B, et al: Induction of amenorrhea during hormone replacement therapy; optimal micronized progesterone dose. A multicenter study, *Maturitas* 19:103, 1994.

Gordon WE, Hermann HW, Hunter DC: Safety and efficacy of micronized estradiol vaginal cream, *South Med J* 72:1252, 1979.

Grady D, Gebretsadik T, Kerlikowske K, et al: Hormone replacement therapy and endometrial cancer risk: a meta-analysis, *Obstet Gynecol* 85:304, 1995.

Greendale G, Barrett-Connor E, Edelstein S, et al: Lifetime leisure exercise and osteoporosis: the Rancho Bernardo study, *Am J Epidemiol* 141:951, 1995.

Grodstein F, Stampfer MJ: Estrogen replacement therapy and cardiovascular disease, *Menopausal Medicine: A newsletter of the American Fertility Society*, 1994, p. 2.

Haas S, Walsh B, Evans S, et al: The effect of transdermal estradiol on hormone and metabolic dynamics over a six-week period, *Obstet Gynecol* 71:671, 1988.

Hegarty V, Stewart B: The cost of calcium supplements, *N Engl J Med* 319:449, 1988 (letter).

Henderson BE, Ross RK, Paganini-Hill A, Mack TM: Estrogen use and cardiovascular disease, *Am J Obstet Gynecol* 154:1181, 1986.

Herrinton LJ, Weiss NS: Postmenopausal unopposed estrogens characteristics of use in relation to the risk of endometrial carcinoma, *Ann Epidemiol* 3:308, 1993.

Hillard T, Whitcroft S, Marsh M, et al: Long-term effects of transdermal and oral hormone replacement therapy on postmenopausal bone loss. *Osteoporos Int* 4:341, 1994.

Hilton P: The use of intravaginal oestrogen cream in genuine stress incontinence, *Br J Obstet Gynaecol* 90:940, 1983.

Hirvonen E, Malkonen M, Manninen V: Effects of different progestogens on lipoproteins during postmenopausal replacement therapy, *N Engl J Med* 304:560, 1981.

Hirvonen E, Salmi T, Puolakka J, et al: Can progestin be limited to every third month only in postmenopausal women taking estrogen? *Maturitas* 21:39, 1995.

Holbrook TL, Barrett-Connor E, Wingard DL: Dietary calcium and risk of hip fracture: 14-year prospective population study, *Lancet* 2:1046, 1988.

Hutchinson TA, Polansky SM, Feinstein AR: Post-menopausal oestrogens protect against fracture of hip and distal radius. A case-control study, *Lancet* 2:705, 1979.

Jaszmann LJB: Epidemiology of the climacteric syndrome. In Campbell S, editor: *The management of the menopause and post-menopause years*, Baltimore, 1976, University Park Press.

Judd HL: Hormonal dynamics associated with menopause, *Clin Obstet Gynecol* 19:775, 1976.

Kelly PJ, Pocock NA, Sambrook PN, Eisman JA: Age and menopause-related changes in indices of bone turnover, *J Clin Endocrinol Metab* 69:9960, 1989.

Kinsey AC, Pomeroy WB, Martin CE, Gebhard PH: *Sexual behavior in the human female*, Philadelphia, 1953, Saunders.

Krailo MD, Pike MC: Estimation of the distribution of age at natural menopause from prevalence data, *Am J Epidemiol* 117:356, 1983.

Krolner B, Toft B, Nielsen SP, Tondevold E: Physical exercise as prophylaxis against involutional vertebral bone loss: a controlled trial, *Clin Sci* 64:541, 1983.

Kronenberg F: Hot flashes: epidemiology and physiology, *Ann N Y Acad Sci* 592:52, 1990.

Leiblum S, Bachmann G, Kemmann E, et al: Vaginal atrophy in the postmenopausal woman: the importance of sexual activity and hormones, *JAMA* 249:2195, 1983.

Lindsay R, Aitken JM, Anderson JB, et al: Long-term prevention of postmenopausal osteoporosis by oestrogen, *Lancet* 2:1038, 1976.

Lindsay R, Hart DM, Clark DM: The minimum effective dose of estrogen for prevention of postmenopausal bone loss, *Obstet Gynecol* 63:759, 1984.

Lindsay R, Hart DM, Purdie D, et al: Comparative effects of oestrogen and a progestogen on bone loss in postmenopausal women, *Clin Sci Mol Med* 54:193, 1978.

Lindsay R, Hart DM, Purdie D, et al: Prevention of spinal osteoporosis in oophorectomized women, *Lancet* 2:1141, 1980.

Lipid Research Clinics Program, Results LRCCPPT: Reduction and incidence of coronary heart disease, *JAMA* 251:351, 1984.

Lobo RA: Estrogen and cardiovascular disease, *Ann N Y Acad Sci* 592:286, 1990.

Longcope C: Hormone dynamics at the menopause, *Ann N Y Acad Sci* 592:21, 1990.

Longcope C, Hunter R, Franz C: Steroid secretion by the postmenopausal ovary, *Am J Obstet Gynecol* 138:564, 1980.

Luckey MM, Meier DE, Mandeli JP, et al: Radial and vertebral bone density in white and black women: evidence for racial differences in premenopausal bone homeostasis, *J Clin Endocrinol Metab* 69:762, 1989.

Magos AL, Brewster E, Singh R, et al: The effects of norethisterone in postmenopausal women on estrogen replacement therapy: a model for the premenstrual syndrome, *Br J Obstet Gynaecol* 93:1290, 1986.

Magos AL, Brincat M, Studd JWW, et al: Amenorrhea and endometrial atrophy with continuous oral estrogen and progestogen therapy in postmenopausal women, *Obstet Gynecol* 65:496, 1985.

Marcus R, Cann C, Madvig P, et al: Menstrual function and bone mass in elite women distance runners: endocrine and metabolic features, *Ann Intern Med* 102:158, 1985.

Masters WH, Johnson VE: *Human sexual response*. Boston, 1966, Little, Brown.

Matkovic V, Chestnut C: Genetic factors and acquisition of bone mass, *J Bone Min Res* 2(suppl 1):329, 1987 (abstract).

Matkovic V, Fontana D, Chesnut C: Influence of calcium on peak bone mass: a 10-month follow-up, *J Bone Min Res* 2(suppl 1):339, 1987 (abstract).

Meldrum DR, Tataryn IV, Frumar AM, et al: Gonadotropins, estrogens, and adrenal steroids during the menopausal hot flash, *Clin Endocrinol Metab* 50:685, 1980 (abstract).

Melis GB, Gambacciani M, Cagnacci A, et al: Effects of the dopamine antagonist Veralipride on hot flushes and luteinizing hormone secretion in postmenopausal women, *Obstet Gynecol* 72:688, 1988.

Nachtigall LE, Nachtigall RH, Nachtigall RD, Beckman EM: Estrogen replacement therapy. I: A 10-year prospective study in the relationship to osteoporosis, *Obstet Gynecol* 53:277, 1979.

Neven P, DeMuylder X, Belle YV, et al: Tamoxifen and the uterus and endometrium, *Lancet* 1:375, 1989 (letter).

Nguyen T, Jones G, Sambrook P, et al: Effects of estrogen exposure and reproductive factors on bone mineral density and osteoporotic fractures, *J Clin Endocrinol Metab* 80:2709, 1995.

Orwoll ES, Ferar J, Oviatt SK, et al: Swimming exercise and bone mass. In Christiansen C, Johanson JS, Riis RJ, editors: *Osteoporosis*, Viborg, Sweden, 1987, Norhaven.

Ottosson UB, Johansson BG, Schoultz BV: Subfractions of high-density lipoprotein cholesterol during estrogen replacement therapy: a comparison between progestogens and natural progesterone, *Am J Obstet Gynecol* 151:746, 1985.

Paganini-Hill A, Ross RK, Henderson BE: Postmenopausal oestrogen treatment and stroke: a prospective study, *Br Med J* 297:519, 1988.

Pang SCE, Lozano K, Cedars MI, et al: Two-year prospective, randomized study of transdermal estradiol (Estraderm patch) use, with and without cyclic progestin (P), in postmenopausal women (PMW) (abstract 64). Presented at the Society for Gynecologic Investigation, 37th Annual Meeting, St Louis, 1990.

Persky H, Dreisbach L, Miller WR, et al: The relation of plasma androgen levels to sexual behaviours and attitudes of women, *Psychosom Med* 44:305, 1982.

Peterson HB, Lee NC, Rubin GL: Genital neoplasia. In Mishell DR Jr, editor: *Menopause: physiology and pharmacology*, Chicago, 1987, Year Book Medical.

Pocock NA, Eisman JA, Yeates MG, et al: Physical fitness is a major determinant of femoral neck and lumbar spine bone mineral density, *J Clin Invest* 78:618, 1986.

Powles TJ: Tamoxifen and oestrogen replacement, *Lancet* 2:48, 1990 (letter).

Ravnikar V: Physiology and treatment of hot flashes, *Obstet Gynecol* 75:3S, 1990.

Reed T: Urethral pressure profile in continent women from childbirth to old age, *Acta Obstet Gynecol Scand* 59:331, 1980.

Ribot C, Tremolliers F, Pouilles J, et al: Preventive effects of transdermal administration of 17 β-estradiol on postmenopausal bone loss: a 2-year prospective study, *Obstet Gynecol* 75:42S, 1990.

Richardson SJ, Nelson JF: Follicular depletion during the menopausal transition, *Am J Obstet Gynecol* 151:746, 1990.

Richardson SJ, Nelson JF: Follicular depletion during the menopausal transition, *Ann N Y Acad Sci* 592:13, 1990.

Richelson LS, Wahner HW, Melton LJ III, Riggs BL: Relative contributions of aging and estrogen deficiency to postmenopausal bone loss, *N Engl J Med* 311:1273, 1984.

Rockwell J, Sorensen A, Baker S, et al: Weight training decreases vertebral bone density in premenopausal women: a prospective study, *J Clin Endocrinol Metab* 71:988, 1990.

Rodriguez C, Calle E, Coates R, et al: Estrogen replacement therapy and fatal ovarian cancer, *Am J Epidemiol* 141:828, 1995.

Rosenberg L, Hennekens CH, Rosner B, et al: Early menopause and the risk of myocardial infarction, *Am J Obstet Gynecol* 139:47, 1981.

Rubin GL, Peterson HB, Lee NC, et al: Estrogen replacement therapy and the risk of endometrial cancer: remaining controversies, *Am J Obstet Gynecol* 162:148, 1990.

Sarrel PM: Sex problems after menopause: a study of 50 couples treated in a sex counseling programme, *Maturitas* 4:231, 1982.

Sarrel PM: Sexuality in the middle years, *Obstet Gynecol Clin North Am* 14:49, 1987.

Sarrel PM: Sexuality and menopause, *Obstet Gynecol* 75:26S, 1990.

Sarrel PM, Whitehead MI: Sex and menopause: defining the issues, *Maturitas* 7:217, 1985.

Schiff I, Tulchinsky D, Cramer D, Ryan KJ: Oral medroxyprogesterone in the treatment of postmenopausal symptoms, *JAMA* 244:1442, 1980.

Semmens JP, Wagner G: Estrogen deprivation and vaginal function in postmenopausal women, *JAMA* 248:445, 1982.

Sherwin BB: Changes in sexual behavior as a function of plasma sex steroid levels in postmenopausal women, *Maturitas* 7:225, 1985.

Sherwin BB, Gelfand MM, Brender W: Androgen enhances sexual motivation in females: a prospective, crossover study of sex steroid administration in the surgical menopause, *Psychosom Med* 47:339, 1985.

Sillero-Arenas M, Delgado-Rodriguez M, Radigues-Canteras R, et al: Menopausal hormone replacement therapy and breast cancer: a meta-analysis, *Obstet Gynecol* 79:286, 1992.

Simkin A, Ayalon J, Leichter I: Increased trabecular bone density due to bone-loading exercises in postmenopausal osteoporotic women, *Calcif Tissue Int* 40:59, 1987.

Sitruk-Ware R, de Palacios PI: Oestrogen replacement therapy and cardiovascular disease in post-menopausal women: a review, *Maturitas* 11:259, 1989.

Spira A: The decline of fertility with age, *Maturitas* 1(suppl):15, 1988.

Stampfer MJ, Colditz GA, Willett WC: Menopause and heart disease, *Ann N Y Acad Sci* 592:193, 1990.

Stanczyk FZ, Shoupe D, Nunez V, et al: A randomized comparison of non-oral estradiol delivery in postmenopausal women, *Am J Obstet Gynecol* 159:1540, 1988.

Stanford J, Weiss N, Voigt L, et al: Combined estrogen and progestin hormone replacement therapy in relation to risk of breast cancer in middle-aged women, *JAMA* 274:137, 1995.

Steinberg KK, Thacker SB, Smith SJ, et al: A meta-analysis of the effect of estrogen replacement therapy on the risk of breast cancer, *JAMA* 265:1985, 1991.

Stevenson J, Whitehead M, Padwick M, et al: Dietary intake of calcium and postmenopausal bone loss, *Br Med J* 297:15, 1988.

Stevenson JC: Pathogenesis, prevention, and treatment of osteoporosis, *Obstet Gynecol* 75(suppl):36, 1990.

Stevenson JC, Cust MP, Ganger KF, et al: Effects of transdermal versus oral hormone replacement therapy on bone density in spine and proximal femur in postmenopausal women, *Lancet* 335:265, 1990.

Stevenson JC, Lees B, Devenport M, et al: Determinants of bone density in normal women: risk factors for future osteoporosis? *Br Med J* 198:924, 1989.

Sullivan JM, Zwagg RV, Hughes JP, et al: Estrogen replacement and coronary artery disease. Effect on survival in postmenopausal women, *Arch Intern Med* 150:2557, 1990.

Thompson SG, Meade TW, Greenberg G: The use of hormonal replacement therapy and the risk of stroke and myocardial infarction in women, *J Epidemiol Community Health* 43:173, 1989.

Tobacman JK, Tucker MA, Kase R, et al: Intraabdominal carcinomatosis after prophylactic oophorectomy in ovarian cancer prone families, *Lancet* 2:795, 1982.

Turken S, Siris E, Seldin D, et al: Effects of tamoxifen on spinal bone density in women with breast cancer, *J Natl Cancer Inst* 81:1086, 1989.

Udoff L, Langenberg P, Adashi E: Combined continuous hormone replacement therapy: a critical review, *Obstet Gynecol* 86:306, 1995.

Vollman RF: *The menstrual cycle*, Philadelphia, 1977, Saunders.

Walsh BW, Sacks FM, Schiff I: Postmenopausal estrogen treatment lowers plasma low-density lipoprotein (LDL) concentrations by accelerating LDL catabolism (abstract 399). Presented at the Society for Gynecologic Investigation, 37th Annual Meeting, St Louis, 1990.

Weiss NS, Ure CL, Ballard JH, et al: Decreased risk of fractures of the hip and lower forearm with postmenopausal use of estrogen, *N Engl J Med* 303:1195, 1980.

Whitehead MI, Fraser D: The effects of estrogens and progestogens on the endometrium: modern approach to treatment, *Obstet Gynecol Clin North Am* 14:299, 1987.

Whitehead MI, Fraser D, Schenkel L, et al: Transdermal administration of oestrogen/progestagen hormone replacement therapy, *Lancet* 335:310, 1990.

Whitehead MI, Hillard TC, Crook D: The role and use of progestogens, *Obstet Gynecol* 75:59S, 1990.

Whitehead MI, McQueen J, King RJB, Campbell S: Endometrial histology and biochemistry in climacteric women during oestrogen and oestrogen/progestogen therapy, *J R Soc Med* 72:322, 1979.

Whitehead MI, Townsend PT, Pryse-Davies J, et al: Effects of various types and dosages of progestogens on the postmenopausal endometrium, *J Reprod Med* 27:539, 1982.

Whittaker PG, Morgan MRA, Dean PDG, et al: Serum equilin, oestrone, and oestradiol levels in postmenopausal women receiving conjugated equine oestrogens ("Premarin"), *Lancet* 1:14, 1980.

Williams D, Voigt B, Fu Y, et al: Assessment of less than monthly progestin therapy in postmenopausal women given estrogen replacement, *Obstet Gynecol* 84:787, 1994.

Witteman JCM, Grobbee DE, Kok FJ, et al: Increased risk of atherosclerosis in women after the menopause, *Br Med J* 289:642, 1989.

Yen SSC, Martin PL, Burnier AM, et al: Circulating estradiol, estrone and gonadotropin levels following the administration of orally active 17β-estradiol in postmenopausal women, *J Clin Endocrinol Metab* 40:518, 1975.

Youngs DD: Some misconceptions concerning the menopause, *Obstet Gynecol* 75:881, 1990.

CHAPTER 7

The Preoperative and Postoperative Visit

ROBERT F. PORGES

THE PREOPERATIVE VISIT
    Establishing Rapport
    History and Physical Examination
    Record Keeping
    Discussion After the Examination

SECOND OPINION
ADDITIONAL RESPONSIBILITIES
    RESULTING FROM THE
    PREOPERATIVE VISIT
THE POSTOPERATIVE VISIT

Practicing obstetrician-gynecologists may expect to spend an increasing proportion of their professional time treating ambulatory patients. The initiating steps taken in the office to prepare a patient for admission to the hospital for surgery are crucial to the success of the venture. For many years clinicians held to the belief that work in one's private office was conducted with less control, scrutiny, and paperwork than activities conducted over a comparable time within a hospital setting. If ever there was truth in that statement, it is less the case today. Office documents are subject to subpoena, and although we do not like to concede that threat of legal action affects the quality of our efforts, work well done and well documented will pay dividends in the distant future when dealing with patient queries and care, lawyers, insurance companies, and regulatory bodies.

Increasingly the interaction between an ambulatory patient and health care providers will require compliance with standardized formats. Medical practices are managed now more frequently by groups of caregivers than by individual physicians.

THE PREOPERATIVE VISIT
Establishing Rapport

Impressions gained from the patient's initial visit tend to persist. Patients expect their physicians to be dressed as professionals. A scrub suit is not appropriate attire for the office. The doctor's hands should be clean and the nails well groomed. One's desk should not be cluttered and the patient should be seated comfortably without glare. The doctor's face should not be hidden in shadow. All but emergency phone calls should be held so that the patient feels she has the physician's full attention and concern.

Although the clientele in any given office or clinic population draws frequently from an economically consistent and predictable range of ethnic backgrounds, initial appearances may not accurately disclose educational background or environmental exposures. It is helpful to know the patient's background, but the doctor should guard against classifying patients according to preconceived stereotypes. Every patient expects and deserves an unvarying display of calm manner, candor, concern, and a sense of responsibility in the individual who is about to be entrusted with her life in the performance of a surgical procedure. The gynecologist should be prepared to respond to this challenge.

History and Physical Examination

The manner in which a medical history is taken, whether by nurse, physician's assistant, physician, or questionnaire, is of consequence in establishing rapport. In certain cases patients may resent discussing intimate details with personnel other than the doctor. The volume of patients seen in an office and community practice will suggest the most appropriate method. The specifics of taking a medical history and performing a physical examination are best described elsewhere; only several generalizations and a few suggestions will be listed here, in the context of their value for a preoperative visit. Language barriers may demand the presence of an interpreter, but patients generally should have the opportunity to speak privately with the doctor, or subtle family dynamics may affect the accuracy of the history. It is imperative to date the onset of symptoms and to clarify what other medical personnel have been consulted and what other health-related facilities have been visited in connection with the particular illness. For example, the necessity to seek out old operative and pathology records makes it important to learn if the patient has used other names in the past.

Evaluating subjective symptoms on an initial visit may be difficult. It may be helpful to ask the woman to compare degrees of pain with other situations in life, such as labor, appendicitis, or even a toothache. Abnormal vaginal bleeding is a frequent symptom in women preparing to have gynecologic surgery. Although it may not be possible to estimate accurately the volume of menstrual bleeding, the patient may usefully act as her own control. If in recent months she has bled longer and more copiously than she is accustomed to, a diagnosis of menorrhagia is warranted. The details should be well documented. When does the patient date the onset, what sort of progression, what events made it better of worse? What about the use of aspirin, or aspirin-containing compounds? What of the role of oral contraceptives? Is an intrauterine device (IUD) in place? Could, perhaps, an IUD be in place without the patient being aware of it? A history of bleeding during or after previous surgical procedures is critical in any preoperative evaluation. Women who have a history of profuse menstrual bleeding and a hematocrit in their mid twenties may have other nongynecologic reasons for anemia, such as thalassemia or bleeding from the gastrointestinal tract, that should not be overlooked. Most patients may expect to receive prophylactic antibiotics during their surgery, so previous reactions to different antibiotics should be carefully recorded. Under most jurisdictions mandatory testing for human immunodeficiency virus (HIV) is not permitted. Although the standard precautions against infection must be applied uniformly, certain information in the history help define a patient's status and may suggest the likelihood of greater risks. Nothing prevents the physician from offering the patient the opportunity to be tested.

Record Keeping

Handwritten notes on office charts are no longer acceptable. Whatever is not already in an electronic form should at the very least be typewritten. All of us have shared the experience of receiving office records from another physician in totally illegible handwriting. As medical practice shifts to larger groups, with multiple caregivers sharing responsibilities, standardized medical record keeping will become imperative. Justification for operative therapy normally originates in the clinic chart and is subject to routine retrieval by insurance companies and government regulatory agencies. Most hospital medical charting soon will become computer compliant, with an option for brief narrative summarization. Office records should be formatted for maximum clarity because it may be anticipated that in the near future some regimentation of office practice will be mandated; standardization of forms will be only the first step. Paradoxically, the universal practice of faxing clinical information, while providing an element of efficiency to communication, has added much clutter to our records and increased the mass of paper.

After a recommendation for surgery the doctor may expect to receive a call from the insurance company. The initial interrogation by a nurse consists of a standard algorithm of data, not unfamiliar to the gynecologist. What are the results of any biopsy? Has the patient been on hormonal therapy? What did the ultrasound show? What is the size of the uterus? Her hematocrit? It is desirable for the doctor's records to list or highlight the answers to these standard questions to make the inevitable process of compliance more efficient. Adherence to such a format will also alert the gynecologist to anticipate a disallowance if certain standard criteria are not being met. Occasionally the indication for surgery may be less conventional, and it may be necessary then for the physician to speak with the insurance company's physician reviewer. For example, although a patient's myomas may not be of impressive size and her hematocrit may be within normal range, her discomfort from menstrual cramping may be truly disabling, despite hormonal or analgesic medication. If insurance coverage is withheld in such a patient the treating gynecologist may wish to formalize the role of the physician representing the insurance company by entering his or her name and state license number in the patient's record.

Only a minority of practicing physicians are able to retrieve the names of patients to whom surgery was recommended but not performed. Did the patient develop an intercurrent illness precluding surgery, did she move to another town, did she elect to be treated medically, or did she die? No patient record is complete without documenting the follow-up of the recommendation for surgery.

Discussion after the Examination

In practice, the history and physical examination in an ambulatory setting are followed by a discussion with the patient, which may also include members of her family or support partners. The physician should lead the discussion to a declaration of a diagnosis or presumptive diagnosis. Depending on the urgency of the patient's complaints and the gravity of the condition, additional diagnostic tests may be required to corroborate a presumptive diagnosis or to rule out other possible diagnoses. If the diagnosis is not certain, a discussion of alternative treatments may or may not be appropriate at this stage. If the diagnosis has been established with reasonable certainty, it is imperative to state the diagnosis to the patient or a member of her family. The declaration of a diagnosis should be made in an even tone and in as reassuring a manner as possible. The physician must recognize when anxiety may interfere with communication, and repetition may be necessary.

The conclusions at the end of this discussion may take several forms. One may recommend medical or surgical management, further testing, consultation with another physician, or routine follow-up. A recommendation for surgical treatment usually will result in ordering presurgical testing and possibly consultation with physicians from other services. From the patient's perspective, she may acquiesce, decline surgical therapy, seek another opinion, or have surgery at another facility. These steps are summarized in Fig. 7-1.

Further discussions with family members, friends, or business associates

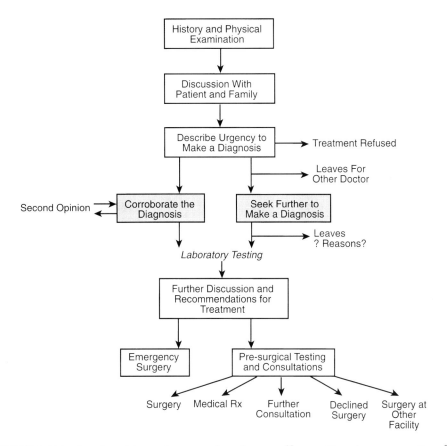

FIGURE 7-1. An algorithm of steps taken in an office setting in preparation for surgery may take the following form: (1) A history is taken, partly by a paramedical individual, partly by the physician. Data are recorded on a prepared form, on a computer screen, or in narrative form. (2) A physical examination, including vital signs, breasts, heart, lungs, abdomen, and pelvis, is done by the physician. Again, the facts are recorded. (3) Next follows a discussion with the patient and perhaps a member of her family concerning the diagnosis. If the diagnosis is clear and unequivocal, one may move next to a discussion of treatment. If the diagnosis is only reasonably clear, one must first prepare the patient for the possible degree of urgency necessary to make the diagnosis. (4) Between this step and the last stage several possible events may have taken place. Endometrial biopsies, computed tomography scans, magnetic resonance imaging, and blood tests may have been done. The patient may have seen another physician for a second opinion, or she may have elected simply not to return. Sadly, most clinicians lack the systems for follow-up of patients seen, in whom surgery was recommended, and who simply do not return or go to the operating room. An analysis of the reasons for attrition would be useful. The patient may have gone to another physician, where surgery may or may not have been done. Medical treatments may have been substituted for operative methods. The patient may have declined surgery for a variety of reasons, such as a different second opinion, fear, inability to take time out of a busy schedule (for an elective procedure), or competing family responsibilities (an ill spouse or child). Initial consultation by the patient with her insurance company is mandated.

that do not include the patient should be undertaken only under special circumstances, and preferably only with the patient's concurrence.

The patient should be led to respond to a surgeon's recommendations, allowing an informed evaluation of the risks, a comparison of the advantages and disadvantages of different operative and medical treatments, and the likelihood of success of the procedure, coupled with the chance of recurrence of the original condition. This is a difficult responsibility for the gynecologist to meet, and one that is carried out with greater or lesser consistency and competence, but certainly without any real outside control. Recently, recommendations have come from committees on quality assurance directed at an exposition of the risk versus benefit ratio. Ideally the dialogue between patient and doctor should be videotaped and analyzed. It is not my recommendation that this be done routinely, although in hindsight, when catastrophic events have occurred, the documentation is always most welcome. Not infrequently the physician may be well advised to probe the reactions of other members of the family or support group regarding their views on the impending surgery. It may be as important to convince the husband of the indications for surgery as the patient herself.

For example, a patient anticipating surgery for a defect in pelvic support needs the best information concerning the likelihood of success or the possibility of failure. No simple answer is available for these patients. Clearly, a physician is proscribed ethically from any guarantees of successful treatments. Most women will have heard from their friends and referring doctors of the distinct possibility of recurrence. Some women have become discouraged from pursuing operative treatment because of the bleak results described in the past. An informed discussion of possible outcomes and complications is required.

There are few indications in gynecology that require emergency surgery. Ruptured ectopic pregnancy, twisted adnexa, profuse hemorrhage from incomplete abortion or an aborting submucous myoma clearly fall into this category. A histologic diagnosis of an early, operable genital malignancy is an urgent indication for treatment in a patient in sufficiently good health whose life span would be compromised by excessive delay. Many other indications are clearly elective, such as dermoid cysts in young women, enlarging myomas in women approaching the menopause, or the discomfort and embarrassment of urinary stress incontinence. In deciding on gradations of severity, physicians must not allow personal biases to influence their recommendations. For example, how urgent an indication is infertility, or the inability to have coitus, or the threat of possible malignancy in a woman with a strong family history of ovarian cancer? It may be anticipated that patient and doctor will perceive the degree of urgency from different points of view. In those instances when a physician's view is at variance with that of his or her patient, as regards for example the indication to conduct an abortion, the physician is responsible to inform the patient of the availability of other facilities in the community or elsewhere. The transaction between a patient and her doctor is always unique. The drama is played out in the doctor's office but today involves hospital administrators, risk management analysts, insurance companies, health maintenance organizations, and federal and state regulators.

A variety of factors interact to determine the outcome of this transaction between patient and doctor. A willing patient and a doctor skilled in an operative procedure plus an available facility within which to do the operation do not alone establish the indication for surgery. Under ideal circumstances surgery results from an accurate history and physical examination by a physician with up-to-date knowledge of the variety of available operative and nonoperative treatments, leading to a diagnosis and recommendation that is perceived by the patient to be in her best interests. There are obvious economic pressures on the doctor to operate. More recently hospitals are under increasing pressure to admit more patients as their volume of patients declines. The needs of teaching services must be met. On the other hand, a physician may be reluctant to operate on a patient if she is deemed "litigious" or if the patient has hepatitis or HIV, which may threaten the physician's health consequent to the performance of surgery.

SECOND OPINION

In the background of every recommendation for surgical treatment for elective surgery has been the question of gain by the physician: a fee for the service. Recognition of this has contributed to an almost universal practice of obtaining a second opinion for the purpose of avoiding unnecessary surgery. Second opinions do not always prevent unnecessary surgery, or necessarily provide a saving to the insurance company. An appropriate referral for a second opinion should be offered by the gynecologist to corroborate a diagnosis or suggested treatment. The referral may serve as a deterrent later to legal action in the event of dissatisfaction or complications. Rather than by another gynecologist, a second opinion may be requested more appropriately of a pathologist in the event of a borderline lesion, or an internist or cardiologist to place in better perspective the balance between risk and benefit in a patient with special medical problems. We may reach a time, under capitated care, when second opinions will be sought by patients to refute the original physician's recommendation that surgery was *not* indicated.

ADDITIONAL RESPONSIBILITIES RESULTING FROM THE PREOPERATIVE VISIT

Same-day admissions have become the rule of the land. Diagnostic uncertainty, extensive medical problems, and special preparatory steps before the actual operation often used to require at least several additional days in the hospital, as did special radiographic studies, consultations with specialists, adjustment of insulin dosages, reduction of hypertension, and bowel preparation. Diagnostic studies must be ordered and coordinated in proper sequence; patients must be counseled regarding the need for the procedures and possible risks of dye studies. The results of each of these tests must be retrieved (often not an automatic event), reviewed, entered into the patient's chart, and the results transmitted to the patient. Medications may need to be adjusted, often in consultation with an internist, ordered from a variety of pharmacies each with different arrangements with insurance companies and health maintenance organizations (HMOs), and reasons for drug modification discussed with the patient or her care partner. The responsibility for virtually all of these preparations has shifted to the doctors' office staff.

The interactions between patient and doctor during a preoperative visit have undergone dramatic transformation. Indications for most elective gynecologic surgical procedures have become more stringent and standardized. A recommendation to admit a patient for an oophorectomy, myomectomy, or hysterectomy, for example, may be expected routinely to be challenged by the patient's HMO or insurance company.

Other factors may come between the patient and the physician. In medium-size towns and in cities patients have until recently enjoyed almost complete freedom of choice in the selection of their physician. Today, the physician being consulted may be the choice of a gatekeeper and not necessarily the physician who has treated other members of the family or friends. A patient's trust and confidence in a physician often precedes her initial office visit, based on the physician's reputation in the community. When reaching a decision for operative intervention, the patient's confidence has always been a vital trump card for the doctor.

After a recommendation for elective surgery, the patient will wish to discuss the situation with her significant other, parent, or guardian. Over the next several days the patient will begin the process of arranging her schedule for surgery. Often, this may result in a second visit, during which the patient will sign the necessary operative consents, appraise the office of her insurance status, and receive specific instructions regarding preoperative testing.

The patient also must be informed of what she may expect at preoperative testing. Blood samples will be drawn, a chest x-ray and electrocardiogram will be taken, the anesthesiologist will interview the patient, and a member of the house staff will introduce himself or herself to the patient. Presurgical testing may be carried out within the hospital, in an ambulatory setting, or at a site remote to the hospital. Under ideal circumstances the admitting hospital assumes a proprietary interest in the performance of presurgical testing and works in cooperation with the doctor's office staff to guarantee timely reporting of results both to the attending gynecologist and the anesthesiologist. Abnormal test results are flagged to help limit unscheduled cancellations of surgery, which leads to less than optimal utilization of operating room time. The additional administrative burdens on the doctor's office staff are substantial.

THE POSTOPERATIVE VISIT

Surgeons are vitally interested in the outcome of their operative procedures based on concern for their patient's welfare, pride in accomplishment, and intellectual curiosity. The physician may find it helpful to use a checklist for mandatory points to be addressed during the postoperative visit. Such a list should include documentation, wound healing, activities, diet, medications and drug reactions, insurance reimbursement, and follow-up.

Perhaps of primary importance is to document the resolution of the preoperative complaints. In the case of excessive bleeding from fibroid tumors of the uterus, one will not need, after removal of the uterus, to deal with the question at great length. If an operation was carried out for urinary stress incontinence or pelvic pain it will be more essential to record any change in symptoms. If objective testing (e.g., urodynamic studies) were carried out preoperatively, one will be interested in repeating some of the same battery of tests, to record again objectively any possible improvement. The indications for repeating such tests are questionable. If a patient, having been operated for urinary stress incontinence, is able to state postoperatively that she is much improved, is it valid to subject her to the risks and expense of testing? An accurate history and physical examination should suffice. For example, does the patient still require protective napkins? Is she able to play tennis without losing urine? Is there an increased tolerance for caffeine? Direct questioning should deal with the specific symptoms that led to the original surgical procedure. Urodynamic testing may need to be repeated in the event symptoms are unchanged or a recurrence develops.

The patient or her care partner should be informed of the actual surgical procedure performed. Details concerning which ovary was removed or whether any ovarian tissue remains should be specifically clarified. Whether an appendix or cervix remains should be stated. The patient should be informed about the prognosis for cure or the likelihood of recurrence. Operative dictations and pathology reports should be forwarded to referring physicians. Within the context of a casual discussion, the response of family members to the patient's recent hospitalization or illness may provide an impression regarding postoperative depression. Clues to the latter also may be gleaned from other historical facts, such as inability to sleep, fatigue, irritability, or reluctance to return to work. Specific referrals may become necessary, although reassurances by the gynecologist regarding the frequency of such symptoms and their common resolution often will provide the basis for a self-fulfilling prophesy. One should recognize that once the stress and fear of an impending operation have passed, the patient's recollection of preoperative events may change, and the original objectives of surgery will be viewed from a different vantage point.

Communication between the hospital record and the doctor's office chart is often poor. The office chart always should contain a copy of the operative dictation and the pathology report. Parenthetically, an operative report dictated more than 24 hours after the surgical procedure has little relevance. The surgeon must develop a routine for carrying out this vital chore at an appropriate time, usually before changing out of one's scrub suit and before talking to members of the patient's family.

The initial postoperative visit is usually scheduled between 2 and 6 weeks after a procedure. Questions are routinely directed toward symptoms related to the operative procedure, such as wound tenderness, bleeding, fever, hot flushes, resumption of normal bowel activity, urinary incontinence, or vaginal discharge. Among the valid concerns for the conscientious surgeon are the appearance and integrity of the wound. Today, prophylactic and therapeutic antibiotics may mask the presence of a wound infection and delay its appearance until after the time of the postoperative visit. Fortunately, wound breakdowns are an infrequent occurrence. When an incision heals by secondary intention the surgeon and the patient will come to know each other well, because of the need for frequent visits to debride and clean the incision site. Incisional hernias generally make an appearance much later than the initial postoperative visit. The patient should be reassured and made to understand that residual symptoms or postoperative discomfort will gradually abate within a reasonable period of time. Women look to their doctors for specific instructions in scheduling resumption of normal activities. Styles of practice vary considerably. Some physicians issue printed instructions on the smallest details; other advise patients, in good conscience, to use their own good judgment. A course between these extremes may be best, taking into careful consideration the nature of the patient's personality, dependence, intelligence, compulsiveness, anxiety, and so on. Often patients avoid asking questions about specific activities, either out of fear, embarrassment, or a false assumption that such activities are forever prohibited. Following most gynecologic surgery it is appropriate for the physician to provide guidelines for resumption of work, exercise, driving, walking up and down stairs, and sex, not necessarily in that order.

Dietary counseling may be in order. A major operative procedure may be recognized by the patient as a significant milestone, allowing changes or modulation of an existing dietary regime. For example, after a hysterectomy, many women will be advised to take hormone replacement, with subsequent increase in weight. It may be valid to point out that the increase in weight comes at a time when a woman's metabolism normally runs down, requiring caloric reduction simply to maintain weight at a stable level. Notwithstanding, hormones are often blamed for the increase in weight.

Medications being taken and prescribed should be reviewed. Did the patient exhibit any allergic reactions to any of her medications while in the hospital, or more specifically to anesthesia? Which medications have been discontinued, which are new, and which are on a maintenance schedule?

Hormone replacement therapy is a controversial subject. For a woman under age 55 who has been surgically castrated, avoidance of hormone replacement is justified only under specific indications, which should be explicitly documented on the record. Many women are sent home from the hospital on maintenance hormonal therapy. The postoperative visit is the appropriate time to discuss the continuation of these medications and to modify the existing regimen, possibly making changes in dosage or route of administration. Associated screening for breast tumors should always be discussed with patients receiving hormone replacement therapy.

Contraceptive guidance should not be overlooked. The postoperative visit often is the last opportunity for the physician to guide the busy woman who will soon return to work and may find valid reasons to miss her doctor's appointments.

The requirements for follow-up vary depending on the original condition. For tumor surveillance, the patient usually will be on a more rigid schedule, which often will be shared with an oncologist or radiation therapist. Whenever a patient is seen by different groups of doctors it is essential to clarify the division of labor (e.g., which group is responsible for ordering a computed tomography scan, doing an internal exam, pap smears, CA-125s). Among groups of physicians who have worked closely together for several years, these items will fall into place routinely. It should not be taken for granted, and the patient should be given an outline of local protocol (who does she call for abdominal pain, a urinary tract infection, neurologic symptoms, etc.?).

Patients with benign diseases must also be followed at regular intervals. It is important to know when fibroids recur after a myomectomy, when endometriomas reappear, when urinary incontinence recurs after surgery, or when the vaginal vault prolapses after a hysterectomy. Without specific instructions for follow-up visits when complications arise or recurrences appear, patients will seek out other doctors for their care. A knowledge of how patients fare over the long term should complement technical virtuosity.

Laboratory follow-up may include, for example, a hematocrit after any operative procedure; chorionic gonadotropin titers after early pregnancy loss and ectopic pregnancies; or urinary cultures after an indwelling catheter. Evaluation of hormonal activity after hysterectomy may be significant. Even in those cases where the patient will be referred back to her regular gynecologist, an additional follow-up visit beyond the first postoperative check is often desirable. Although this may take place within 4 to 6 months, one must recognize that this interval of time is insufficient to evaluate the success of operations for pelvic support defects or urinary incontinence.

The most sensitive discussions at the time of the postoperative visit concern complications that may have occurred as a direct result of surgery. These incidents may include some from which the patient has recovered completely and that are of no lingering significance, others from which she may reasonably be expected soon to recover, and others of a serious and permanent nature that will result in lasting damage. Examples include excessive loss of blood and the need for transfusions; hoarseness after traumatic endotracheal intubation; inadvertent endotracheal intubation of the esophagus, with tardy recognition and resultant brain damage; fistula formation, with the need for subsequent repair; wound infections and dehiscence; and myocardial infarction. One could describe many more. A frank exposition of the facts, consistent with information available in the hospital record, is helpful. One must be extremely cautious in accepting blame for a complication beyond recognizing that accidents are often unavoidable. At the merest hint of litigation, dissatisfaction on the part of the patient, or a bad outcome, the physician is well advised, in fact *required*, to communicate promptly with his or her insurance carrier and the hospital risk-management committee.

Discussions will arise regarding the doctor's fee. The physician may complain that payment of the fee is overdue. The patient may complain that the fee is excessive. The patient may plead hardship, to which the doctor may respond in a number of ways. A schedule of payments over a period of time may be worked out, or the physician may refer the patient to the office manager. Reduction of a patient's fee, as a courtesy, should never be presented to suggest that the treatment was flawed or as an admission of blame. On the other hand, reducing a patient's fee in response to conditions of hardship will in no way hurt the doctor's reputation in the community.

A desire to maintain a close bond with our patients must be tempered by the understanding that patients who reside at an inconvenient distance may be cared for as well by their family physicians or internists. Referring a patient back to her source is proper etiquette. Referrals to other physicians are made more appropriately by the original referring doctor.

BIBLIOGRAPHY

ACOG Technical Bulletin no 111: *Prophylactic oophorectomy*, Dec 1987.

ACOG Technical Bulletin no 136: *Ethical decision making in obstetrics and gynecology*, Nov 1989 (available through ACOG Resource Center, 409 12th Street, SW, Washington, DC 20024-2188).

Evaluation and management documentation guidelines, Medicare News Brief 95-6, May 1995.

Gambone JC, Lench JB, Slesinski MJ, et al: Validation of hysterectomy indications and the quality assurance process, instruments and methods, *Obstet Gynecol* 73:1045, 1989.

Jacobs JA: Preoperative evaluation of the gynecologic patient. In Jacobs JA, Gast MJ, editors: *Practical gynecology*, Norwalk, Conn, 1994, Appleton & Lange.

Standards for obstetric-gynecologic services, ed 7, Washington, DC, 1989, American College of Obstetricians and Gynecologists.

CHAPTER 8

Subjective Disorders: Dysmenorrhea, Chronic Pelvic Pain, and Premenstrual Syndrome

JOHN F. STEEGE

Although they are probably different from each other in etiology, the disorders discussed in this chapter present similar dilemmas to the clinician, hence their discussion together. Dysmenorrhea, chronic pelvic pain, and premenstrual syndrome have in common significant difficulties in assessment because the severity of symptoms in each case defies objective measurement. Evaluation relies extensively on clinical judgment, and treatment is often multifactorial, especially in more severely affected women.

DYSMENORRHEA

The discovery of prostaglandins and their role in the physiology of dysmenorrhea radically changed the diagnosis and treatment of this common disorder. Before this discovery, the literature emphasized the role of psychologic factors in discomforts associated with an otherwise "normal" physiologic process. Medications that reduce prostaglandin production or block their actions are so effective that such considerations are of clinical interest primarily when pain itself is refractory to treatment or the behavioral impairment associated with the pain seems disproportionate.

Clinical Features

Primary dysmenorrhea. In the absence of pelvic pathology, painful menstrual cramps are termed *primary dysmenorrhea*. About 25% of women report severe menstrual cramps, and about 10% of women regularly miss work because of dysmenorrhea, at significant economic cost. It is most common in younger women, declining in prevalence after 30 years of age.

Dysmenorrhea is usually described as cramping pain and most often can be readily distinguished by the patient from bladder or intestinal cramps. Radiation to the lower portion of the back and anteromedial aspect of the thighs is common. Intrauterine pressure during cramps may reach 120 to 150 mm Hg, significantly above the levels seen in active labor.

Painful menstruation usually begins when regular ovulatory cycles become established. Most often, cramps are worst during the first 24 to 48 hours and rapidly taper thereafter. Primary dysmenorrhea is often but not always relieved by vaginal delivery. Dysmenorrhea that gradually worsens in severity or duration over time is often a sign of organic pathology.

Secondary dysmenorrhea. Menstrual cramps occurring in the presence of organic disease are termed *secondary dysmenorrhea*. Any of the associated organic conditions may mimic primary dysmenorrhea by appearing in teenagers, and cramps may certainly have both primary and secondary components.

Etiology

Primary dysmenorrhea. Excessive uterine contractions are associated with increased production and release of prostaglandins, primarily prostaglandin (PG) $F_{2\alpha}$. Increased production of leukotrienes and vasopressin may play a role, as may diminished release of prostacyclin.

Cervical stenosis may aggravate menstrual discomfort, but only as an acquired condition secondary to infection, cervical trauma, or cryotherapy.

Secondary dysmenorrhea.

Endometriosis. Although menstruation may indeed be painless in the presence of even severe endometriosis, the majority of women with this disease report progressively worsening dysmenorrhea. The severity of pain does not correlate with the amount of disease present, which perhaps attests to the complexity of both endometriosis and pain perception itself. In an

individual patient, however, the return of dysmenorrhea after treatment c.
warn of regrowth of disease.

Pelvic adhesions. Increased dysmenorrhea is seen in association with
chronic pelvic inflammatory disease (PID) and postsurgical adhesive
disease. A physiologic mechanism for this is not apparent. In the case of
PID, cyclic alterations in immunologic defenses may occur, but the
relationship of these changes to dysmenorrhea is uncertain because clinical
studies have not detected regularly occurring increases or changes in
intrauterine or intrapelvic bacterial populations in association with
dysmenorrhea.

Adenomyosis. In women in the fourth and fifth decades of life,
increasing dysmenorrhea is often associated with the presence of endometrial glands deep within the myometrium, or adenomyosis. It is uncertain
whether this alters prostaglandin production or stimulates increased
myometrial activity on a more mechanical basis. A significant premenstrual
increase in uterine size may suggest the presence of this condition.

Leiomyomas. Uterine fibroids have long been associated with increased
menstrual pain, although the mechanism is uncertain.

Other. Cervical stenosis, flexion of the cervix on the uterus, and
retroversion of the uterus have been anecdotally mentioned as causes of
dysmenorrhea, with uncertain documentation. Logically, any significant
obstruction to this flow could increase the pain because increased volume
of menstrual flow increases menstrual cramps.

Management

Nonsteroidal antiinflammatory drugs. Since their introduction over the
past two decades, nonsteroidal antiinflammatory drugs (NSAIDs) have
changed dramatically the treatment of dysmenorrhea (Table 8-1). Further,
their success compelled revision of prevailing etiologic theories, with
deemphasis of psychologic factors. To be fair, it is unclear why some women
produce excess prostaglandins in the endometrium, and a brief review of
the stimuli that can augment the prostaglandin synthetic pathway (including stress and many of its chemical mediators) leaves room for the
hypothesis that such overproduction may be in part mediated by psychophysiologic factors. However, the therapeutic success of these agents allows
the clinician to surrender the search for an etiologic connection between
psychologic events and dysmenorrhea, instead separately directing attention to physical and emotional complaints as it seems clinically appropriate.

With less potent NSAIDs such as aspirin, beginning treatment several
days before the onset of menses seems to improve results, but at the potential cost of increased gastric irritation. More potent agents, such as
mefenamic acid, are often effective even if dosage begins when menstruation starts.

TABLE 8-1. Nonsteroidal antiinflammatory drugs commonly prescribed for dysmenorrhea

Drug	Loading dose	Maintenance dose	Frequency
Ibuprofen	–	200-800 mg	q4h
Naproxen	500 mg	250 mg	q6-8h
Mefenamic acid	500 mg	250 mg	q6h
Aspirin	–	650 mg	q4h

Oral contraceptives. Steroid contraceptives are highly effective: they reduce or eliminate cramps in up to 80% of users. When they are otherwise appropriate for contraceptive purposes, oral contraceptives (OCs) are the birth control method of first choice for women with dysmenorrhea.

If OCs or NSAIDs fail to relieve dysmenorrhea, or if cramps progressively worsen after a time of good relief over months or years, the clinician should suspect endometriosis. At the same time, good relief of dysmenorrhea by these agents does not eliminate the possibility that endometriosis may be present.

Laparoscopy. Although initially intended as a diagnostic instrument, the laparoscope has matured into a powerful therapeutic device as well. Laser ablation of endometriosis is probably a reasonable sequel to laparoscopic diagnosis, although trials (open or blind) comparing this method with standard hormonal treatment are lacking.

In the patient with dysmenorrhea refractory to the agents discussed previously and with a laparoscopically negative pelvis, laser ablation of the medial two thirds of each uterosacral ligament proximal to the uterus (laparoscopic uretosacral nerve ablation [LUNA] procedure) provides significant relief at 1-year follow-up in 60% to 70% of patients in open trials and 45% in one single-blind controlled trial. In general, the long-term effects of this procedure on pelvic support are unknown, although two cases have been reported of uterine prolapse after the LUNA procedure.

Calcium channel blockers. Agents such as nifedipine have been beneficial in preliminary trials but are not yet first-line agents. Their use should probably remain investigational at present.

Nonpharmacologic methods.

Exercise. Although controlled studies have failed to support the idea that exercise helps, many individuals report relief with running or other forms of physical exertion. As a usually harmless approach that may have other benefits and may serve as a coping method, exercise merits an attempt.

Acupuncture and acupressure. One trial using stimulation in "nonsense" areas as a control reported relief of dysmenorrhea for a year following weekly acupuncture therapy for 3 months. The authors report the "well-known" observation that acupuncture during menstruation makes the pain worse, hence they avoided treatments during the menstrual week of each month.

Transcutaneous electrical nerve stimulation. Recent studies report positive results with high-frequency electrical stimulation applied via external lower abdominal electrodes. About one third of patients require no additional medication, and many of the remainder notice decreased medication needs. The expense involved and cumbersome nature of the instrument make it useful mainly for those who obtain no relief from reasonable levels of medications or who strongly prefer not to use medication.

Transcutaneous electrical nerve stimulation (TENS) probably works both by inducing endorphin release and by overloading connections in the dorsal horn of the spinal cord, thus blocking propagation of nociceptive signals from the pelvis (see the discussion of the gate theory of pain perception later in this chapter).

Cognitive-behavioral therapy. Recent theorists have emphasized the importance of cognitive self-statements in pain modulation. For example, if, in reaction to the anticipation of menses or their actual beginning, a woman thinks the pain is likely to progressively worsen, interfere with activities and relationships, and signal the advance of disease (e.g., endometriosis), the intensity of the pain may increase. Structured approaches to interruption of continuing loops of negative self-statements may be a valuable coping skill and may reduce pain on a physiologic basis.

Psychotherapy. Gone are the times when severe dysmenorrhea was thought to represent rejection of one's femininity, unconscious hatred of men, and the like. However, the event of severe cramps may take on significant meaning in the context of psychopathology. For example, it is now well established that women who have endured sexual abuse are more likely to suffer as adults from sexual dysfunction, depression, and other psychiatric disorders, as well as chronic pelvic pain. Although an association with increased dysmenorrhea has not yet been demonstrated, such a finding would not be surprising. Psychotherapy may be of value for these accompanying difficulties and may help the dysmenorrhea at the same time. The clinician faced with a psychiatrically distressed patient should hesitate, however, before ascribing all the patient's discomfort to her emotions.

Summary

Primary dysmenorrhea is associated with the production of excess $PGF_{2\alpha}$ by the endometrium. Secondary dysmenorrhea is associated with endometriosis, pelvic adhesions, and uterine fibroids. Prostaglandin inhibitors relieve dysmenorrhea in 80% to 90% of patients. Diagnostic laparoscopy should be considered in the woman with dysmenorrhea refractory to OCs and

NSAIDs. Progressive dysmenorrhea is often a sign of organic pathology. Alternative treatments include calcium channel blockers, acupuncture and acupressure, TENS units, biofeedback, and individual psychotherapy in selected cases.

CHRONIC PELVIC PAIN

After about 4 to 6 months of chronic constant or intermittent pelvic pain, pain can become an illness in itself. A review of the mechanisms of pain perception will provide needed background for discussing evaluation and treatment.

Theories of Pain Perception

Cartesian theory. In the 16th century, Descartes proposed the existence of specific pain fibers that carried pain signals from the periphery to the brain. His theory assumes that the severity of pain will be proportional to tissue damage. Although this model may explain much of acute pain behavior, it falls well short of explaining the experience of chronic pain. For example, several studies have recently documented that the pain of endometriosis is not related (either directly or inversely proportionate) to the anatomic progression of the disease. Our theoretical understanding of pain perception must therefore be expanded.

Gate-control theory. The work of Melzack and colleagues proposed the existence of a spinal cord system responsible for filtering incoming signals, now called nociceptive (somehow negative), from the periphery (Fig. 8-1). This theory recognizes that single fibers dedicated to pain perception have not been found and that nociception is a complex integration of a variety of signals. Moreover, the degree to which these signals traverse the spinal cord and ascend to the brain may be influenced by impulses or neurotransmitter-mediated modulating signals coming down to the spinal cord "gate" from higher centers in the brain.

Information transfer is thus bidirectional. This allows for the possibility that psychologic processes may play a direct physiologic role in influencing these modulating systems (Fig. 8-1), thus incorporating physical and psychologic processes into a single network of events.

A person who has had pain for 6 months or longer may thus appear depressed. Depression and pain may have become inextricably involved, making it difficult and probably clinically useless for the clinician to decide which came first.

Cognitive theories. As mentioned earlier, recent literature questions the completeness of the gate theory and suggests that conscious thought processes or cognitions may be important not only in influencing behavior and relationships but also in modulating levels of pain more directly, perhaps even on a physiologic basis.

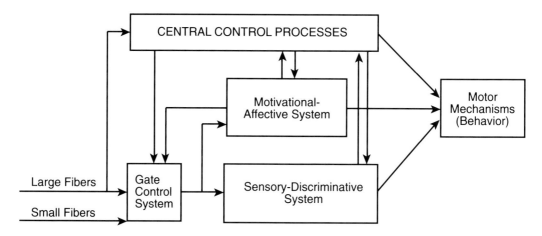

FIGURE 8-1. The gate-control theory of pain perception.

This formulation does not directly contradict gate theory, but rather expands it and opens new treatment avenues. For example, understanding the patient's own thoughts as she experiences pain on a daily basis may reveal her attributions about the pain's cause as well as demonstrate that anxious rumination (about the meaning of the pain, etc.) may increase pain levels. Under the supervision of a psychologist or other mental health professional, the patient may successfully employ cognitive treatments such as thought stopping, progressive relaxation, and directed imagery.

Contribution of Tissue Damage

Endometriosis. The first symptom of significant endometriosis is often increased dysmenorrhea. As the disease advances, the duration and severity of the pain often progress to the point of being present the majority of the time. Again, the severity of the pain does not offer a clue to the amount of disease when comparing one patient with another, but progressive increases in pain severity and duration within the same patient often mark the advance of disease. One must temper this with the observation that the fear of worsening disease or of recurrent disease after treatment may increase pain levels. For example, I have evaluated many women for recurrent pain years after complete hysterectomy and adnexectomy for endometriosis. Of those laparoscoped, only a small minority prove to have recurrent disease. In the vast majority, postoperative adhesions and significant (sometimes morbid) fear of disease seem to account for the pain.

Pelvic adhesions. In the patient with chronic pain, the site of adhesive disease correlates well with the site of pain, but the intensity is unrelated to the amount of adhesions present. Nociceptive signals from the damaged tissue seem subject to modulation at the spinal cord level and interpretation in higher centers. Although adhesions are most likely stable anatomically after a few months following injury (surgery, infection, etc.), the intensity of associated pain may progress. After about 6 months of this experience, complex relationships among physical, emotional, and cognitive factors may exist and require comprehensive treatment.

Pelvic support. Problems with pelvic relaxation are common in the sixth and seventh decades of life, but most pain clinic attenders are in the third and fourth decades. The woman with pelvic support problems rarely describes her discomforts in terms of pain. Instead, she usually complains of heaviness, pressure, dropping sensations, aching, and so on. More intense discomfort (pain) may occur when, in an attempt to hold in prolapsing organs, the levator plate becomes tense and tender during daily activities and intercourse. Fear of (or actual) loss of urinary control during coitus may impair physiologic sexual response, causing vaginal dryness and frictional dyspareunia.

Other. Beard, Reginald, and Wadsworth suggest that overfilling, or congestion, of the pelvic venous system causes chronic dull aching pain that worsens premenstrually, at the end of the day, after prolonged standing, and after nonorgasmic coitus. The problem is likely to be partly anatomic because it is usually present in multiparous women and may occasionally be unilateral. Good radiologic studies in awake women have documented increased pelvic venous diameter in those affected. Psychophysiologic factors may also contribute, as indicated by a high comorbidity with psychologic distress and the observation that, although medroxyprogesterone may help to some degree by eliminating the menstrual cycle, the best long-term results follow psychotherapy in conjunction with menstrual cycle suppression.

Chronic pelvic pain may arise from excess mobility of the pelvic organs (universal joint or Allen-Masters syndrome), attributed to childbirth or other traumatic causes of tears of the ligamentous (especially broad ligament) uterine supports. As highly subjective physical examination findings, these changes are difficult to document rigorously. Because surgery has been the traditional primary treatment, controlled studies have not been possible.

Psychologic Factors

Personality. Disorders of personality, especially borderline personality, are more prevalent among severe chronic pain patients in general and pelvic pain patients in particular. In primary care, however, such patients are less common, and the label of personality disorder should not be applied to every angry patient by her frustrated physician. People who have had difficulties maintaining satisfactory relationships and function in life, in part because of subsyndromal personality problems, may nevertheless be more vulnerable to nociceptive signals from tissue damaged by endometriosis, infection, or surgery. Unmet dependency needs may lead them to seek external solutions such as medications and further surgery, rather than rely on their own coping skills.

History of sexual abuse. As noted in the discussion of dysmenorrhea, women who have been sexually abused in childhood have many problems in adult life, and pelvic pain is certainly among them. When such a history is documented, the clinician and patient together must then judge whether the feelings surrounding these events remain intense enough to be intruding on the present. If so, psychotherapeutic help may be indicated. If not, although the memories may be painful, further emotional work in this area may not be beneficial. In either case, it is impossible to know whether these events are directly relevant to the present pain and hence demand attention, or whether they contribute to a psychologically vulnerable substrate acted on by subsequent physical or emotional events.

The treatment of pelvic pain in a woman with a history of abuse should include all the reasonable medical, surgical, and mental health modalities that would be offered to any patient. Because the treatment literature on the sequelae of abuse is disappointing, mental health assistance to deal with the abuse issue should be separately and thoughtfully considered.

Depression. The biochemical systems regulating mood (endorphins, serotonergic systems, etc.) are important factors in pain perception. This link may explain why people with chronic pain may become depressed, and people with a chemical (perhaps genetic) vulnerability to depression may develop chronic pain more often in response to illness. When sufficiently severe, depression warrants concomitant evaluation and treatment.

Diagnostic Strategies

Recognizing a chronic pain syndrome. The following are six common characteristics of a chronic pain syndrome:

1. Duration of 6 months or longer
2. Incomplete relief by most previous treatments
3. Significantly impaired physical function at home or work
4. Signs of depression (sleep disturbance, weight loss, loss of appetite)
5. Pain out of proportion to pathology
6. Altered family roles

Many people have pain for longer than 6 months without developing the other changes listed; they might be described as having chronic pain, not a chronic pain syndrome. The less fortunate, perhaps those with fewer coping skills and family and social supports, may slide little by little into a chronic pain syndrome, as behaviorally and psychologically defined here. The more flagrant pain behaviors (e.g., obvious medication abuse, losing a job) are easy to spot. Earlier detection, by looking for the signs listed, may allow easier treatment.

The first three signs are self-explanatory but may require direct questioning to detect. Of the signs of depression, sleep disturbance is usually the first to appear. Careful questioning is needed to distinguish awakening because of pain from awakening that just happens. In the true vegetative sign, the person usually cannot get back to sleep even if pain is relieved (by medication or other means).

The alteration of family roles is perhaps the most important of those mentioned. Alterations include changed responsibilities for household, children, finances, and so on. Initially intended as helpful, they may diminish the patient's self-esteem in the long run and gradually reduce her interactions with the family to little more than checking on her pain. Over time, this covertly reinforces the complaint of pain and may give it unintended value as a means of maintaining connection with other family members.

Simultaneous medical and psychologic evaluation. When the aforementioned markers of chronic pain syndrome are present, one should avoid attempting to discover how much of a pain problem is physical and how much is psychologic because it is almost always impossible to do anything but guess. Rather, it is useful to ask two separate questions:
1. Is there physical disease that requires medical or surgical treatment?
2. Is there emotional or psychologic distress that requires treatment?

It is useful to directly state that the precise connection between these two cannot be measured because this may help diminish the patient's fear that she will be told it is "all in her head." She may then be more open to sharing personal and emotional concerns. When sensitive personal questions are asked before all physical factors have been evaluated, the patient is likely to be less defensive. At this stage, a mental health consultant will have a better chance of developing rapport with the patient and will be a more helpful collaborator when needed later on.

History taking. The site, duration, pattern during activities, relationship to position changes, and association with bodily functions are important. For example, pain that is focal and positional is more often associated with adhesive disease; pain that is absent in the morning but worsens progressively during the day may be associated with pelvic congestion.

The chronology of the pain is critical, especially when it has come to affect more and more areas over time. As a chronic pain syndrome develops, the physiologic systems that deal with pain signals may "wear out"; pain may spread over a progressively larger area despite stable organic pathology. Interpreting this change in physiologic terms will make sense to the patient and has substantial biologic validity.

From a cognitive perspective, it is invaluable to discern the patient's ideas (as well as her family's ideas) about what started it and what it will do in the future. Fears of cancer can be discovered even when this diagnosis was never even remotely considered by the clinician. Less dramatic but equally powerful attributions of causality may emerge, such as pelvic infection from sexual acts remote in time, arguments with a spouse, or even divine retribution.

Physical examination. Standard techniques of abdominal and pelvic examination will not be reviewed here. Rather, I will point out particular additional procedures that help to identify somatic versus visceral sources for pain and further help isolate particular visceral contributions.

Musculoskeletal sources merit consideration, both because of their ubiquity and because gynecologists are not typically taught how to detect them. Gentle fingertip palpation of the abdominal wall can detect such trigger points in the musculature. Guiding a patient through contraction-relaxation sequences of the abdominal muscles may reduce the discomfort of the examination and indicate the patient's degree of control over muscle tension. If focal abdominal wall pain is aggravated by having the patient elevate her head (flexing the rectus muscles), there is probably an intrinsic abdominal wall source.

Similar principles should guide the pelvic examination. Have the patient contract and relax the vaginal introitus in a manner similar to that used with the abdominal wall. Single-digit palpation of the levator plate and piriformis muscles may elicit tenderness compatible with the label of pelvic floor tension myalgia. This condition is often present as the sequel to some other pelvic pain but can become a problem in itself. (Discomfort is usually felt as pelvic pressure and radiation pain to the sacrum near the insertions of the levator plate muscles.)

During the bimanual portion of the examination, any tender areas should be palpated separately with the vaginal and abdominal hands before using both hands simultaneously. This prevents misinterpreting abdominal wall pain as arising from the adnexa. Adnexal thickening and mobility, pelvic relaxation, coccygeal tenderness, and foci of pain that reproduce dyspareunia (e.g., along the urethra) should be noted. Gentle cotton swab palpation may detect areas of sensitivity compatible with vestibulitis in the introitus or trigger points higher in the vagina.

Laboratory tests.

Imaging studies. In the case of chronic pain syndrome, we have already established that intensity of pain does not correlate well with the extent of organic pathology. It follows that if the physical examination is relatively benign, extensive imaging most often adds little to the database needed before laparoscopy is performed. This is especially true in the absence of symptoms or signs pointing to a specific organ system (e.g., blood in stools). If the patient has had multiple previous surgeries, detailed studies such as magnetic resonance imaging (MRI) and computed tomography (CT) are often misleading because of postoperative artifact. A potential exception is a transvaginal ultrasound done by a gynecologist in conjunction with a bimanual examination, but even this widely employed test seems to offer more in the case of acute pain than it does in evaluating chronic pain.

Psychologic tests and interviews. In an attempt to distinguish physical and psychologic causes for pain, many authors have administered standardized psychometric tests such as personality tests (Minnesota Multiphasic Personality Inventory [MMPI]) and indices of depression (Beck Depression Inventory, Hamilton Depression Scale). In some studies more abnormalities can be detected in women without physical pathology at laparoscopy; in other papers women with organic disease who have had pain for a long time appear equally distressed. Psychometric tests are most useful when interpreted by a psychologist who has interviewed the patient; they best serve as a way to better understand the patient's strengths and weaknesses rather than as a way to decide who needs surgery.

Laparoscopy. The art of operative laparoscopy has leapt forward during the past two decades. New techniques and new terminology (e.g., pelviscopy) imply new magic to physician and public alike. Laparoscopy should be liberally performed for diagnostic purposes, and ablation of endometriosis and lysis of adhesions are no doubt useful procedures. Unfortunately, the premature surgical procedure reinforces the idea that pain is "hardwired" to pelvic pathology. In chronic pain, an illness qualitatively different from acute pain, the available evidence clearly argues against this notion. When a chronic pain syndrome is clinically evident in a patient, results of laparoscopic treatment alone are much less impressive, despite comparable pathology. For the patient with the clinical markers of chronic pain syndrome listed previously, the complete workup as described should be done before proceding with laparoscopy.

Management

General principles. A complete evaluation of chronic pain syndrome often reveals a number of contributing factors, such as bladder irritability, irregular bowel function, poor posture, and emotional and relationship stresses, in addition to laparoscopically-visualized pathology. Treating each component in turn is common practice but often ends in frustration because each treatment addresses only part of the problem. Simultaneous treatment often begins with disquieting polypharmacy, but allows better relief. Close follow-up at regularly scheduled visits will allow gradual tapering of medications over time. Planned visits also provide support and a coping mechanism for the patient without having the pain complaint reinforced by requiring that the patient repeatedly feel bad enough to call up for another appointment time.

Specific principles. With the use of long-term narcotics, some euphoria often continues long after the analgesic effect has diminished. Other medications should be used instead and prescribed in a continuous, non–pain-contingent fashion. This eliminates the need for the patient to demonstrate continued or increased pain to justify the use of medication to herself or her family; the pain behaviors are not reinforced.

Antidepressants, particularly the tricyclics, may potentiate the effects of analgesics in chronic pain syndrome even when used at doses below those usually employed in the treatment of depression (e.g., amitriptyline 50 mg qhs [at bedtime]). New agents such as fluoxetine (Prozac) hold promise because of their infrequent side effects, but they have not been extensively evaluated in chronic pain.

Surgery. Several surgical techniques are applicable to the patient with chronic pain syndrome. Laparoscopy may be both diagnostic and therapeutic, as discussed previously, and laser uterosacral nerve ablation may help the dysmenorrhea component of pain in about half of women. Presacral neurectomy is a useful adjunct to infertility surgery in the patient with central pelvic pain but is rarely justified in the patient not already undergoing surgery for some other reason. It will not relieve pain in the adnexae or lateral regions of the pelvis.

Hysterectomy for pain limited to the uterus resulted in good relief in 78% of patients in one study, but relief was not related to the presence of pathology. In another group the frequency of hysterectomy for chronic pain was dramatically reduced by the availability of pain clinic treatment. Compared with results in these tertiary care populations, the vast majority of women in the primary care setting feel satisfied with the results of hysterectomy for pelvic pain. This population should be further investigated to better understand the prevalence of chronic pain syndrome and its impact on surgical results. Clearly, chronic pain is a complex matter in which surgery plays only a limited role.

Alternative treatments. Biofeedback, TENS units, relaxation training, and individual and couples counseling all have their appropriate roles in individual cases, but none is clearly applicable or effective enough to support its automatic use in cases of chronic pelvic pain. In keeping with the approach outlined earlier, if problems requiring counseling are discovered, they should be addressed along with offering appropriate surgical approaches; cause-effect relationships are difficult to demonstrate, even in retrospect when psychologic assistance works.

Summary

In the case of chronic pain, discomfort is not proportional to tissue damage. The gate-control theory takes this observation into account and integrates physical and psychologic factors in a single theory of pain perception. A high percentage of women with chronic pelvic pain have been sexually abused at some time in their lives. Personality disorders, depression, and other psychiatric problems are more common in women with chronic pelvic pain. The six clinical hallmarks of a chronic pain syndrome are as follows:

1. Duration of 6 months or longer
2. Incomplete relief by previous treatments
3. Diminished physical function
4. Vegetative signs of depression
5. Pain not proportional to tissue damage
6. Altered roles within the family

When these hallmarks are seen, psychologic evaluation should accompany physical evaluation.

General management principles include the following:

• Treat all symptomatic organ systems simultaneously.
• Schedule regular office visits.

Specific management principles include the following:

• Do not prescribe narcotics.
• Prescribe analgesics in a non–pain-contingent fashion.
• Use antidepressants.

Laser/operative laparoscopic adhesiolysis is useful but less effective in those with a chronic pain syndrome, regardless of the degree of physical pathology.

The frequency of hysterectomy in patients with chronic pain can be reduced with pain management techniques.

PREMENSTRUAL SYNDROME

Both positive and negative physical and emotional changes may occur premenstrually in some women. Studies of women without clinically significant symptoms have generally failed to show important changes in cognitive, sensory, neurologic, or neuropsychologic functioning during the premenstrual days, but several recent studies suggest that subtle changes may occur in highly symptomatic women. More important from a clinical perspective are treatment studies showing that several pharmacologic agents can be of significant benefit in a woman experiencing negative premenstrual symptoms. The present discussion will focus on those premenstrual changes that are clinically problematic.

Definition

Premenstrual syndrome (PMS) may be defined as a group of somatic and affective symptoms occurring during the luteal phase and abating shortly after the onset of menstruation. Behavioral and cognitive changes are also frequently noted, although recent etiologic formulations might suggest that these are sequelae to the affective and anxiety changes. The major distinction between PMS and more traditionally characterized disorders of mood is the cyclicity seen in PMS. Qualitatively, the problems of anxiety, irritability, depression, crying spells, mood swings, sleep disturbance, appetite changes, changes in libido, and so on are similar to those seen in mood disorders and anxiety. The physical symptoms present premenstrually vary in intensity but do not necessarily parallel the emotional changes; they may have separate etiologies despite appearing concurrently.

Prevalence

Probably the vast majority of women notice some identifiable premenstrual physical change, traditionally called molimina. Noticeable emotional changes probably occur in about 25% of women and reach clinically significant levels in about 5% to 7%. Epidemiologic studies in Europe and the United States have yielded similar prevalence figures. The peak prevalence is in the thirties, with a slight decline noted in the forties age group; it does not correlate with marital status, education level, race, or culture.

Theories of Etiology

Psychosocial theories. Perhaps the most controversial discussions of PMS in recent years have centered around the issue of whether negative emotional and cognitive premenstrual changes really occur at all or whether their existence has been essentially manufactured by a culture and medical establishment that negatively views women (in general) and menstruation (in particular). Recent studies seem to have sufficiently documented the existence of the phenomenon, although they certainly have not settled the question of whether a biologic basis for premenstrual changes exists. Ruble's studies showed that the reporting of subjective premenstrual symptoms is subject to the power of suggestion, but it seems unlikely that these forces account entirely for the PMS phenomenon. The dramatic response to serotonergic antidepressants strongly suggests that PMS (in its more severe forms) is a variation on the theme of neurotransmitter dysregulation that seems to cause most biologic depression.

Biologic psychiatric theories.

Endorphins. Reid and Yen and, concurrently, Halbreich and Endicott suggested that premature dropping of endorphin levels might produce premenstrual symptoms. Endorphin antagonists can produce symptoms of anxiety in normal volunteers, and the symptoms of endorphin withdrawal are somewhat similar to those seen in PMS. However, several studies have failed to show a plausible time course of endorphin changes in symptomatic women that would fit the usually pattern of PMS symptoms.

Serotonin. Antiserotonergic drugs produce irritability and altered behaviors in monkeys. Serotonin levels were lower in the luteal phase of women with PMS in one study, and platelet binding of imipramine (an alleged marker for serotonergic systems in the brain involved in the regulation of mood) has been found to be cyclically lower in women with PMS in two studies. Several controlled therapeutic trials of fluoxetine (Prozac) showed it to have a positive effect on women with severe premenstrual depression. Other selective serotonin reuptake inhibitors (SSRIs) are also widely used to treat PMS.

Substantial clinical evidence supports a link between depression and PMS. Women with PMS have a significantly higher prevalence of personal histories of a depressive episode and family histories of depression. Of hospitalized psychiatric patients, those with depression have a higher prevalence of premenstrual symptoms compared to women with other diagnoses.

Taken together, these observations suggest that women with severe premenstrual symptoms may have an alteration of central serotonergic systems. These systems, similar to those which are strongly suspected to cause depression, are modulated by a menstrual cycle that is itself hormonally normal.

Endocrine theories. The following is a short (and no doubt incomplete) list of endocrine etiologic theories that have each enjoyed a flurry of interest, only to fade in the absence of sufficient data: estrogen excess, progesterone deficiency, increased estrogen/progesterone ratio, aldosterone excess, testosterone excess, dehydroepiandrosterone (DHEA) sulfate excess, and prolactin excess. Some disturbance of the thyroid axis may be present based on the observation that thyrotropin-releasing hormone (TRH) stimulation tests are abnormal in about 8% to 10% of women with PMS. However, the results do not vary in a consistent direction and yield scattered abnormalities similar to those seen in depressed patients.

Neuroendocrine reactivity. Neuroendocrine reactivity (release of epinephrine and norepinephrine) and cardiovascular reactivity (pulse and blood pressure) may be increased in some women with PMS, although the data on this point are preliminary and mixed. These more dramatic physiologic responses to stressful stimuli may contribute to adverse-feeling states and self-perceptions that may reinforce cyclic premenstrual changes. The relationship of these proposed changes in reactivity to serotonergic systems is uncertain.

Metabolic theories.

Glucose metabolism. Diabetic control may be more difficult premenstrually, but it is uncertain whether this stems from hormonally mediated changes in glucose metabolism or altered dietary patterns resulting from emotional changes. Glucose tolerance does not regularly change premenstrually in normal women or those with PMS. However, there remains the possibility that neuroendocrine responses to otherwise normal shifts in glucose levels may be greater in women symptomatic premenstrually.

Salt and water balance. Careful studies have failed to show true premenstrual increases in body weight that are independent of changes in caloric intake. Similarly, although renin, angiotensin II, and aldosterone levels increase in the luteal phase, they do so equally in women with and without PMS. Total body sodium and water do not increase, but some studies support the hypothesis that perceived bloating sensations may be due to a decreased colloid osmotic pressure that results in shifting of fluid into the interstitial space.

Miscellaneous theories.

Prostaglandins. Both underproduction of PG_1-series prostaglandins and excess production of PG_2-series compounds (by virtue of the strong association of PMS with dysmenorrhea) have been suggested as causes of premenstrual symptoms. Evidence for both remains indirect. Therapeutic trials of dietary supplements of linoleic acid have alleged benefit, but the clinical importance based on the degree of improvement seen is doubtful. Several trials of NSAIDs that are prostaglandin inhibitors have shown beneficial effects.

Vitamins. Several anecdotal reports allege etiologic roles for deficiencies of vitamins A, B_6, and E, although direct measurements have failed to document deficiencies. Therapeutic trials and clinical surveys evaluating B_6 have yielded mixed results. Vitamin E improves mastalgia in some reports. Special multivitamin preparations with labeling that suggests special benefits for the PMS sufferer are essentially without scientific support.

Ovarian infection. A trial of doxycycline for therapeutic use seemed effective in relieving PMS. However, the often-noticed changes in bowel function that occur with antibiotic use may obviate the apparent "blinded" nature of the study.

Yeast overgrowth. Mentioned for the sake of completeness, the notion that overgrowth of *Candida* in the bowel may cause PMS (as well as chronic fatigue syndrome and a host of other maladies) enjoys little scientific support. No adequate blinded therapeutic trials of anticandidal regimens have been carried out.

Diagnosis

A careful clinical history or symptom checklist will take inventory of the symptoms most troublesome to an individual. Once listed, the symptoms must then be rated prospectively on a daily symptom record of some type to determine the degree of cyclicity present. Questionnaire and clinical history methods that rely on recall only overestimate the degree of cyclicity in about 30% to 40% of cases.

Premenstrual stress is not particularly associated with any other gynecologic disease except dysmenorrhea, although a possible association with endometriosis has been suggested. Several studies note a higher prevalence of postpartum depression in the histories of women with PMS, but the data are conflicting.

The physical and pelvic examinations are important as part of a general health survey since symptoms from other illnesses (e.g., glaucoma, diabetes, allergies) may at times worsen in the luteal phase and make the patient suspect a PMS component. In a similar fashion, screening laboratory values are useful, but no peripheral sex steroid, gonadotropin, electrolyte, trace element, or other blood levels have been found to diagnose PMS.

Differential Diagnosis

Depression. As mentioned previously, significant evidence exists to support the theory that a central disorder of serotonergic systems involved with mood regulation may result in premenstrual emotional changes, especially those involving depression. Depending on the severity of symptoms reported, some formal evaluation for depression is often warranted. Psychometric inventories (Beck Depression Inventory, Hamilton Depression Scale, Zung Depression Scale) are widely used in research studies and may have some utility in general clinical practice. Their best use is in conjunction with a clinical interview by an experienced mental health professional. This often is accomplished best when introduced early in the evaluation process because it allows the development of rapport before all medical treatment avenues have been exhausted. The decision of whom to refer, as in the case of chronic pelvic pain, is sometimes difficult but can be made with reasonable accuracy after a modicum of clinical experience.

Anxiety disorders. Recent epidemiologic research suggests that many people suffering from depression have substantial accompanying anxiety. Many studies of PMS have shown that women with severe premenstrual anxiety do not return to follicular-phase baselines comparable to asymptomatic controls. The debate is then whether they are experiencing premenstrual exacerbation of a mild generalized anxiety disorder or whether the disorder is truly limited to the luteal phase. Examples occur of both patterns. Anxiety per se has been less completely studied, probably because it is difficult to find research subjects with symptom profiles free of depression.

There is some evidence that links PMS to panic disorder (a type of anxiety disorder). In a study of women without histories of true panic episodes, carbon dioxide inhalation (a commonly used experimental stimulus that can provoke a panic episode in a susceptible individual) provoked panic attacks in 9 of 14 women with PMS regardless of the cycle phase of the study. This would suggest some central vulnerability to anxiety that is not limited to the luteal phase but may be modulated by otherwise normal fluctuations in gonadal steroid hormones.

Marital discord. Women attending PMS clinics are frequently accompanied or sent by partners anxious to resolve ongoing conflict in their relationships and eager to document a hormonal etiology for the problems. The issues raised in anger premenstrually are most often indicative of significant individual or relationship issues, even if the apparent precipitant may seem trivial. Many complain of "exploding over nothing" (child's behavior, etc.), but important issues, such as sharing responsibility, affection, and so on, are often part of these disputes. Structured marital inventories (e.g., Dyadic Adjustment Scale, Locke-Wallace Marital Adjustment Scale) can be useful in detecting problem areas and require little time to complete. Again, depending on the severity of the problems discussed, participation by a mental health professional may be additive. One should avoid trying to assign a degree of blame for marital problems on hormone changes; rather, suggest that regardless of cause, major marital discord needs professional help to get better.

Drugs and alcohol. Alcohol abuse is more common in women with PMS. It is unclear whether this begins as a way of treating dysphoria premenstrually or whether this is part of the comorbidity with depression and anxiety in general. Regardless, when control of alcohol intake is a problem, appropriate treatment is indicated rather than hoping that treatments aimed at PMS alone will resolve the problem. Fewer data are available on the use of drugs by women with PMS, but prudent inquiry is probably appropriate.

Treatment

In this area the medical and lay literature are in agreement that the least intrusive and expensive treatments should be tried first, moving on to more involved therapies only when more conservative measures fail. With the etiology uncertain, all treatments are to be regarded as treatments, not cures. Early clarification of this point is useful in establishing realistic expectations.

Beyond this initial point of agreement, opinions diverge widely, depending on the theoretic bias of the proponents. The following discussion lists treatments in a hierarchy as suggested previously and attempts to distinguish those with and without scientific support.

Diet and nutritional supplements. Recent studies show that carbohydrate intake boosts serotonin levels. These results may provide a clue to the carbohydrate cravings often reported. Being able to withstand these cravings by sticking to a diet emphasizing complex carbohydrates and protein may be effective as a coping skill rather than on a biochemical basis. Clearly this is an area needing more research; however, no credible evidence exists at the present time for the therapeutic benefit of one dietary program over another. For general clinical use, it seems prudent to recommend regular intake from the basic food groups, emphasis on complex rather than simple sugars, modest salt control, and abstention from caffeine-containing beverages. Much has been said about the evils of chocolate, but the caffeine and theobromine content in chocolate are small in comparison with coffee and caffeinated soft drinks. Caffeine precipitates panic episodes in those with panic disorder; this lends indirect support to the idea of caffeine restriction in PMS (see the section on differential diagnosis earlier in this chapter).

A general multivitamin that includes a B-complex supplement may be prudent, especially in women needing improvement in general dietary balance. If B_6 is used, the dose should be restricted to 100 mg per day or less in view of the sensory neurotoxicity documented in the chronic use of B_6 doses as low as 200 mg per day. Many vitamin supplements labeled in ways that suggest special efficacy in PMS result in consumption of 300 mg per day or more when taken as directed.

Exercise. Clinical observations have long suggested that aerobic exercise may help PMS, and several recent research studies are consistent with this idea. Transient increases in central endorphin production after exercise might alter mood, even if premature endorphin withdrawal cannot be demonstrated to be a cause of PMS. At a psychologic level, a prescribed break from daily responsibilities that seem overwhelming is certainly beneficial.

Lifestyle changes. At least in women attending a PMS clinic, we often observe a pattern of putting personal and relationship needs last on the priority list; these are often omitted in the course of the daily mechanics of life. Although probably not etiologic, this pattern may result in accumulated frustrations and unmet needs that can only aggravate premenstrual emotional liability. Perhaps one of the greater benefits of attention to the problem is helping couples refocus on the more important emotional priorities in their lives. In that effort, the attitude and perceptions of the partner are obviously as central to the problem as those of the woman with symptoms.

It may be useful, whenever possible, to attempt to schedule difficult or emotionally stressful tasks or experiences at times when symptoms are expected to be less. In addition, we find that many symptomatic women need encouragement to delegate responsibilities to other family members, especially children.

Diuretics. This is probably the class of drugs most widely prescribed for premenstrual discomforts. In the experience of most PMS clinics, edema, weight gain, and the like are seldom reasons for significant disability. These symptoms do not vary in proportion to emotional changes and therefore probably have a separate etiology. Judicious use of potassium-sparing diuretics may be warranted in selected individuals but should not be expected to have an effect on emotional complaints.

Prostaglandin inhibitors. Ibuprofen relieves luteal-phase pelvic discomforts and mastalgia, and it may also improve emotional symptoms to some extent. It is uncertain whether emotional improvement is a direct effect or secondary to the relief of pain. This therapy seems to work best in women who also have severe dysmenorrhea. Other NSAIDs no doubt work in similar fashion.

Hormone supplements. Starting with Dalton, many clinicians have used supplemental progesterone to treat PMS. Because progesterone has central effects such as sedation, it could have an anxiolytic effect. Unfortunately, multiple controlled trials have failed to demonstrate a benefit in women with PMS. There remains the possibility that premenstrual changes may be biochemically diverse in ways not yet understood, and hence a subpopulation may exist that benefits from progesterone supplementation. Perhaps studies of the clinical and biochemical characteristics of progesterone responders would clarify this question. For the present time, a trial of progesterone may not be unreasonable for the patient strongly invested in this approach, but the serotonergic drugs seem a better choice in general for the patient with symptoms that last for more than a week.

Other hormonal supplements such as luteal estrogen have been mentioned periodically in the literature but have not been studied extensively. It is important to recognize that because alterations of sex steroid profiles have not been documented in PMS, any hormone used must be presented as a medication, not a replacement of a deficiency.

Anovulation. It seems clear that any method that eliminates corpus luteum function helps PMS. The choice of method hinges on relative cost, toxicity, and other patient needs.

Oral contraceptives. In general, OC users have lower levels of premenstrual symptoms than do nonusers. For the patient who has tolerated OCs well in the past, the appearance of premenstrual symptoms should not make the clinician hesitant to use them again. In view of the evidence that vitamin B_6 may eliminate the depression seen in some OC users, I usually prescribe 50 mg of B_6 along with OCs for anyone with any premenstrual dysphoria. This method is clearly most appropriate for the patient needing contraception as well.

Danazol (Danocrine). High-dose Danocrine (800 mg/day) eliminates menstrual cyclicity in most women, although the toxicity is usually greater than most women can tolerate. Low-dose regimens (200 mg/day) may be helpful while not entirely interrupting the cycle. The mechanism for this effect is uncertain.

Gonadotropin-releasing hormone agonists. Available by monthly injection or nasal inhalation, these agents first provoke a release of gonadotropins, but then shut down their production and eliminate the menstrual cycle. One study demonstrated that this eliminates PMS, but it is debatable whether patients experiencing resulting amenorrhea were truly blinded to the nature of the medication. With continued use, significant amounts of calcium loss occur, making it necessary to add back some type of estrogen replacement. To avoid endometrial overstimulation (and perhaps hyper-plasia), concomitant progestin must be given. Most patients tolerate this well, although the use of the progestin may provoke the return of PMS symptoms in some. In view of the great expense involved and the biologic intrusiveness of completely eliminating the menstrual cycle, common sense would seem to relegate this approach to those not responding to other treatments.

Surgery. Removal of the ovaries eliminates their cyclicity. Only rarely is this approach indicated in the absence of some other medical indication for the procedure. Several studies suggest that hysterectomy and bilateral salpingo-oophorectomy are effective in those remaining asymptomatic during prolonged (1 year) trials of ovarian suppression, but it seems that many subjects in these trials had not had adequate trials of psychophar-macologic agents before proceeding to surgery. The implications of these studies are therefore less clear, especially in view of the more recent availability of SSRIs.

Psychotropic drugs.

Alprazolam. As an anxiolytic with some antidepressant effects, this drug is attractive for PMS treatment; indeed, its efficacy has been demonstrated in several studies. It can be addictive when used for prolonged periods. We therefore use it for patients requiring a week or less of medication, and we generally recommend low doses such as 0.25 mg or 0.5 mg three times daily or less often. In practice the availability of the medication is a coping device in itself, and many women find that they need it only once or twice a day.

Nortriptyline. Therapeutic trials of the classic tricyclic antidepres-sants are conspicuously absent from the literature, which suggests that they may not work well or that the side effects are poorly tolerated in this population. A recent report, however, suggests that nortriptyline may be helpful.

Fluoxetine. As a popular serotonergic antidepressant, this drug has appeal for treating PMS. Several studies showed dramatic relief of PMS, which makes it a good choice for women with symptoms lasting long enough to make it worthwhile to take medication continuously. As a practical matter, this deemphasizes the differential diagnosis of depression because pharmacologic management may be the same. However, the gynecologic clinician should always be alert to the presence of severe depression (including suicidal ideation, present in up to 20% of women seen in referral settings) and insist on psychiatric management in such cases.

Summary

Moderate or severe premenstrual mood changes affect about 5% to 7% of reproductive-age women. Premenstrual mood changes likely are due to an alteration in central serotonergic systems. Diagnosis is made by prospective symptom charting. Symptoms should be limited to the luteal phase, with prompt improvement after the onset of menstrual flow. The differential diagnosis includes mood and anxiety disorders, personality disorders, and marital discord. Women with PMS have a higher prevalence of drug and alcohol abuse problems. Effective treatments include diet, exercise, lifestyle changes aimed at stress reduction, mild diuretics, prostaglandin inhibitors, and drugs that eliminate ovulation. Effective psychotropic drugs include alprazolam for symptoms of short duration and fluoxetine (and other SSRIs) for symptoms of longer duration. Progesterone supplementation, despite its popularity, has little scientific support for claims of efficacy.

BIBLIOGRAPHY

Akerlund M, Stromberg P, Forsling MD: Primary dysmenorrhea and vasopressin, *Br J Obstet Gynaecol* 86:484, 1979.

Andersch B, Hahn L: Progesterone treatment of premenstrual tension—a double-blind study, *J Psychosom Res* 29:489, 1985.

Andersch B, Milsom I: An epidemiologic study of young women with dysmenorrhea, *Am J Obstet Gynecol* 144:655, 1982.

Andersch B, Wenderstam C, Hahn L, et al: Premenstrual complaints: 1, prevalence of premenstrual symptoms in a Swedish urban population, *J Psychosom Obstet Gynecol* 5:39, 1986.

Beard RW, Reginald PW, Wadsworth J: Clinical features of women with chronic lower abdominal pain and pelvic congestion, *Br J Obstet* 95:153, 1988.

Brayshaw ND, Brayshaw DD: Thyroid hypofunction in premenstrual syndrome, *N Engl J Med* 315:1486, 1986.

Budoff PW: The use of prostaglandin inhibitors for the premenstrual syndrome, *J Reprod Med* 28:469, 1983.

Casper RF, Hearn MT: The effect of hysterectomy and bilateral oophorectomy in women with severe premenstrual syndrome, *Am J Obstet Gynecol* 162:105, 1990.

Casson F, Hahn PM, Van Vugt DA, et al: Lasting response to ovariectomy in severe intractable premenstrual syndrome, *Obstet Gynecol* 162:99, 1990.

Chuong CJ, Coulam CB, Kao PC, et al: Neuropeptide levels in premenstrual syndrome, *Fertil Steril* 44:760, 1985.

Dalton K: *The premenstrual syndrome and progesterone therapy*, ed 2, Chicago, 1984, Year Book, Medical.

Dawood MY: Hormones, prostaglandins and dysmenorrhea. In Dawood MY, editor: *Dysmenorrhea*, Baltimore, 1981, Williams & Wilkins.

Dawood MY: Dysmenorrhea and prostaglandins: pharmacological and therapeutic considerations, *Drugs* 122:42, 1982.

Dawood MY: Ibuprofen and dysmenorrhea, *Am J Med* 77:87, 1984.

Dawood MY, Ramos J: Transcutaneous electrical nerve stimulation (TENS) for the treatment of primary dysmenorrhea: a randomized crossover comparison with placebo TENS and ibuprofen, *Obstet Gynecol* 75:656, 1990.

Demers LM, Hahn DW, McGuire JL: Newer concepts in dysmenorrhea research: leukotrienes and calcium channel blockers. In Dawood MY, McGuire JL, Demers LM, editors: *Premenstrual syndrome and dysmenorrhea*, Baltimore, 1985, Urban & Schwarzenberg.

Dennerstein L, Spencer-Gardner C, Gotts C, et al: Progesterone and the premenstrual syndrome: a double-blind cross over trial, *Br Med J* 290: 1617, 1985.

Endicott J, Halbreich U, Schacht S, et al: Premenstrual changes and affective disorders, *Psychosom Med* 45:519, 1981.

Farquhar CM, Rogers V, Franks S, et al: A randomized controlled trial of medroxyprogesterone acetate and psychotherapy for the treatment of pelvic congestion, *Br J Obstet Gynaecol* 96: 1153, 1989.

Fedele L, Arcaini L, Parazzini F, et al: Stage and localization of pelvic endometriosis and pain, *Fertil Steril* 53: 155, 1990.

Freeman E, Rickels K, Sondheimer SJ, et al: Ineffectiveness of progesterone suppository treatment for premenstrual syndrome, *JAMA* 264:329, 1990.

Gambone JC, Reiter RC: Nonsurgical management of chronic pelvic pain: a multidisciplinary approach, *Clin Obstet Gynecol* 33:205, 1990.

Goldstein DP, Choikony C, Emans JS: Adolescent endometriosis, *J Adolesc Health Care* 1:37, 1980.

Good MC, Copas PR, Doody MC: Uterine prolapse after laparoscopic uterosacral transection. A case report, *J Reprod Med* 37:995, 1992.

Halbreich U, Endicott J: Possible involvement of endorphin withdrawal or imbalance in specific premenstrual syndromes and postpartum depression, *Med Hypotheses* 7:1045, 1981.

Halbreich U, Endicott J, Schact S, et al: The diversity of premenstrual changes as reflected in the premenstrual assessment form, *Acta Psychiatr Scand* 65:46, 1982.

Halliday A, Bush B, Cleary P, et al: Alcohol abuse in women seeking gynecologic care, *Obstet Gynecol* 68:322, 1986.

Harrison WM, Sandberg D, Gorman JM, et al: Provocation of panic with carbon dioxide inhalation in patients with premenstrual dysphoria, *Psychiatr Res* 27:183, 1988.

Horrobin DF: The role of essential fatty acids and prostaglandins in the premenstrual syndrome, *J Reprod Med* 28:465, 1983.

Keye WR Jr, Trunnel EP: A biopsychosocial model of premenstrual syndrome, *Int J Fertil* 31:259, 1986.

Kresch AJ, Seifer DB, Sachs LB, et al: Laparoscopy in 100 women with chronic pelvic pain, *Obstet Gynecol* 64:672, 1984.

Landau RL, Lugibihl K: The catabolic and natriuretic effects of progesterone in man, *Recent Prog Horm Res* 17: 249, 1961.

Lichten EM, Bombard J: Surgical treatment of primary dysmenorrhea with laparoscopic uterine nerve ablation, *J Reprod Med* 32:37, 1987.

Lundeberg T, Bondesson L, Lundstrom V: Relief of primary dysmenorrhea by transcutaneous electrical nerve stimulation, *Acta Obstet Gynecol Scand* 64: 491, 1985.

Magos AL, Studd JWW: Assessment of menstrual cycle symptoms by trend analysis, *Am J Obstet Gynecol* 155:271, 1986.

Melin P, Akerlund M, Vilhardt H: Antagonism of the myometrial response to oxytocin and vasopressin synthetic analgesics, *Dan Med Bull* 26:126, 1989 (questionnaire).

Melzack R: Neurophysiologic foundations of pain. In Sternbach RA: *The psychology of pain*, New York, 1986, Raven Press.

Mira M, McNell D, Fransen IS, et al: Mefenamic acid in the treatment of premenstrual syndrome, *Obstet Gynecol* 68:395, 1986.

Moos RH: The development of a premenstrual distress questionnaire, *Psychosom Med* 30:853, 1969.

Muse KN, Cetel NS, Futterman LA, et al: The premenstrual syndrome. Effects of "medical ovariectomy," *N Engl J Med* 311:1345, 1984.

Neighbours LE, Clelland J, Jackson JR, et al: Transcutaneous electrical nerve stimulation for pain relief in primary dysmenorrhea, *Clin J Pain* 3:17, 1987.

O'Brien PMS, Craven D, Shelby C, et al: Treatment of premenstrual syndrome by spironolactone, *Br J Obstet Gynaecol* 86:142, 1979.

Oian P, Tollan A, Fadnes HO, et al: Transcapillary fluid dynamics during the menstrual cycle, *Am J Obstet Gynecol* 156:952, 1987.

Pariser SF, Stern SL, Shank ML, et al: Premenstrual syndrome: concerns, controversies and treatments, *Am J Obstet Gynecol*, 153:599, 1985.

Pary GJ, Bredesen DE: Sensory neuropathy with low dose pyridoxine, *Neurology* 35: 1466, 1985.

Rapkin AJ: Adhesions and pelvic pain: a retrospective study, *Obstet Gynecol* 68: 13, 1986.

Rapkin AJ, Edelmuth E, Chang LC, et al: Whole blood serotonin in premenstrual syndrome, *Obstet Gynecol* 70: 533, 1987.

Reid RL, Yen SSC: Premenstrual syndrome, *Am J Obstet Gynecol* 139:85, 1981.

Roy-Byrne PP, Rubinow DR, Moban MC, et al: TSH and prolactive response to TRH in patients with premenstrual syndrome, *Am J Psychiatry* 144:480, 1987.

Rubinow DR, Roy-Byrne P: Premenstrual syndromes. Overview from a methodologic perspective, *Am J Psychiatry* 141:163, 1984.

Ruble DN: Premenstrual symptoms. A reinterpretation, *Science* 197:291, 1977.

Rudy TE, Kerns RD, Turk DC: Chronic pain and depression: toward a cognitive-behavioral mediation model, *Pain* 35:129, 1988.

Sampson GA: Premenstrual syndrome: a double-blind controlled trial of progesterone and placebo, *Br J Psychiatry* 136:209, 1975.

Sandahl B, Weinstein U, Andersson KE: Trial of calcium antagonist nifedipine in the treatment of primary dysmenorrhea, *Arch Gynecol* 227:147, 1979.

Sarno AP Jr, Miller EJ, Zundblad EG: Premenstrual syndrome: beneficial effects of periodic, low-dose danazol, *Obstet Gynecol* 70:33, 1987.

Schaumburg H, Kaplan J, Windebank A, et al: Sensory neuropathy from pyridoxine abuse. A new megavitamin syndrome, *N Engl J Med* 309:445, 1983.

Sinaki M, Merritt JL, Stillwell GK: Tension myalgia of the pelvic floor, *Mayo Clin Proc* 52:717, 1977.

Slocumb J: Neurological factors in chronic pelvic pain: trigger points and the abdominal pelvic pain syndrome, *Am J Obstet Gynecol* 149:536, 1984.

Smith S, Rinehard JS, Ruddock VE, et al: Treatment of premenstrual syndrome with alprazolam: results of a double-blind placebo-controlled randomized cross over clinical trial, *Obstet Gynecol* 70:37, 1987.

Steege JF, Blumenthal J: The effects of aerobic exercise and strength training on premenstrual symptoms in middle-aged premenopausal women, *J Psychosom Res* 37:127, 1993.

Steege JF, Stout AL: Resolution of chronic pelvic pain after laparoscopic lysis of adhesions, *Am J Obstet Gynecol* 165:278, 1991.

Steege JF, Stout AL, Somkuti S: Chronic pelvic pain in women: toward an integrative model, *Obstet Gynecol Survey* 48:95, 1993.

Stenchever MA: Symptomatic retrodisplacement, pelvic congestion, universal joint, and peritoneal defects: fact or fiction? *Clin Obstet Gynecol* 33:161, 1990.

Stone AB, Pearlstein T, Brown W: Fluoxetine in the treatment of late luteal phase dysphoric disorder, *Psychopharmacol Bull* 26:327, 1990.

Stout AL, Steege JF, Dodson WC, et al: Relationship of laparoscopic findings to self-report of pelvic pain, *Am J Obstet Gynecol* 164:73, 1991.

Stovall TG, Ling FW, Crawford DA: Hysterectomy for chronic pelvic pain of presumed uterine etiology, *Obstet Gynecol* 75:676, 1990.

Toth A: *Vibramycin therapy for premenstrual syndrome (PMS).* Presented at the Society for Gynecologic Investigation, Toronto, 1986.

Walker E, Katon W, Harrop-Griffiths J, et al: Relationship of chronic pelvic pain to psychiatric diagnoses and childhood sexual abuse, *Am J Psychiatry* 145:75, 1988.

Watts JE, Butt WR, Edwards RL: A clinical trial using danazol for the treatment of premenstrual tension, *Br J Obstet Gynaecol* 94:30, 1987.

Wong WH, Freedman RL, Levan NE, et al: Changes in the capillary filtration coefficient of cutaneous vessels in women with premenstrual tension, *Am J Obstet Gynecol* 114:950, 1972.

Wood SH, Mortola JF, Chan YF, et al: Treatment of premenstrual syndrome with fluoxetine: a double-blind, placebo-controlled, crossover study, *Obstet Gynecol* 80:339, 1992.

Yikorkala O, Dawood MY: New concepts in dysmenorrhea, *Am J Obstet Gynecol* 130:833, 1978.

York R, Freeman E, Lowery B, et al: Characteristics of premenstrual syndrome, *Obstet Gynecol* 73:601, 1989.

PART TWO

SPECIFIC CONDITIONS

CHAPTER 9

Clinical Approach to Breast Disease

ROGER E. MOE

The incidence of breast cancer is four times as high as that of cancer of the uterus and is increasing at the rate of 1% to 1.5% annually. Approximately one out of nine women will get breast cancer within their lifetime. So this is indeed a formidable challenge to the clinician. But there is a reward for assiduous attempts at early diagnosis. The earliest forms of breast cancer are just under 100% curable, a fact that does not apply to numerous other diseases that do not carry the ominous label of cancer (such as diabetes, coronary artery disease, rheumatoid arthritis, regional ileitis, and so on). Moreover, a variety of therapeutic modalities are effective against breast cancer, unlike some other kinds of cancer (such as carcinoma of the pancreas). Fortunately, most breast disease is not cancer. Among patients referred to our surgical breast clinic, there are at least five times as many patients with benign breast problems as with cancer. On the one hand, benign breast problems can becloud the detection of breast cancer; on the other, cancer can have the same clinical features as benign breast disease. So it behooves the clinician to have a system for clinical decision making that can sift through the presentations of breast disease to have a reasonable likelihood of sorting out the breast cancer. Certainly, the goal of a clinician is to correct symptoms presented by the patient, whether or not these pertain to cancer. But in the background lurks the possibility of cancer, related or not to the overt signs and symptoms in the patient.

At this time, technology is not the practical limiting factor in early diagnosis or therapy. Clinical decision making and interpretation of physical findings have a considerable way to go before technology becomes the main impediment to progress. Clinical decision making is often incomplete, and technology often is not used to its maximum capability. This chapter simplifies decision making, provides insight into the details and context of clinical findings, and points out some limitations of technology that must be taken into account.

The largest overall impact on reducing morbidity and mortality from breast cancer will be population-based measures such as mammography. The main problem here is to get more and more women into mammography surveillance—even to get at least one baseline set of mammograms. But to the clinician, the main problem is to interpret breast symptoms and signs on a day-to-day basis. Clinicians often bring to this task an inaccurate concept of the tissue inside a breast, along with obfuscating terminology such as "fibrocystic disease," which makes the diagnostic process more difficult.

PHYSICAL EXAMINATION

In our clinic, when I am about to begin the physical examination, most patients immediately proceed to lie back on the examining table, thus indicating that they are not used to being examined while in the upright posture. This means that the role of inspection as a part of physical examination is minimized. While the patient is in the sitting posture with hands on hips, breast surfaces should be inspected with an oblique light to look for the shadows of skin indentations or dimpling and other telltale signs of breast disease. One is not looking for lumps that protrude from the skin—these are late signs of locally advanced disease. Rather, one is looking for minor degrees of skin traction, such as an indentation similar to a fingerprint or for traction effects that shorten the breast on one side or pull the nipple out of position, which indicates a process of internal fibrosis, benign or malignant. One is also looking to see whether both nipples protrude normally or whether they point normally or may be deviated on one side. One also looks for discoloration with erythema of the skin or for increased redness or crusting of one nipple as in Paget's carcinoma of the end of the nipple. The arms of the patient are then raised toward the ceiling, sometimes eliciting subtle skin traction signs with this change in posture, or by pressing the hands together or pressing the hands on the hips to contract the pectoralis muscle, thereby bringing out skin traction.

During inspection, it is often the case that one breast is larger than the other. Indeed, it is surprising that this doesn't happen more often in paired organs on a physiologic basis. Although unilateral breast enlargement certainly can occur with locally advanced cancer, this is mostly a developmental or a hormonal physiologic response. Other types of developmental findings on inspection are smooth curvilinear fullness several centimeters in diameter behind either pectoral muscle in the axilla (a sign of ectopic breast tissue), sometimes with a rudimentary nipple overlying it. The same findings can occur at the caudal end of each breast in the axis of the nipple or sometimes down the abdomen toward each groin, the embryologic milk line.

Also while the patient is sitting, the axillary lymph nodes are examined. Each nipple is examined between the clinician's thumb and index finger, not looking for a nipple discharge but for an internal thickening inside the nipple such as a little lump similar to a BB or a thickening similar to a piece of twine. The normal nipple usually flattens to about 3-mm thickness. Note that milk ducts do not usually open onto the areola, so the areola itself is not a principal focus of interest—the central ducts of the nipple are the main concern. Palpation of the breast is then carried out with the patient lying supine and the arms elevated above the head to flatten out the breast tissue on the chest. (As a generalization, bimanual examination of the breast itself while the patient is sitting up is an unrewarding maneuver.) All areas of the breast are then systematically covered with the palpating fingers, both the fingertips and the palmar broad surfaces of the fingers. The fingertips are "walked" across the breast surface rather than examining the breast surfaces in a series of "pokes" and picking the fingers up off the breast each time to change location; the poking and lifting method of examination leaves many intervals of tissue unexamined. Whether the clinician uses a motion such as a circular motion is a matter of personal preference but is unnecessary. There is a concept in the minds of some clinicians that a lump may "move around." I have never seen this happen, and I cannot conceive of any way in which it can happen because all the internal tissue is attached and secured in place—not free to change location except insofar as the contour of the breast changes with posture or as the position of the breast moves on the chest wall.

CLINICAL FEATURES OF INTERNAL BREAST TISSUE

Normal breasts have normal lumps (Figs. 9-1 and 9-2). Adipose tissue, immediately under the skin and in front of the fibroglandular tissue, is a tissue that is made up normally of lumps — it is not smooth like butter. There are hundreds of such normal lumps in normal breasts. Adipose lumps are not usually noticeable in thin patients, but in obese patients they may be as large as a Ping-Pong ball (although not actually round). Adipose lumps tend to be flat on the surface of each lump, elliptical in outline in the plane that parallels the breast surface, with noticeable ridgelike edges on palpation. Details such as the shape and size of these lumps are found with the tips of the examining fingers, not the flats or the palmar surfaces of the fingers. These adipose lumps are somewhat smaller in the upper part of the breast above the transverse axis at the level of the nipple and more prominent but less numerous in the caudal part of the breast, especially in the lower inner quadrant. In the lower inner quadrant, the background fibroglandular tissue is minimal, so the adipose lumps are especially discernible against the underlying chest wall. Moreover, postmenopausal patients often have a distinct transverse ridge of fat in the caudal edge of the breast, immediately above the inframammary crease. This aggregation of adipose tissue is often palpable as a mass transversely oriented along the caudal edge of the breast, but this is not abnormal. When biopsied, one sees only normal fat. Why this aggregation of fat has more consistency or density than other areas of adipose tissue above it in the breast is unknown.

Just below the layer of subcutaneous adipose tissue, the superficial surface of this internal fibroglandular tissue is not flat and smooth during palpation; instead it is like the surface of a lake in a mild breeze, with numerous waves or ridges and points and with fluted indentations or troughs between the ridges. These waves and ridges, known as Cooper's ligaments, extend up through the fat to the skin for attachment (see Figs. 9-1 and 9-2). These are not ligaments — they are merely extensions of the normal fibroglandular tissue. In any event, they are palpable. Some patients normally have considerably more surface fluting of the fibroglandular tissue than other patients. This fluted surface characteristic becomes more accentuated during pregnancy. These surface flutings are the lumps that are said to "come and go" on a cyclic basis; however, they do not come and go. As stated, they are structural features, and they do not disappear. They merely become more evident or less evident, more easily palpable or less easily palpable, with changes in the consistency of the internal fibroglandular tissue during changes in the hormonal effects on the breast in the menstrual cycle. In other words, the same structural features are easily discerned before menses and may be difficult to discern after menses, but they are still present. These surface flutings are more noticeable in the upper

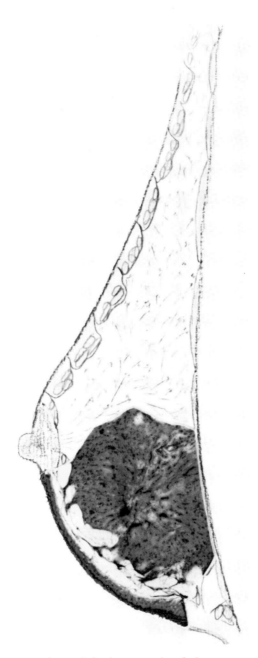

FIGURE 9-1. Diagram and partial photograph of the cut surface of a breast showing skin, then adipose tissue, with deeper fibroglandular tissue. Normal breasts have normal lumps of adipose tissue along with surface irregularities of fibroglandular tissue. Note the small size of the epithelial elements as compared with the overall scale of the breast.

Tissue portion prepared and provided courtesy of Dr. Hanne Jensen, Davis, California.

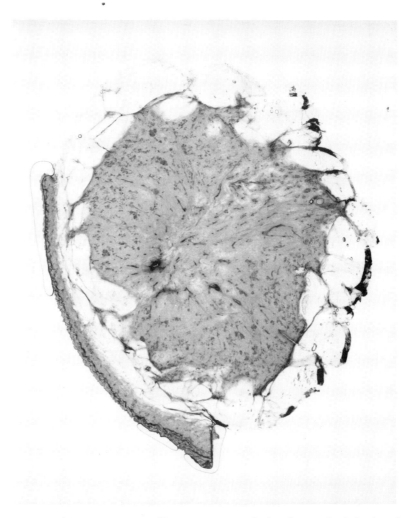

FIGURE 9-2. A large specimen of breast tissue with the skin at the left, then fat, and then fibroglandular tissue, nearly actual size. Use a hand lens to see details of the darkened ductal and lobular elements. Relate the size of the various tissue components to physical examination and to mammograms.

Normal tissue prepared with subgross method and provided courtesy of Dr. Hanne Jensen, Davis, California.

outer quadrant of the breast than in other quadrants because that location is where the volume of the internal fibroglandular tissue is greatest. Those surface flutings become camouflaged by adipose tissue in obese patients.

Frequently, when asked about past breast problems, patients make statements such as "I have lumpy breasts," or "I have fibrocystic disease," or "I have cysts." Sometimes the patient says she had this since her late teens. With further questioning, it usually turns out that she went to a doctor for a physical examination and she was told as a teenager that she had fibrocystic disease. This clinical assessment of a teenager usually indicates an inaccurate clinical interpretation. If a doctor has a mental image of multiple cysts in a teenager, that will almost always be wrong. A single macrocyst in a teenager is rare. I have never seen multiple cysts in a teenager. What happens is that the teenage patient typically has a thin subcutaneous adipose layer beneath the skin and compact fibroglandular tissue deep to the adipose layer, with the normal surface irregularities of the fibroglandular tissue easily discernible on palpation. The structural irregularities are frequently interpreted as fibrocystic disease, nodules, or some other such label—a label other than normal.

In a thin patient during the reproductive years, it is important to have a mental image of the scale (the relative size) of the elements of epithelial tissue within the internal fibroglandular tissue of the breast. Fig. 9-2 reveals the epithelial elements, which are darkly stained with hematoxylin to contrast with the lighter translucent fibrous supporting tissue. The small size of these epithelial elements clearly shows that they are not palpable to the examiner's fingers, that it is not possible to discern the epithelium or glandular component of the internal tissue distinctly from the fibrous supporting tissue, that these epithelial elements are much smaller than the normal adipose lumps and surface irregularities previously described, and that the small size of these epithelial elements prevents a description of them in mammograms. Mammograms do not distinguish the density of fibrous supporting tissue and epithelial elements. Therefore one cannot palpate a breast and talk about "glandular tissue," and one cannot look at a mammogram and make precise descriptions of the epithelium by using words similar to those used by pathologists who see this tissue with a microscope. In mammograms, one can only indirectly assess the character of the epithelium. It is essential to keep in mind this concept of scale—the small size of the epithelial elements as compared with the aggregation of other tissue components within the breast when doing a physical examination or when looking at mammograms; this will improve one's accuracy and form a clinical impression or diagnosis while reducing the use of ambiguous, "pseudoprecise" terminology. To strengthen this mental picture of the internal breast tissue, it is most helpful to participate in or closely observe surgical breast operations to see and palpate the internal tissue with its several components and to pay close attention to the normal tissue and its detailed characteristics—irregularities, tissue colors, consistency, and so on. Unless this is done, inaccurate interpretation of physical findings will probably continue.

Notice in Fig. 9-2 that most of the internal tissue of the breast is fibrous supporting tissue, a tissue that is not the source of the usual breast cancers; epithelial tissue, which does generate breast cancers, is a lesser component of the internal tissue. One cannot tell by palpation whether the epithelial tissue is exuberant and proliferative or whether it is sparse and quiescent. The patient with dense internal tissue may have epithelium that is not much more abundant than in a male patient, with few or poorly developed lobules. Another patient with dense internal tissue may have florid development of the epithelium with abundant and extensive lobules. Keep in mind that it is the epithelium that generates breast cancers, except for rare cancers of mesenchymal origin.

After menopause, when ovarian hormonal stimulation falls off, internal fibroglandular tissue regresses and is replaced by adipose tissue (unless the patient is receiving exogenous hormones). Exogenous hormones may maintain the fibroglandular tissue; this should be taken into account during physical examination or when interpreting mammograms.

To reiterate, interpretation of the internal fibroglandular breast tissue by means of palpation is done by using the fingertips to determine the shape, consistency, and size of the lumps normally found in the breast in order to look for one or more abnormal lumps. The size of breast lumps noticed on self-examination is easily followed in a reproducible fashion by using the tip of the index finger as a ruler. Use of the same finger in this way thus gives one a frame of reference so that changes in size can be reasonably determined. On the other hand, use of the broad palmar surfaces of the fingers over each quadrant of the breast gives an impression as to the "sameness" of the many discernible lumps. There will be hundreds of such lumps, but interpretation of broad areas gives one the impression that these lumps are diffusely similar in any given quadrant and therefore likely to be normal. When the self-examiner or the clinician questions a lump that is different from the others, the next decision is whether this tissue is abnormal. This decision is made by the clinician—not the patient. The patient should consult a clinician when a question arises. On evaluation, the clinician does not need to think of the tissue in terms of being suspicious, worrisome, or otherwise. If the clinician concludes that an area of tissue is abnormal, this tissue needs a diagnosis—not a conjectural label.

If the clinician is not sure about whether an area is thickened or different in a part of the breast, the most sensitive method to help the interpretation is to do simultaneous mirror-image palpation bilaterally. This maneuver often convinces the clinician that there is an asymmetric thickness in one breast as compared with the other. The clinician can then get further details by palpating with the index finger of each hand simultaneously (bimanually) around the perimeter of the area in question—this will often delineate soft lumps that are otherwise hard to palpate such as a fluid-filled macrocyst that is not tense or tightly filled. The method of using both index fingers in apposition (not in contact) bimanually is often considerably more rewarding than merely pushing about over the surface of the breast with three or four fingertips.

Abnormal lumps such as cysts often have a rounded arciform contour. This is a contour different from that of the adipose lumps, which have already been described. It is helpful to pay some attention to details of contour of what turns out to be a known cyst and to compare those details on palpation with the details of prominent fat lumps found in the lower inner quadrant. This helps sharpen one's clinical acuity.

During palpation, with the patient supine and her arm up over her head to flatten out the fibroglandular tissue of the breast, one is not palpating for "a cancer" per se. Breast cancers are often much too small to palpate, or they are camouflaged by 1 to 2 cm or more of overlying normal tissue, or they have characteristics identical to normal tissue. Yes, cancer may be hard, with poorly defined margins and tethered skin overlying it, but it may also be identical to the features of a benign rounded fibroadenoma, small or large, soft or firm. Also, cancers can be shaped like a spider or can be in the form of a sheet that can cover 4 or 5 cm and still be difficult to discern. One can never tell by palpation that an abnormal area is not a cancer; furthermore, one can never tell by clinical examination or available technology that there is no cancer, that "there is nothing to worry about." One can conclude only that no evidence of a cancer is found if a clinical evaluation is normal.

DISPOSITION IN THE EVENT OF ABNORMAL TISSUE

It is important that the charted record include a diagram of where the abnormality is and its actual measurements. Inaccurate estimated measurements and lack of diagrams compromise one's ability to assess changes in an area of tissue over a period of time. Moreover, a description of breast abnormalities is facilitated by valuable illustrations in Barth's atlas.

What typically happens when an area of abnormal tissue is encountered during clinical evaluation is that the patient is advised to return again after her next menstrual period for reevaluation to see whether the lump or thickening has gotten smaller or has gone away. In the meantime the patient is sent for mammograms. Sometimes the mammograms do not confirm any specific abnormalities, and because a cancer is not seen, nothing further is done. In other instances the patient is referred for surgical evaluation because of mammographic abnormalities. One mistake that occurs all too frequently is that an abnormal lump has been palpated, but the mammogram does not show the lump; thus, the lump is not dealt with. A palpable lump needs a definitive diagnosis whether or not it is found by mammography. Mammograms are in no way tantamount to a microscopic evaluation. A negative mammogram in no way guarantees that there is no cancer. In yet other instances, the gynecologist may do a needle aspiration for cells or fluid in the area of tissue in question and then refer the patient.

In our experience, when one finds a clearly abnormal area of tissue in the breast, this abnormal area seldom becomes smaller or goes away after the next menstrual period. Such an area of tissue is perhaps more likely to regress in a teenager, in a patient in her early twenties, and sometimes during pregnancy because the hyperplasia of pregnancy is not always a uniform process.

Needle Aspiration Biopsy

There is little reason why the gynecologist cannot proceed promptly with a needle aspiration when a definite abnormality is initially found. This is more efficient than waiting until other tests and evaluations are done, and the cost is relatively low. For example, if a lump is found, raising the question of a cyst, aspiration with the use of a needle and syringe may produce fluid, eliminate the lump, and yield a prima facie diagnosis as well. If one can palpate a lump, it can be needled and does not require ultrasound to tell one that the lump contains fluid. We have not seen substantial harm caused by a needle aspiration, but we certainly have seen untoward consequences from failure to diagnose a thickening when needle aspiration might have indicated much earlier the presence of a cancer that later became obvious.

Needle aspiration of a thickening or lump can yield further information beyond the simple presence or absence of fluid. The necessary equipment for this procedure is shown in Fig. 9-3. The first step is to apply an iodine solution to the skin. Next, local anesthesia is injected into the skin with a 30-gauge needle. The lesion is then fixed under two fingers of one hand, and with the other hand a 21-guage needle is inserted through the skin using a 20-cc syringe in an Aspir-Gun handle (Fig. 9-4). No vacuum is applied until the needle is up against the lesion; then full vacuum is applied, and the needle is passed three or four times through the lesion. *Release the vacuum completely before removing the needle from the breast. Do not aspirate the contents of the needle into the barrel of the syringe.* After removing the needle from the breast, detach the needle from the syringe and remove the syringe from the aspirating gun (Fig. 9-5). Then pull some air into the syringe, reattach the needle to the syringe, place the bevel of the needle down against the microscope slide surface, and expel the air through the needle to blow out the needle contents onto the slide; repeat this process with the other slide. Then pick up the two slides and touch the two surfaces together with the aspirated material between the slides (Fig. 9-6). *Do not make a smear with the slides.* The slides are touched together for contact only and then dropped into a bottle of alcohol fixative for delivery to cytology. This procedure should be done expeditiously to avoid artifacts from air-drying and smearing. More details of aspiration biopsy are found in the book by Frable, *Thin-needle aspiration biopsy* (see the Bibliography).

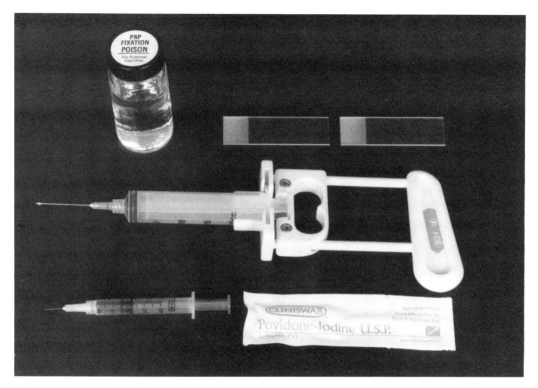

FIGURE 9-3. Necessary equipment for needle aspiration cytology: iodine swab and local anesthesia needle at the bottom, syringe and needle in an aspirating handle, microscope slides, and alcohol fixative (ethynol, 95%, methcual, 5%).

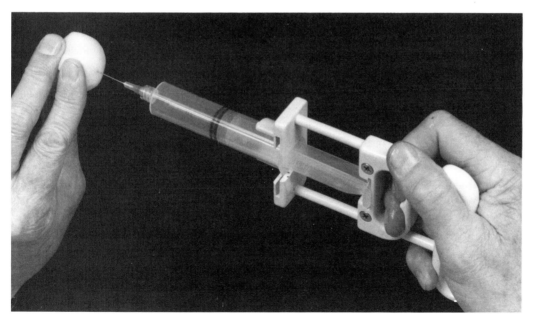

FIGURE 9-4. Process of needle aspiration of a lump. The aspirating handle is pulled into the vacuum position when the needle is at the lump itself, and not until.

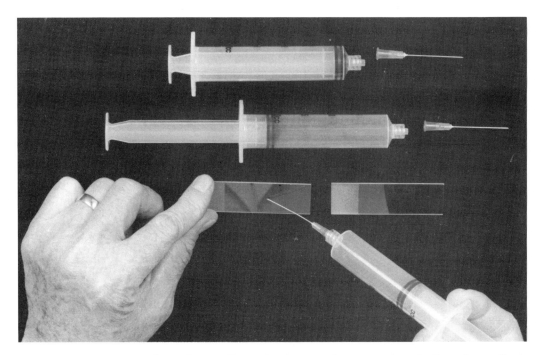

FIGURE 9-5. Steps in needle aspiration cytology, continued. *Top,* A needle is detached from a syringe. *Middle,* Air is pulled into the syringe. *Bottom,* The needle reattached and contents expelled with air from the syringe onto the microscope slide.

Indications for a biopsy after needle aspiration are as follows:
1. Old blood (dark color) in the lump
2. No fluid
3. Residual thickening after aspiration of fluid
4. Several recurrences of fluid in a cyst that had been previously aspirated
Other potential reasons to carry out a biopsy include early recurrence of a cyst, such as in a few weeks, which implies an active epithelial secretory process of some sort (possibly neoplastic). (Recurrence of a lump the same day or the day after fluid was removed usually means that the aspirating needle hit a blood vessel that filled the cavity with blood.) Another indication for a biopsy is a patient inappropriate for the type of pathology; that is, lumps such as cysts are usually estrogen related, and an elderly woman or a patient whose ovaries have been removed should not develop cysts unless she is receiving exogenous estrogens. An elderly patient not receiving exogenous estrogens who is still developing a cyst should probably undergo a biopsy to rule out an unsuspected cancer.

Another reason for doing an early needle aspiration in an area of abnormal tissue is that a report that is positive for malignancy from a laboratory with experienced cytopathologists is highly accurate. In over a

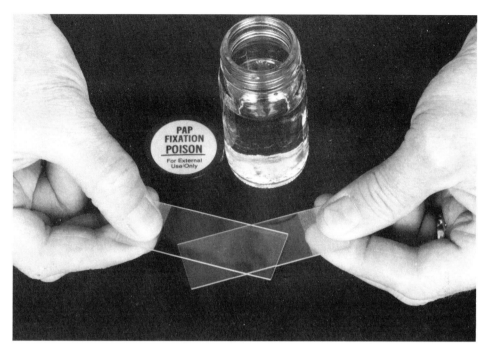

FIGURE 9-6. Microscope slide surfaces with the content of the needle are touched together but not smeared; the slides are then dropped into the PAP fixative bottle.

thousand needle aspiration cytologies, we have never had a false-positive result for a breast malignancy, although false-negative results for malignancies are encountered often enough that a negative report for malignancy is disregarded. In the latter instance, all one knows about is the contents of the needle, not the character of all the residual tissue in the thickening in the breast. Heterogeneous histologic characteristics commonly occur within abnormal breast tissue; the aspirating needle can easily miss a cancer that is present.

Mammography

As a generalization, when abnormal tissue is encountered in a breast examination or when the patient has symptoms, mammography should be undertaken (Fig. 9-7). (This is not the same issue as screening mammography in the patient with no symptoms or no findings.) Exceptions apply to teenagers, probably also to patients in their early twenties, and to pregnant patients—mammograms are unlikely to be useful in patients in their teens or early twenties. Typically, the density of normal tissue in these age groups makes it unlikely that an abnormal shadow would be seen in mammograms; moreover, the probability of a cancer would be low. Only microscopy of tissue from an open biopsy settles the diagnosis.

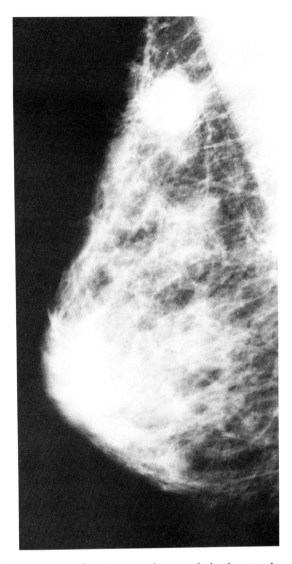

FIGURE 9-7. Mammogram showing an abnormal shadow in the upper portion of the breast. The abnormal shadow has irregular streaky edges almost diagnostic of breast cancer in a 52-year-old woman with 19 lymph nodes positive.

The use of mammograms in instances where abnormal tissue has been found is not predicated on the idea that mammograms may tell the clinician that a biopsy is unnecessary. On the contrary, if there is an area of tissue abnormal by palpation, mammograms do not obviate the need for a diagnosis. Mammograms do not generally lead to a definitive diagnosis. However, mammograms may well display other abnormal tissue either in the same breast or in the opposite breast that is unsuspected by the clinician. Also, mammograms may show a collection of microcalcifications indicating a substantial potential for malignancy, which should expedite further

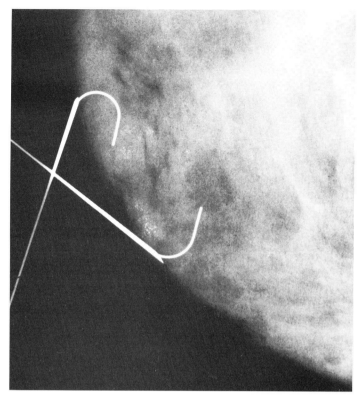

FIGURE 9-8. Portion of a dense mammogram from a 30-year-old female with extensive noninvasive breast cancer in an area shown by speckled white spots adjacent to the two Homer needles inserted for guidance at the time of a biopsy. Microcalcifications can be seen in tissue that is too dense to demonstrate abnormal shadows.

diagnostic tests (Fig. 9-8). Finally, even when mammographic evidence of malignancy is high, the clinician may gain a valuable impression of the extent of the disease, possible multiplicity, and other information that bears on management of the case.

When mammography has been requested and the report is received, the gynecologist frequently does not have the opportunity to see the actual mammograms. If any abnormalities are described in the mammogram report, it is helpful to have the patient carry her own mammograms back to the gynecologist's office when the patient comes in for reevaluation. In looking at the mammograms, one of the first things to consider is the concept of usefulness. How useful is a given mammogram in this particular patient? In other words, how likely is it that one could expect to find a cancer in mammograms for that particular patient? When one sees extensive diffuse dense fibroglandular tissue throughout the mammograms, their usefulness is compromised both for diagnosis and for surveillance. Cancers are not made of cells that are a new type of tissue in the breast. Cancers consist of alterations in cells that are normally found within the breast, so cancer cells do not stand out against a background of other fibroglandular cells that are not cancer. Looking for a cancer on the basis of an abnormal shadow that is in mammograms of a breast already very dense is like looking for a polar bear in a snowstorm. A sizeable cancer can be present but not evident. Remember that cancers arise from epithelium, not mesenchymal tissue; mammograms do not distinguish between epithelium and its accompanying fibrous tissue. Only the microscope does this. This is an inescapable limitation of mammograms and must be kept in mind, although it does not undercut the fact that mammograms are by far the best technology for displaying cancers clinically. Nonetheless, only a microscope yields definitive details about the character of epithelium in the breast tissue. Anything less than microscopy, with the exception of withdrawing fluid from a lump that is a cyst and having the cyst disappear, is educated conjecture.

The earliest indications of potential breast cancer in mammograms are tiny white dots similar to grains of salt or even smaller, called microcalcifications (Figs. 9-9 and 9-10). The number of microcalcifications within a square centimeter of tissue has a direct bearing on the likelihood of cancer. Microcalcifications are found in 60% to 70% of breast cancers, and the average cancer displays around 30 to 35 calcifications within a square centimeter. In contrast, when five or fewer microcalcifications are found in a square centimeter, these have not been found to be cancers unless even a single calcification displays a linear branch pattern.

These calcifications are tiny focal precipitates that occur within milk ducts or next to them for reasons unknown. Microcalcifications are not intrinsically part of a malignant process. Numerically, more biopsy speci-

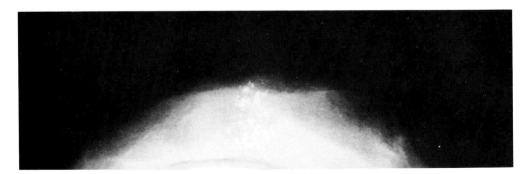

FIGURE 9-9. Mammogram showing part of a cephalocaudal view just over the edge of an augmentation Silastic implant, with a prominent group of microcalcifications shown as white specks toward the nipple.

mens for microcalcifications in mammograms are benign than malignant. With invasive ductal carcinoma and noninvasive carcinoma, microcalcifications are apt to be in or next to malignant ducts; with lobular carcinoma the situation is different. The microcalcifications are more apt to be associated with benign tissue near a lobular carcinoma or a lobular carcinoma in situ rather than in the cancer itself. Microcalcifications are like the license plates on cars—license plates do not tell what kind of a car it is. But when microcalcifications in mammograms are grouped within a square centimeter as mentioned earlier, they do indicate that there appears to be a concentration of milk glands that may be proliferating and possibly malignant. Therefore a biopsy and microscopy would be indicated. Microcalcifications can be found not only in mammograms with an average level of density but also in mammograms that are of greater than usual density for age and parity of the patient. Recall that dense mammograms are less useful in searching for other characteristics of malignancy. Therefore microcalcifications are a particularly valuable feature of mammography, including dense mammograms. Generally, these microcalcifications are not displayed by ultrasound.

When the gynecologist sees a report of microcalcifications, the question then follows as to whether or not these calcifications are grouped within a square centimeter and how many calcifications there are. Are there any linear or branched calcifications suggestive of cancer? Also, have these calcifications been previously seen on mammograms and are the calcifications increasing in number, staying the same, or decreasing? An increasing number of calcifications suggests the need for a biopsy.

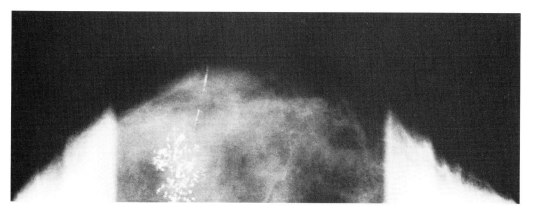

FIGURE 9-10. Same patient as in Fig. 9-9 with the augmentation implant pushed aside as well as cone compression of the breast tissue for better detail. There are light calcifications in an area of invasive breast cancer and a streak of noninvasive breast cancer extending all the way into the nipple, thus precluding breast preservation.

Generally, the number of calcifications is slow to change over a period of months, such as a 6-month interval. Ordinarily it is not particularly fruitful to obtain follow-up mammograms in only 2 or 3 months to count calcifications. As a generalization, open biopsies are advisable for six or eight or more microcalcifications grouped within a square centimeter, even though the probability of finding cancer is substantially lower than when larger numbers of calcifications are grouped. For six to eight microcalcifications in a square centimeter, the probability of finding an early cancer is about 16% to 18%.

MACROCYSTS OF THE BREAST

This category of breast disease is probably as poorly understood as any inasmuch as it represents a clinical category that is often diagnosed by conjecture, and when actually diagnosed is often managed with a rather casual attitude. It is common for a patient to announce that she has "cystic breasts" without having any proof from techniques such as needle aspiration of fluid, ultrasound, or actual biopsies to document cysts. The impression of cystic breasts often comes from the misinterpretation of normal clinical irregularity found by palpation of breasts that have normally large adipose lumps or by palpation of normally prominent structural ridges and troughs in the surface of fibroglandular tissue during the reproductive years. With increasing use of ultrasound, especially newer equipment with higher frequencies, the accuracy of diagnosing a fluid-filled breast cavity approaches 85% or 90%. (This is not to say that ultrasound assessment of nonfluid components of the breast for early cancer has that high an accuracy.) Accordingly, many clinicians are satisfied with an ultrasound diagnosis of a fluid-filled cavity or cyst as the explanation for a mammographic shadow, with no further action taken. This discussion will suggest that a somewhat more cautious clinical policy may be in order.

At the outset, it is important to define the pathology that is being discussed here. Macrocysts are defined as cysts that are 3 mm and greater in measured diameter, visibly and palpably discernible in gross tissue specimens, and objectively verified officially with measurements in pathology reports or verified by aspiration of fluid from the breast by using a syringe and needle. These are unambiguous criteria. There is a body of literature describing the clinical sequence of events in patients with this disease. This definition of macrocyst does *not* include cases in which dense mammograms have been labeled fibrocystic disease by the radiologist; pathology reports containing a variety of benign changes, often with no cysts at all, that the pathologist has labeled fibrocystic disease or cystic mastitis; and the patient with normally abundant compact breast tissue in the reproductive years.

Palpation

Usually the patient or the clinician has discovered a lump by palpation. Fewer than half of the population of patients with actual macrocysts have pain or tenderness. Palpable lumps that are cysts have certain features helpful to the clinician in making a diagnosis. In the first place, a cyst has a smooth, curved, arclike surface, which is different from the features of adipose lumps described earlier. Some of these smooth round lumps from cysts are soft and difficult to discern, whereas other lumps from cysts are firm and rubbery because of the increased pressure of the contents of the cysts. Soft cysts can be most accurately defined during palpation by using the two index fingers along the periphery of the cyst on opposite edges of the cyst. Using the index fingers to make the cyst rock or move a bit helps define the size. Sometimes a cyst is located on the back wall of the breast and is camouflaged by overlying tissue. In that setting, one can sometimes perceive a deep-lying rounded contour by eliciting a rocking motion of the rounded contour between the two index fingers, and this rocking motion conveys a smooth, slippery sensation to the examiner's fingers. Most of the time there will only be one or two such lumps in one breast. A smaller percentage of these patients have three or four lumps in one or both breasts. These lumps tend to be located closer to the areola in any quadrant than to the periphery of the breast. Moreover, when more than one of these lumps occurs, their size tends to differ considerably. (For example, one lump might be 3 cm in diameter, another lump 1 cm in diameter, and still another lump a different dimension.) The key point here is that palpation of a large number of similar lumps in both breasts is not characteristic of bona fide cystic disease with actual macrocysts. Breasts with hundreds of lumps palpable through an extensive area on both sides do not present the picture of macrocysts. Such diffuse irregularity with a carpet of lumps is almost certainly the normal structural character of a given breast.

Aspiration of Fluid

Cancer within a cyst is rare, although breast cancer in patients who have or have had macrocysts is not rare. Only one in over a thousand macrocysts that have been aspirated turns out to reveal breast cancer. Common clinical practice is to discard fluid specimens. However, some fluid specimens are sent for cytologic evaluation. These are the specimens that are the color of old blood, a dark chocolate brown; fluid from a cyst that has recurred several times; or fluid from a postmenopausal patient, a patient who is not expected to form macrocysts because of low estrogen levels. Sometimes one is not sure about the presence of old blood in cyst fluid. This fluid might be almost black, for example. In such an instance, one can drop some of this fluid onto a piece of white gauze, which often demonstrates that the fluid is in fact a dark green rather than dark brown, and the fluid should also be tested for occult blood by using a Hemoccult test, the same as is done under other circumstances for fecal specimens. Macrocyst fluid can be gray, straw colored, pea green, slate green, clear, or turbid. Cancer can exist with any of these colors. But when there is evidence of old blood in the cyst, as opposed to fresh red blood from the trauma of a needle hitting a small blood vessel, this means that there is an epithelial ulceration of some sort in the cyst, benign or malignant. It might be added that these indications for a cytologic examination of the fluid are also indications for open biopsy of such a cyst. Negative cytologic findings would not prevent the need for an open biopsy of the cyst with old blood in it, for example. Positive cytologic results, on the other hand, would clearly confirm the need for an open biopsy and the need for current mammograms to look for the extent of local pathology or the presence of other lesions.

Open Biopsy

Open biopsy would also be indicated if the aspirating needle of a palpable lump did not yield fluid or if there still was some residual palpable thickening. Indeed, normally when a palpable macrocyst is aspirated successfully and the fluid removed, not only is the lump gone, but the lump is replaced by a palpable, saucerlike depression.

Ultrasound

If a mammogram reveals a nonpalpable round shadow with a smooth border consistent with a cyst, it is reasonable to request ultrasound evaluation and aspiration of the shadow under ultrasound guidance in an attempt to eliminate the shadow and to confirm the impression of a cyst. In some clinics, ultrasound capability is sufficiently sophisticated to determine whether the wall of a macrocyst is smooth and thin or potentially thicker or irregular; this degree of sophistication or technologic capability certainly is not found everywhere. Some ultrasonographers inject air into the cyst cavity after aspiration to aid demonstration of the character of the lining of the cyst. In our clinic, we have seldom seen the need for this. Indications for cytologic evaluation of the fluid at aspiration under ultrasound guidance or for subsequent open biopsy are the same as those already discussed. It is not clear just how well ultrasound evaluation can differentiate between a cyst containing old blood and one with other kinds of fluid. If one merely makes an ultrasound diagnosis of a cyst and does not verify this, one must realize that the probability of overlooking a cancer is small—but is not zero. Whether a cyst is aspirated or not, follow-up evaluation with mammography or ultrasound should be scheduled, perhaps in 2 to 4 months. If the cyst recurs or never was actually eliminated, it should be dealt with again by aspiration or by open biopsy.

Ultrasound may reveal multiple cysts in both breasts, and one cannot eliminate all these cysts from a practical standpoint. At the same time, the body of literature about macrocysts comes largely from the time before the advent of mammography and ultrasound technology, when it was not found to be necessary to do larger operations to eliminate cysts that were not clinically evident. Indeed, many such patients went through a physiologic remission when they went through menopause.

Risk

The preceding comments describe a basic clinical approach to macrocysts of the breast, but the whole picture is not quite that simple. There is a subpopulation of patients with macrocyst who have a somewhat higher risk for breast cancer than others, and one such subpopulation is patients whose mothers have a history of breast cancer. Such patients have been reported by Dupont and Page to incur an increased risk of two to three times for future breast cancer. On the other hand, patients who proceed to get breast cancer are not limited to that subpopulation with a positive family history, so other methods of sorting out macrocyst patients with a higher risk for breast cancer would certainly be in order.

One of the key points to be understood about macrocysts is that the fluid contents are not just inert, inactive, and inconsequential collections of watery material. On the contrary, macrocyst fluid contains a complex array of secretory products, electrolytes, and other substances. Especially notable are a variety of hormones, some of which can be found in high concentrations; glycoproteins of several types; and biologic growth factors. These substances interact with contiguous epithelium and mesenchymal tissue in autocrine and paracrine pathways, and some of these substances get into the circulatory system and are found in peripheral blood samples. For example, Bradlow, Schwartz, Fleischer, and others described the hormonal contents of macrocysts and found that cortisol, progesterone, testosterone, and dihydrotestosterone had concentrations in cyst fluid similar to the concentrations in plasma. However, 17-ketosteroids and estrogen sulfates were present in high concentrations in cyst fluid. Also, Haagensen and Mazoujian found several glycoproteins in macrocyst fluid, one of which they also found in the peripheral blood of some patients, with increased blood levels corresponding to the activity of some androgen-controlled breast cancers and even existing within such breast cancers as shown by immunocytochemistry. This glycoprotein is apparently secreted by apocrine epithelium, a metaplastic type of epithelium commonly found lining macrocysts. The fluid in macrocysts also contains mitogens. At least one of these mitogens has been identified by Tapper, Gajdusec, Moe, and colleagues as epidermal growth factor, one of the biologic growth factors found in a variety of normal tissues but also present in breast cancers. Preliminary data suggest that the level of epidermal growth factor in macrocyst fluid shows a statistically significant correlation with parameters of increased risk for future breast cancer. Epidermal growth factor binds to epidermal growth factor receptor, one of the protein receptors not only found in breast cancer but also associated with more aggressive forms of breast cancer. Cells that respond to epidermal growth factor must possess an epidermal growth factor receptor, and this receptor also binds at least two other ligands, one of which is transforming growth factor α. This growth factor may be involved in cell transformation to a malignant phenotype. There are other growth factors besides epidermal growth factor in macrocyst fluid. This area of investigation is just evolving, but it is likely that in the near future macrocyst fluid will preferably be assayed for biologic parameters rather than be simply discarded.

In the minds of many clinicians, macrocysts of the breast are pictured as large numbers of cavities similar to those in Swiss cheese. However, we probably see only six or eight patients a year with disease that extensive and advanced.

In any event, when a lump is palpated and judged to be abnormal, it needs a diagnosis. Should the next step be to send the patient for ultrasound evaluation? No! If you can palpate a lump, you can aspirate the lump with a syringe and needle and settle the issue right then. This is both less expensive and more efficient than always sending the patient for an ultrasound test. If fluid is obtained and the lump is gone, then what is the next step? A follow-up physical examination should be scheduled in 2 to 4 months, and the patient should be instructed to return earlier if she detects another lump. Mammograms are indicated if these have not been done.

NIPPLE DISCHARGE

Most nipple discharge that is clinically significant occurs spontaneously—it is not manually expressed. Patients are often taught to do self-examination, including squeezing their nipples to see whether there is any fluid. Many parous women in the reproductive years have physiologic, manually expressible nipple discharge that is not considered to be abnormal. The epithelium inside the breast is composed of tubes or ducts that are not dry—they normally contain some fluid. It is not surprising that this should be expressible in some women. Accordingly, I do not instruct patients to try to express nipple fluid during self-examination; palpation of the nipples is done to search for abnormal thickening of the central ducts.

Occasionally, spontaneous nipple discharge occurs on a physiologic basis. This can be a reflex action during a hot shower, can happen with a parous female who has a reflex action on seeing a baby, and can occur with certain medications or sometimes with trauma. Spontaneous nipple discharge is sometimes loosely referred to as galactorrhea. Technically, *galactorrhea* means a spontaneous discharge of milk. A spontaneous milky discharge may indicate a pituitary adenoma, particularly in a patient who has headaches, visual disturbances, and menstrual abnormalities. This type of patient should have a gynecologic evaluation, a serum prolactin test, and referral to an endocrinologist.

For spontaneous discharge that does not appear to be galactorrhea, the next step is to decide whether this appears to be a surgical or a hormonal physiologic problem. If the patient is taking exogenous medications, these are screened for side effects, including nipple discharge. Assuming that this is not the case, considerations pointing to a possible surgical procedure are visible changes in a nipple, especially a shiny red color or a raw weeping surface on the end of the nipple, or a palpable thickening in the nipple or in the breast. Nipple discharge from a single site in one nipple is more apt to be a surgical problem than bilateral nipple discharge from various ductal openings. Nipple discharge from multiple ductal openings implies a physiologic source involving multicentric epithelial hyperplasia probably with a hormonal basis. However, discharge issuing from one duct, regardless of the color of the discharge, is more apt to be a focal surgical lesion. Cancer can occur with any color of nipple discharge, although a bloody nipple discharge indicates a higher risk of cancer. But even with a bloody nipple discharge, cancer is not at the top of the diagnostic list. In order of likelihood, bloody nipple discharge is related to multifocal epithelial hyperplasia, referred to as epitheliosis; to an intraductal papilloma, benign; or to a cancer. Presumably, in one of these forms of epithelial hyperplasia an ulceration has occurred with subsequent bleeding. The color of the nipple discharge can vary in much the same way as the colors previously mentioned for macrocysts. Reasons for these different colors are unknown.

Mammograms should be requested for patients with spontaneous nipple discharge. Some patients demonstrate overt radiologic abnormalities or more subtle findings such as microcalcifications that are concentrated in a particular area. If the opening from a milk duct with discharge can be identified, cannulation of the milk duct by the radiologist can be carried out and mammograms used to study the appearance of dye injected into the duct to look for abnormalities such as a papilloma. Occasionally such lesions are found. In other cases, the dye may not even reach the offending lesion because of obstruction from debris in the duct.

Cytologic evaluation of the nipple discharge should also be obtained. A Hemoccult test is useful to test for blood if the color of the nipple discharge is only suggestive. In most instances, a bloody nipple discharge warrants referral to a surgeon for an open biopsy through a periareolar approach. The color of dark blood helps identify the duct in question at the time of surgery, and insertion of a piece of 0-nylon through the end of the nipple into the duct can be helpful to use as a follower. In other instances, a palpable mass may be present, so a biopsy specimen is taken directly from that site.

When a biopsy is undertaken because of nipple discharge from a lesion that cannot be discerned by physical examination or by mammography, a blind resection of the central ducts deep to the nipple over a 2- to 3-cm distance may be performed. Because the milk ducts radiate out from the nipple in an orderly fashion, similar to the numbers on the face of a clock, sometimes one can get an impression of the sector of the breast from which the discharge comes by palpating the tissue around the areola in a sequential fashion and looking for a point at which the discharge is elicited. This would then provide a clue as to which direction to dissect out from the nipple. Central duct resection may be an appropriate approach for patients who are in their late thirties and forties and who have had children and are finished nursing. This may not be a satisfactory approach for younger patients in their early thirties or earlier in the absence of some localizing findings. On one hand, resection of the central ducts deep to the nipple can be followed by nipple numbness, malfunction, and distortion. On the other hand the actual source of the discharge may not be included within the specimen. Nipple discharge can indeed be stopped with this kind of a surgical procedure, but unless an objective focus of pathology is found in a tissue specimen, the actual source of the discharge may be left behind within the breast. There would be no way to know this, and thus there might be a false sense of security created. Such a patient must be kept under surveillance, then, in the event that the pathologist does not find an obvious lesion in the inspected specimen. For young patients, resection of the central ducts may be an unsatisfactory procedure, so whenever possible considerable effort should be expended by the surgeon in trying to identify a specific portion of the central ductal system that might contain the offending lesion. Just that portion of the ducts should be resected in a radial direction, instead of transecting and removing all the central ducts. Such a radial approach is considerably less likely to lead to complications of nipple appearance and function.

Special mention should be made of bloody nipple discharge that occurs during pregnancy. Haagensen described a personal series of such patients and observed that, to his knowledge, cancer did not evolve in any of his cases. Not much information is available on this subject because the number of such cases is small. Certainly, if there are any clinical findings such as a palpable mass or features of nipple lesions, these require a biopsy whether the patient is pregnant or not. But in the absence of localizing findings, these patients are generally managed by serial observation and physical examination only. So far, bleeding in these cases has been self-limited. One is hesitant to subject the patient and the fetus to irradiation from mammography. If mammography is attempted, the abdomen must be carefully shielded with a lead apron. For bloody nipple discharge during pregnancy, it is important to carefully determine when this discharge began. I have seen at least one case in which a young pregnant patient with a bloody nipple discharge turned out to have a cancer, but it is important to note that her bloody discharge first began 2 or 3 months before she was pregnant.

How this self-limited bloody nipple discharge during pregnancy occurs is not known. Presumably, the changes during pregnancy involve rapid proliferation of the epithelium, and for some reason, a focal ulceration might develop; however, this is only conjecture.

SKIN ERYTHEMA

Visible erythema of the skin of the breast, the areola, or the nipple can occur for a variety of reasons. Erythema of the breast skin is most often due to inflammatory changes caused by infection. Erythema of the areola by itself is most often due to a dermatitis (such as a contact dermatitis or eczema). Erythema of the nipple is more often due to Paget's carcinoma. The earliest changes of Paget's carcinoma are not ulceration and crusting—they are reddening of the end of the nipple with thinned-out, almost transparent epithelium. Such an observation alone warrants referral to a surgeon for a nipple biopsy.

Skin erythema resulting from benign inflammatory changes has a distinctive clinical picture. In postmenopausal elderly patients, the degree of erythema may be somewhat pale, and the underlying process is apt to be a chemical inflammation characterized by periductal mastitis, apparently from effects of the ductal contents getting into the surrounding tissues. In such patients the process occurs in dilated or ectatic ducts and then goes through a sequence of periductal inflammatory changes and later fibrosis that are reflected on nearby skin with edema of the dermis, sometimes with traction effects and other characteristics strongly suggesting cancer. This process requires mammograms and a biopsy to document the nature of the problem.

Erythema caused by inflammatory changes of acute infection tends to occur in younger patients, especially those who are lactating. These changes are sometimes seen in teenagers who have never been pregnant. The presumed source of this infection is exogenous oral contamination through the nipple. The skin erythema of acute mastitis from infection involves only one sector of the contiguous breast extending out from a segment of the periphery of the areola. Beneath this erythema, which is often bright red, tender, and painful, is a region of palpable induration within the tissue that is oriented centrally toward the axis of the nipple. Such an area of inflammation caused by infection is often so tender that the patient will hardly allow herself to be examined, and there may be some throbbing. Exquisite tenderness and throbbing of this sort has not been a characteristic of cancer. If such erythema and induration form a sort of island or are located out in the tissue away from the nipple, the diagnosis of infection must be suspect, and needle aspiration cytology and potentially open biopsy should be done. Mammograms may not be feasible because of the degree of tenderness in the breast.

Also, if the erythema of the skin extends 360° around the areola and particularly if it occupies the dependent third of the breast, one immediately should think of an inflammatory carcinoma rather than an infection. The milk ducts inside the breast are not interconnected through the periphery of the breast, so infection does not travel in a 360-degree distribution; infection has a radial distribution. The erythema of inflammatory carcinoma may be pale or red, and there is usually palpable dermal thickening. This type of breast is not exquisitely tender like that caused by acute infection, although there may be some degree of palpably increased skin temperature. Whether the patient is lactating, pregnant, or nonpregnant, 360-degree circumferential skin erythema of the breast may indicate cancer. Needle aspiration cytology of the internal breast tissue can be carried out, but in this setting referral to a surgeon for open biopsy is preferable so that a larger sample of the tissue can be obtained for frozen section and immunocytochemical tests. The biopsy sample should include a piece of the dermis to look for lymphangitic spread of cancer cells. Inflammatory carcinoma represents only 1% to 3% of breast cancers, so most clinicians may not have encountered these changes before. The patient is apt to be treated with antibiotics for infection, sometimes for a month or two, delaying the discovery of a fast-moving cancer. Certainly if antibiotics are used for a presumed infection, there should be a clear improvement within 5 or 7 days; lack of obvious improvement should bring into question the diagnosis of infection.

INFECTION

Most breast infections are not seen in a surgical clinic. These are more commonly encountered in lactating females in the obstetric clinic. Infection ordinarily responds promptly to treatment with antibiotics for gram-positive organisms. In a patient with acute erythema, pain, and induration as seen in the surgical clinic, the main problem is whether an abscess already exists and requires open drainage under general anesthesia. An abscess can be 2 or 3 inches deep within a breast in the central axis of the nipple and can be difficult to determine by palpation. With local anesthesia, aspiration can be attempted, but because of the viscid nature of the contents of an abscess, a relatively large needle, such as a number 18, should be used in conjunction with an aspirating pistol grip on the syringe to develop maximum vacuum. The specimen should be sent for a culture to check for both aerobes and anaerobes, even if no abscess fluid is obtained. Not all the infections are due to gram-positive organisms. Walker, Edmiston, Krepel, and others found that breast abscesses also have a major anaerobic component. If an abscess is not defined, the patient can be treated with an antibiotic such as cephalexin (Keflex), starting with a loading dose of 500 mg four times a day for the first 2 days, then going to twice a day. If a prompt response is not obtained and a needle aspiration has not been done, a needle aspiration should be carried out under sterile precautions for evaluation of possible anaerobic infection.

The most common problem of infections is recurrence resulting from inadequate treatment. If there is an abscess, this should be drained under general anesthesia, a rubber drain sutured in place for several weeks (until the drain is pushed out of the cavity inside), and systemic antibiotics used. If there is no abscess, antibiotic treatment should be continued for at least 2 weeks. A course of only 7 or 8 days is likely to be insufficient for the infections seen in a surgical clinic.

BREAST PAIN

The most common type of breast pain and tenderness is cyclic premenstrual pain during the reproductive years, which is referred to as mastalgia. For practical purposes, I do not include patients who have had such symptoms less than 7 to 10 days. When cyclic pain and tenderness occur for 10 days or more in a menstrual cycle, the degree of pain becomes considerable, particularly in the patient who has this distress throughout the month. The actual mechanism by which this pain arises is unknown. Biopsy specimens do not show inflammatory features, edema, or any other specific features in most patients. Indeed, in a patient in psychiatric services who was suicidal and had severe breast pain, open breast biopsy showed mostly fibrous supporting tissue with little epithelium and certainly no epithelial hyperplasia. There was no inflammation. This patient was determined to be anovulatory and had dramatic relief of her pain with the use of a progestin. She became able to play tennis again, ride horses again, and pick up her children, each of which she had become unable to do previously.

Such pain is clearly of a hormonal nature; it correlates with the menstrual cycle, sometimes beginning on the actual day of ovulation, and then gets worse until menstruation. For some reason, many patients have this type of pain in only one breast; however, it still must be hormonal in nature. These symptoms have often been imputed to cystic mastitis or fibrocystic disease. On one hand, a large percentage of these patients have never had documented cysts, and on the other hand, at least 50% of patients who do have documented macrocysts do not have pain. I have discussed this type of pain with clinicians in our pain clinic and in our neurosurgery department, but the physiologic explanation of the pain remains abstruse.

Kuttenn, Fournier, Sitruk-Ware, and colleagues and the Marseilles group have written a number of papers on breast pain and described mastalgia in a setting of anovulation and low progesterone levels during the luteal phase of the menstrual cycle. In women who have had their ovaries surgically removed or gone through menopause and who have persistent breast pain and tenderness, one should think of exogenous estrogens or obesity, a setting in which levels of endogenous estrogens are elevated. Dietary factors such as caffeine intake have also been implicated by Minton and others. Clinical evaluation should include a current pelvic examination to look for ovarian pathology as well as a breast examination. If the patient has not had recent mammograms, these should be done, providing that the degree of tenderness allows mammograms to be performed. The purpose of these mammograms is to search for associated breast pathology—these mammograms will not usually delineate the source of such pain. Blood tests of endogenous hormone levels are not usually carried out, although they would be in order if there were signs of androgen excess or other relevant physiology. Blood tests or hormone levels are difficult to interpret because of the well-known variability seen during menstrual cycles.

Clinical evaluation usually turns up no specific findings. The clinician can reassure the patient that these cyclic symptoms are not an indication of breast cancer. This does not mean a breast cancer cannot exist—it means that these symptoms, in general, are not those of a breast cancer. The kinds of pain that make one think of a breast cancer involve a localized tightening or pulling sensation or a localized burning or itching inside the breast. The latter symptoms warrant referral to a surgeon for an assiduous search for cancer, including physical examination, mammograms, and sometimes even a blind biopsy.

When the patient is reassured that her cyclic symptoms are not characteristic of cancer, she may need no further treatment. The clinician also inquires about potential sources of stress, such as a divorce, a move from another city, loss of a job, or any other contributory source that can affect ovulatory function. If such a source of stress is found, this can be explained to the patient, with the expectation that the symptoms will be alleviated when the stress remits. Moreover, some patients can anticipate remission of the symptoms if menopause is imminent. Some patients have less breast pain and tenderness if they eliminate caffeine from their diet or in some instances if they take exogenous vitamin E, 400 to 600 U daily. There is no way to predict which patients will experience some improvement in their symptoms and which will not. Those patients with severe pain and tenderness may warrant a trial of hormonal manipulation. The least expensive medication (and one of the more physiologic) is medroxyprogesterone acetate given in doses of 20 mg daily from about day 5 through day 25 of the menstrual cycle. Danazol, a weak androgen, can be tried, but should not be used in the high doses used for diseases such as endometriosis. It can be started at doses of 50 mg to 100 mg daily after determining that the patient is not pregnant, potentially increasing the dose after a month's trial if the lower dose is not beneficial. The other medicines that have been used include bromocriptine and tamoxifen. Unfortunately, all of these hormonal medications have side effects that patients do not appreciate, and they are expensive. The most common side effects are a 5- to 7-lb weight increase that persists and sometimes depression or other symptoms. The use of danazol or tamoxifen can cause menstrual changes as well. There is no simple solution applicable to all patients.

BREAST CANCER IN YOUNG PATIENTS

More and more breast cancers are being found in young patients, and this is of particular importance to gynecologists. Patients below the age of 35 years have not been included in recommendations for screening asymptomatic patients with mammography, for example. Among 700 of my breast cancer patients, 150 were under the age of 40 years, some as young as 17, with no abrupt falloff in incidence at an arbitrary age (such as 35 years). Ninety percent of the breast cancers in women under the age of 35 years are first detected as a palpable lump, and a delay in diagnosis is common in this age group because clinician's expect the changes to be benign. These are not the patients who are undergoing mammograms, and some calcifications unexpectedly are found that reveal early noninvasive breast cancer. When a lump is already palpable, the patient often has a late stage I or stage II invasive breast cancer. These young patients between the ages of 25 and 35 years are three to four times as likely to have a first-degree family member with breast cancer as compared with the broader population.

My experience with these patients applies to those who were referred to a surgical clinic for a variety of reasons. In these young patients who develop breast cancer and have had mammograms, two thirds of those cancers found in the past 5 years and 80% of those found in the last 1 to 2 years had abnormal mammograms. Abnormalities such as microcalcifications or an abnormal shadow push the clinician toward early referral to a surgeon for a biopsy as opposed to cases where no mammograms are done. The technology of mammography has improved even in the last few years, so past experiences with mammography may not reflect the current potential of this procedure. In our breast clinic, symptomatic patients 25 years of age and older undergo mammograms, and patients who have a mother who developed breast cancer in her 30's get baseline mammograms at 25 years of age and older even if they are not symptomatic. This is not to say that women in these age groups in the general population should be treated in the same way. For the time being at least, young patients in our breast clinic receive earlier mammographic surveillance in an effort to better the distressing figure of 90% of breast cancers not being detected until palpable.

BREAST CANCER IN PREGNANT PATIENTS

Discovery of early breast cancer in pregnant patients is impeded by its rarity, by the density of fibroglandular tissue that is normal in young patients, by the increased density and volume of fibroglandular proliferation in pregnancy, and by the hesitation to use diagnostic mammography with its possible radioactive effect on the fetus. Likewise, pregnant patients frequently get the types of benign breast diseases incurred by nonpregnant patients. It is not surprising that the rare inflammatory carcinoma is treated as a breast infection or that a rounded breast cancer is clinically determined to be a benign fibroadenoma. (Indeed, a benign fibroadenoma can be stimulated to enlarge considerably during pregnancy).

Petrek reviewed the problems of diagnosing breast cancer in pregnant patients, citing delays both by the patient and the clinician that average 3 to 7 months. At Memorial Sloan-Kettering Cancer Center, the median size of these cancers is 3 cm (already stage II). Fewer than 20% of those cancer patients were diagnosed and treated during pregnancy. Nearly 50% of the patients who had a mass documented during pregnancy were diagnosed and treated in a 12-week interval *after* pregnancy. By the same token, Lichter and Lippman collected reports of 465 patients with pregnancy-associated breast cancer and observed that 65% to 85% of pregnant or lactating females had positive axillary lymph nodes as compared with 45% to 50% of nonpregnant patients.

The initial diagnostic issue in pregnant patients is most frequently a palpable indurated area or a lump. There is no reason to pursue a diagnosis less expeditiously in a pregnant patient than in a nonpregnant patient. Such a palpable abnormality can be aspirated by using a syringe and needle and obtaining a cytologic study if the lump is solid. If fluid is aspirated and the lump is gone, follow-up examination should be done in 1 to 2 months. On the other hand, if the lump is solid, the patient should be referred after needle aspiration to a surgeon for evaluation regardless of the cytologic report. This is obvious when the cytologic findings are positive for cancer, but negative cytologic results should not be trusted as fully representative of the lesion—a needle core biopsy or an open biopsy should be considered. Mammograms should be obtained (using lead to shield the fetus) if the cytologic study is positive; if the findings are negative, it is not essential to have a mammogram ahead of time when an open biopsy is planned because the lesion will be diagnosed anyway. Ultrasound may be informative, however, because features of malignancy can often be defined from benign features in dense breast tissue. If for some reason a biopsy of a lump is not undertaken, ultrasound is recommended. On the other hand, when mammograms are done, features of malignancy (such as grouped micro-calcifications) point to the need for a prompt biopsy, but the absence of mammographic features of malignancy does not in any way justify a pronunciation that there is no cancer, or that "there is nothing to worry about." An open biopsy or a core needle biopsy of an abnormal breast lump should not be delayed because of negative mammograms or because of hesitation to get mammograms when the patient is pregnant.

Mammograms are not used for screening purposes in pregnant patients for a variety of reasons, one of which is risk of radiation effects on the fetus. When mammograms are indicated, the abdomen of the mother should be carefully shielded with lead, and well-calibrated low-dose mammography equipment should be used. Petrek discussed radiation risks in rodents and humans: The risk of congenital anomalies in the fetus after irradiation is much lower beyond the 8-week period early in pregnancy when organo-genesis occurs. Beyond 30 weeks of gestation, congenital anomalies after irradiation are believed to be extremely rare. Another potential problem is future carcinogenesis in the offspring after irradiation, the risks of which are controversial but small. I do not know of a report linking fetal damage to mammography in a well-shielded pregnant patient.

Diagnostic considerations for postpartum lactating patients differ little from those for pregnant patients except the issue of mammographic radiation effects no longer applies. Mammographic details are more likely to be obscured in a lactating breast than in a nonlactating breast, but ultrasound is still helpful. When there is a palpable lump in a lactating breast, it is worth the patient asking whether it goes away during nursing, which would suggest a galactocele that empties and later refills with milk. Likewise, physical examination soon after the patient nurses her baby may facilitate evaluation of a lump in question. Needle aspiration of a lump should be undertaken. If milk is obtained in the syringe and the lump is gone, no biopsy is needed. Cancer in a galactocele would be a medical curiosity. A galactocele can be expected to refill with milk, however, so this lump will probably continue to recur with repeated aspirations; thus repeated aspirations are not necessary. If the lump is solid or does not go away the first time with aspiration, cytologic studies can be obtained, and the patient should be referred to a surgeon.

In lactating patients an open biopsy can readily be done with local anesthesia, just as in a pregnant patient. At biopsy, removal of fibroglandular tissue in a radial direction can minimize damage to contiguous milk ducts because these ducts travel in a radial direction. Suture ligation of the remaining fibroglandular tissue at the side of the biopsy cavity toward the nipple and of any visibly leaking milk ducts generally leaves a dry operative field not requiring a drain. Wound closure with buried sutures and application of a transparent plastic dressing (such as Tego-Derm) to the skin incision are all that is required. Nursing can proceed as scheduled with this type of closure, and the plastic is left in place for 5 to 7 days. Occasionally a streak of blood appears in the milk at the nipple; this simply represents access of some blood from the wound into a transected milk duct.

BREAST BIOPSIES

Needle aspiration biopsies have been mentioned earlier; this is an expeditious diagnostic technique that should be used more often than it is to reduce the amount of conjecture that often delays definitive diagnosis. A positive needle aspiration cytology report from an experienced cytologist is highly accurate. But a confirmatory open biopsy and frozen section is recommended at the time of major surgery such as a mastectomy because even one false-positive result in a thousand will have unfortunate sequelae. Particularly during pregnancy, proliferative benign changes can be difficult to differentiate from a papillary carcinoma. Even so, according to Preece, Hunter, Duguid, and coworkers, needle aspiration biopsy can detect about 90% of breast cancers in symptomatic patients. In addition to high sensitivity, they and others describe a specificity over 99% (a very low false-positive rate).

Use of a cutting needle to obtain a core of breast tissue for permanent histologic sections has increased. This is most frequently done during mammography or ultrasound evaluation. Stereotactic mammographic control is accurate for accessing nonpalpable lumps either by needle core biopsy or fine needle aspiration. Ultrasound guidance of needle core biopsies also is now done frequently. The advantage of needle core biopsies (number 14 needle) is that a core of tissue is obtained for paraffin sections. A diagnosis of invasive cancer, in situ cancer, or benign disease can be made. Thus unnecessary open biopsies can often be avoided, saving health care costs.

Regarding open biopsy of the breast, this chapter is not intended to be a technical manual of how to do the procedure. The reason is that both breast cancer biology and treatment considerations are more and more complex. Possible eventualities must be anticipated and the conduct of the procedure modified according to the surgical pathology that is seen and felt in conjunction with the biologic parameters that desired by those who plan treatment (Figs. 9-11 and 9-12). Almost anyone can do the mechanical steps in a biopsy; the mechanical steps are not the most challenging part of the procedure (although the patient may have a different point of view). Those who do breast biopsies should be trained to recognize the meaning of the tissue colors, architecture, and consistency and to recognize the subtleties that require extending the procedure here or there, where to mark the tissue, what special studies to order, and when to prepare frozen sections. It is

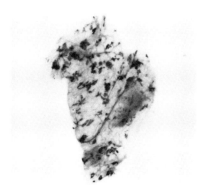

FIGURE 9-11. Breast biopsy specimen, actual size. Note the darkly stained epithelial elements with lobular hyperplasia, seen best with a hand lens.

Tissue prepared and provided courtesy of Dr. Hanne Jensen, Davis, California.

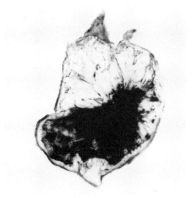

FIGURE 9-12. Breast biopsy specimen, actual size. A dark mass of invasive breast cancer has irregular streaky edges. Compare with the shadow in Fig. 9-7.

Tissue prepared and provided courtesy of Dr. Hanne Jensen, Davis, California.

common for us to see referred patients for breast preservation therapy using primary irradiation, for example. One dictum is to try to have surgical margins free of cancer in the biopsy site to minimize the risk of local recurrence. But when we observe the histologic sections, the edges of the surgical specimen may not have been covered with ink at the time of surgery. After the pathologist cuts the specimen into smaller pieces to fit onto tissue slides, cancer is often seen at a cut edge in a microscopic section; it is impossible to tell whether the edge is an outer margin (cut by the surgeon) or an inner margin (cut by the pathologist). The patient must then undergo surgery for wider local excision. Moreover, even when the surgical margins are free of cancer, suitable for breast preservation, marker clips may not have been left in the breast around the perimeter of the biopsy cavity at the time the biopsy was done. These metal vascular clips are visible on x-ray films, so the radiation oncologist can see exactly where to guide the higher dose of irradiation to the tumor bed. For the radiation oncologist simply to look at the skin incision as a guide can be misleading as to just where surgery was done. So these and other considerations must be anticipated at the time of biopsy.

The large majority of our patients undergo biopsy with local anesthesia and intravenous sedation, including careful monitoring with continuous electrocardiographic tracing, continuous oxygen saturation, and automatic blood pressure readout. Usually, cosmetic incisions concentric to the areola are used. With careful hemostasis, drains are not used. A rubber drain may prevent some (but by no means all) hematomas. The skin is closed with buried sutures, and a plastic dressing is applied. All cancer specimens should be analyzed for estrogen and progesterone receptor proteins, preferably by immunocytochemistry. Other tests are desirable, such as monoclonal antibody labeling of Her-2/neu protein product, p53 protein, and cell proliferation. Detailed information about biologic parameters is provided by McGuire's group at San Antonio; by Lippman; by Bacus, Goldschmidt, Chin, and coworkers, and by Howell and Millis.

For specimens that might contain early noninvasive cancer, a frozen section is not done. In this setting the pathologist looks for even tiny foci of invasive cancer that coexists and affects management. Thus the whole tissue specimen goes into permanent histologic sections, whereas in frozen sections some of the tissue is trimmed off first in the microtome to make a flat surface for tissue sections. Invasive cancer could be trimmed off inadvertently and lost in that process.

RISK FACTORS FOR BREAST CANCER

A practical method of simplifying decision making regarding risk is to sort out risk factors into major and minor factors. Major risk factors are those that call for action or special consideration by the clinician; minor risk factors are those that do not indicate special action by the clinician. Without going into an extensive discussion, I consider only two major risk factors; a history of premenopausal breast cancer in first-degree relatives (mother, sister, daughter); and second, histologic documentation of tissue features indicating increased risk for breast cancer. These are two settings where the subjects of counseling for special surveillance or for prophylactic surgery arise. In contrast to these major risk factors, minor risk factors include such things as nulliparity, late first pregnancy, early menarche, late menopause, and obesity; the clinician cannot do much about these things, and a decision for or against something like a biopsy for the usual indications is not swayed one way or the other by minor risk factors.

One of the useful sources of information on risk from family history is a review by Williams and Osborne. This information is compiled in terms of lifetime risk in a concise fashion appropriate for general clinicians. Levels of observed lifetime risk in family studies done by others approach 50% in some instances. Examples are:

- the risk to a patient who has a sister with premenopausal bilateral breast cancer
- a mother and sister both with premenopausal breast cancer, bilateral in one of these
- two sisters both with premenopausal breast cancer, one bilateral

When the patient's mother and sister both had premenopausal breast cancer (not bilateral), the observed risk was about 33%. The levels of risk just mentioned warrant a consideration of prophylactic bilateral mastectomy or at least careful surveillance. These patients should preferably be referred to an academic clinical genetics unit for detailed analysis of the family pedigree. There are pedigrees with unique cancers or multiple kinds of cancer where the risk approaches 100%. Moreover, these issues of risk include cancers other than just breast cancer, and special health care of other relatives may be warranted. Thus genetic consultation is recommended.

Evaluation by a surgeon is also important for a patient with high familial risk. There may already be an existing clinical problem that requires attention. The surgeon must determine how effectively the patient can be followed by surveillance—how useful physical examination and mammograms are in a given patient, what previous breast problems there were, what histologic details are available, and so forth. The patient must know what would be involved in a bilateral mastectomy (probably with cosmetic reconstruction).

Hereditary breast cancers are incurred at earlier ages and are more likely to be multicentric or bilateral than sporadic nonhereditary breast cancers. Hereditary breast cancers occur most frequently in the forties but can even occur in the twenties.

These high-risk patients should be taught monthly self-examination around 20 years of age, followed by annual physical examinations by the doctor. I favor baseline mammograms at the age of 25, repeated in 3 years, then going to annual mammograms sometime between the ages of 30 to 35. Physical examinations should become more frequent, at about 6-month intervals, by the ages of 28 to 30. Prompt biopsy should be performed for any physical or mammographic abnormalities in these patients. There is no role for "watching." Genetic counseling should be sought sometime between the ages of 25 to 30.

Besides familial risk, the other major risk factor stems from documented breast biopsy microscopic findings. It is of interest, however, that high risk levels from histologic findings are not nearly as high as the higher levels of familial risk. Page and Dupont describe three categories of increased risk for future invasive breast cancer. Slightly increased risk (1.5 to 2 times that of the general population) corresponds to moderate and florid epithelial hyperplasia without atypia. Moderately increased risk (4 to 5 times) applies to atypical hyperplasia. (Keep in mind that this is histologic atypia, not the atypia of a class II cytologic report.) Also, this atypia is severe atypia with some but not all of the features of noninvasive carcinoma. High risk (about 10 times) pertains to noninvasive or in situ ductal and lobular carcinoma. These risk levels are not lifetime risk levels and are reported differently from those mentioned earlier for familial risk. These histologic risk levels are relative risk, not lifetime risk. They usually mean a comparison of the patient with women of the same age in the general population or some other specified group. One does not use these multiples to multiply lifetime risk to get absolute risk. Absolute risk is sought in specific articles by Page and Dupont.

Patients with severe atypia or carcinoma should be referred to a surgeon if the biopsy was done by someone else. Also, it may be unwise to treat such patients, with estrogens after menopause. Although the role of pharmaceutical estrogens appears to be nil or extremely low for increasing risk of invasive breast cancer in the general population, there may be undefined subpopulations who have increased risk, given that endogenous estrogen stimulates most of the biologic growth factors found in breast cancer (although this has not been investigated with pharmaceutical estrogens). Again, these patients with increased histologic risk should be doing monthly self-examinations and getting annual mammograms and physical examinations at 6- to 12-month intervals.

PREVENTIVE HEALTH CARE AND SCREENING

There is no definite way to prevent breast cancer. As far as diet is concerned, women are advised to pursue the same dietary measures that would be generally beneficial. This includes a low-fat, low-red-meat, high-fiber, high-fish diet, including vegetables from the cabbage family.

The only proven way to detect the earliest forms of breast cancer on a systematic basis is with mammography. Noninvasive breast cancer or precancerous changes may be incidental findings when more prominent benign changes are biopsied after palpation by the patient or by the clinician. Technologies such as thermography or diaphonography are not useful for detecting noninvasive cancer. Moreover, ultrasound does not reliably demonstrate the microcalcifications that are so helpful in detecting nonpalpable lesions in mammograms.

Years ago, the well-known Health Insurance Plan of Greater New York (HIP) study of 31,000 women between the ages of 40 and 64 years showed a significant reduction in mortality after screening with mammograms and physical examinations as compared with a control group. After an 18-year follow-up, there continues to be a 25% reduction in mortality, and this applies to women under the age of 50 as well as those over 50 years of age, according to Strax.

Over 275,000 women between the ages of 35 and 74 years were studied in the breast cancer detection demonstration project with mammography and physical examination, recently discussed by McClelland and Pisano and by Byrd and Hartmann. A third of the cancers discovered were in women under the age of 50 years, and a third of these were detected by mammography alone (as compared with 13% by physical examination alone). Patients who had cancers smaller than 1 cm had a survival rate over 90% after 10 years of follow-up. The patients in this study were also taught breast self-examination. A group of these women who continued breast self-examination and got cancer had a 5-year survival rate of 78% as compared with 61% for a group with cancer who had not continued self-examination. Also, in the HIP study, among patients who had cancer at intervals between the annual evaluations, those patients who had been taught self-examination had cancers with features as favorable as those found by mammography; those with interval cancers who did not practice self-examination got cancers resembling those of patients not receiving mammograms. (About 15% of the cancers overall were interval cancers.)

Feldman, Carter, Nicastri, and coworkers reported that among 996 cancer patients, those patients who had been doing breast self-examination had smaller cancers and one-third fewer positive lymph nodes than did patients not doing self-examination. Similarly, Huguley, Brown, Greenberg, and others studied 2093 patients with breast cancer and showed a 15% higher 5-year survival rate in those patients doing self-examination as compared with those not doing self-examination. Suitable instructions for self-examination are provided by Tyrer and Granzig, and commercial videos are available as well.

The main problem in screening is the lack of mammography use for various reasons on the part of both patients and doctors. Numerous guidelines for mammography have been published. But too many patients have not had any mammograms at all until a lump is felt. Even one set of baseline mammograms for patients 35 years of age and over will detect cancers at the same rate as the rate for a first visit in published screening studies. Mammography should be done for any symptomatic breast patient — this is not screening. We are seeing more and more breast cancer in young patients, so I favor baseline mammograms between the ages of 25 and 30 years for patients with major risk factors. Otherwise, I favor mammograms at the age of 40 years, with subsequent frequency depending on what is found. After negative mammograms, these would be repeated at

1- or 2-year intervals, depending on the patient. Tabar and Dean described the results of a Swedish screening study using only a single mammographic view without physical examination at 2-year intervals in women aged 40 to 49 years and at 33-month intervals for women aged 50 to 74 years. By the end of about 6 years there was a 31% reduction in mortality from breast cancer in the study group. This was a randomized controlled trial. Also, a Nijmegen study used a single-view mammogram at 2-year intervals in eight rounds of screening over 40,000 women. The sizes of the cancers detected by screening were smaller than those detected clinically for all age groups. Moreover, the number of ductal carcinomas in situ detected by screening younger women was significantly greater than the number detected by screening older women. For women over 50 years of age, cancers detected by screening had a more favorable stage distribution than clinically detected cancers (although this was not the case for women under 50). Thus even a small number of mammographic screening events can be valuable. If one wishes to apply mammographic screening only to those patients with risk factors for breast cancer, keep in mind that nearly 75% of patients who get breast cancer do not have known risk factors and only about 15% of patients with breast cancer have a positive family history, one third of which is hereditary.

BIBLIOGRAPHY

Bacus SS, Goldschmidt R, Chin D, et al: Biological grading of breast cancer using antibodies to proliferating cells and other markers, *Am J Pathol* 135: 783, 1989.

Barth V: *Atlas of diseases of the breast*, Chicago, 1979, Year Book Medical.

Bradlow HL, Schwartz MK, Fleischer M, et al: Hormone levels in human breast cyst fluid. In Angeli A, Bradlow HL, Dogliotti L, editors: *Endocrinology of cystic breast disease*, New York, 1983, Raven Press.

Byrd BF, Hartmann WH: Breast cancer detection epoch, *Semin Surg Oncol* 4:221, 1988.

Dupont WD, Page DL: Risk factors for breast cancer in women with proliferative breast disease, *N Engl J Med* 312:146, 1985.

Feldman JG, Carter AC, Nicastri AD, et al: Breast self-examination, relationship to stage of breast cancer at diagnosis, *Cancer* 47:2740, 1981.

Frable WJ: *Thin-needle aspiration biopsy*, Philadelphia, 1983, Saunders.

Haagensen DE, Mazoujian G: Relationship of glycoproteins in human breast cystic fluid to breast carcinoma. In Angeli A, Bradlow HL, Dogliotti L, editors: *Endocrinology of cystic breast disease*, New York, 1983, Raven Press.

Homer MJ: Localization of nonpalpable breast lesions with the curved-end retractable wire: leaving the needle in vivo, *AJR Am J Roentgenol* 151:919, 1988.

Howell A, Millis RR: Cellular aspects of breast cancer: workshop report, *Eur J Cancer Clin Oncol* 24:21, 1988.

Huguley CM, Brown RL, Greenberg RS, et al: Breast self-examination and survival from breast cancer, *Cancer* 62: 1389, 1988.

Jensen HM: Breast pathology, emphasizing precancerous and cancer-associated lesions, *Commentaries Res Breast Dis* 2:41, 1981.

Kuttenn F, Fournier S, Sitruk-Ware R, et al: Progesterone insufficiency in benign disease. In Angeli A, Bradlow HL, Dogliotti L, editors: *Endocrinology of cystic breast disease*, New York, 1983, Raven Press.

Lichter AS, Lippman ME: Special situations in the treatment of breast cancer. In Lippman ME, Lichter AS, Danforth DN, editors): *Diagnosis and management of breast cancer*, Philadelphia, 1988, Saunders.

Lippman ME: Steroid hormone receptors and mechanisms of growth regulation in human breast cancer. In Lippman ME, Lichter AS, Danforth DN, editors: *Diagnosis and management of breast cancer*, Philadelphia, 1988, Saunders.

McLelland R, Pisano ED: Issues in mammography, *Cancer* 66:1341, 1990.

Minton JP, Abou-Issa H: Nonendocrine theories of the etiology of benign breast disease, *World J Surg* 13:680, 1989.

Page DL, Dupont WD: Histopathologic risk factors for breast cancer in women with benign breast disease, *Semin Surg Oncol* 4:213, 1988.

Petrek JA: Breast cancer and pregnancy. In Harris JR, Hellman S, Henderson CI, et al, editors: *Breast diseases*, Philadelphia, 1987, Lippincott.

Petronella PGM, Holland R, Jan HCLH, et al: Age-specific effectiveness of the Nijmegen population-based breast cancer–screening program: assessment of early indicators of screening effectiveness, *J Natl Cancer Inst* 86: 436, 1994.

Preece PE, Hunter SM, Duguid HLD, et al: Cytodiagnosis and other methods of biopsy in the modern management of breast cancer, *Semin Surg Oncol* 5:69, 1989.

Saez RA, McGuire WL, Clark GM: Prognostic factors in breast cancer, *Semin Surg Oncol* 5:102, 1989.

Strax P: Mass screening to reduce mortality from breast cancer, *Semin Surg Oncol* 4: 218, 1988.

Strax P: The Health Insurance Plan of New York study: clinical aspects, *Cancer* 64(suppl):2641, 1989.

Tabar L, Dean PB: The present state of screening for breast cancer, *Semin Surg Oncol* 5:94, 1989.

Tapper D, Gajdusec C, Moe R, et al: The identification of a unique biologic tumor marker in human breast cyst fluid and breast cancer tissue, *Am J Surg* 159:473, 1990.

Tyrer LB, Granzig WA: Instructing patients in self-examination of the breast, *Clin Obstet Gynecol* 18:175, 1975.

Walker AP, Edmiston CE, Krepel CJ, et al: A prospective study of the microflora of nonpuerperal breast abscess, *Arch Surg* 123:908, 1988.

Williams WR, Osborne MP: Familial aspects of breast cancer: an overview. In Harris JR, Hellman S, Henderson CI, et al, editors: *Breast diseases*, Philadelphia, 1987, Lippincott.

CHAPTER 10

Management of Vulvar Diseases

LOUIS A. VONTVER

Complaints referable to the vulva are common in office practice. Patients have a vulvar itch, pain, or irritation or discover a lump and are justifiably concerned. Most of these concerns can be relieved by diagnosis and treatment in the ambulatory setting.

Initially the differential diagnosis of vulvar abnormalities is made by history and gross visualization. What are the symptoms? How long have they lasted? What has been done to treat them? What are the physical signs? The vulvar skin and mucous membranes can respond in only one of a few ways. Therefore many etiologic factors may cause the same type of response, such as itching, burning, pain, redness, whiteness, lichenification, blistering, and ulcers. The vulvar skin is also richly supplied with sweat and sebaceous glands. It has a moist environment with an increased concentration of skin bacteria. Therefore lesions that appear characteristic on dry surface skin elsewhere may not have the same appearance on the vulva.

The history and examination are followed by specific tests such as a wet mount of vaginal secretions, potassium hydroxide (KOH) scrapings of vulvar skin, dark-field preparations, cultures, and liberal use of biopsy samples for microscopy or immunocytochemistry. Most of these tests are easily performed. By using history, physical examination, and indicated tests, most vulvar abnormalities can be diagnosed and successfully treated. However, some are obscure, persistent, chronic, recurrent, and resistant to many alternative therapies. Patients with such abnormalities are often difficult to manage. They frequently have tried over-the-counter remedies, seen many physicians, and become discouraged, feeling that their problem is undiagnosable and untreatable. They tend to lose confidence in their health care providers. The use of untried or "shotgun" remedies, some of which are sensitizing, may add to their problem. Therefore one should try to make a definitive diagnosis as early as possible. Avoid treating over the telephone for a suspected disorder or using a shotgun therapeutic approach. Most often, a careful examination results in a precise diagnosis and permits a specific therapy. Even if it does not, the physician is usually able to reassure the worried patient with a persistent vulvar complaint that she does not have a serious disease such as cancer or a sexually transmitted disease (STD).

Some patients have chronic complaints of vulvovaginal symptoms but repeated negative findings on examination, culture, biopsy, and microscopy. These patients have a significantly higher incidence of depression and anxiety than do women with similar complaints who have diagnostic findings on their examinations. Significant depression may underlie vulvovaginal complaints that persist in the absence of any pathologic finding. Psychologic and psychosocial assessment and care should be considered for such patients.

Some general preventive and therapeutic rules apply in most cases of vulvar complaints. Keep the vulvar area clean and dry. Use cotton undergarments that allow better ventilation. Avoid perfumed and colored toilet tissues, douches, and tight clothing. Do not use known sensitizing substances such as benzocaine preparations for topical anesthesia. Even K-Y jelly, which contains parabens, may aggravate or create symptoms in patients who are paraben sensitive. A primary goal is to stop the itch-scratch cycle that frequently perpetuates whatever problem is present. Much can be done to help resolve recurrent vulvar complaints by establishing rapport and working closely with the patient and by seeking appropriate consultation as indicated.

ANATOMY

The vulva, or female external genitalia, includes the mons pubis, labia majora and minora, hymen, clitoris, vestibule, urethral meatus, and Bartholin's and Skene's gland ducts (Fig. 10-1). The vulva is covered by stratified squamous epithelium that becomes thicker, more keratinized, and more pigmented the farther it is from the vaginal introitus. The labia majora contains fatty tissue and many skin appendages, hair follicles, sebaceous glands, sweat glands, and blood vessels, which may form varicosities. The vulvar fat pad atrophies after menopause (Fig. 10-2). The labia minora are located between the labia majora and the vaginal introitus. They form the prepuce anteriorly, and contain many sebaceous glands (but no hair follicles or sweat glands). The clitoris is a short, erectile organ that is less than 1 cm in diameter. If its diameter is greater than this, clitoromegaly may be diagnosed. The vestibule is the area extending from the clitoris to the

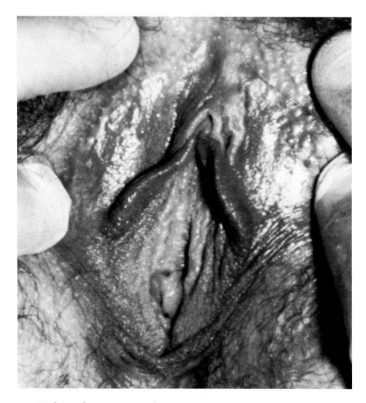

FIGURE 10-1. Vulva of a menstrual-age woman.

posterior fourchette, into which the urethra, vagina, and Bartholin's gland's ducts open. The vestibule's distal, outer boundary is the inner labia minora and the hymeneal ring is its inner, proximal boundary. Skene's glands are periurethral glands that open into the distal portion of the urethra or just outside the urethral orifice. Occasionally paramesonephric or mesonephric duct remnants persist as far distally as the vulva and can give rise to cysts, usually in the upper and middle third of the vulvar area. Ectopic breast tissue may cause solid masses in the labia majora.

In children the labia are smaller and flatter, and the hymen may take one of several forms (Figs. 10-3 and 10-4). These should be recognizable by the

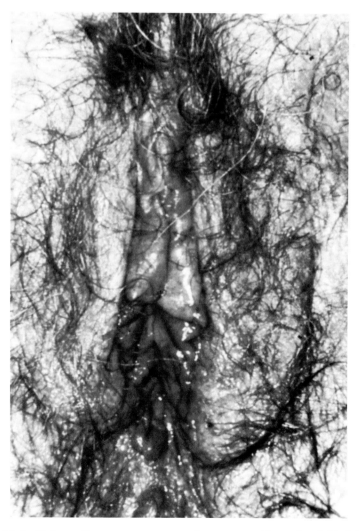

FIGURE 10-2. Vulva of a postmenopausal woman. Note the labial folds and decreased amount of fat in the labia majora.

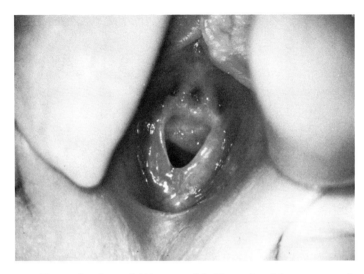

FIGURE 10-3. Normal vulva of 1¾-year-old. Note the thin, symmetric, crescent-shaped hymen.

Courtesy of Dr. Mary Gibbons, Harborview Sexual Assault Center.

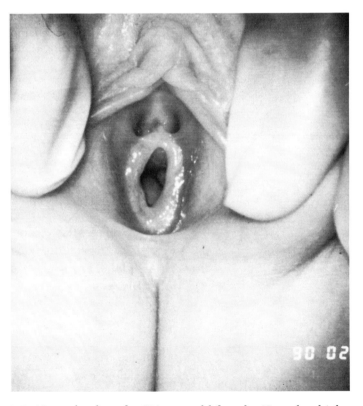

FIGURE 10-4. Normal vulva of a 2¼-year-old female. Note the thick, prominent, symmetric annular hymen and prominent urethral supporting bands.

Courtesy of Dr. Mary Gibbons, Harborview Sexual Assault Center.

clinician so that normal variance is not confused with changes caused by trauma.

Local factors of heat, friction, occlusion, and normal moisture may modify the morphology of abnormalities. Hyperkeratosis may appear pale, and blisters may rupture easily and therefore not be recognized as such.

ABNORMALITIES ARISING FROM ANATOMIC STRUCTURES IN THE VULVA

Vulvar varicosities are common. They are frequently seen during pregnancy, but most of these resolve after delivery. After menopause, they may become prominent concomitant with the loss of the fatty tissue in the labia majora. They produce swelling and a sensation of fullness and usually require no treatment other than support. Occasionally ligation is necessary.

Several types of cysts may be seen on the vulva. Epidermal or sebaceous cysts are caused by local sequestration of epidermis. Usually no treatment is required. Mucocysts may arise from the minor vestibular glands in the vestibule or from mesonephric duct remnants that extend as far distally as

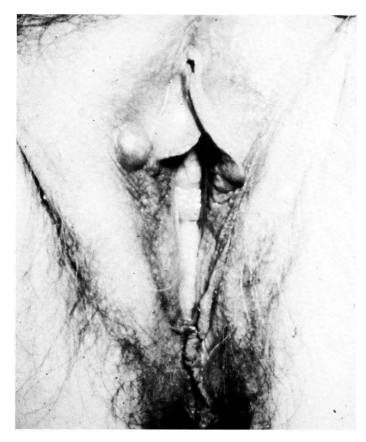

FIGURE 10-5. Gross appearance of hidradenoma of the vulva.

From Jones HN, Wentz AC, Burnett LS: In *Novak's textbook of gynecology*, ed 11, Baltimore, 1988, Williams & Wilkins.

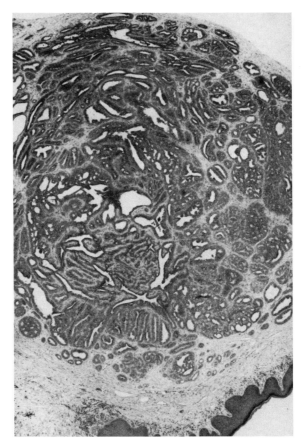

FIGURE 10-6. Hidradenoma. The complex glandular architecture can be confused with an infiltrating carcinoma under low power.

the vulva. Inguinal and pudendal hernias may also extend into the vulva and may or may not transilluminate. Occasionally a patent processus vaginalis (canal of Nuck) can cause intermittent or persistent swelling. They may be first noted if a patient develops ascites and the patent lumen fills with the ascitic fluid. The fluid-filled canal of Nuck usually transilluminates. A concurrent inguinal hernia may be present in up to one third of the cases of patent canal of Nuck. Because of this possibility, such cysts should be opened and explored with definitive repair of any fascial defects.

Solid masses of the vulva include rare tumors such as hidradenoma arising from sweat glands (Fig. 10-5), aberrant breast tissue located at the caudal end of the milk line, granular cell tumor (previously called granular cell myoblastomas but now renamed because they are derived from nerve sheaths), and more commonly fibromas and lipomas that arise from the vulvar connective and fatty tissue. The latter must be differentiated from hernias. Having the patient stand and cough while palpating the inguinal

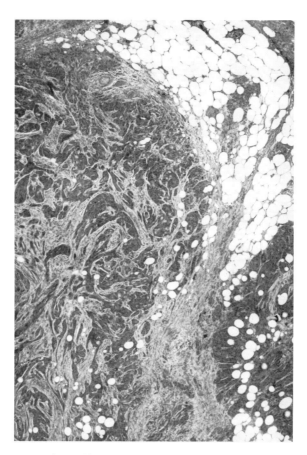

FIGURE 10-7. A granular cell tumor with an infiltrating border. This appearance may be confused with cancer unless one observes it at higher magnification.

and femoral canals may reveal a fascial dcfcct. If found, the hernia should be reduced and the defect surgically repaired. Treatment for most subepithelial solid masses should be excision. They are rarely malignant.

Although uncommon, hidradenoma and granular cell tumors are important because these benign lesions can each be mistaken for malignancies when examined microscopically, hidradenoma because of its architecture (Fig. 10-6) and granular cell tumor because of its invasive appearance caused by an infiltrating border (Fig. 10-7). The cytology is benign in both cases. Granular cell tumors should be widely excised because they are not encapsulated and tend to recur locally if not completely removed.

URETHRAL MEATAL ABNORMALITIES

The caruncle is a common urethral meatal abnormality (Fig. 10-8). It is a benign, strawberry-colored mass usually found on the posterior wall of the urethral meatus. It is composed of granulation-like tissue and is found most frequently during the postmenopausal years. It may be asymptomatic or cause pain or bleeding. Management may include biopsy to eliminate the rare case of carcinoma, if any such diagnostic question exists. It is then treated with systemic or topical estrogens. If no resolution occurs, the tissue may be destroyed by cryotherapy, electrodesiccation, or excision, either by knife or laser.

Urethral prolapse is circular eversion of the urethral mucosa through the external meatus. It is rare and tends to occur either in the premenarchal or postmenopausal age range. In children it is usually asymptomatic but may cause bleeding. In the postmenopausal years, urinary symptoms of nocturia, urgency, dysuria, and frequency are most common. Local estrogen therapy, with or without systemic antibiotics, is recommended initially. If prolapse persists, surgical intervention may be necessary. Tying a purse-string suture over the prolapsed tissue against an indwelling catheter is a simple, effective therapeutic technique.

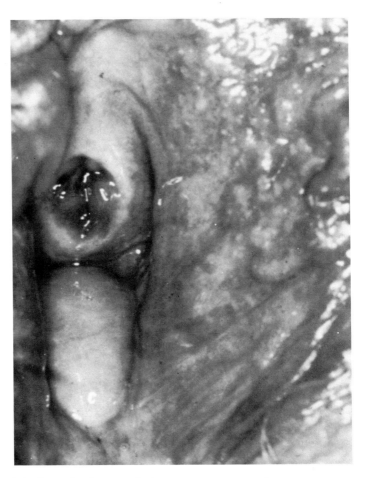

FIGURE 10-8. A urethral caruncle in a postmenopausal woman.

TRAUMATIC INJURIES

Trauma to the highly-vascular vulva can cause lacerations that bleed freely and require cleansing and suture. As with any penetrating injury, tetanus boosters should be given if needed (if not immunized within the last 7 years). Blunt trauma may result in a vulvar hematoma that is usually self-limiting (Fig. 10-9). The swelling may mask severe damage to the pubic bone or cause urethral occlusion. Because finding the bleeding source after incision is often difficult and may result in an infection, initial treatment should be compression with ice. If the hematoma expands in spite of pressure, incision and ligation of the bleeding vessel should be employed. A urethral catheter is often needed to allow voiding.

Sexual abuse may cause bruises and tearing of the introital tissues (Fig. 10-10). Painting the tissue with 1% toluidene blue and wiping it off with K-Y jelly (Fig. 10-11), which does not sting, aids in the detection of small epithelial defects such as fissures around the introitus or anus if sexual abuse is suspected. Inspection of the perineum with a colposcope can also help identify small lesions. Viewing the area with a Woods lamp in a dark room with dark adaptation may detect the fluorescence of dried semen. Knowledge of variations of normal pediatric vulvar anatomy prevents misdiagnosing a normal anatomic variant as an old injury.

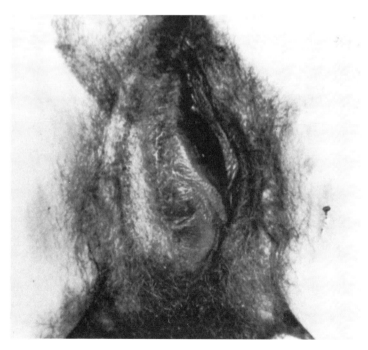

FIGURE 10-9. A vulvar hematoma caused by a straddle injury. Urethral catheterization was necessary to permit voiding.

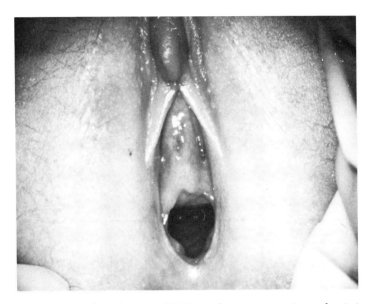

FIGURE 10-10. Vulva of an 8-year-old. Note the asymmetric and minimal rim of hymeneal tissue with absence of hymen posteriorly, consistent with the patient's history of sexual abuse.

Courtesy of Dr. Mary Gibbons, Harborview Sexual Assault Center.

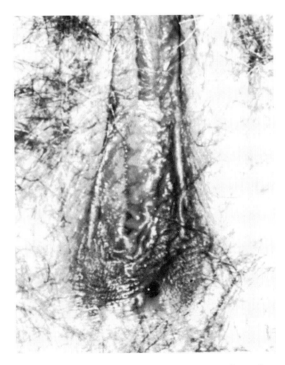

FIGURE 10-11. A small epithelial defect in the posterior fourchette is demonstrated by toluidene blue staining. It was not visible before staining.

INFECTIONS
Vaginal Infections Causing Vulvar Symptoms

When discharge occurs from a vaginitis, the vulva often becomes irritated, particularly in the area of the posterior fourchette, the perineal body, and the perianal area. The cause of erythema and itching or pain in these areas can often be resolved by performing a wet mount of the vaginal secretions to diagnose *Monilia, Trichomonas,* or bacterial vaginosis and treating it properly. Even if there is no obvious vaginitis, one should evaluate the vaginal secretions in cases of vulvar itching or burning because the symptoms may be due to an occult vaginitis. Occasionally, a culture or Gram stain is revealing when a wet mount is not, especially for yeast. The sensitivity of a wet mount will only permit detection of 10^4 or 10^5 organisms/ml in vaginal secretions. When one organism is seen per high-powered field in a wet mount, its concentration is approximately equal to 10^5 organisms/ml of secretion.

Usual therapy for yeast infection is vaginal application of an imidazole cream or suppository (see Chapter 11). Recently, oral fluconazole in a single 150-mg oral dose has been used to treat vaginitis with great success. It may prove equally useful for treating the vulva. So far side effects from this compound have been low, although reports of nausea, vomiting, diarrhea, abdominal pain, and headache can occur with even a single dose, and anaphylaxis has been reported.

Yeast Infections of Vulvar Skin

In some women, particularly those receiving long-term antibiotics or those with diabetes, immunodeficiency, or obesity, cutaneous yeast infections of the vulvar skin may occur. Clinically, a symmetric red area with satellite pustules may be evident (Fig. 10-12). Often a concomitant yeast vaginitis is found. A vaginal wet mount and a scraping from the vulvar skin placed on a slide and heated with 20% KOH for microscopic examination are useful for diagnosis. If the clinical picture is strongly suggestive of candidiasis but the KOH preparation of the skin scraping is negative, a culture of the scrapings on Nickerson's or Sabouraud's media can be used. Tinea cruris caused by dermatophytic fungi or erythrasma caused by bacteria may present similar symptoms and findings. Usually the lesions from *Candida* are symmetric, whereas those from tinea cruris are not. Tinea cruris may also be diagnosed by KOH scrapings or culture. Treatment for vulvar candidiasis is by application of an imidazole cream or lotion one to two times a day, 1% gentian violet applied weekly for 2 or 3 weeks, or both. These treatments are effective for tinea cruris as well. Adequate topical treatment of cutaneous yeast infections often takes several weeks and should be continued for several days after the acute condition is resolved. In resistant cases, ketoconazole (200 mg daily) can be given orally if one recognizes the side effects of therapy, which include thrombocytopenia, leukopenia, and hepatotoxicity. Liver function tests and blood counts should be monitored. Fluconazole is safer than ketoconazole and may become an important drug for cutaneous yeast therapy.

Non-*albicans* species of yeast, particularly *Candida glabrata* and *Saccharomyces cerevisiae,* are resistant to most topical applications with the exception of butoconazole. The in vitro potency of the oral medication fluconazole against species other than *Candida albicans* is poor. Therefore if a patient fails to respond to therapy and is shown to have persistent vaginitis caused by yeast, one should consider susceptibility testing before further treatment.

Erythrasma is a rare condition that is easily confused in a clinical setting with yeast infection; however, it is caused by bacteria. It is usually asymptomatic, but it may flare in chronic disease states such as diabetes

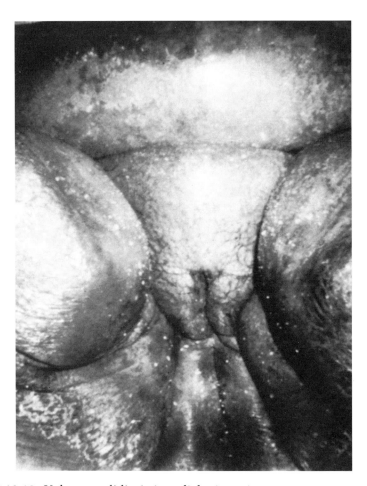

FIGURE 10-12. Vulvar candidiasis in a diabetic patient.

and therefore further mimic a yeast infection. A diagnosis is made by its orange fluorescence under Wood's lamp. The fluorescence is due to the porphyrins in *Corynebacterium minutissimum*, which is the causative organism. Erythrasma is treated with erythromycin. It should be considered if what appears to be a yeast infection does not respond to adequate therapy.

Bartholin's and Skene's Duct Abscesses

Occasionally the Bartholin's gland ducts, or more rarely the Skene's gland ducts, may become occluded, and a cyst will form that may be entirely asymptomatic. In a menstrual-age woman, this requires no therapy. However, if it becomes infected and is fluctuant (Fig. 10-13), drainage is the recommended procedure. If the infected area is not yet fluctuant, hot soaks should be used before incision, which can usually be done in the office with local 1% lidocaine (Xylocaine). A medial incision is made near the original Bartholin's gland duct orifice. A small incision allows placement and retention of a Word catheter, which usually provides adequate drainage until the drainage tract reepithelializes and prevents closure and abscess recurrence. If the incision is too large, the inflated Word catheter will fall out. The

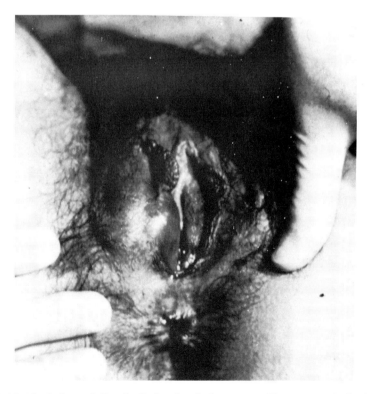

FIGURE 10-13. Infected Bartholin's gland duct cyst. Treatment is incision and drainage.

organisms found are usually facultative gram-negative rods or mixed infections with anaerobic and facultative organisms. Rarely, gonococci may be isolated. If the abscess is isolated, drainage alone is adequate, but if there is surrounding cellulitis or systemic symptoms, antibiotics should be given.

If the area is too painful for local anesthetic, a transrectal pudendal block can be administered to provide excellent anesthesia for incision and drainage (Fig. 10-14). Other treatments such as marsupialization (excising a portion of the abscess wall and stitching it open) or total excision are best performed after the acute abscess has resolved or in recurrent cases. They should be done in a surgical setting.

Any Bartholin's duct abscess occurring in a postmenopausal woman should be excised because acute infection is rare in that age group. Underlying Bartholin's duct carcinoma should be considered. If present carcinoma can be discovered by a total excision of the mass.

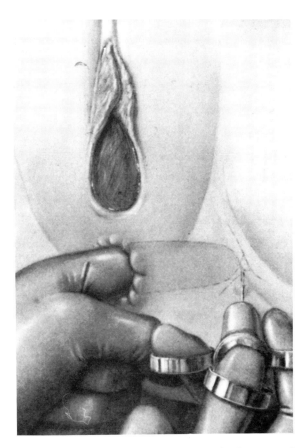

FIGURE 10-14. Transperineal pudendal anesthetic. The finger in the rectum guides the needle and avoids tender areas on the vulva.

From Bonica J: *Principles and practice of obstetrics: analgesia and anesthesia,* Oxford, 1967, Blackwell Scientific.

Skene's duct abscess, which is rare, should be incised and drained during the acute inflammatory stage. This can also be done under local anesthetic.

Parasites

Scabies or lice may also infect the vulva. Both cause itching of the hair-bearing skin of the vulva, including the mons pubis. With scabies, careful examination reveals excoriated areas often associated with similar lesions in the interphalangeal webs of the fingers and on the wrists. Lice may be seen as small, dark (blood-filled) organisms near hair follicles, often associated with eggs (nits) cemented to the hair shaft. Diagnosis may be made by placing a drop of mineral oil on the area and scraping vigorously with a scalpel blade. The mineral oil prevents the organism from being lost during the scraping. The parasite may also be picked off carefully with a small needle using mineral oil as described. The removed organism may be placed on a slide and observed under low power. Lice have six legs with claws (Fig. 10-15), and scabies have a rounded body with small protuberances near the head (Fig. 10-16). Both parasites may be treated with permethrin (Nix).

Pinworms may cause itching of the perianal area and perineal body. They can be diagnosed by collecting ova from the perianal skin on

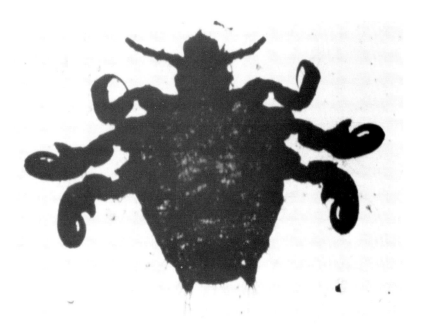

FIGURE 10-15. The pubic louse has been described as a freckle that moves. Small numbers of them may be found with a careful search of the hairy regions of the pubis.

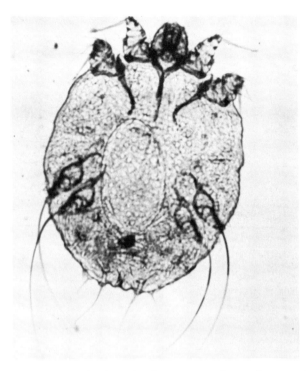

FIGURE 10-16. Scabies may be found in burrows in the epidermis. The fecal pellets are also diagnostic and sometimes more easily found.

cellophane tape. The patient should place the tape sticky side out around the index finger and roll it over the anal area after arising in the morning. The tape picks up eggs from the skin. It is then placed sticky side down on a glass slide and taken to the laboratory for examination. If one member of a family has pinworms, they are frequently found in others. If diagnosed, pinworms are treated with 100 mg mebendazole in one dose. This drug should not be used during pregnancy.

Molluscum Contagiosum

Molluscum contagiosum is a relatively uncommon infection of the skin caused by a pox virus. It can be sexually transmitted and has an incubation period of 15 to 50 days. It causes small, pearly, umbilicated, papular epithelial lesions, usually on the lower part of the abdomen, inner aspect of the thighs, and external genitalia (Fig. 10-17). Except for palpable nodularity, they are generally asymptomatic. Treatment includes curettage, cryotherapy, electrocautery, or laser therapy. Curetting out the central core with a 20-gauge needle, followed by application of silver nitrate or simple cleansing, yields excellent results. At least one report documents the frequent occurrence of keloid scars after CO_2 laser treatment for molluscum. Less expensive treatment modalities should be used preferentially.

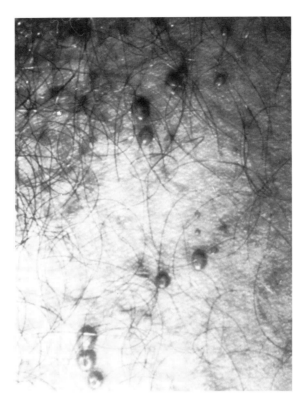

FIGURE 10-17. Molluscum contagiosum. Note the shiny umbilicated nodules. Those without umbilication have been called water warts.

Human Papillomavirus Infections

Vulvar warts have been known for centuries and were initially thought to be present in only a small portion of the population. With the recognition of subclinical human papillomavirus (HPV) infection, greater awareness of HPV in general, more frequent sampling, and use of better detection methods, HPV infection has been found in a progressively higher percentage of both men and women (Tables 10-1 and 10-2). Human papillomavirus is often found in multiple sites, such as the vulva, anus, cervix, and urethra.

There is compelling evidence that subclinical genital HPV infection exists in a majority of all adults. These infections are asymptomatic, and these patients do not have grossly visible warts, so the presence of HPV is not detected by routine clinical evaluation. As stated, HPV is multifocal. If it is detected in one genital area, such as the cervix, it will probably be found on the vulva also if the search is diligent. Over 80% of women who have vulvar infection have been shown to have cervical infection (and vice versa). At least 70% of male partners of HPV-infected women have been shown to have genital HPV.

TABLE 10-1.   Efficacy of common clinical methods to detect HPV

Method	Sensitivity	Specificity
Inspection	Low	Moderate
Colposcopy	Low	Low
Cytology	Low	Low
Histology	Low	Low

Adapted from Koutsky L, Galloway D, Holmes K, et al: *Epidemiol Rev* 10:122, 1988.

TABLE 10-2.   Efficacy of HPV DNA hybridization methods to detect HPV

Method	Sensitivity	Specificity
Dot blot	Moderate	Moderate
In situ	Moderate	Moderate
Southern blot	Moderate	High
Polymerase chain reaction	High	High

Adapted from Koutsky L, Galloway D, Holmes K, et al: *Epidmiol Rev* 10:122, 1988.

Human papillomavirus is a double-stranded deoxyribonucleic acid (DNA) virus that is about 50 to 55 nm in diameter and contains about 8000 nucleotide base pairs. It has been classified into at least 80 different types on the basis of its DNA homology. New types are discovered regularly. A new type is defined as one that has less than 50% DNA homology with any other type by DNA reassociation tests. More accurate testing is showing greater homology between types than is evident with the reassociation tests; however, the reassociation test is still being used for classification. As better methods of classification are developed, we may see a change in HPV type designation.

The HPV genome can be divided into early and late regions on the basis of when the various genes act in the process of viral replication and structural formation. The early-region genes encode for proteins required to initiate the process of replication, and the late-region genes encode for viral structural capsid proteins. After an initial infection of the basal epithelial cells, noncapsulated HPV DNA can lie dormant with few copies of DNA per cell. During this time, HPV DNA is difficult to detect, particularly in small specimens that contain relatively few cells, because most methods used clinically cannot find small amounts of HPV DNA; thus HPV infection is not clinically evident at all during this time. Complete viral particles with protein capsids are formed only in differentiated cells in the upper layers of the epidermis. As emphasized earlier, the more sensitive the methodology used, the better the chance the virus will be found. Also the more frequently the virus is looked for, the more frequently it is found (Table 10-3). Increasing data attest to the high prevalence of so-called high-risk

TABLE 10-3. Increased detection of HPV by using repeated tests

Subject	Test	N	Positive First Test (%)	Number of Tests	Total positive (%)
Normal females	PCR*	20	25	10–12	90
Prostitutes	FISH*	56	21	06	82
Normal females	PCR	91	42	02	57
CIN*	FISH	39	79	02	89

CIN, Cervcal intraepithelial neoplasia; *FISH*, filter in situ hybridization; *PCR, polymerase chain reaction.*

HPV infections in clinically normal individuals. With diligent search using sensitive tests, HPV DNA 16 is found in many totally asymptomatic normal women.

Current studies using sensitive and specific techniques such as the polymerase chain reaction or immunologic response to the HPV proteins have demonstrated genital HPV in 70% to 90% of normal adult populations. Human papillomavirus has been found in 30% of children, and HPV DNA has been found in 17% of swabs from underwear of patients with lower genital HPV, even when using relatively insensitive techniques. Human papillomavirus infection has also been demonstrated at birth, and fomites have been shown to contain HPV DNA. For all these reasons one cannot always attribute genital warts to sexual contact.

Because of the frequency with which HPV is found it is hard to believe the presence of HPV alone is sufficient to cause cancer. However, the sensitive tests may have false-positive results if extreme care is not exercised in their performance, and therefore the high prevalence may be overestimated. Also, HPV DNA can transform infected cells, and portions of HPV DNA have been found both integrated and episomally in carcinomas. Therefore we must remain aware of the association of HPV with dysplasia and carcinoma while awaiting further evidence of a cause-effect relationship. A current theory, based on accumulated evidence, is that HPV infection is not sufficient by itself for the development of neoplasia. With our present knowledge, attempts to treat asymptomatic subclinical HPV infections are not warranted because we know that treatment does not eradicate the virus and we cannot prove that it decreases the occurrence of cancer.

Although a lot has been written about HPV typing, especially in cases of cervical HPV, the predictive value of finding a given type resulting in future development of cancer is low. The cost of typing is high and as yet is not clinically useful or cost-effective.

Clinically visible condylomas on the vulva appear as small, warty growths and can vary from individual rough polypoid lesions (Fig. 10-18, *A*) to large cauliflower-appearing masses (Fig. 10-18, *B*). When examined

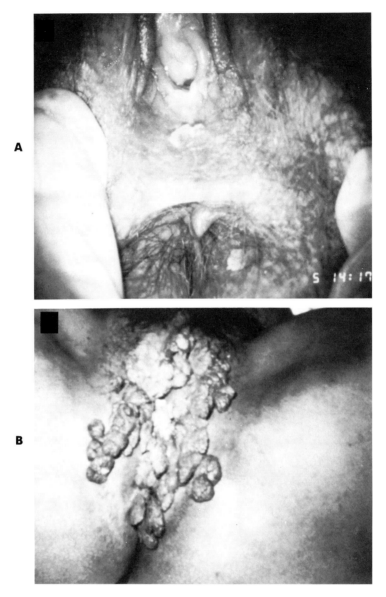

FIGURE 10-18. A, Small wart in the posterior fourchette and perianal area. **B,** Large warts covering the perineum.

microscopically warts are papillomas with hyperkeratosis, acanthosis, and elongated rete ridges (Fig. 10-19). Many warts on the vulva are not visible to the naked eye but appear only after prolonged (5 to 15 minutes) application of 3% acetic acid, followed by colposcopy. Often white epithelium will appear with small, punctate microcapillaries or cobblestone granulation (Fig. 10-20). The cobblestone thickening is difficult to distinguish from vulvar intraepithelial neoplasia (VIN) and multiple biopsies may

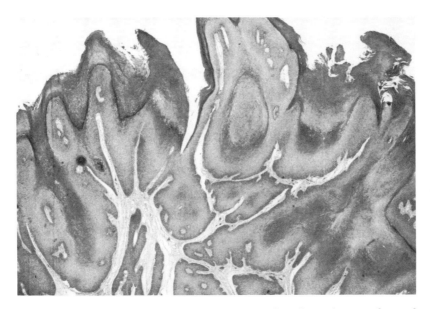

FIGURE 10-19. A low-power microscopic view of a clinical wart shows hyperkeratosis, acanthosis, and papillary folds.

be necessary. Filaments or spikes (asperities) may also be seen. Most of these patients are totally asymptomatic, but some have significant symptoms of itching, burning, and other types of pain. Because of the frequency of HPV without manifestations, it has been difficult to absolutely ascribe any specific syndrome to subclinical infection.

Although there are many treatments for visible genital warts, no therapeutic regimen currently exists that eradicates the wart virus. Expensive or toxic therapies or procedures that are extremely painful or result in scarring should be avoided. Eradication of visible warts can be done inexpensively in the office by applications of podophyllin, trichloroacetic acid, electrocautery, cryocautery, or liquid nitrogen. A 0.5% solution of podofilox for careful self-treatment has also been used with some success. Electrodesiccation and cryotherapy appear more effective than podophyllin or trichloroacetic acid. None of the treatments are highly successful in the long term, with visible warts recurring in at least 25% of patients. Subclinical HPV DNA remains in most if not all cases.

Laser therapy is more expensive but can also be used in the office to eradicate visible warts. Recurrences are frequent. Human papillomavirus DNA in the plume and splatter from laser ablation of warts has raised concern that the intact wart virus can be spread in the environment and perhaps infect those who are treating the patient. The likelihood of spread is low if good filters and masks are used; but because routine testing is not sensitive and we cannot grow the virus in tissue culture to be sure of HPV

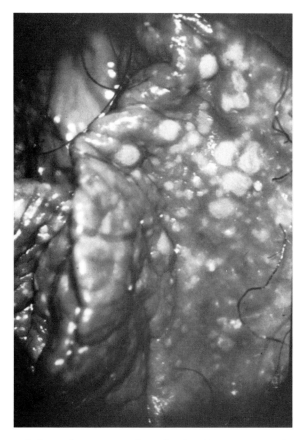

FIGURE 10-20. Subclinical wart manifested only after acetic acid staining. Note the fine, cobblestone appearance within the areas of white epithelium.

DNA infectivity, we should be cautious. Recent data show a significant increase in nasopharyngeal warts in laser surgeons compared with the general population. Certainly adequate devices for removing smoke and splatter should be available in any laser treatment facility, whether in the office or hospital. Laser ablation of the visible wart does not eliminate HPV DNA in surrounding normal-appearing tissue.

Recently the use of topical creams of α-interferon or local or systemic injections of α-interferon in varying doses and application has been reported. As with most studies of treatment, gross changes in genital warts were used as a measure of effectiveness. When using this criterion, clearance rates of from 0% to 80% have been reported with recurrences of 0% to 25%. The regimens using injection result in a high incidence of systemic reaction consisting of flulike syndrome with fever, chills, headache, myalgias, nausea, and fatigue. Leukopenia and abnormal liver function can occur, but they have reverted to normal function when therapy is stopped. As with other treatment modalities, there is no evidence that interferon destroys HPV DNA or intact virus in adjacent cells.

Topical fluorouracil (5-FU) (5% Efudex) has been used both vaginally and on the vulva, but application more than one time a week is often associated with severe burning and desquamation of tissue. Because the effects of 5-FU are not manifested for 5 to 7 days, even daily observation while applying the medication is not adequate to prevent these severe side effects, and this drug should not be used routinely.

In summary, it is best to treat visible HPV lesions on the vulva with simple, cost-effective methods. Efforts to treat subclinical infections are not indicated with the present level of knowledge about HPV. Such patients should be reassured and followed on their regular schedule. If associated dysplasia or VIN is present, it should be removed or destroyed.

Herpes Simplex Virus Infection

Genital herpes simplex virus (HSV) type II infections are often manifested on the vulva. The primary acquisition occasionally causes severe lesions (Fig. 10-21) and systemic symptoms (fever, myalgia, headache) that last for 10 to 20 days. Recurrent episodes cause less severe lesions and little or no systemic manifestations (Fig. 10-22). The duration of the blisters and ulcers

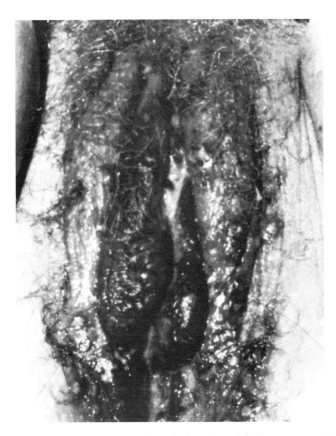

FIGURE 10-21. A severe primary vulvar infection with herpes type II.

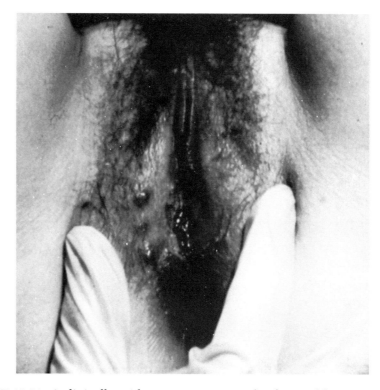

FIGURE 10-22. A clinically evident recurrent episode of genital herpes type II. No systemic symptoms were noted.

of recognized recurrent disease is usually from 1 to 10 days. The recurrent episodes are due to reactivation of HSV from a latent state in dorsal root ganglia. Recurrent lesions may arise in any skin surface supplied by that nerve distribution. Herpes simplex virus type I may also occur on the vulva, but recurrences are much less frequent.

Both primary and recurrent disease are often asymptomatic. Therefore the prevalence of HSV type II infection in the general population is greater than originally supposed. The prevalence of serologic evidence of infection with HSV II ranges from less than 1% in people under 15 years of age to a little over 20% in people 30 to 44 years of age, and it increases only slightly thereafter. In a study of women attending a sexually transmitted disease clinic, 48% had either serologic or virologic evidence of genital herpes. Of those with HSV II antibodies, 78% had no historical, clinical, or virologic evidence of genital herpes and were identified only by the serology. The accumulating evidence clearly shows that a significant proportion of women with genital herpes recognized neither their acquisition of the disease nor any episodes of recurrence. Also the vulvar lesions in some of these patients were atypical in that they had erythema, fissures, or furuncle-like indurated lesions rather than an ulcer. At least 50% of people infected with genital HSV have asymptomatic infection or minor symptoms and do not recognize them as HSV, although they can be shown to have HSV by serology in quiescent periods or by culture techniques if an asymptomatic lesion is found. Persons who have asymptomatic shedding of HSV are more apt to spread the virus because they do not know that they have it or that the lesions are active. Persons with asymptomatic genital HSV type II infection can learn to recognize minor symptoms of their recurrences if they receive detailed instructions of the mild clinical signs and symptoms. The symptoms are often limited to recurrent itching or small, hard-to-see fissures in the vulvar skin. The classic presentation of crops of blisters, ulcers, and eschar are easy to identify, but this sequence is present only in a minority of cases.

Herpes simplex virus should be considered in any patient with recurrent episodes of vulvar itching or irritation that cannot be otherwise explained. A high level of suspicion in looking for lesions and rubbing the vulva with a cotton applicator to detect small, hard-to-see, painful areas may be rewarding. Herpes simplex virus may also be confused with vestibular vulvitis, which causes similar signs and symptoms but is more constant. An HSV culture helps resolve some of these cases. However, HSV culture will be negative in many cases because of its low sensitivity, especially as the lesions heal. Attempts to culture HSV from crusting lesions or normal vulvar epithelium have an extremely low yield, whereas culturing unroofed vesicles or pustules has a high success rate. Herpes simplex virus serology using Western blot may be helpful in detecting antibodies to HSV type II. This helps determine whether HSV exposure has occurred but does not definitely indicate that the vulvar symptoms noted are due to HSV. Complement fixation (CF) antibody testing is less useful because of its cross-reaction with HSV type I, which is much more common. If HSV causes prolonged ulceration, evaluating for human immunodeficiency virus (HIV) and immune system integrity is appropriate.

Intravenous (IV) acyclovir is used to treat severe primary HSV infection. Oral acyclovir, 200 mg five times a day, is given for treatment of recurrent episodes or moderate primary disease. Acyclovir (200 mg two to five times daily) may be used to suppress recurrences for up to 3 years. Most recurrences do not require therapy, but if they are severe or the patient does not wish to have recurrences during a certain period of time, suppressive therapy is beneficial. Acyclovir does not eliminate the latent virus in the dorsal root ganglia, nor does taking it decrease reactivation after the drug is stopped. Acyclovir should not be used in pregnancy unless the benefits clearly outweigh the risks. Prevention of cesarean delivery may be an example.

Syphilis

The differential diagnosis for ulcerative lesions of the vulva should include syphilis, which is becoming more prevalent. Other causes of ulcers include herpes and carcinoma, as well as more unusual ulcerative diseases of the vulva such as Behçet's disease, Crohn's disease, pemphigus, and tuberculosis. A purified protein derivative (PPD) and chest film to rule out tuberculosis is warranted in high-risk populations. As a rule of thumb any ulcerative lesion that does not heal within 2 weeks should undergo biopsy.

Because syphilitic primary chancres heal spontaneously, dark-field preparations from vulvar ulcers should be done to rule out this treatable disease. A dark-field preparation can be easily prepared by abrading and squeezing the lesion to promote serous discharge. The discharge is then applied to the surface of a clean glass slide. A coverslip that has been prepared with a wall of petrolatum (Vaseline) around all its edges is placed over the wet discharge to protect a thick film of the serous discharge, which will not dry out while being transported and studied with a dark-field microscope. The Vaseline wall is formed around the coverslip by spreading a thin layer of Vaseline on the hand and scraping it with each edge of the coverslip. Serology for syphilis should also be done and repeated at least twice at 6-week intervals to allow adequate time from the appearance of the initial chancre to conversion to a positive test result. Serology should be done not only for patients with vulvar ulcers but also for those with STDs or erythematous skin lesions, especially if they involve the palms and soles.

Treatment for early syphilis (of less than 1 year's duration) is benzathine penicillin, 2.4 million units intramuscularly (IM) in one dose. For allergic, nonpregnant patients, doxycycline (100 mg orally two times a day for 2 weeks) may be used. Patients should be monitored both clinically and serologically at 3 and 6 months, with the expectation of quantitative serologic test results declining at least fourfold during that time. If such decline does not occur, patients should be reevaluated, including cerebrospinal fluid (CSF) examination, and retreated as indicated. Patients with other stages of syphilis should be managed as appropriate for their stage with specific counseling for other conditions such as pregnancy or HIV.

Other Sexually Transmitted Diseases

Several other STDs may cause ulcers of the vulva. Chancroid, which is associated with painful inguinal adenopathy, is diagnosed by culture for *Haemophilus ducreyi*. Lymphogranuloma venereum (LGV) is caused by *Chlamydia trachomatis* and results in inguinal adenopathy, which is its most common clinical manifestation. Aspiration and culture of fluctuant lymph nodes are a prime diagnostic method for both chancroid and LGV. Aspiration should be done with a large (18- or 20-gauge) needle for ease of aspiration. It should be done through the intact skin to prevent fistulas. Granuloma inguinale causes coalescing ulcers. It is due to *Calymmatobacterium granulomatis,* which forms the Donovan bodies seen in phagocytes. It is rare in the United States.

Human immunodeficiency virus may be an etiologic factor in cases of persisting or overwhelming secondary infections such as yeast or HSV. Also, HIV-infected women may have genital ulcers that are negative for HSV and chancroid and on dark field. A primary HIV lesion should be considered when vulvar ulcers are present in a woman with a positive HIV serology. Ulcerative lesions of the genitalia from any cause appear to predispose to infection with HIV by enhancing contact. Counseling and testing for HIV should be offered to any person with high-risk behaviors such as IV drug abuse, homosexuality, bisexuality, or sexual contact with multiple or IV drug–abusing partners.

Hidradenitis Suppurativa

Hidradenitis suppurativa is a chronic relapsing inflammatory disease of the apocrine sweat glands that occurs in the axilla, groin, and external genitalia and perianal region. In the early stages, there is nonspecific inflammation, but it does not respond well to treatment with antibiotics or to incision and drainage; it therefore has multiple remissions and exacerbations resulting in extensive involvement of the vulva and perineum with chronic inflammation, induration, and discharging sinuses (Fig. 10-23). In later stages the

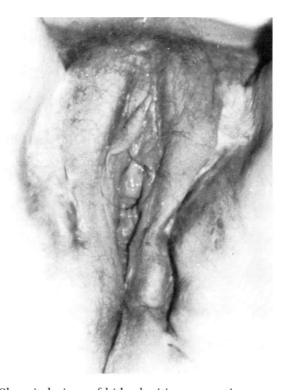

FIGURE 10-23. Chronic lesions of hidradenitis suppurativa.

only beneficial treatment is surgical excision with skin grafting. It can be mistaken for other chronic granulomatous diseases, but biopsy shows only a diffuse chronic inflammatory response with involvement of the sweat glands. Treatment with isotretinoin for several weeks at a dose of 1 mg/kg/day has been reported to result in some improvement and may be worth attempting before surgical excision. Isotretinoin is contraindicated in pregnancy. Blood counts and liver function tests should be followed during the treatment period.

VULVAR PAIN
Vulvar Vestibulitis

Another irritative, inflammatory lesion of the vulva is vulvar vestibulitis, which has also been known as vestibular adenitis and focal vulvitis. The term *vestibular adenitis* is incorrect because the inflammation is not confined to the minor vestibular glands. Currently the cause is unknown.

The prevalence of vulvar vestibulitis and the normal variation and sensitivity of vulvar vestibular skin was studied in unselected patients from a general gynecologic practice. In 210 consecutive patients, 15% had significant vulvar discomfort. Of patients with significant vulvar vestibular pain, 50% had developed it in their teens. The remainder developed it after delivery or some vaginal infection. There was a strong similar family history in the first group, whereas the latter group had no family association.

Vulvar vestibulitis is diagnosed by a history of persistent (6 months or more), moderate to severe pain localized in the vestibule without other significant physical findings and with no other known reason for the discomfort. The pain is demonstrated by gently rubbing the vestibule with a cotton swab, which causes pain significantly out of proportion to the physical findings (Fig. 10-24). Painful areas of the vestibule may appear slightly erythematous, but biopsy reveals only a nonspecific inflammatory infiltrate. Studies for yeast or HSV are negative. In spite of the minimal physical findings, women with this complaint can suffer much discomfort and undergo significant changes of lifestyle with complete avoidance of intercourse, tampon use, and tight clothing. Often the patients have seen many physicians and have been treated with numerous antifungal creams, steroidal preparations, and other emollients without relief. They frequently have been told that their pain is psychosomatic.

The general therapeutic measures for vulvar complaints described earlier are beneficial, and occasionally a bland ointment will have success; however, no treatment has been universally efficacious. Because nearly half of the significant symptoms resolve intermittently, it is hard to imply a cause-effect relationship for any therapy. Assuring patients that they are not imagining the symptoms and are not the only persons with this disorder is often of major benefit. Friedrich reported an approximately 60% success

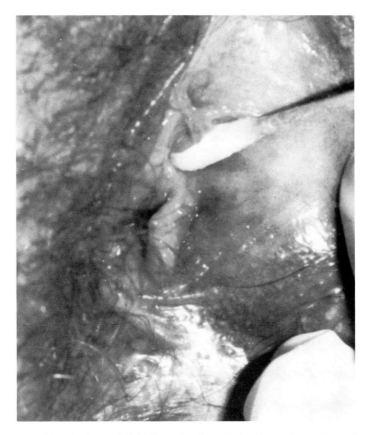

FIGURE 10-24. Vestivular vulvitis. Despite the minimal physical signs, the area was exquisitely painful to light touch.

rate for surgical removal of the vestibule in extremely severe cases, but this should be used only as a last resort. Laser therapy has generally not been effective, although reports of its use continue to be published, usually without long-term follow-up. Interferon has been helpful in some cases, but the long-term effectiveness is unknown at this time. Injections of 1 million units of α-interferon are given sequentially around the vulva three times a week for 4 weeks (Fig. 10-25). A recent study has evaluated the effect of progressive rehabilitation of pelvic floor musculature with the use of twice-daily exercises. The initial results are encouraging: relaxation and stability of pelvic muscles was accompanied by a decrease in subjective pain reports and an increase in the resumption in coitus. This treatment result persisted for a 6-month follow-up period. If this treatment is substantiated by further studies or practice it may provide an important therapeutic modality for this disturbing entity. Regardless of other therapy, counseling and psychologic support give great comfort to the patients, and viscous lidocaine may offer temporary symptomatic relief.

Essential Vulvodynia (Burning Vulva Syndrome)

Vulvodynia is an inclusive, descriptive term defined as chronic vulvar discomfort characterized by burning but not itching. If the patient feels like scratching, vulvodynia should not be diagnosed. Several different subsets of vulvodynia have been described, including the vulvar dermatoses, infections such as papillomatosis or candidiasis, and vulvar vestibulitis, which all have distinguishing diagnostic features and should be diagnosed as such. Essential vulvodynia is therefore diagnosed when other syndromes or diseases have been excluded. Before making a diagnosis of essential vulvodynia (or burning vulva syndrome [BVS]), a thorough history and physical examination should be done, including cultures for *Candida* and acetic acid application for vulvar colposcopy to search for specific etiologies. Patients with essential vulvodynia have

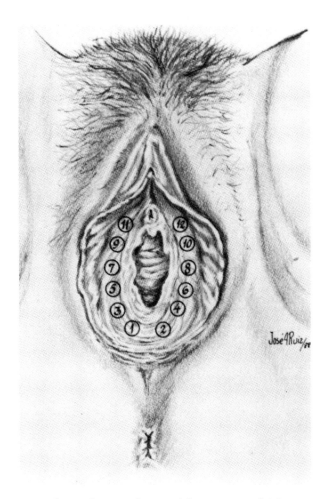

FIGURE 10-25. Interferon therapy for condylomatous vulvitis.

From Horowitz BJ: *Obstet Gynecol* 73:447, 1989.

been treated with tricyclic antidepressants, which have been successful in some cases, particularly if clinical depression is manifested. However, they may cause sleepiness. Drugs such as the serotonin uptake inhibitors (e.g., trazodone) have fewer side effects. They appear to be most useful in patients over age 40. Alcohol injection is not indicated in vulvar syndromes characterized by burning, although it may be helpful for entities that cause significant itching in which other treatments have failed.

SYSTEMIC DISORDERS
Crohn's Disease

Some dermatologic findings of the vulva are due to systemic conditions such as Crohn's disease, which can cause vulvar swelling and ulcers (Fig. 10-26). Sinuses may develop later. It is diagnosed by biopsy and a history of concomitant bowel involvement, although rarely the vulvar manifestation

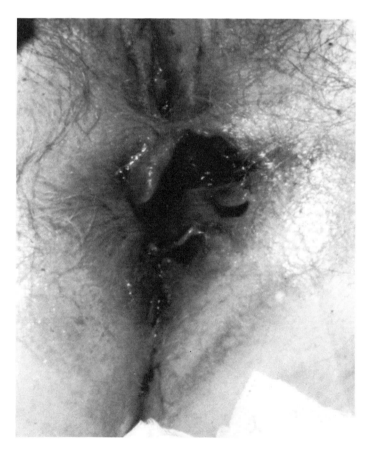

FIGURE 10-26. Crohn's disease in a young woman with severe perianal lesions and vulvar ulcers.

may occur before bowel symptoms become prominent. Crohn's disease of the vulva may be confused with several other ulcerative lesions, including Behçet's. Diseases causing granulomatous inflammation of the vulva, such as LGV, granuloma inguinale, syphilis, tuberculosis, and *Actinomyces* and fungal infections, should be included in the differential diagnosis. Biopsy reveals numerous confluent granulomas in the dermis. If the patient is acutely and severely ill, necrotizing fasciitis, which is an acute, extensive infective necrosis of superficial tissues leading to a severe toxic, systemic reaction, should be considered (Fig. 10-27). With necrotizing fasciitis there is microscopic vascular thrombosis in the absence of major vascular occlusion. It requires extensive immediate debridement to prevent overwhelming sepsis. With Crohn's disease, the patient is usually not severely ill, nor is there evidence of a rapidly progressing necrotizing process. In a patient who is not systemically ill, hidradenitis suppurativa may be the reason for large nonhealing ulcers. A definite diagnosis is made by culture, biopsies, or other appropriate tests. Usual treatment of Crohn's disease is corticosteroids. Metronidazole has been effective in some cases in which steroids have failed.

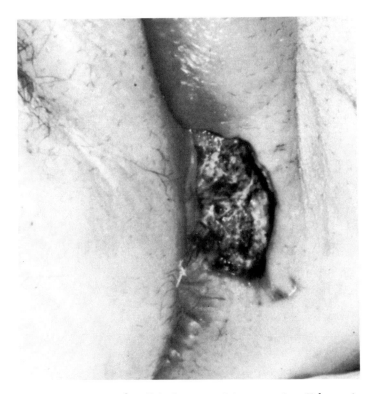

FIGURE 10-27. Necrotizing fasciitis in an episiotomy site. Edema involved the labia. It also extended onto the anterior abdominal wall.

Behçet's Syndrome

Behçet's syndrome is a rare systemic disease characterized by polyarthritis, uveitis, and urethritis with oral and often genital mucous membrane lesions. Recent diagnostic criteria for Behçet's syndrome are oral ulceration plus any two of the following: genital ulcers, eye lesions (uveitis), skin lesions (erythema nodosum), or pathergy (sterile pustule in 24 to 48 hours at the site of a needle stick). It is rare in women and usually spontaneously regresses. It is probably overdiagnosed because few patients meet the strict criteria. In true cases ophthalmologic consultation should be obtained because of the risk of blindness if the eyes are involved. The etiology is unknown, but it may be due to vasculitis because nonspecific perivascular depositions of immune globulins and complement complexes may be found. A recent study showed increased thrombo modulin in patients with active Behçet's. It is also elevated in patients with other active collagen diseases. Treatment for Behçet's is with corticosteroids and azathioprine or other immunosuppressive therapy. It may be distinguished from gonococcal arthritis by negative gonococcal cultures and failure to respond to penicillin.

Because several dermatologic conditions, such as Behçet's syndrome and lichen planus, involve the oral mucous membranes and eyes as well as the genitalia, these areas should be evaluated by history and physical examination when there is a question about the etiology of a vulvar lesion.

NONNEOPLASTIC EPITHELIAL DISORDERS

Nonneoplastic epithelial disorders are some of the most common lesions of the vulva. They were called dystrophies of the vulvar skin and mucosa, and they may be asymptomatic or cause symptoms of itching and burning. They also have been known by various nonspecific terms such as leukoplakia or kraurosis vulvae. In 1975 the International Society for the Study of Vulvar Disease adopted a classification of the dystrophics to facilitate diagnosis and study. The 1975 classification is as follows:
1. Hyperplastic dystrophy (without atypia or with atypia)
2. Lichen sclerosis
3. Mixed dystrophy (without atypia or with atypia)

However, because lesions with atypia were judged inappropriate to be classified as nonneoplastic, and also because many lesions classified as hyperplastic dystrophy are a result of an irritative dermatitis caused by an itch-scratch cycle, a new classification was proposed based on a combination of gross and histopathologic changes. This classification was approved in 1989 and is as follows. Nonneoplastic epithelial disorders of the vulvar skin and mucosa:
1. Squamous cell hyperplasia (formerly hyperplastic dystrophy)
2. Lichen sclerosis
3. Other dermatoses

When mixed epithelial disorders occur, as happens frequently, each diagnosis should be reported (for example, lichen sclerosis and squamous cell hyperplasia). If atypical cells are present, VIN should be noted separately.

A comparison of the two classifications minimizes the confusion that is apt to occur during the transition. Pathologists may use either or both classifications. Speak directly to the pathologist to resolve sematic differences in diagnostic classification and description.

Squamous Cell Hyperplasia

The hyperplastic lesions may be lichenified (having pronounced or accentuated skin markings) and may have highly variable gross appearances caused by vulvar moisture, scratching, and medications that have

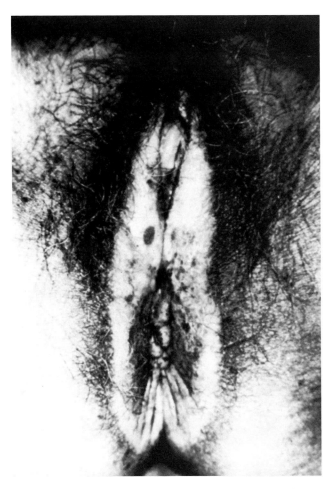

FIGURE 10-28. Chronic changes seen in squamous cell hyperplasia. Many of these are due to the constant scratching.

been used (Fig. 10-28). Often the areas are white and thickened, with fissures and excoriation. Thickened areas require biopsy specimens to make the diagnosis and to rule out carcinoma. Pathologic examination of squamous cell hyperplasia reveals hyperkeratosis, a thick epithelial layer of squamous cells with parakeratosis, and often an inflammatory response in the dermis (Fig. 10-29). Diagnosis is made by biopsy of several areas, particularly those where there is ulceration or induration. A few patients also have intraepithelial neoplasia, so biopsy of the clinically most-concerning areas is important. Biopsy should be repeated occasionally during follow-up if there is persistent or newly developed ulceration or thickening. If there is no atypia, subsequent development of carcinoma is not likely.

Treatment of squamous cell hyperplasia is aimed at stopping the itch-scratch cycle. If the vulva is macerated and wet, Burow's solution applied for 30 minutes three or four times a day helps dry it. Application of a potent corticosteroid preparation or a mixture of betamethasone valerate and crotamiton, an antipruritic (seven parts 0.1% valisone, three parts 10% Eurax), may be applied twice a day for 3 to 4 weeks as described by Friedrich. Prolonged use of these preparations causes atrophy of the tissues and occasionally creates a thin, fragile epithelium susceptible to trauma and infection that may cause symptoms similar to the original hyperplasia. Therefore close observation and an individualized decrease in frequency or potency of steroid application is important in long-term management.

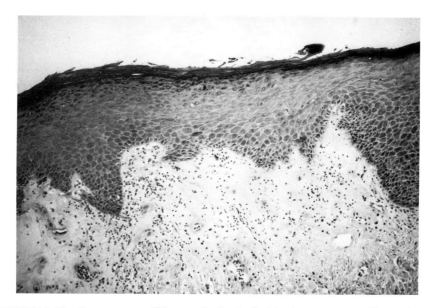

FIGURE 10-29. Squamous cell hyperplasia. Individual squamous cells are benign.

Lichen Sclerosis

Lichen sclerosis (LS) is a specific disorder of the vulva that is also found in nongenital sites. Although most common in the elderly, it can occur at all ages and may be misdiagnosed as a residual of trauma or sexual abuse in children. It has been called lichen sclerosis et atrophicus, but the term *atrophicus* has been dropped because the epithelium is metabolically active, although it appears atrophic (Fig. 10-30). The epithelium probably differentiates early, which gives LS its thin appearance. Lichen sclerosis may be asymptomatic or cause itching or pain. The epithelium often has a thin, finely wrinkled appearance with frequent midline fissures. In late stages, the vulva may become flat, with stenosis of the introitus, obliteration of the labia, and fusion over the clitoris. Lichen sclerosis has a classic microscopic appearance, with thin epithelium, hyperkeratosis, and vacuolization of the basal cells (Fig. 10-31). Directly beneath the epidermis, a layer of pink-staining, collagenous, homogeneous tissue is found that usually has a layer of chronic inflammatory cells beneath it. Areas of LS and hyperplastic epithelium are often juxtaposed.

There has been a recent change in the first choice therapy for lichen sclerosis. A high-potency steroid cream (clobetasol proprionate 0.05% b.i.d. for 12 weeks) has been used and its effectiveness compared with the effectiveness of testosterone and progesterone preparations. The clobetasol-

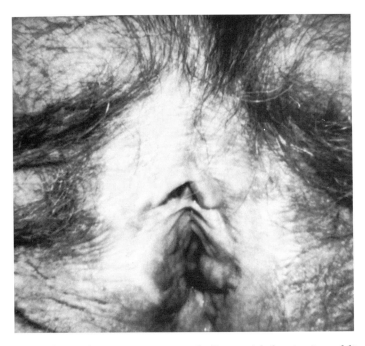

FIGURE 10-30. Thin, white-appearing epithelium with beginning obliteration of the labia minora.

treated patients had improved histology, a reduction in epidermal atrophy, and quicker clinical response. This improvement has been maintained with lower or less-frequent doses. However, there is the potential for true steroid atrophy, and the patients should be followed closely. Earlier treatments for LS were by testosterone proprionate, 2% in petrolatum applied two to three times a day for several months. The dosage may be decreased for maintenance, which is often required for years. If severe itching is present, a cortisone cream is useful. For a few women, topical testosterone causes increased libido, which they may find unacceptable. More frequently patients complain of severe burning from the testosterone application. Topical application of progesterone, 2% in petrolatum two to four times a day, is helpful for some of these patients. If severe itching of either LS or squamous cell hyperplasia cannot be relieved by topical medication, injection of absolute alcohol, 0.2 ml, at the intersections of a 1-cm grid drawn on the vulva may provide relief (Fig. 10-32). Alcohol injections should not be used for symptoms of burning.

Other Dermatoses

Dermatologic conditions found on the vulva include many of the dermatologic diseases that affect skin anywhere on the body. Lichen planus is a relatively common papulosquamous disorder of unknown etiology that may cause ulcerative lesions, especially in the vagina, and should also be considered in any patient with erosive vulvar disease. Differential diagnoses

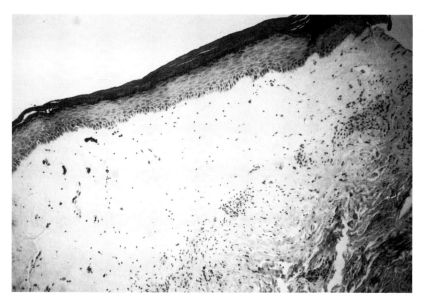

FIGURE 10-31. Photomicrograph of lichen sclerosis. Note the thin epithelium and homogeneous collagenous layer directly beneath it.

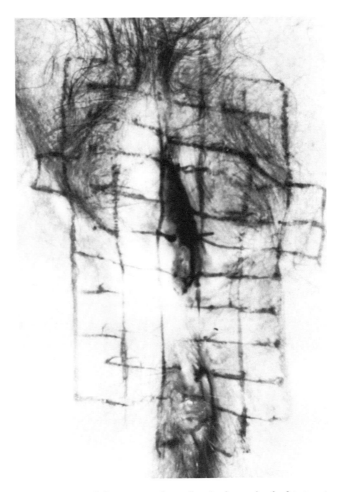

FIGURE 10-32. A 1-cm grid drawn on the vulva before alcohol injection therapy for intractable itching due to a mixed lichen sclerosis and squamous cell hyperplastic lesion.

include ulcers caused by infection, Crohn's disease, Behçet's disease, pemphigoid, pemphigus, epidermolysis bullosa, Stevens-Johnson syndrome (severe erythema multiforme), and burns such as those caused by 5-FU. Diagnosis of many of these syndromes is aided by the concomitant finding of characteristic lesions in other areas of the body. Lichen planus has a characteristic lacelike reticular pattern that is commonly found on the buccal mucosa. It is diagnosed by biopsy. Treatment is not highly effective but includes topical oral and intralesional steroids. Oral retinoids, griseofulvin, and cytotoxic agents have also been used.

Other dermatoses include intertrigo, contact dermatitis, and seborrheic dermatitis. Intertrigo is inflammation from sweat and friction, usually found in folds of skin. It is treated by keeping the skin folds clean, dry, and separated. Hair dryers on low or cool settings are useful to dry the skin surfaces after careful cleansing. The use of mild topical steroids such as 1% hydrocortisone cream and relief from or protection against secondary infection by yeast and bacteria speed resolution. Contact dermatitis is an allergic response to a contact substance such as the perfume contained in soap. Treatment is to discover and avoid the allergenic substance and topical application of a mild corticosteroid while preventing secondary infection. Seborrheic dermatitis is occasionally found in the genital area, but it is more common on the scalp and ears. Seborrheic dermatitis is also treated with low-potency topical corticosteroids.

Psoriasis and pemphigus can also be found on the vulva. Psoriasis has silvery scaling that may be found in the pubic area and on the labia majora but not on labia minora or mucosa. Diagnosis of psoriasis is greatly assisted by finding classic lesions on extensor surfaces such as the knees and elbows. Pemphigus is a serious rare bullous autoimmune disease that may cause erosions of the vulvar and vaginal mucous membranes. Biopsy for IgG deposition in the intercellular space of the epidermis should be done. Psoriasis and pemphigus may be best managed with the help of a dermatologist.

NEOPLASTIC OR PREMALIGNANT LESIONS
Vulvar Intraepithelial Neoplasia

Vulvar intraepithelial neoplasia is approximately one tenth as common as cervical intraepithelial neoplasia. It appears to be more prevalent than in the past, although increased recognition is in part responsible. It may be found in women of all ages, cases having been reported in teenagers, but it is most common in the late twenties or early thirties. It appears to be increased in HIV-positive patients and in patients who have had organ transplants, especially if the transplant was done at an early age. The predominant clinical symptom is pruritus. Lesions are usually multifocal. Approximately one third are pigmented with melanin diffused throughout the epithelium. They may therefore appear clinically either as pigmented or white thickened areas (Fig. 10-33). Colposcopy of the vulva after staining it with 3% to 5% acetic acid for several minutes is a good method of determining where to take biopsy samples. Vulvar intraepithelial neoplasia often has a slightly granular appearance on colposcopy. It usually also stains with toluidine blue. Biopsy of multiple sites is important to establish the diagnosis and to distinguish VIN from areas of subclinical HPV infection, which may coexist. Microscopically, biopsy specimens of VIN reveal nuclear clumping, atypical mitosis, individual cell keratinization, and corps ronds (Fig. 10-34).

There is still disagreement about the frequency with which these lesions progress to vulvar cancer, but progression is generally thought to be low. The multifocal pattern is different from most invasive vulvar carcinoma,

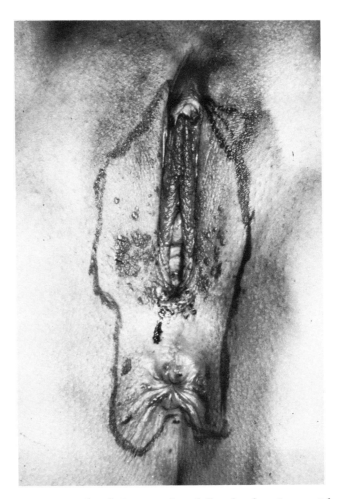

FIGURE 10-33. An example of pigmented multifocal vulvar intraepithelial neoplasia in a young woman.

which is usually unifocal and tends to occur at a much later age. However, there is general agreement that VIN should be conservatively treated by wide local excision.

Other modalities of destructive therapy have been used, including cryotherapy, laser, and 5-FU. However, all of these have the disadvantage of creating significant discomfort and vulvar ulceration and not having tissue for pathologic examination. Because new vulvar lesions of VIN occur after treatment in 30% to 50% of cases, patients should be followed regularly by visual and tactile examination of the vulva with colposcopy or inspection with a magnifying glass after acetic acid or toluidine blue staining to detect any such recurrences. If a woman has VIN, carefully evaluate the cervix, vagina, and perianal area for other intraepithelial

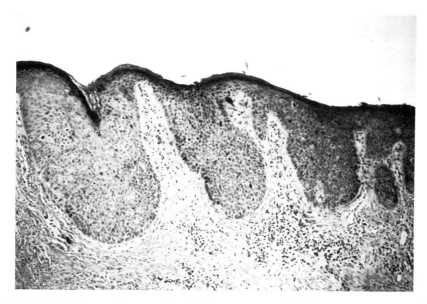

FIGURE 10-34. Photomicrograph of vulvar intraepithelial neoplasia.

neoplastic processes, which are more likely to be found than in a normal population.

If you suspect a lesion on the vulva of being an invasive carcinoma, its diameter should be precisely measured with a centimeter rule for accurate staging. Measurement should be done before biopsy. If the lesion is under 2 cm, the biopsy should be excisional because treatment protocols of vulvar carcinoma may be modified by small differences in depth of invasion. It may be difficult to determine the exact diameter and depth of invasion after a lesion has been partially biopsied.

Paget's Disease

Paget's disease of the vulva is a rare neoplasm that may be confused with other erythematous lesions, especially yeast infections (Fig. 10-35). It should be considered particularly in elderly women who have persistent redness of the vulvar area. The diagnosis is made by biopsy (Fig. 10-36). Paget cells in the epidermis have a tendency to spread locally beyond the limits of the clinical disease. They also are occasionally associated with an underlying carcinoma, so one should palpate the involved skin carefully for any thickening that may herald such an event. If an indurated or thick area is felt, it should be specifically biopsied (some advocate thin-needle aspiration) to rule out underlying carcinoma. Treatment is by wide local excision using frequent frozen sections to be sure that the extent of the lesion is included in the resection because the Paget cells tend to extend beyond clinically defined margins.

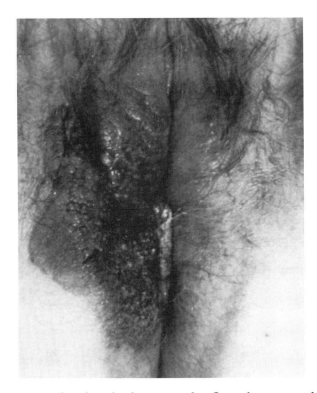

FIGURE 10-35. Note the sharply demarcated inflamed area on the right labia. Biopsy revealed Paget's disease that extended beyond the clinical margins at the time of excision.

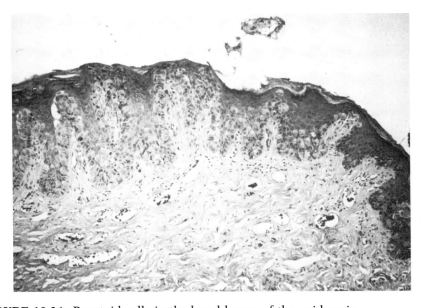

FIGURE 10-36. Pagetoid cells in the basal layers of the epidermis.

PIGMENTED LESIONS

Melanocytes containing melanin cause several different pigmented areas on skin.

1. Freckles have the normal number (approximately 1 melanocyte for every 20 to 30 basal cells) of melanocytes with increased melanin resulting from increased exposure to the sun. They are not usually found on the vulva.

2. Lentigo is simply an increased number of normal melanocytes found in the basal layer of the epithelium. Lentigo is benign and found commonly on the vulva (Fig. 10-37).

3. Nevi contain melanocytes in nests. Nevi are further divided by the position of these melanocytes in the skin. In junctional nevi the melanocytes are only in the basal layer of the epidermis. In compound nevi the melanocytes are contained within both the basal layer and the dermis. In the intradermal nevi the melanocytes are only within the dermis. Vulvar nevi are common and benign (Fig. 10-38).

4. Melanomas have atypical melanocytes with or without increased pigmentation (Fig. 10-39).

Melanin-producing cells cause pigmented areas of the vulva, just as they do in other areas of the body. Although the vulva contains only 2% of the body's skin, 3% to 5% of melanomas originate in this area. This leads some authorities to suggest that melanomas have a predilection for the vulva and

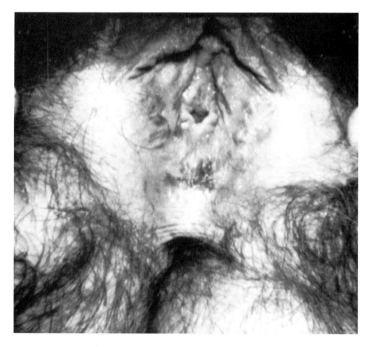

FIGURE 10-37. Lentigo found on the perineal body.

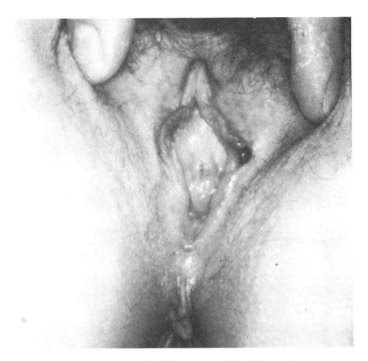

FIGURE 10-38. A well-circumscribed nevus on the labia minora.

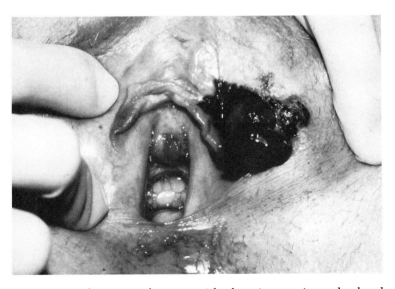

FIGURE 10-39. A malignant melanoma with elevation, an irregular border, deep pigmentation, and asymmetry.

TABLE 10-4. Clinical signs that increase the probability of melanoma

A. *Asymmetry,* when one half of the lesion is unlike the other half
B. *Border,* irregular with scalloped edges
C. *Color,* a disorderly arrangement of various shades of brown, gray, white, or blue
D. *Diameter* over 6 mm
E. *Elevation* above the surrounding skin surface
F. in*F*lammatory response accompanied by itching, weeping, or bleeding
G. *Growth* evidenced by a recent change in size

to recommend removal of all pigmented areas from the vulva because it is difficult to tell exactly what they are (i.e., lentigo, nevus, or melanoma) without histologic verification. However, if all vulvar pigmented lesions were removed, a great number of women would have unnecessary biopsies. It seems reasonable to excise suspicious pigmented areas for histologic review. A helpful mnemonic for assigning suspicion of melanoma to a pigmented lesion is A, B, C, D, E, F, G (Table 10-4).

In a study of 222 skin lesions, seven of eight malignant melanomas were detected clinically when three or more of the signs were present. The most significant clinical sign was the irregular border, which was found in all eight melanomas. Large size and irregular pigmentation were the next most significant factors. The presence of any of the seven signs should lead to a biopsy of any pigmented area of the vulva while recognizing that many will be lentigo, nevi, seborrheic warts, or other unusual and usually benign lesions such as angiomas. Vulvar melanomas are more common in white women than black women and have an overall survival of about 50% in the United States; however, melanomas with less than 0.76 mm of penetration (Breslow's first stage) have an excellent prognosis. Some pigmented raised lesions will be VIN, as discussed earlier. Excisional biopsy of a pigmented lesion should be deep enough to allow assessment of the depth of invasion if it is a melanoma.

VULVAR BIOPSY TECHNIQUES

Because the diagnosis of many vulvar lesions depends on biopsy and because vulvar biopsy is often done in the office, it will be discussed here briefly.

Vulvar biopsy is usually done under local anesthesia, such as 1% lidocaine (Xylocaine) with or without epinephrine. By using a 30-gauge needle and slow infiltration of several cubic centimeters of anesthesia, the discomfort from injecting anesthesia can be minimized. Full-thickness biopsy specimens should be obtained. A Keye's punch (Fig. 10-40) or a standard large biopsy forceps such as Tischler punch (Fig. 10-41) will provide adequate full-thickness specimens. Bleeding can usually be stopped

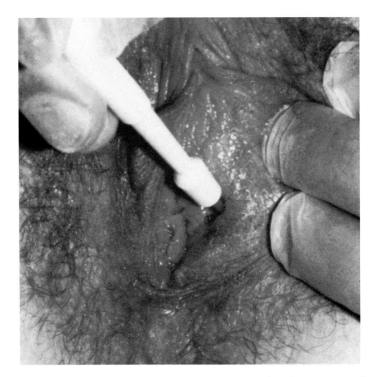

FIGURE 10-40. Biopsy of the vulva with a Keye's punch. After cutting the circular biopsy specimen, it is lifted with forceps and excised from the subcutaneous tissue with scissors.

by pressure and application of silver nitrate or Monsel's solution. If excess bleeding occurs from a small biopsy sample, a suture of 4-0 chromic or 3-0 plain gut suture on a cutting needle will stop the bleeding and allow healing without premature separation and without the irritation of longer-lasting polyglycolic suture. A cutting needle should be used because vulvar skin makes penetration with a tapered needle difficult. For larger elliptical excisional biopsy specimens, which should be taken along skin lines if possible, closure with longer-lasting suture is preferred.

CONCLUSION

Adequate history, examination, and appropriate tests rapidly diagnose most vulvar disorders. Listening carefully to the patient's concerns and developing a good working relationship enhances the physician's ability to care for all vulvar abnormalities, especially those that are resistant to diagnosis and therapy or are recurrent. Liberal use of biopsy specimens often provides diagnoses and if not usually allows the physician to reassure patients that they do not have a life-threatening disease. Use benign inexpensive prophylactic measures, and avoid shotgun therapy in the absence of definitive diagnoses. In those cases that are chronic and resistant to therapy,

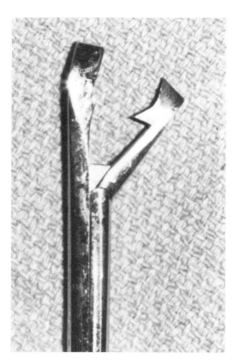

FIGURE 10-41. Tischler punch biopsy. This alligator biopsy forcep will obtain a full-thickness specimen that can be easily oriented.

the patient can usually be helped by a persistent, conscientious, thorough partnership approach using numerous diagnostic techniques and liberal consultation.

BIBLIOGRAPHY

American College of Obstetricians and Gynecologists: Technical Bulletin No. 139, Jan 1990.

Bergen S, DiSaia P, Liao SY, et al: Conservative management of extramammary Paget's disease of the vulva, *Gynecol Oncol* 33:151, 1989.

Bergeron C, Ferenczy A, Ritchart R: Underwear: contamination by human papilloma virus, *Am J Obstet Gynecol* 162:25, 1990.

Berth-Jones J, Graham-Brown R, Burns DA: Lichen sclerosus, *Arch Dis Child* 64:1204, 1989.

Bhatia NM, Bergman A, Broem E: Advanced hydradenitis suppurativa of the vulva: a report of three cases, *J Reprod Med* 29:436, 1984.

Birkeland SA, Storm HH, Lamm LU, et al: Cancer risk after renal transplantation in the nordic countries 1964-1986, *Int J Cancer* 60:183, 1995.

Boden E, Rylander E, Evander M, et al: Papilloma virus infection of the vulva, *Acta Obstet Gynecol Scand* 68:179, 1989.

Bonica J: *Principles and practice of obstetrics: analgesia and anesthesia,* vol 1, Oxford, 1967, Blackwell Scientific.

Bracco G, Carli P, Sonni L, et al: Clinical and histological effects of topical treatment of vulvar lichen sclerosis: a critical evaluation, *J Repro Med* 38: 37, 1994.

Brown CF, Gallup DG, Brown VM: Hydradenitis suppurativa of the anogenital region: response to isotretinoin, *Am J Obstet Gynecol* 158:12, 1988.

Centers for Disease Control: Sexually transmitted diseases treatment guidelines, *MMWR Morb Mortal Wkly Rep* 42:RR-14, 1993.

Clouser K, Friedrich EG: A new technique for alcohol injection in the vulva, *J Reprod Med* 31:971, 1986.

Coates JB, Hales JS: Granular cell myoblastoma of the vulva, *Obstet Gynecol* 41:796, 1973.

Dalziel K, Millard P, Wojnarowska F, et al: The treatment of vulvar lichen sclerosis with a very potent topical steroid (clobetasol proprionate 0.05%) cream, *Br J Dermatol* 124:461, 1991.

Droegemueller W: Benign gynecologic lesions. In Droegemueller W, Herbst AL, Mishell DR, et al, editors: *Comprehensive gynecology*, St Louis, Mosby, 1992.

Duhra P, Paul CJ: Metastatic Crohn's disease responding to metronidazole, *Br J Dermatol* 119:87, 1988.

Edwards L: Vulvar lichen planus, *Arch Dermatol* 125:1677, 1989.

Ferenczy A, Bergeron C, Richart R: Human papilloma virus DNA in CO_2 laser generated plume of smoke and its consequences to the surgeon, *Obstet Gynecol* 75:114, 1990.

Friedman M, Gaul D: Keloid scars as a result of CO_2 laser for molluscum contagiosum, *Obstet Gynecol* 70: 394, 1987.

Friedrich EG: *Vulvar disease*, ed 2, Philadelphia, 1983, Saunders.

Friedrich EG: Vulvar dystrophy, *Clin Obstet Gynecol* 28:178, 1985.

Gibson PE, Gardner SD, Best SJ: Human papilloma virus types in anogenital warts of children, *J Med Virol* 30:142, 1990.

Glazer HI, Rodke G, Swencionis C, et al: Treatment of vulvar vestibulitis syndrome with electromyographic biofeedback of pelvic floor musculature, *J Reprod Med* 40:283, 1995.

Gloster HM, Roenigk RK: Risk of acquiring human papilloma virus from the plume produced by the carbon dioxide laser in the treatment of warts, *J Am Acad Dermatol* 32:436, 1995.

Goetsch M: Vulvar vestibulitis prevalence and historic features in a general gynecologic practice population, *Am J Obstet Gynecol* 164:1609, 1991.

Hoffman MS, Roberts WS, Lapolla JP, et al: Recent modifications in the treatment of invasive squamous cell carcinoma of the vulva, *Obstet Gynecol Surv* 44:227, 1989.

Horowitz BJ: Interferon therapy for condylomatous vulvitis, *Obstet Gynecol* 73:446, 1989.

Husseinzadeh N, Newman NJ, Wesseler TA: Vulvar intraepithelial neoplasia: a clinicopathologic study of carcinoma in situ of the vulva, *Gynecol Pathol* 33:157, 1989.

International Study Group for Behçet's Disease: Criteria for diagnosis of Behçet's disease, *Lancet* 335:1078, 1990.

Jenison SA, Yu X, Valentine JM, et al: Evidence of prevalent genital type human papilloma virus infections in adults and children, *J Infect Dis* 162: 60, 1990.

Johnson MA, Bloomfield PI, Bevan IS, et al: Analysis of human papilloma virus type 16 E6E7 transcription in cervical carcinomas and normal cervical epithelium using polymerase chain reaction, *J Gen Virol* 71:1473, 1990.

Johnson RE, Nahmias A, Magder L, et al: A seroepidemiologic survey of the prevalence of herpes simplex type II infection in the United States, *N Engl J Med* 321:7, 1989.

Jones HN, Wentz AC, Burnett LS: Benign diseases of the vulva and vagina. In Jones HN, Wentz AC, Burnett LS, eds: *Novak's textbook of gynecology*, ed II, Baltimore, 1988, Williams & Wilkins.

Kaufman RH: Establishing a correct diagnosis of vulvovaginal infection, *Am J Obstet Gynecol* 158:986, 1988.

Keefe M, Dick DC, Wakeel RA: A study of the value of the seven point checklist in distinguishing benign pigmented lesions from melanoma, *Clin Exp Dermatol* 15:167, 1990.

Kirby PK, Kiviat N, Beckman A, et al: Tolerance and efficacy of recombinant human interferon gamma in the treatment of refractory genital warts, *Am J Med* 85:183, 1988.

Korn AP, Autry M, DeRemer PA, et al: Sensitivity of the Papanicolaou stain in human immunodeficiency virus infected women, *Obstet Gynecol* 83:401, 1994.

Koutsky L, Ashley R, Holmes K, et al: The frequency of unrecognized type II herpes simplex infection among women, *Sex Transm Dis* 94:90, 1990.

Koutsky L, Galloway D, Holmes K, et al: Epidemiology of genital human papilloma virus infections, *Epidemiol Rev* 10:122, 1988.

Koutsky LA, Stephens CE, Holmes KK, et al: Underdiagnosis of genital herpes by current clinical and viral isolation procedures, *N Engl J Med* 326:1533, 1992.

Kraus SJ, Stone KM: Management of genital infection caused by human papilloma virus, *Rev Infect Dis* 12(suppl):620, 1990.

Krebs HB: Treatment of extensive vulvar condylomata accuminata with topical 5 fluorouracil, *South Med J* 83:761, 1990.

Kucera PR, Glazer J: Hydrocele of the canal of Nuck: a report of four cases, *J Reprod Med* 30:439, 1985.

Kulski JK, Demeter T, Rakoczy P, et al: Human papilloma virus coinfections of the vulva and uterine cervix, *J Med Virol* 27:244, 1989.

Langenberg A, Benedetti J, Jenkins J, et al: Development of clinically recognizable genital lesions among women previously identified as having "asymptomatic" herpes simplex virus type II infection, *Ann Intern Med* 110:882, 1989.

Larson J, Peterson C, Weismann K: Prolonged application of acetic acid for detection of flat vulval warts, *Dan Med Bull* 37:286, 1990.

Lauber A, Souma M: Use of toluidine blue for documentation of traumatic intercourse, *Obstet Gynecol* 60:644, 1982.

McKay M: Vulvodynia vs. pruritus vulvae, *Clin Obstet Gynecol* 28:123, 1985.

McKay M: Subsets of vulvodynia, *J Reprod Med* 33:695, 1988.

McKay M: Vulvodynia: a multifactoral clinical problem, *Arch Dermatol* 125:256, 1989.

McKay M: Dysesthetic "essential" vulvodynia: treatment with amitriptyline, *J Reprod Med* 38:9, 1993.

Minkoff HL, DeHovitz JA: Care of women infected with the human immunodeficiency virus, *JAMA* 266:2253, 1991.

Nystatin Multicenter Study Group: Therapy of candidal vaginitis: the effect of eliminating intestinal *Candida*, *Am J Obstet Gynecol* 155:651, 1986.

O'Duffy D: Behçet's syndrome, *N Engl J Med* 322:326, 1990.

Ohdama S, Takano S, Miyake S, et al: Plasma thrombomodulin as a marker of vascular injuries in collagen vascular diseases, *Am J Clin Pathol* 101:109, 1994.

Oral fluconozol for vaginal candidiasis, *Med Lett* 36:81, 1994.

Pao CC, Lin CY, Maa JS, et al: Detection of human papilloma viruses in cervical vaginal cells using polymerase chain reaction, *J Infect Dis* 161:113, 1990.

Pride GL: Treatment of large lower genital tract condylomata accuminata with topical 5 fluorouracil, *J Reprod Med* 35:384, 1990.

Reeves W, Arosemena J, Garcia M, et al: Genital human papilloma virus infection in Panama City prostitutes, *J Infect Dis* 160:599, 1989.

Richardson DA, Haji SN, Herbst AL: Medical treatment of urethral prolapse in children, *Obstet Gynecol* 59:69, 1982.

Ridley CM: Dermatologic conditions of the vulva, *Baillieres Clin Obstet Gynaecol* 2:317, 1988.

Ridley CM, editor: *The vulva*, New York, 1988, Churchill Livingstone.

Ridley CM, Frankman O, Jones ISC, et al: New nomenclature for vulvar disease—report of the Committee on Terminology of the International Society for the Study of Vulvar Disease, *J Reprod Med* 35:483, 1990.

Riva J, Sedlace KT, Cunnane M, et al: Extended carbon dioxide laser vaporization in the treatment of subclinical papilloma virus infection of the lower genital tract, *Obstet Gynecol* 73:25, 1989.

Scully RE, Mark EJ, McNeely W: Weekly clinical pathologic exercises: case records of the Massachusetts General Hospital, June 19, *N Engl J Med* 320:1741, 1989.

Sobol JD, Vazquez J, Lynch M, et al: Vaginitis due to saccharomyces cerevisiae: epidiomology, clinical aspects, and therapy, *Clin Infect Dis* 16:93, 1993.

Sobel JD, Brooker D, Stein GE, et al: Single oral dose fluconazole compared with conventional clotrimazole topical therapy of Candida vaginitis, *Am J Obstet Gynecol* 172:1263, 1995.

Spitzer M, Krumholz B, Seltzer V: The multicentric nature of disease related to human papilloma virus infection of the female lower genital tract, *Obstet Gynecol* 73:303, 1989.

Stewart DE, Whelan CI, Fong IW, et al: Psychosocial aspects of chronic, clinically unconfirmed vulvovaginitis, *Obstet Gynecol* 76:852, 1990.

Stone KM, Becker TM, Hadgu A, et al: Treatment of external genital warts: a randomized clinical trial comparing podophyllin, cryotherapy, and electrodessication, *Genitourin Med* 66:16, 1990.

Thomas R, Barnhill D, Bibro M, et al: Hidradenitis suppurativa: a case presentation and review of the literature, *Obstet Gynecol* 66:592, 1985.

Weinstock MA: Malignant melanoma of the vulva and vagina in the United States: patterns of incidents in population based estimates of survival, *Am J Obstet Gynecol* 171:1225, 1994.

Whitley RJ, Gnann JW Jr: Acyclovir: a decade later, *N Engl J Med* 327:782, 1992.

Yazici H, Pazarli H, Barnes C, et al: A controlled trial of azathioprine in Behçet's syndrome, *N Engl J Med* 322:281, 1990.

Young L, Bevin I, Johnson MA, et al: The polymerase chain reaction: a new epidemiologic tool for investigating cervical human papilloma virus infection, *Br Med J* 298:14, 1989.

CHAPTER 11

Diagnosis and Treatment of Vaginitis

DAVID A. ESCHENBACH

Depending on the population, three major causes of vaginitis exist: bacterial vaginosis, formerly called nonspecific vaginitis (40% to 50%); candidiasis (20% to 30%); and trichomoniasis (20% to 30%). An additional 5% of women have an inflammatory vaginitis that has not been well characterized. The number of women who have a vaginal discharge caused by cervicitis has not been well studied in comparison to vaginitis, but cervicitis is underdiagnosed, and the addition of women with cervicitis to these data would alter these proportions. In addition, the number of cases of trichomoniasis has dropped in the past several years, and this infection may be less common than indicated.

Despite a limited number of causes, physicians often have difficulty establishing an accurate diagnosis of vaginitis. Vaginitis is frequently overdiagnosed among women who actually have normal flora and misdiagnosed as one cause when another is present. An accurate diagnosis is the most important factor in determining therapeutic success. Diagnostic difficulties probably account for the largest number of women who continue with symptoms after therapy, although persistent vaginitis is also caused by therapeutic failures, sexual reacquisition, nonsexual recurrence, drug resistance, and depressed cellular immunity. The frequent failure to relieve symptoms leads to a high rate of both patient and physician frustration.

Persistent symptoms often lead to patients being dissatisfied with their physicians and switching to new physicians. Persistent symptoms also lead to high costs for repetitive visits in managed health care systems. Thus it may be doubly rewarding and particularly cost-effective to refer patients with persistent symptoms to individuals with particular experience in vaginitis.

COMPONENTS OF NORMAL VAGINAL DISCHARGE

Vaginal discharge is mainly composed of water together with electrolytes, microorganisms, epithelial cells, and organic compounds—fatty acids, proteins, and carbohydrates. Vaginal fluid is largely derived from serum transudate in vaginal capillary beds that seep through intercellular channels. Smaller amounts of fluid are derived from Bartholin's glands, cervix, endometrium, and fallopian tubes.

Cellular elements represent sloughed cells from both cervical columnar and vaginal squamous epithelium. White blood cells (WBCs) are usually present only in small numbers, although this number may increase slightly in the secretory phase of the menstrual cycle.

Estrogen and the pH are two important factors that influence the types of organisms present in the vaginal flora. Vaginal lactic acid content provides an acidic pH of less than 4.5 in adult women. Lactic acid is produced from the metabolism of both lactobacilli and vaginal epithelial cells. The low pH favors the growth of acidophilic organisms such as lactobacilli and inhibits the growth of most other bacteria. The presence of lactobacilli appears to be central in limiting the growth of most other bacteria. Lactobacilli are also capable of producing hydrogen peroxide, which, together with peroxidase and a halide ion, forms a potent system to kill bacteria, particularly the frequent isolates that lack catalase.

NORMAL VAGINAL MICROORGANISMS

An average of 5 to 10 microorganisms are recovered from the vagina, although repeated sampling could undoubtedly recover even more individual species. The vagina has a unique flora. The most prominent facultative microorganisms are species of lactobacilli, corynebacteria, and streptococci and *Staphylococcus epidermidis* and *Gardnerella vaginalis* (formerly called *Haemophilus vaginalis*). Each of the listed individual facultative microorganisms can be found in 40% to 80% of women. *Escherichia coli*, the most common virulent coliform microorganism, can be recovered from about 20% of women. Group B streptococci are present in about 15% to 20% of women. The most prominent anaerobic microorganisms are pepstreptococci, *Bacteroides* species, anaerobic lactobacilli, and eubacteria, which together are recovered from virtually all and individually are recovered from 20% to 60% of women. *Candida albicans*, the most common yeast microorganism, is present in 5% to 10% of women. *Mycoplasma hominis* is present in 20% to 50% and *Ureaplasma urealyticum* in 50% to 70% of sexually active asymptomatic women.

However, despite the large number of species present in vaginal flora, in patients with a lactobacillus-dominant flora, about 95% of the bacteria in the vagina are lactobacilli. Thus in most women the nonpathogenic lactobacillus is the dominant bacteria. In women with lactobacillus-dominant flora, potential pathogens such as *E. coli* or group B streptococci may consist of less than 1% of the total bacterial count in the vagina.

MECHANISMS OF VAGINAL INFECTION

When the complex balance of microorganisms changes, potentially pathogenic endogenous microorganisms that are part of the normal flora—for example, *C. albicans* in cases of candidiasis and *G. vaginalis* and anaerobic bacteria in the cases of bacterial vaginosis—proliferate to a concentration that causes symptoms. At present, little is known about factors that contribute to the overgrowth of normal flora. Pathogenic exogenous microorganisms can also cause infection, and most of these are sexually transmitted, such as *Trichomonas vaginalis*, *Neisseria gonorrhoeae*, and *Chlamydia trachomatis*.

DIAGNOSIS

Diagnosis of vaginitis cannot be based solely on the presence or absence of symptoms. A wide range of symptoms occurs among women with vaginitis that provides a large overlap with the symptoms that occur in women with no vaginitis. Thus physical and laboratory parameters and not symptoms must be used to establish a diagnosis of vaginitis.

The diagnosis of vaginitis is largely based on microscopic criteria. The specificity of detecting trichomonads, clue cells, or hyphae is virtually 100%. However, the sensitivity of identifying any of these three microscopic features by wet mount is only about 80% under ideal circumstances and is much lower with inexperienced microscopists. Algorithms based solely on symptoms are unacceptably inaccurate in any modern medical setting. If a diagnosis cannot be established with certainty, a repeat examination should be made several days later for symptomatic women with suspected vaginitis (to make a specific diagnosis) and symptomatic women with a presumed normal discharge (to further exclude vaginitis). Two examinations with normal findings would theoretically raise the diagnostic accuracy in both categories to 96% (80% + [0.80 × 20]). The use of this plan should reduce the physician's tendency to exclude vaginitis after one "normal examination" among symptomatic women with infection while reassuring the symptomatic woman with normal findings on both examinations that no infection is present.

Physical Examination

Vulvar appearance. The vulva should be inspected for the geographic erythema or fissures that can occur with candidiasis and for the white epithelium of lichen sclerosis. A thin vaginal discharge is often present at the introitus among women with trichomoniasis or bacterial vaginosis. Patients with excessive vulvar tenderness should be scrutinized for vestibulitis, particularly if they have pain from penetration with intercourse.

Appearance of vaginal discharge. Normal vaginal discharge is usually white and clumpy and pools in the vagina. In contrast, the discharge from bacterial vaginosis is gray, homogeneous, and watery, with the appearance of skim milk, and is present on the anterior and lateral vaginal walls. The characteristics of vaginal discharge are also sufficiently different to be helpful in an initial classification attempt (Fig. 11-1). However, a specific diagnosis cannot be made solely from the appearance of the discharge alone because many patients do not have the "typical" appearance.

Cervical appearance. During the early estrogen-dominant phase of the menstrual cycle, a clear mucus endocervical discharge is normally present. In the later progesterone phase of the cycle, cervical mucus is thick, scant, or not visible. Vaginal discharge on the ectocervix must be wiped from the cervical portio with a cotton swab to exclude a purulent appearance from vaginal discharge. However, the presence of a purulent discharge in the endocervical canal at any point should prompt a diagnosis of cervicitis. *N. gonorrhoeae* and *C. trachomatis* are present in about half of women with cervicitis. With cervicitis, frequently endocervical bleeding may occur from swabbing from excessive friability of the columnar epithelium.

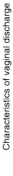
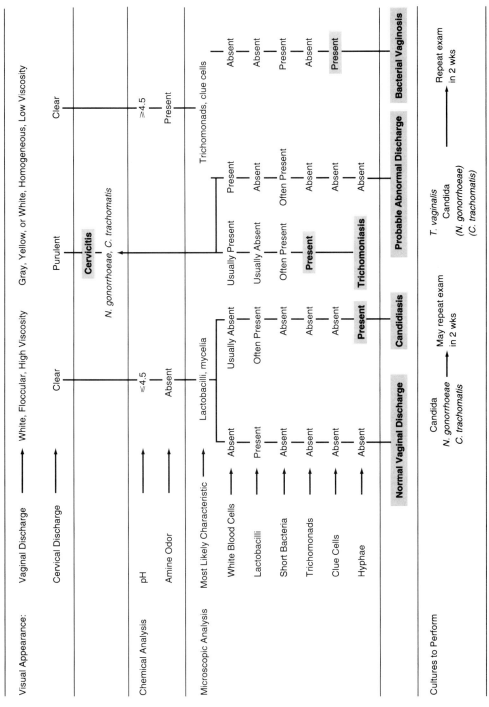

FIGURE 11-1. Systematic determinations useful to diagnosis of the causes of a vaginal discharge.

From Eschenbach DA: In Galask RP, Larsen B, editors: *Infectious diseases in the female patient*, New York, 1986, Springer-Verlag. Used by permission.

Office Analysis

Simple office analysis of the vaginal discharge is helpful and inexpensive. Results allow the placement of patients in one of the two major diagnostic categories (Fig. 11-1).

pH. The pH should be tested by placing a drop of the vaginal discharge on pH paper. Cervical mucus must be avoided because it has a basic pH. The pH is 4.5 or less among women with candidiasis and a normal vaginal discharge. The pH is increased above 4.5 in women with trichomoniasis, bacterial vaginosis, and patients with an inflammatory normal vaginal discharge. However, a normal pH virtually excludes bacterial vaginosis.

Amine odor. Normal vaginal fluid mixed with a drop of 10% potassium hydroxide (KOH) on a glass slide does not provide an odor. A fishy amine odor occurs in women with bacterial vaginosis and in many women with trichomoniasis. The odor is caused by the volatilization of amines, such as putrescine, cadaverine, and trimethylamine, which are by-products of anaerobic metabolism.

Microscopic Analysis

A small amount of vaginal discharge is mixed with normal saline on a glass slide and covered with a coverslip. A large amount of vaginal discharge is mixed with 10% KOH, checked for odor, and covered with a coverslip. The microscopic examination should be performed within a few minutes of preparing the slide. Based on the previous appearance and chemical determinations, the most likely characteristic to be identified by microscopy is sought (see Fig. 11-1). The most likely features present in patients with a pH $\leq$ 4.5 and no amine odor is lactobacillus indication, normal flora, or hyphae in patients with candidiasis. By contrast, the microscopists would search for clue cells or trichomonals in patients with a pH > 4.5 and an amine odor. Systematic analysis of several microscopic features is the key to an accurate diagnosis.

White blood cells. A few WBCs can be present in the vagina as a result of physiologic cervical discharge, particularly premenstrually, but normally the number of WBCs does not exceed the number of vaginal epithelial cells. A large number of WBCs suggests trichomoniasis, cervicitis or occasionally candidiasis. As mentioned previously, 5% of women with vaginitis have inflammatory vaginitis characterized by a pH > 4.5, red vaginal spots, purulent discharge, and, on microscopy, a large number of WBCs, no lactobacilli, other small rod or cocci morphotypes, and parabasal cells.

Lactobacillus morphotypes. The discharge of women with either candidiasis or a normal discharge usually contains a predominance of large, gram-positive rods. These rods can be seen on wet mount preparation. The large rods, which represent lactobacilli, are present in normal and candida discharge and are usually decreased in number or absent in patients with bacterial vaginosis and trichomonas (Figs. 11-2 and 11-3).

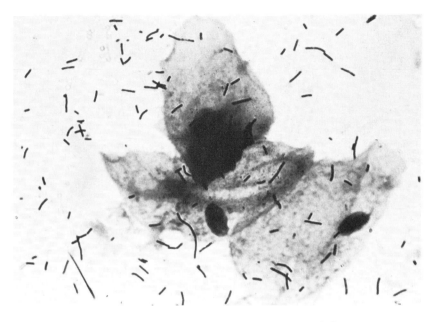

FIGURE 11-2. Gram stain of vaginal discharge obtained from a woman with normal *Lactobacillus*-dominant flora where only large-rod *Lactobacillus* morphotypes are present (1000 × power).

Courtesy of Sharon Hillier, PhD.

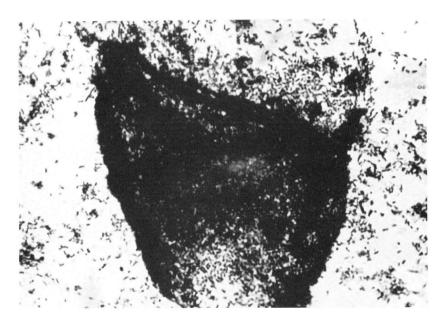

FIGURE 11-3. Gram stain of vaginal discharge obtained from a woman with bacterial vaginosis where a variety of bacterial morphotypes are present, including small straight rods, curved rods, and cocci. Considerably more bacteria are present on this slide than on the slide of normal *Lactobacillus* flora in Fig. 11-2 (1000 × power).

Courtesy of Sharon Hillier, PhD.

Short bacteria morphotypes. In contract to patients with normal lacto-bacillus flora, those with bacterial vaginosis have a predominance of short rods or cocci and none or only a few lactobacillus morphotypes. These small bacteria are often numerous in bacterial vaginosis.

Trichomonads. The trichomonad is a motile, flagellated microorganism that is slightly larger than a WBC. Fully motile trichomonads are easily identified by their characteristic undulating swimming motions. However, WBCs often inhibit their mobility. In about 20% of women with trichomo-niasis, motile trichomonads are not observed under low (100×) power, but the beating flagella can be detected under the 400× objective. About half of women with trichomoniasis on culture have too few trichomonads to be detected by direct microscopy. Fortunately, most of these patients are asymptomatic.

Clue cells. The clue cell is a vaginal epithelial cell to which such a large number of bacteria attach that the cell border is obscured and has a serrated appearance (Fig. 11-4). Clue cells are most objectively identified by noting

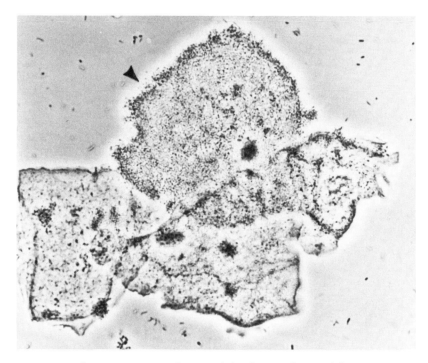

FIGURE 11-4. Saline wet mount of vaginal discharge obtained from a woman with bacterial vaginosis. A clue cell is present in the figure *(arrow)*. The clue cell is an epithelial cell to which so many bacteria are attached that the cell border has a serrated appearance. In contrast, two normal epithelial cells with a clear outline of the cell border are present to the left and below the clue cell.

From Vontver LA, Eschenbach DA: *Clin Obstet Gynecol* 24:453, 1981. Used by permission.

the absence of a straight cell border through the $400 \times$ objective. In women with bacterial vaginosis, 5% to 50% of the vaginal epithelial cells are clue cells.

Hyphae. Hyphae are identified in the 10% KOH solution. Hyphae have a characteristic branching appearance that is usually identified in the $100 \times$ objective. The entire surface of the coverslip should be scanned, because even in symptomatic women, hyphae may be clumped in only one area of the slide.

Gram stain. Vaginal Gram stains can be used in place of the wet mount to detect WBCs, predominant flora, and yeast forms. The Gram stain is not useful for detecting trichomonads. Patients with bacterial vaginosis have a predominance of small gram-negative bacillus flora (*Gardnerella* species, anaerobes) and a relative absence of large gram-positive bacilli (*Lactobacillus* morphotypes). The Gram stain is more sensitive than the wet mounts in identifying *Candida*.

Vaginal Cultures

Vaginal cultures are of limited benefit to diagnose vaginitis. Cultures should be used only in specific circumstances. Cultures for *N. gonorrhoeae* and *C. trachomatis* should be obtained in any woman with a purulent cervical exudate. Gonorrhea and chlamydia infection are also common among women with trichomoniasis.

Vaginal cultures for *Candida* are also useful in women with suspected candidiasis but normal KOH preparations. *Candida* cultures should be obtained from women without hyphae on the KOH smear but with pruritus, an erythematous vulvar rash, or vulvar fissures or white plaques from patients unresponsive to antifungal medication.

Trichomonal cultures can be obtained in cases of a purulent vaginal discharge when repeated microscopic examinations fail to identify the organism. Wet mounts identify only 50% to 70% of asymptomatic women with trichomoniasis. However, these cultures are not readily available.

Vaginal cultures for *G. vaginalis*, other normal vaginal flora bacteria, or genital mycoplasmas are of almost no benefit in making a diagnosis of vaginitis. These organisms are isolated from about 50% of asymptomatic women without vaginitis, so their presence correlates poorly with vaginitis or bacterial vaginosis.

PHYSIOLOGIC VAGINAL DISCHARGE

About 10% of women who complain of vaginal discharge have a physiologic increase in the amount of normal cervical mucus or normal vaginal fluid exudate. Women with a physiologic discharge usually have no vulvar abnormalities and a vaginal discharge that is white and floccular (contains clumps of epithelial cells). The discharge is thick and tends to pool in the inferior portion of the vagina. The vaginal and cervical epithelial surfaces are a normal pink color. The pH of normal discharge is usually less than 4.5, and there is no amine odor when KOH is applied (see Fig. 11-1). At microscopy, no clue cells, trichomonads, or mycelia are seen, and only a few WBCs and short bacteria are present. The most striking microscopic finding is an abundance of vaginal epithelial cells and large rods representing normal gram-positive lactobacilli (see Fig. 11-2).

Cervical mucus can cause a large amount of discharge, particularly in women with a large area of cervical columnar epithelium. Such women typically have excessive discharge midcycle. Examination of the cervix at midcycle reveals a large amount of clear cervical mucus and usually a large area of columnar epithelium on the cervix. Gram stain of the cervical discharge reveals only an occasional WBC. The microscopic appearance of vaginal discharge in these women is that of the physiologic vaginal discharge. Cervical gonococcal and chlamydia cultures should be obtained to exclude their presence.

Women with a physiologic discharge should be reassured that the discharge is normal and therapy is not needed. Symptomatic patients who suspect they have infectious vaginitis should be reexamined in 1 to 2 weeks. Long-term use of tampons should be avoided to prevent vaginal ulceration. Although the practice should generally be discouraged, some women insist on douching, in which case mild vinegar solutions or water should be used. However, the repeated drying effect of multiple douches may actually increase the amount of discharge, and douching with commercial preparations frequently may cause abnormal shifts in vaginal flora. Douching should be actively discouraged because of its link with salpingitis. Antimicrobial regimens should not be administered to women with a physiologic vaginal discharge because of their cost, ineffectiveness, propensity to cause candidiasis, and most important because their failure creates unneeded concern when the discharge persists after repeated therapy. Cryocautery, laser cautery, electrical cautery, and silver nitrate application treatment of a normal columnar epithelium is usually unnecessary.

CANDIDIASIS

C. albicans causes 80% to 90% of vaginal fungal infections. Other *Candida* species and *Torulopsis* cause the remainder. These saprophytic fungi can be isolated in small numbers in 5% to 20% of asymptomatic women. Symptoms usually result only when these organisms proliferate in large numbers.

Infrequent Acute Infection

Topical azole therapy remains the first choice for the treatment of infrequent acute candidiasis. Azoles inhibit ergosterol (and membrane) synthesis and have a fungistatic effect. *Candida* are in turn killed by the host lymphocytes through cell-mediated immune mechanisms. Only a limited fungicidal effect can be achieved by a high concentration of azoles, which produce direct membrane damage. Topical azoles are effective, well tolerated, and relatively inexpensive. Products currently marketed include buconazole (Femstat), clotrimazole (Gyne-Lotrimin, Mycelex), miconazole (Monistat), and terconazole (Terazol). A variety of doses and forms are available (Table 11-1). For some preparations, the dosing has been increased to twice daily, or the dose has been increased from 100 mg to 200 mg while concurrently reducing the length of medication from 7 to 3 days. Cure rates of the 3-day course have been equal to longer courses. Short-term cure rates (7 to 30 days) with topical azoles used for 3 to 7 days are usually 80% to 90%. There is no suggestion that the cure rates differ among various different azoles or between suppository versus cream form.

I do not recommend single-dose therapy because clinical experience suggests that 1-day courses are less effective than published reports indicate. This may be explained in part by the tendency to include in studies women with symptoms that are mild or of short duration and women with no prior candidiasis. Additionally, usually only short-term clinical cure rates (7 to 30 days) are reported; higher mycologic failure rates occur at 30 days among patients given a single dose compared with a longer course of therapy. The association of increased clinical candidiasis with higher rates of candida recovery is unclear; patients may not have been followed long enough.

The oral azole fluconazole makes oral medication a safe choice for a vaginal candidiasis. A one-time 150-mg oral dose is effective for patients with mild to moderate symptoms. This drug has become popular. Short-term use is without liver toxicity, a problem that prevented widespread use of azole. However, the dose often must be repeated in 4 to 5 days among highly symptomatic patients in whom failure rates otherwise exceed local

TABLE 11-1. Recommended azole regimens for the treatment of vulvovaginal candidiasis

Azole	Intravaginal dose	Duration
Butoconazole (Femstat)	2% cream hs*	3 days
Clotrimazole (Gyne-Lotrimin, Mycelex)	100-mg tablet bid*	3 days
	100-mg tablet hs	7 days
	1% cream hs	7 days
Miconazole (Monistat)	200-mg suppositories hs	3 days
	100-mg suppositories hs	7 days
Terconazole (Terazole)	80-mg suppositories hs	3 days
	0.4% cream hs	7 days

*bid, twice a day; hs, at bedtime.

therapy. However, concern exists that widespread use will eventually lead to resistance.

Topical polyene therapy consisting of nystatin has been largely replaced by topical azole treatment. Nystatin is well tolerated and inexpensive, but cure rates of 50% to 80% are lower than those of azoles. Thus nystatin is a second-line choice in treating vaginal candidiasis.

Boric acid capsules (600 mg or boric acid in "0" size gelatin capsules) inserted twice daily for 14 days provides clinical cure rates similar to the topical azoles. The boron ion has not been detected in blood, and boric acid is inexpensive and well tolerated. However, boric acid can produce esophageal ulcers if inadvertently swallowed, and the preparation should be stored in bottles with childproof caps, kept in a locked medicine cabinet, and used with caution if small children are present in the household. Because of unproven fetal safety, boric acid should not be used in pregnancy. Gentian violet treatment is effective for the treatment of candidiasis, but the staining of clothing and skin limits its use to the rare case unresponsive to other medication. Potassium sorbate and povidone iodine have limited effectiveness against candidiasis.

Local *Candida* therapy is usually well tolerated, and reactions are unusual. Occasionally, increased vaginal irritation occurs. Patients should immediately stop and change to a different preparation. Most of these irritations result from "inactive" compounds in the cream vehicle.

Rapidly Recurrent Infection

Patients may have the return of symptoms a few days after completing a course of medication. A lack of compliance is the most common reason for the return of symptoms. Resistance of *Candida* to antifungal medication is uncommon. Patients with a rapid recurrence have candidiasis documented by a potassium hydroxide wet mount or a culture. Medication should be changed to eliminate the possibility of a drug reaction. Patients without objective evidence of *Candida* but with persistent symptoms after these corrective measures should be scrutinized for vaginitis or vulvitis caused by conditions other than candida. Neurodermatitis, lichen plants, lichen sclerosis, burning vulvar syndrome, and minor vestibular gland inflammation should be considered when patients originally diagnosed to have *Candida* fail to respond to appropriate treatment.

Drug resistance is unusual. Patients usually have a reduction of symptoms while on therapy but a rapid recurrence of symptoms once medication is stopped. *Candida albicans* is almost uniformly sensitive to all azoles and makes up over 90% of the fungi that produce vaginitis. Drug resistance is more common among unusual fungi such as *C. glabrata*, *C. torulopsis*, *C. tropicalis*, and other non-*albicans* species. Possible resistance should be considered if these fungi are present. Terconazole treatment may be tried because it has greater activity than other azoles against *C. glabrata* and *C. tropicalis*. Second, patients should be switched to the nonazole nystatin. Gentian violet therapy may also be of benefit. In rare instances none of the topical medications are effective in eliminating vaginal fungi, and azoles or nystatin must be given every 2 or 3 days to suppress rather than eliminate resistant fungi.

Reasons for Failure

Treatment failures have been so infrequent for candidiasis that systematic studies have not been performed to determine the causes of treatment failure. Additionally, the follow-up period is usually too short (30 days or less) to accurately assess the frequency of failures. Compliance failure, pseudofailure caused by a reaction to the vehicle, and drug resistance have been mentioned. Two other prominent theories of treatment failure require discussion.

The first theory is that recurrent vaginal candidiasis results from gastrointestinal tract *Candida. Candida* organisms are found in higher rates in the oral cavity and gastrointestinal tract of patients with candidiasis than in controls. However, most patients carry *Candida* in the gastrointestinal tract without developing vaginal candidiasis, and in longitudinal studies vaginal candidiasis has not been related to gastrointestinal *Candida*. Oral therapy has provided mixed results. Oral nystatin has not had a dramatic effect, although a slight but statistically significant reduction in subsequent *Candida* vulvovaginitis occurred in the group receiving oral nystatin compared with placebo. Recently, 4 ounces of lactobacillus-containing yogurt eaten twice daily has also provided some significant reduction in recurrence. Unfortunately, experience suggests a limited effect of oral therapy.

The second theory envalues sexual transmission of recurrent candidiasis. Male sexual partners of patients with vaginal candidiasis have higher rates of genital colonization than controls. Sexual transmission probably does occur for the small number (estimated to be 10% to 15%) of males who have *Candida* balanitis concurrent with their partner's vaginal candidiasis. However, only 20% of male sexual partners are colonized with *Candida*, and treatment of males has not decreased vaginal candidiasis for the female. Males may become passively colonized by the female and appear to play a limited rate in recurrent vaginal candidiasis.

Adjunctive Treatment

Temporary reduction of vulvar symptoms occurs with a sitz bath followed by superdrying of the skin with a hair dryer using the low heat setting. Topical azole creams can also be prescribed for direct vulvar use, but little information is available on the effectiveness of this therapy over vaginal therapy alone.

Abandonment of tight, poorly ventilated clothing may help prevent reinfection. Dietary measures to reduce high carbohydrate levels has been of some benefit to a subset of patients with a history of developing candidiasis shortly after ingesting unusually high amounts of sugar. Among diabetics, candidiasis treatment is usually not successful until the diabetes is controlled. The avoidance of foods made from yeast has been popularized, but scientific documentation of effectiveness is absent. Yeasts present in food are not the species that cause vaginitis, and yeasts that cause vaginitis are so prevalent in the environment and the skin that it is difficult to believe that a yeast-free diet influences vaginal candidiasis. Cessation of antibiotic therapy can be considered, when possible, in a small number of patients on chronic antimicrobials. Cessation of oral contraceptive therapy is controversial and probably of limited benefit.

Chronic (Frequently) Recurrent Infection

Recently a significant subset of patients has been identified with chronic or frequently recurrent (at least four annually) episodes of vaginal candidiasis. These patients represent a significant number of patients with vaginal candidiasis attending certain clinics.

It is not clear whether these patients have a limited immunologic defect from lymphocytes incapable of killing their *Candida* or other reasons for recurrence. Recurrence is not related to unusual or drug-resistant strains of *Candida*, and few are diabetic or taking oral contraceptives, immunosuppressive drugs, or antibiotics. Women with frequent recurrences of vaginal candidiasis or candidiasis that does not respond to treatment should be considered for human immunodeficiency virus (HIV) testing. However, almost no women will have HIV or any other commonly recognized factor that predisposes patients to candidiasis.

Frequently symptomatic disease can be difficult to manage. An important breakthrough in the treatment of frequently recurrent candidiasis has been the recognition that suppressive rather than curative therapy is in order. Suppressive antimicrobial therapy has been successfully used to treat chronic recurrent urinary tract infection, and this principal has been applied to chronic recurrent candidiasis. An initial therapeutic dose of a standard intravaginal antimycotic agent or 400 mg of oral ketoconazole is given daily for 14 days. This is followed by a maintenance dose of antifungal therapy daily for 6 to 12 months. Potential liver toxicity and expense limits ketoconazole use. Practical maintenance regimens include biweekly or topical boric acid or azole administration. In the only controlled published report, ketoconazole produced a recurrence rate at 6 months of 70% for those on placebo versus 5% for those on daily ketoconazole (Table 11-2). Ketoconazole is not recommended for maintenance because of potential liver toxicity. Recurrence of vaginal can-

TABLE 11-2. Recurrent vulvovaginal candidiasis related to 6 months of prophylactic ketoconazole therapy

Recurrent *Candida* infection	Treatment group	Placebo group
6 months (on prophylaxis)		
Candida positive	3/21 (14%)	15/21 (71%)
Symptomatic vulvovaginitis	1/21 (5%)	15/21 (71%)
12 months (6 months postprophylaxis)		
Candida positive	12/21 (57%)	16/21 (76%)
Symptomatic vulvovaginitis	10/21 (48%)	16/21 (76%)

Data from Sobel JD: *N Engl J Med* 315:1455, 1986.

didiasis may resume at the same rates as was present before suppression when maintenance therapy ceases.

Treatment in Pregnancy

Systemic absorption of either azoles or nystatin from the vagina is so limited that both can be safely used during all trimesters of pregnancy. Boric acid fluconazole and ketoconazole should not be used during pregnancy. Compared with nonpregnant women, candidiasis in pregnancy is more resistant to treatment, is more likely to relapse, and thus responds better to more prolonged therapy (7 to 14 days) than 1- to 3-day therapy.

TRICHOMONIASIS

Trichomonas vaginalis is a ubiquitous sexually transmitted anaerobic parasite. It has been associated with vaginitis, atypical cytologic smears, and other sexually transmitted infection (up to half of women with gonorrhea also have trichomoniasis). Only 50% of the women infected with trichomonads are symptomatic.

T. vaginalis can be recovered from the prostatic fluid of up to 70% of male contacts of women with trichomoniasis. A significant number of men carry the organism for a prolonged time, although some men are cured without treatment. Male contacts are particularly likely to harbor trichomonads (>60%) if they are examined within 6 days of their last exposure, but 33% of male contacts carried trichomonads from 6 to over 60 days after the last exposure. The organism was present in 14% to 60% of male contacts of women with trichomoniasis in 19 studies, which confirms sexual transmission and the need to treat male partners.

Symptomatic women characteristically complain of a profuse, malodorous, often uncomfortable vaginal discharge that causes both internal and external dysuria. A sense of vulvar-vaginal fullness and even lower abdominal tenderness may also be present. Symptoms typically exacerbate around menses. *T. vaginalis* is considered to be an agent that causes only lower genital tract infection (the vagina, Bartholin glands, urethra, periurethral glands, and bladder of women and the urethra and prostate of men).

On examination, the vulva may be slightly edematous, and the vulva and vagina may be covered with a gray, green, or yellow, purulent, frothy, odorous discharge. The classic discharge is present in only about one third of women. Small areas of subepithelial hyperemia of the vagina and cervix usually require colposcopy for identification, but occasionally the areas are identified on the cervical epithelium (strawberry cervix) by the naked eye.

Metronidazole Therapy

Metronidazole is the only effective drug approved for the treatment of trichomoniasis in the United States. Oral therapy provides adequate levels of medication not only for vaginal, but also for periurethral, urethral, and bladder infection.

Recommended treatment consists of 2 g of metronidazole given as a stat one-time dose or 500 mg of metronidazole given twice daily for seven days (Table 11-3). A 250-g, three-times-daily regimen for 7 days has been most frequently studied, but the half-life of metronidazole supports the use of the 500-mg dose twice daily over the three-times-daily regimen. The stat and the 7-day regimens are equally effective for the treatment of uncomplicated trichomoniasis, but the stat dose is preferred because of increased compliance over the 7-day regimen. Cure rates of over 95% are usually reported with either regimen, particularly when male sexual partners also receive treatment.

Nausea, the most common side effect, occurs in 5% to 25% of patients. A metallic taste, cephalgia, dizziness, and dark urine also occur with metronidazole use. Patients should be advised not to drink alcohol for 24 hours after the last metronidazole dose because of a disulfiram-like effect that produces nausea when alcohol is concomitantly ingested.

Mutagens have been identified in the urine of women taking metronidazole. At present, metronidazole must be considered a weak carcinogen

TABLE 11-3. Recommended regimens to treat trichomoniasis*

Type of infection	Metronidazole dose	Administration	Duration
Uncomplicated infection			
Recommended	2 g	Oral	Single dose
Alternative or for a repetitive failure	500 mg	Oral	bid for 7 days
Documented treatment failure	1 g	Oral	bid for 7–14 days
	500 mg	Vaginal	bid for 7–14 days

*Sexual partner should be concomitantly treated.

capable of producing DNA damage. This has produced concern of increased rates of cancer among former metronidazole users. Two relatively small retrospective studies have shown no relationship between metronidazole and cancer. Rates of some cancers were slightly increased among metronidazole users compared with controls but with relative risks less than 2. However, the studies are too small to detect an effect at less than a twofold-increased risk. Weak carcinogens often are associated with risk ratios lower than 2. Data are also incomplete because of short follow-up (3 to 11 years) compared with up to a 30-year latency period of clinical cancer. Studies of the relation of cancer to metronidazole are of too short a duration to address this issue with certainty. Thus one must remain concerned about the potential carcinogenic effect of metronidazole.

Sexual Partner Therapy

Concomitant male sexual partner therapy is recommended to effectively treat this sexually transmitted infection. About 75% of male contacts of women with trichomoniasis acquire the microorganism. Approximately one third of infected males appear to have spontaneous cures, but clear evidence exists for the treatment of male sexual partners. Female cure rates are increased 10% to 25% when the male is also treated. A 97% cure rate has been reported with both the 2-g and the 7-day regimen when incarcerated women were treated without reexposure to male partners. Male therapy also reduces spread of trichomonas to other females. Because they are usually asymptomatic, males may resist the notion of therapy.

Treatment of Asymptomatic Women

About 50% of women with trichomoniasis are asymptomatic. The asymptomatic form of the infection is related to low concentrations of trichomonads and to individual patient differences in the recognition of symptoms. Asymptomatic women detected with trichomoniasis should be offered therapy to reduce sexual transmission. Therapy should also be given to patients with atypical inflammatory Papanicolaou smears and *T. vaginalis*.

Treatment Failure

A possible failure of compliance should be sought in patients who initially received the 7-day regimen. Patients with persistent trichomoniasis can also have sexual reinfection, and both they and their partners should be retreated with the 7-day regimen. Cure rates after retreatment remain high with the standard regimens.

T. vaginalis remains susceptible to metronidazole over 35 years of use. However, resistance of *T. vaginalis* to metronidazole has now been reported in a small number of patients even after two to three times the usual dose of drug. A general correlation exists between in vitro susceptibilities and clinical cure rates, but clinical and laboratory efficacy do not correlate as well for *T. vaginalis* as for bacterial susceptibility testing. Nevertheless, the mean in vitro susceptibility of *T. vaginalis* from women resistant to standard metronidazole therapy was about eight times higher than the susceptibility of standard isolates.

Patients who fail to respond to the usual doses of metronidazole, who have been compliant, and who have not been reexposed to male partners should be treated with an increased dose of drug. These cases have been infrequent, and a uniform treatment regimen has not yet been established. One regimen I found to be helpful is given in Table 11-3. In general, patients who failed standard therapy responded to a 2-g daily oral dose of metronidazole given with a 1000-mg intravaginal dose of metronidazole over 7 to 14 days. Most patients have considerable nausea when given 3 g or more of metronidazole daily, but they are usually able to complete treatment. Intravenous administration has been used for clinically resistant cases, but this regimen is expensive, toxic, and probably unnecessary because oral metronidazole is well absorbed. Infectious disease specialists should be consulted when high doses of metronidazole are required. Administration of 4 to 6 g or more of metronidazole daily has been associated with seizures and a potential of disabling peripheral neuropathy.

Treatment in Pregnancy

Treatment of trichomoniasis with metronidazole in pregnancy is controversial. Despite two reports of an association of *T. vaginalis* with prematurity, there is little evidence that the microorganism ascends into the uterus or placenta or to the neonate. At present, treatment in pregnancy is justified for symptoms but not to reduce premature birth. Metronidazole has been administered to a large number of pregnant women, but outcome data are available for only a modest number of patients. Metronidazole has not been associated with a recognized teratogenic or other adverse neonatal effect, with the exception of two small reports associating congenital anomalies with metronidazole use during the first trimester. Metronidazole has both a mutagenic and carcinogenic potential. Although the magnitude of these effects is not certain, there is reason for concern about injudicious or widespread use of metronidazole in pregnancy.

Several modifications of therapy are possible during pregnancy. Treatment should be avoided in the first trimester, when the neonate is most susceptible to the effects of drugs. Treatment can be considered for patients with moderate or severe symptoms in the second and third trimester. Clotrimazole may temporarily reduce symptoms, although actual cure is rare. Asymptomatic or minimally symptomatic patients should not receive treatment during pregnancy but can receive a 2-g dose of metronidazole on the day of delivery. Levels of drug in breast milk are equal to serum levels, and breast-feeding can be delayed for 24 hours to limit levels present in breast milk. In summary, because of concerns over the weak carcinogenic potential of metronidazole, its use should be limited during pregnancy.

BACTERIAL VAGINOSIS

Bacterial vaginosis results from an overgrowth of both anaerobic bacteria and *G. vaginalis*, formerly called *Haemophilus vaginalis*. Although the microbiology of this infection is complex, consistent microbiologic findings are now being reported. It is now recognized that *G. vaginalis* is commonly present in the vagina of normal women; 40% of asymptomatic women without vaginitis have *G. vaginalis* recovered from the vagina. It is recovered from more than 95% of women with bacterial vaginosis (BV). Among women with BV, the *G. vaginalis* concentration increases 10 to 100 times to 10^5 to 10^8 colony-forming units (CFU) per cc of vaginal fluid compared to normal women.

Similar increases in anaerobic flora occur among women with BV. The prevalence of detectable anaerobic bacteria increases from 50% in normal women to over 95% in women with BV. This increased prevalence is undoubtedly due to the increased concentrations of anaerobes among women with BV. In women with BV, compared with normal women, the concentration of total anaerobic bacteria increases 10 to 100 times to reach levels of 10^5 to 10^7 CFU per cc of vaginal fluid. The most common anaerobes are members of the *Bacteroides, Peptostreptococcus*, and *Mobiluncus* species.

Lactobacilli are infrequently identified by Gram stain or wet mount in women with BV. The relatively acidity (pH < 4.5) in the vagina in normal women is increased in women with BV because of this shift from a lactobacillus-dominant flora to one dominated by other bacteria. The vast majority of lactobacilli isolated from normal women are facultative, and the majority of lactobacilli isolated from women with BV are anaerobic. The factors that influence the presence of lactobacilli in the vagina are largely unknown.

The most common characteristic symptom is a fishy vaginal odor that occurs spontaneously or after intercourse. The odor is caused by the volatilization of amines, notably putrescine, cadaverine, and trimethylamine, which are produced by bacterial metabolism. This amine odor often increases with menses and after intercourse when the amines are disassociated from protein by alkalinization.

A high concentration of potentially virulent anaerobic bacteria might be expected to cause other morbidity. Bacterial vaginosis has recently been associated with postcesarean endometritis, postcesarean wound infection, prematurity, and posthysterectomy infection.

Diagnosis

A false-positive diagnosis is the most common cause for a failure to successfully treat bacterial vaginosis. Most patients who are believed to have failed treatment do not have bacterial vaginosis; they have a normal lactobacillus-dominant flora associated with either an excessive discharge or odor, or they have cervicitis or some other lower genital tract infection.

Bacterial vaginosis can be diagnosed by clinical or Gram stain criteria. Clinical criteria include the presence of at least three of the following four characteristics of the vaginal discharge: a thin "skim milk" appearance, a pH $\geq$ 4.5, a fishy amine odor with the addition of 10% potassium hydroxide to the discharge, and clue cells by microscopy. Lactobacilli dominate vaginal flora of patients with a normal vaginal discharge. Gram stain criteria use a relative increase in the number of gram-negative rods and positive cocci that occurs in bacterial vaginosis compared with gram-positive rods that represent *Lactobacillus* in normal discharge.

Because *G. vaginalis* is present in approximately half of patients without vaginitis, its recovery by culture is not a specific finding for the diagnosis of bacterial vaginosis. Cultures for *G. vaginalis* are also not useful when making a diagnosis of bacterial vaginosis after antibiotic therapy because half of patients successfully treated for bacterial vaginosis still have *G. vaginalis*.

All pregnant symptomatic patients and asymptomatic patients undergoing invasive genital surgery (induced abortion, hysterectomy) should be treated. The optimal timing of therapy before surgery has not received study but is probably 1 month before or 1 to 2 days before surgery. Treatment 1 to 3 weeks before surgery is associated with a temporary overgrowth of other pathogens in the vagina that may increase the risk of infection by these bacteria. Pregnant patients with prior preterm birth and bacterial vaginosis should be treated because metronidazole is effective in reducing the increased rate of preterm birth in this group. Data are accumulating that suggest pregnant patients with bacterial vaginosis but without a prior preterm birth should also be treated to prevent preterm birth.

First-Choice Therapy

Several antimicrobial regimens provide cure rates of 85% to 95%. These regimens include metronidazole 500 g taken orally twice daily for 7 days; clindamycin 300 mg taken orally twice daily for 7 days; and two intravaginal regimens, 0.75% metronidazole gel inserted twice daily for 5 days and 2% clindamycin cream inserted nightly for 7 days. Local regimens are associated with fewer side effects because the dose of antibiotic is low compared with oral therapy.

Second-Choice Therapy

Two regimens that provide cure rates of 80% to 85% are metronidazole 2 g taken orally at one time and amoxicillin/clavulanic acid 500 mg three times daily for 7 days.

Third-Choice Therapy

Third-line regimens have minimal efficacy in the treatment of bacterial vaginosis. Ampicillin or amoxicillin (500 mg, three or four daily oral doses) cures bacterial vaginosis in only 30% to 45% of patients. Ciprofloxacin taken orally (500 mg three times per day) and triple sulfa vaginal cream used twice daily for 7 days provide cure rates of only 20% to 50%. Generally, these regimens should not be used.

Ineffective Therapy

Several drugs have been ineffective in treating bacterial vaginosis. These drugs include erythromycin, tetracycline, doxycycline, and several intravaginal products (povidone-iodine, acetic acid gel, and lactobacillus).

Male Therapy

Bacterial vaginosis has frequently been suspected of being a sexually transmitted condition, although no direct proof exists. Because recurrent infection is common, some authors advocate treatment of male partners. There are now four randomized trials in which metronidazole therapy of male sexual partners of women with bacterial vaginosis had no effect on the subsequent recurrence of bacterial vaginosis in the female. Male partner treatment should not be included in the usual treatment of bacterial vaginosis. More research is required on the cause of recurrence.

Frequently Recurrent Bacterial Vaginosis

Cure rates are high when first- or second-choice drugs are used, but a group of women either have rapid or repetitive recurrent infection. The cause of recurrent infection has not been elucidated, but one obvious possibility is the emergence of resistant bacteria. Patients with rapidly recurrent infection should be empirically switched to a different antimicrobial agent to account for possible resistance (e.g., from metronidazole to clindamycin). For patients who recur after changing antimicrobials, I give an intravaginal preparation of metronidazole or clindamycin for 3 weeks followed by intravaginal therapy every third day for 3 additional weeks. The latter part of the regimen is designed to inhibit bacteria from causing bacterial vaginosis while allowing lactobacilli to recolonize the vagina. A few patients who note recurrences associated with intercourse benefit from taking a tablet of metronidazole each time they have intercourse.

Complications

Bacterial vaginosis is a condition in which unusually high concentrations of potentially virulent bacteria are present in the vagina. It is not surprising to find that invasion of these bacteria into the upper genital tract as a result of surgery or pregnancy causes infection. The reported relative risk of these infections is provided in Table 11-4. About 15% of patients have bacterial vaginosis, so the importance of bacterial vaginosis on these infections is substantial. Generally, the rate of preterm delivery increased 1.5 to 2 times among those with bacterial vaginosis compared with those without in seven studies. Amniotic fluid and chorioamnion infection and histologic chorio-amnionitis have been related to bacterial vaginosis. Bacteria associated with bacterial vaginosis are common isolates from the amniotic fluid and chorioamnion of women in premature labor. Metronidazole given for 7 days to women with both bacterial vaginosis and prior preterm labor significantly reduced the rate of preterm delivery in the present pregnancy.

Postpartum endometritis after both cesarean section and vaginal delivery is associated with bacterial vaginosis. This elevated rate of endometritis occurs despite the use of prophylactic antibiotics for cesarean delivery. About two thirds of the endometrial isolates in patients with postpartum endometritis are those bacteria that are found at high concentrations in women with bacterial vaginosis.

Cuff cellulitis after abdominal hysterectomy occurs in about 35% of women with and 10% of those without bacterial vaginosis. Pelvic inflammatory disease after induced abortion is increased in patients with bacterial vaginosis, and this infection is reduced by treatment with metronidazole. The link between bacterial vaginosis and spontaneous pelvic inflammatory disease is not well established.

ATROPHIC VAGINITIS

Atrophic vaginitis is a symptomatic vaginal inflammatory condition caused by estrogen-deficient vaginal epithelium. Symptoms include vaginal bleed-

TABLE 11-4. Complications associated with bacterial vaginosis

Complication	Approximate relative risk
Preterm delivery	1.5-2.0
Amniotic fluid infection	2.0-2.5
Chorioamnionitis	3
Histologic chorioamnionitis	2.5
Postpartum endometritis	
Postcesarean section	6
Postvaginal delivery	2
Postabortion pelvic inflammatory disease	2.5-3
Postabdominal hysterectomy	3.5

ing and soreness, external dysuria, pruritus, and dyspareunia. The diagnosis of atrophic vaginitis can be confirmed by finding a smooth, pale pink vaginal surface without rugae and a predominance of parabasal cells on a vaginal smear. Moderate vulvar irritation may be present. The discharge is usually slight, the vaginal pH is greater than 5. Microscopy usually reveals an absence of organisms, including lactobacilli, although the bacteriology of atrophic vaginitis has not been well defined. Neoplasm, foreign bodies, and other infectious causes of the symptoms should be excluded. Atrophic vaginitis is treated with topical estrogens, which thicken the vaginal epithelium and reduce the susceptibility of the surface to infection. Estrogen cream can be inserted into the vagina once daily for 2 weeks and then every other day for 2 weeks. In the majority of patients, estrogen therapy can be completely stopped without recurrence of symptoms. Because vaginal estrogens are readily absorbed, prolonged vaginal use of estrogen has the same disadvantages as systemic use in the postmenopausal woman, and therapy is not usually necessary beyond 4 weeks for the majority of patients.

CERVICITIS

Cervicitis is a common finding among sexually active women. Although cervicitis can result in a vaginal discharge, it is often present without symptoms. *C. trachomatis, N. gonorrhoeae,* and *Herpesvirus hominis* are related to cervicitis.

The diagnosis can be made by clinical or microscopic criteria. Clinical criteria include a grossly visible yellow or white mucopus in situ or in the endocervix on a cotton swab from the endocervix, often with a columnar epithelium that is friable and bleeds easily on contact. Microscopic criteria consist of finding 10 or more polymorphonuclear leukocytes in areas of the most dense inflammation on a Gram stain of cervical mucus. About one third of women with cervicitis do not have grossly visible mucopus, yet there are 10 WBCs or more per field identified by Gram stain.

Cultures should be obtained for both *C. trachomatis* and *N. gonorrhoeae.* Recently *C. trachomatis* antigen detection by fluorescent staining or enzyme-linked immunoabsorbent assays can also be used to detect *C. trachomatis. C. trachomatis, N. gonorrhoeae,* or both have been isolated in approximately half of women with mucopurulent cervicitis. The cause of the remaining cases has yet to be determined. Tetracycline, 500 mg four times daily, or doxycycline, 100 mg twice daily for at least 7 days, is the recommended treatment. Virtually all cases of cervicitis with chlamydia or gonorrhea respond to antibiotic treatment, but some cases without either organism do not respond. The cause and the appropriate treatment of the cervicitis in these women remain to be determined. Destruction of the columnar epithelium by cryocautery, laser therapy, or conization should be limited to women without chlamydia or gonorrhea who remain symptomatic despite adequate antibiotic therapy.

OTHER CAUSES OF VAGINAL DISCHARGE

Approximately 5% of women with vaginitis have one of a variety of heterogeneous vaginal conditions. Some women have bacterial vaginitis characterized by a constellation of a purulent discharge, patches of submucosal erythema, and a pH greater than 4.5. Microscopically there is a large number of WBCs, parabasal cells, small bacteria, and no lactobacillus or clue cells. I find that patients have responded to 2% clindamycin or cephalothin cream on alternate days with hydrocortisone suppositories used intravaginally for 21 days. Recurrence rates are moderately high. This group of women has findings suggestive of desquamative inflammatory vaginitis.

BIBLIOGRAPHY

Amsel R, Totten PA, Spiegel CA, et al: Nonspecific vaginitis: diagnostic criteria and microbial and epidemiological association, *Am J Med* 74:14, 1983.

Balsdon MJ, Tobin JM: Recurrent vaginal candidosis: prospective study of effectiveness of maintenance miconazole treatment, *Genitourin Med* 64:124, 1988.

Beard CM, Noller KL, O'Fallon WM, et al: Lack of evidence for cancer due to use of metronidazole, *N Engl J Med* 301:519, 1979.

Bisschop MPJM, Merkus JMWM, Scheygrond H, Van Cutsem J: Cotreatment of the male partner in vaginal candidosis: a double-blind randomized control study, *Br J Obstet Gynaecol* 93:79, 1986.

Block E: Occurrence of trichomonas in sexual partners of women with trichomoniasis, *Acta Obstet Gynecol Scand* 38:398, 1959.

Bradbeer CS, Mayhew SR, Barlow D: Butoconazole and miconazole in treating vaginal candidiasis, *Genitourin Med* 61;:270, 1985.

Brundin J: The effect of miconazole on vulvovaginal candidiasis in pregnant and non-pregnant patients and their partners, *Int J Gynaecol Obstet* 14:537, 1976.

Brunham RC, Paavonen J, Stevens CE, et al: Mucopurulent cervicitis: the ignored counterpart in women of urethritis in men, *N Engl J Med* 311:1, 1984.

Como JA, Dismukes WE: Oral azole drugs as systemic antifungal therapy, *N Engl J Med* 33:263, 1994.

Eschenbach DA: Lower genital tract infections. In Galask RP, Larsen B, editors: *Infectious diseases in the female patient*, New York, 1986, Springer-Verlag.

Eschenbach DA, Critchlow CW, Watkins H, et al: A dose duration study of metronidazole for treatment of nonspecific vaginitis, *Scand J Infect Dis Suppl* 40:73, 1983.

Eschenbach DA, Hillier S, Critchlow C, et al: Diagnosis and clinical manifestations of bacterial vaginosis, *Am J Obstet Gynecol* 158:819, 1988.

Eschenbach DA, Hillier SL: Advances in diagnostic testing for vaginitis and cervicitis, *J Reprod Med* 34(supple 8):555, 1989.

Friedman GD: Cancer after metronidazole, *N Engl J Med* 302:519, 1980 (letter).

Gardner HL, Dukes CD: *Haemophilus vaginalis* vaginitis, *Am J Obstet Gynecol* 69:962, 1955.

Gravett MG, Nelson HP, DeRouen T, et al: Independent association of bacterial vaginosis and *Chlamydia trachomatis* infection with adverse pregnancy outcome, *JAMA* 256:1899, 1986.

Hager WD, Brown ST, Kraus SJ, et al: Metronidazole in vaginal trichomoniasis: seven day vs. single-dose regimens, *JAMA* 244:1219, 1980.

Hardy PH, Hardy JV, Well EE, et al: Prevalence of six sexually transmitted agents among pregnant inner-city adolescents and pregnancy outcomes, *Lancet* 2:333, 1984.

Hill GB, Eschenbach DA, Holmes KK: Bacteriology of the vagina. In Mardh PA, Taylor-Robinson D, editors: *Bacterial vaginosis*, Stockholm, 1984, Almquist and Wiksell.

Hillier SL, Krohn MA, Rabe LK, et al: The normal vaginal flora, H_2O_2-producing lactobacilli, and bacterial vaginosis in pregnant women, *Clin Infect Dis* 16(suppl. 4):S273, 1993.

Hillier SL, Krohn MA, Watts DH, et al: Microbiological efficacy of intravaginal clindamycin cream for the treatment of bacterial vaginosis, *Obstet Gynecol* 76:407, 1990.

Hillier SL, Lipinski CM, Briselden AM, Eschenbach DA: Efficacy of intravaginal 0.75% metronidazole gel for the treatment of bacterial vaginosis, *Obstet Gynecol* 81:963, 1993.

Hillier SL, Martius J, Krohn M, et al: A case-control study of chorioamnionic infection and chorioamnionitis in prematurity, *N Engl J Med* 319:972, 1988.

Hilton E, Isenberg HD, Alperstein P, et al: Ingestion of yogurt containing *Lactobacillus acidophilus* as prophylaxis for candidal vaginitis, *Ann Intern Med* 116:353, 1992.

Horowitz BJ, Edelstein SW, Lippman L: Sexual transmission of *Candida*, *Obstet Gynecol* 69:883, 1987.

Huggins GR, Preti G: Volatile constituents of human vaginal secretions, *Am J Obstet Gynecol* 126:129, 1976.

Jerve F, Berdal TB, Bohman P, et al: Metronidazole in the treatment of nonspecific vaginitis, *Br J Vener Dis* 60:171, 1984.

Krieger JN: Trichomoniasis in men: old issues and new data, *Sex Transm Dis* 22:83, 1995.

Kutzer E, Oittner R, Leodolter S, Brammer KW: A comparison of fluconazole and ketoconazole in the oral treatment of vaginal candidiasis; report of a double-blind multicentre trial, *Eur J Obstet Gynecol Reprod Biol* 29:305, 1988.

Lebherz T, Guess E, Wolfson N: Efficacy of single versus multiple dose clotrimazole therapy in the management of vulvovaginal candidiasis, *Am J Obstet Gynecol* 153:965, 1985.

Lossick JG: Single-dose metronidazole treatment for vaginal trichomoniasis, *Obstet Gynecol* 56:508, 1980.

Lossick JG: Treatment of *Trichomonas vaginalis* infections, *Rev Infect Dis* 4(suppl):S801, 1982.

Lossick JG, Muller M, Gorrell TE: In vitro drug susceptibility and doses of metronidazole required for cure in cases of refractory vaginal trichomoniasis, *J Infect Dis* 153:948, 1986.

Lyng J, Christensen J: A double-blind study of the value of treatment with a single-dose tinidazole to partners of females with trichomoniasis, *Acta Obstet Gynecol Scand* 60:199, 1981.

McLennon MT, Smith JM, McClennon CE: Diagnosis of vaginal mycosis, trichomoniasis. Reliability of cytologic smear, wet smear and culture, *Obstet Gynecol* 40:231, 1972.

McNellis D, McLeod M, Lawson J, Pasquale SA: Treatment of vulvovaginal candidiasis in pregnancy: a comparative study, *Obstet Gynecol* 50:674, 1977.

Miles MR, Olsen L, Rogers A: Recurrent vaginal candidiasis: importance of an intestinal reservoir, *JAMA* 238:1836, 1977.

Milne JD, Warnock DW: Effect of simultaneous oral and vaginal treatment on the rate of cure and relapse in vaginal candidosis, *Br J Vener Dis* 55:362, 1979.

Morales WJ, Shorr S, Albritton J: Effects of metronidazole in patients with preterm birth in preceding pregnancy and bacterial vaginosis: a placebo-controlled, double-blind study, *Am J Obstet Gynecol* 171:345, 1994.

Muller M, Lossick JG, Gorrell TE: In vitro susceptibility of *Trichomonas vaginalis* to metronidazole and treatment outcome in vaginal trichomoniasis, *Sex Transm Dis* 15:17, 1988.

Nugent RP, Krohn MA, Hillier SL: Reliability of diagnosing bacterial vaginosis is improved by a standardized method of Gram stain interpretation, *J Clin Microbiol* 29:297, 1991.

Nyirjesy P, Seeney SM, Terry-Grody MH, Jordan CJ: Chronic fungal vaginitis: the value of culture, *Am J Obstet Gynecol* 173:820, 1995.

Nystatin Multicenter Study Group: Therapy of candidal vaginitis: the effect of eliminating intestinal *Candida*, *Am J Obstet Gynecol* 155:651, 1986.

Odds FC: Candida *and candidosis*, Baltimore, 1979, University Park Press.

Pereyra AJ, Lansing JD: Urogenital trichomoniasis: treatment with metronidazole in 2002 incarcerated women, *Obstet Gynecol* 24:499, 1964.

Peterson WF, Stauch JE, Ryder CO: Metronidazole in pregnancy, *Am J Obstet Gynecol* 94:343, 1966.

Piot P, Van Dyck E, Godts P, VanderHeyden J: A placebo-controlled, double-blind comparison of tinidazole and triple sulfonamide cream for the treatment of nonspecific vaginitis, *Am J Obstet Gynecol* 147:85, 1983.

Proost JM, Maes-Dockx RM, Nelis MD, Cutsem JM: Miconazole treatment of mycotic vulvovaginitis, *Am J Obstet Gynecol* 112:688, 1972.

Roe JFC: A critical appraisal of the toxicology of metronidazole. In Phillips I, Collier J, editors: *Metronidazole*, London, 1979, Academic Press.

Sobel JD: Recurrent vulvovaginal candidiasis: a prospective study of the efficacy of maintenance ketoconazole therapy, *N Engl J Med* 315:1455, 1986.

Sobel JD, Brooker D, Stein GE, et al: Single oral dose fluconazole compared with conventional clotrimazole topical therapy of *Candida vaginitis*, *Am J Obstet Gynecol* 172:1263, 1995.

Soper DE, Bump RC, Hurt WG: Bacterial vaginosis and trichomoniasis vaginitis are risk factors for cuff cellulitis after abdominal hysterectomy, *Am J Obstet Gynecol* 163:1016, 1990.

Spiegel CA, Amsel R, Eschenbach DA, et al: Anaerobic bacteria in nonspecific vaginitis, *N Engl J Med* 303:601, 1980.

Swedberg J, Steiner JF, Deiss F, et al: Comparison of single dose versus one week course of metronidazole on symptomatic bacterial vaginosis, *JAMA* 254:1046, 1985.

Thin RN, Leighton M, Dixon MJ: How often is genital yeast infection sexually transmitted? *Br Med J* 2:93, 1977.

Van Slyke KK, Michel VP, Rein MF: Treatment of vulvovaginal candidiasis with boric acid powder, *Am J Obstet Gynecol* 141:145, 1981.

Vejtorp M, Bollerup AC, Vejtorp L, et al: Bacterial vaginosis: a double-blinded randomized trial of the effect of treatment of sexual partners, *Br J Obstet Gynaecol* 95:920, 1988.

Vontver LA, Eschenbach DA: The role of Gardnerella vaginalis in nonspecific vaginitis, *Clin Obstet Gynecol* 24:439, 1981.

Watts DW, Krohn M, Hillier SL, Eschenbach DA: Bacterial vaginosis as a risk factor for postcesarean endometritis, *Obstet Gynecol* 75:52, 1990.

Witkin SS: Inhibition of *Candida*-induced lymphocyte proliferation by antibody to *Candida albicans*, *Obstet Gynecol* 68:696, 1986.

Wølner-Hanssen P, Krieger JN, Stevens CE, et al: Clinical manifestations of vaginal trichomoniasis, *JAMA* 261:571, 1989.

CHAPTER 12

Acute Pelvic Inflammatory Disease

PÅL WØLNER-HANSSEN

DEFINITION

The Centers for Disease Control and Prevention (CDC) has described pelvic inflammatory disease (PID) as a spectrum of inflammatory disorders of the upper genital tract among women. Pelvic inflammatory disease includes any combination of endometritis, salpingitis, tuboovarian abscess, and pelvic peritonitis. The anatomic limits of the infection in a single case are difficult to determine without invasive procedures. When using endometrial biopsy and laparoscopy, one can achieve a more specific diagnosis. There is no generally accepted histopathologic definition for endometritis, but the presence of a certain number of plasma cells in endometrial biopsies is usually used as one criterion for endometritis. Characteristic alterations of the fallopian tubes define acute salpingitis; these include erythema, edema, purulent exudate, and fresh adhesions. In the following, I will use *PID* as a general term for pelvic infection. For cases in which laparoscopy or endometrial biopsy has been performed, I will use the term *salpingitis* or *endometritis*.

EPIDEMIOLOGY

Between 1979 and 1988, an annual mean of 420,000 initial office visits for PID were estimated from data reported to the National Disease and Therapeutic Index (NDTI). Over this period the rate of office visits remained unchanged. The annual mean number of hospitalizations for acute PID was 167,800 (National Hospital Discharge Survey). According to one estimate, 10% to 15% of U.S. women will have at least one episode of PID in their reproductive life. The rate of hospitalization for PID decreased 36% from 1983 to 1988. This trend may reflect milder forms of PID in recent years, an actual decrease in the incidence of PID, or both.

These data are uncertain for several reasons. Few reported cases of PID have been verified by laparoscopy (12%), even when 42% of hospitalized cases of acute PID underwent abdominal surgery; the NDTI does not survey visits to emergency rooms and sexually transmitted disease (STD) clinics. Socioeconomic factors might have caused a drift of certain patient groups from private physicians' offices to emergency rooms. Therefore the NTDI survey may have missed a considerable portion of PID cases. The incidence trends for PID during the past years are unclear.

ETIOLOGY

There is general agreement that pathogens recovered directly from the fallopian tubes are etiologic agents in acute salpingitis. In routine clinical evaluation, few U.S. physicians sample the tubes because they are not easily accessible. Clinicians who do sample the fallopian tubes with a laparoscope often achieve negative cultures in obvious acute salpingitis. The reason for this is speculative. Tubal specimens may contain low numbers of organisms, or immune defenses may have damaged the microorganisms to the point where they are unable to grow in culture media. For these reasons, most authors rely on culture specimens from the cervix, endometrium, cul-de-sac, urethra, or rectum. The presumption is that pathogenic organisms isolated at these sites are identical to the ones infecting the tubes. This may be true for *Chlamydia trachomatis* and *Neisseria gonorrhoeae*, but not for anaerobic or facultative microorganisms. Anaerobic or aerobic microorganisms belong to the normal vaginal and cervical flora. Isolation of these organisms from the cervix or endometrium is therefore not helpful in defining the etiology of PID.

Most U.S. studies have shown a predominant role of *N. gonorrhoeae* as an etiologic agent in acute PID. In Europe, *C. trachomatis* is more common in PID than *N. gonorrhoeae*. In a recent study from Seattle, we isolated *N. gonorrhoeae* from any genital site in 51% and *C. trachomatis* in 40% of women with confirmed acute PID. We recovered both organisms from 21% of the women. Nine out of ten women with salpingitis and endometritis had infection with either microorganism in the genital tract. In a study from

New York, 45% of women with acute PID had *C. trachomatis*, and 36% had *N. gonorrhoeae* in the genital tract. Some women with acute PID have growth of anaerobic or facultative microorganisms with or without *C. trachomatis* or *N. gonorrhoeae* in the tubes. The most important non-STD organisms implicated in acute PID are *Escherichia coli* and different bacteroides and peptococci species. *Mycoplasma hominis* often colonizes the vagina, but whether *M. hominis* can cause PID is uncertain. It is unusual to isolate this organism from the fallopian tubes.

Thus different organisms can cause acute PID. Some authors have therefore suggested that PID is a polymicrobial disease. In a single case, however, it is unusual to isolate more than one bacterial strain from the tubes. At the time of diagnosis, the particular strains infecting the tubes are unknown in most cases. Treatment must therefore include an antibiotic regimen with a broad spectrum.

RISK FACTORS AND RISK MARKERS

Risk factors and risk markers are important for at least two reasons. First, knowledge of risk factors may help the clinician in his or her diagnostic considerations. Second, elimination of risk factors might prevent PID. For a woman to develop PID, at least two events must occur. First, she must be infected with the microorganisms causing PID. Second, the microorganisms must spread to the fallopian tubes and infect them. These two events correlate to different risk factors.

Risk factors for the acquisition of *N. gonorrhoeae* and *C. trachomatis* are those associated with sexual activity. Examples of known risk factors for STDs are low socioeconomic status, age at first intercourse, number of partners, and use of no birth control methods. A possible relationship between STDs and ''partner-choosing'' behavior needs more study. Women choosing high-risk partners probably will be more exposed to STDs than will those being critical with their choice of partner.

The relationship between *C. trachomatis* infection and oral contraceptive use deserves special comment. Several studies have shown that oral contraceptive users are more often culture positive to *C. trachomatis* than nonusers are. However, it is not clear whether oral contraceptive users more often get *C. trachomatis* or whether *C. trachomatis* is easier to isolate from infected oral contraceptive users. Cervical ectopy is a condition in which columnar endocervical mucosa cover a part of the face of the cervix. *C. trachomatis* prefers columnar cells. Oral contraceptive users are more likely than nonusers to have cervical ectopy. Thus oral contraceptive users may be more susceptible to chlamydial infection because of the exposed columnar cells on the cervix. However, in cervical ectopy, higher numbers of chlamydial elementary bodies might be reproduced, thus making an infection easier to identify.

Among already-infected women, risk factors for developing PID are those related to spread of the microorganisms to the upper genital tract. The intrauterine device (IUD) is thought to promote spread of microorganisms to the upper genital tract. A recent review of the World Health Organization's IUD clinical trial data revealed that among 22,908 IUD insertions and 51,399 woman-years of follow-up, the risk of PID was increased by a factor of 6 during the first 20 days after insertion, but thereafter PID was an infrequent event (it is therefore recommended that IUDs be left in place up to their maximum lifespan). Use of IUDs is associated with PID unrelated to sexually transmitted infection, suggesting that IUD insertion helps introduce otherwise harmless endogenous microorganisms from the lower to the upper genital tract.

Recently, we found an association between vaginal douching and acute PID. This association increased with the frequency of douching. Women who douched three or more times per month had a risk of PID 3.6 times higher than did those who douched less than once per month. A later, population-based study confirmed these findings. Women who douched at least once a week had an estimated risk of PID equal to 3.9 compared with those who douched less often. Vaginal douching is a habit of many low-income, less-educated U.S. women. Few other risk factors for PID are changeable. Physicians should therefore discourage women from regular douching.

At the same time as oral contraceptive use increases the risk of positive *C. trachomatis* culture, it reduces the risk of PID. Among women with acute salpingitis, those using oral contraceptives had milder tubal disease than did those using no birth control method or an IUD. The possible protective effect of oral contraceptive use is limited to women infected with *C. trachomatis* and is stronger with longer use of oral contraceptives. Nevertheless, to prescribe oral contraceptives as protection against PID is unwarranted. Oral contraceptives provide no protection against gonococcal PID and may promote chlamydial infection.

SIGNS AND SYMPTOMS

Lower abdominal pain is a principal but not mandatory symptom of acute PID. The intensity of pain is variable. Some women have excruciating pain. For example, when the infection has spread to the liver capsule (perihepatitis, or Fitz-Hugh–Curtis syndrome), severe right-upper abdominal pain may occur. Some patients with PID have no pain at all. In several studies of infertile women, investigators asked women with adnexal scarring whether they have had PID in the past. Less than half of the women answered yes to this question. The term *silent PID* was coined for this apparently asymptomatic PID. In a recent study, infertile women were asked not only if they had had PID, but if they had sought medical advice for *any* abdominal pain in the past. Not more than 1 in 10 of those with adnexal or perihepatic scarring had no history of abdominal pain. Thus *silent* PID seems to be overstated, and physicians should follow the CDC recommendations of maintaining a low threshold of diagnosis for PID.

Abdominal pain associated with PID is often continuous, sometimes with crampy exacerbations. The pain usually is bilateral. In women with only right-sided pain, the differential diagnosis to appendicitis is difficult. Pain caused by pelvic infection usually lasts for less than 3 weeks. Women with acute PID may have had pain for a longer period, but one should seriously consider other conditions for women with chronic abdominal pain.

Patients with acute PID may report several genital and extragenital symptoms (Table 12-1). Nausea and vomiting are symptoms that should disqualify the patient from outpatient therapy. Irritation of the peritoneum covering the gut and the bladder probably causes diarrhea, dysuria, and frequency in some women with PID. Menorrhagia (heavy or long menstrual bleeding) is a sign of endometritis. A recent onset of increased menstrual bleeding in a young, sexually active woman therefore supports a presumptive diagnosis of upper genital tract infection. Increased or malodorous discharge may reflect cervicitis or vaginitis unrelated to PID.

On pelvic examination, adnexal tenderness, uterine tenderness, and cervical motion tenderness are nonspecific but typical signs of acute PID. Adnexal tenderness is usually bilateral but may be unilateral. Adnexal masses can be caused by tuboovarian abscesses, ovarian tumors, or cysts. It is difficult to decide whether a palpable mass is an abscess. For this reason, women with PID and palpable masses need inpatient treatment under the presumption that they have tuboovarian abscesses.

Clinicians commonly expect fever in women with acute PID. This is not surprising because fever has been one of the inclusion criteria in several published studies. However, in studies with less strict criteria for enrollment but with strict criteria for the final diagnosis of pelvic infection, fever is an uncommon sign of PID. Only 20% of women with chlamydial salpingitis had

TABLE 12-1. Symptoms and signs in women with acute chlamydial salpingitis

Sign or symptom	Frequency (%)
Abnormal bleeding	50
Increased discharge	68
Dysuria	21
Nausea, vomiting	31
Diarrhea	5
Fever	24
Erythrocyte sedimentation rate > 15 mm/hr	76
White blood cell count > 10^{10}/L	44

Adapted from Wølner-Hanssen P, Mårdh PA, Svensson L, et al: *Obstet Gynecol* 61:299, 1983.

fever in one study. Of women infected with *C. trachomatis* and with clinical evidence of acute PID but without confirmation of acute salpingitis, 21% had fever. Among women with acute salpingitis of any etiology, only one third had a temperature above 38°C.

Purulent cervical discharge is another sign of acute PID among women with abdominal pain. Grossly purulent cervical mucus or the presence of more than 10 polymorphonuclear leukocytes per 1200× field of Gram-stained cervical mucus indicates cervicitis. However, no good data are available that relate cervical mucopus to acute PID. Clear cervical mucus does not rule out PID in a woman otherwise suspected of having the disease.

The pelvic infection may spread to the liver capsule and cause perihepatitis (Fitz-Hugh–Curtis syndrome). Of PID cases, 4% to 12% also have perihepatitis. Women with perihepatitis experience a sudden onset of severe right-upper abdominal pain. The pain gets worse with deep breathing, coughing, laughing, or movement of the torso. The onset of upper abdominal pain often coincides with the lower abdominal pain but may occur up to 14 days after the lower abdominal pain. Traditionally, investigators believed that perihepatitis was a complication of gonococcal PID. However, in cases of PID with perihepatitis that were reported during the last decade, *C. trachomatis* was equally important. In fact, perihepatitis among women with acute salpingitis is significantly associated with serum antibodies to the 60-kD chlamydial heat shock protein (Money and others, unpublished data). On laparoscopy, fibrinous, approximated adhesions between the anterior liver surface and the adjacent abdominal wall plus erythema of the surrounding peritoneum indicate acute perihepatitis. In older cases of perihepatitis, there are violin string and filmy adhesions between the liver and the anterior abdominal wall or diaphragm.

SEQUELAE

The two most significant sequelae after acute salpingitis are infertility and tubal pregnancy. The reasons for infertility after acute salpingitis are persistent periadnexal adhesions and distal tubal occlusion preventing ovum pickup. During tubal infection, ciliated cells of the tubal mucosa may get lost or damaged. After the infection, ciliated cells do not recover. As a result, the tubes cannot transport a fertilized ovum fast enough to reach the uterine cavity at the time of scheduled implantation. This may lead to infertility in some cases and tubal pregnancy in other cases. A long-term follow-up study identified the risks of infertility and ectopic pregnancy caused by tubal damage. Briefly, after a single episode of acute salpingitis, 8% remained infertile. The infertility risk increased sharply with each new episode of salpingitis. After three or more episodes of salpingitis, 40% were infertile. The severity of tubal inflammation also correlated with the infertility risk. After a single episode of mild salpingitis, only 0.6% were infertile, whereas after a single episode of tuboovarian abscesses 21% were infertile. The risk of ectopic pregnancy after acute salpingitis is between 7 and 10 times that in women who never have had salpingitis. After one episode of acute salpingitis, about 9% of pregnancies will be ectopic. After two or more episodes, 15% of pregnancies will be ectopic. Thus in a pregnant woman with a history of repeated episodes of acute salpingitis, one should be highly suspicious of ectopic pregnancy. Moreover, one must counsel a patient with acute salpingitis about how to reduce the chance of recurrences.

CLINICAL APPROACH

Different nonspecific signs and symptoms are often the basis of a clinical diagnosis of PID. Not surprisingly, the clinical diagnosis is often erroneous. Clinicians confuse acute PID with other conditions, including ectopic pregnancy, appendicitis, ovarian cysts, and urinary tract infections. Many women thought to have acute PID have no laparoscopic evidence of disease. Some of these women may have endosalpingitis, endometritis, or just cervicitis. A classic Swedish study showed that only two thirds of women suspected of having acute salpingitis had the disease. We confirmed these figures in a later Seattle study. Thus one important attitude in the office management of PID is to keep in mind that the diagnosis might be wrong.

A thorough history is important. Inquire in detail about location, duration, character, and pattern of abdominal pain. For example, unilateral right-sided pain may suggest appendicitis, ruptured ovarian cyst, twisted adnexa, or ectopic pregnancy. Instant onset of unilateral pain during intercourse is typical for a ruptured ovarian cyst; a gradual onset of pain over several hours with pain moving from the epigastric area to the right lower quadrant may suggest appendicitis. Gradually increasing pain in the right and left lower abdominal quadrants is more typical for PID. One should ask patients for risk factors, including previous PID, symptomatic or new sexual partner, or recently introduced IUD. To differentiate between infection and pregnancy, a thorough bleeding history may be helpful.

On physical examination, external abdominal palpation will help localize the disease process and detect peritonitis. During a bimanual pelvic examination one can define adnexal and cervical motion tenderness and search for adnexal masses. Palpable adnexal masses may reflect pelvic abscesses or "innocent" ovarian cysts. Inspection of the cervix helps identify cervicitis. A purulent cervical discharge suggests cervicitis. A combination of lower abdominal pain, adnexal tenderness, and purulent cervical discharge strongly suggests acute PID. A lack of cervical discharge does not rule out PID. Right upper abdominal direct and rebound tenderness suggests perihepatitis. One should measure the oral temperature. Fever is a reason to hospitalize a woman with acute abdominal pain.

An important initial management decision when caring for a woman with acute PID is to determine if she needs inpatient therapy. Inpatient treatment probably has several advantages over outpatient treatment: better compliance with therapy, better monitoring of the disease process, sexual abstinence, and better opportunity for the clinician to give advice for future disease prevention. No investigators have randomized patients between inpatient and outpatient therapy to study whether the aforementioned beliefs are true or not. It is, moreover, not known whether the infertility prognosis is better after inpatient therapy. Some clinicians would like to admit every woman with possible acute PID. In the United States inpatient therapy for every case of PID is unrealistic. The CDC has therefore put together recommendations for when to select inpatient therapy. One should admit patients with possible PID if the diagnosis is uncertain. One should admit patients who might have appendicitis or ectopic pregnancy, those who have a pelvic mass (possible abscess) or right upper abdominal pain, and women who might not tolerate ambulatory therapy (those with nausea and vomiting, fever, peritonitis, severe abdominal pain). If a patient does not respond to ambulatory therapy (no improvement after 48 hours of follow-up), it is better to admit her than continue outpatient therapy. Patients who do not seem reliable should also be admitted (Table 12-2).

Women with an IUD in situ should have the device removed. Some authors have recommended removal of the IUD at a 48-hour follow-up visit; others recommend immediate removal. The former hope to reduce the chance of flushing endometrial bacteria into the system while removing the IUD. This idea might be a good one. However, patients with acute PID are often not reliable and may not return for follow-up visits. Therefore, this author recommends immediate removal of the IUD.

TABLE 12-2. Situations in which hospitalization of patients with acute pelvic inflammatory disease is indicated

1. The diagnosis is uncertain
2. Surgical emergencies such as appendicitis and ectopic pregnancy cannot be excluded
3. Pelvic abscess is suspected
4. The patient is pregnant
5. The patient has human immunodeficiency virus infection
6. The patient is an adolescent
7. Severe illness precludes outpatient management
8. The patient is unable to follow or tolerate an outpatient regimen
9. The patient has failed to respond to outpatient therapy
10. Clinical follow-up within 72 hours of starting antibiotic therapy cannot be arranged

Adapted from Centers for Disease Control: *MMWR* 42:78, 1993.

Nevertheless, one should schedule a 2-day follow-up visit for all ambulatory PID patients. There are at least three reasons for scheduling this follow-up visit: to reevaluate the diagnosis, to find out whether the patient tolerates and adequately responds to ambulatory therapy, and to discuss her progress in convincing her partner to get examined. Also, schedule a further visit after completion of therapy to repeat cultures and to make sure that the patient is improving. If the patient still has significant pain, one should consider laparoscopy. I do not recommend further antibiotic therapy for abdominal pain after a complete course of adequate antibiotics unless laparoscopy has shown ongoing infection. It is often forgotten that we give antibiotics to kill bacteria, not to relieve pain. After adequate antibiotic therapy, one has probably eradicated any pathogenic bacteria in the upper genital tract.

LABORATORY TESTS

The most important laboratory test is a rapid and sensitive pregnancy test. This test should be performed liberally for young women with acute abdominal pain to differentiate between pregnancy-related and pregnancy-nonrelated conditions.

Another useful test in the evaluation of women with PID is serum C-reactive protein (CRP). Elevated values suggest inflammation of some sort. Erythrocyte sedimentation rate (ESR) and white blood cell count (WBC) are insensitive and nonspecific tests for PID. For example, in one study 36% of women with acute salpingitis had a normal ESR, and 31% of those without confirmed salpingitis had an elevated ESR. Of women with acute chlamydial salpingitis, 70% had normal WBC compared with 68% of those who did not have salpingitis. In cases of acute PID, there is no correlation of ESR, CRP, or WBC with the degree of inflammation and with the enlargement of the tubes (Eschenbach and others, unpublished data) (Table 12-3).

Broad-spectrum antibiotic treatment has to start before culture results are available. Therefore the main advantages of microbiologic workup are to confirm the suspected diagnosis, to add weight to the recommendation

TABLE 12-3. Tests recommended for women with suspected pelvic inflammatory disease

Pregnancy test
Oral temperature
Microscopy of Gram-stained cervical mucus
C-reactive protein
Cervical culture for *N. gonorrhoeae*
Cervical culture, antigen detection test, or polymerase chain reaction for *C. tra-chomatis*

of partner treatment, and to educate the patient about her disease. Minimal microbiologic workup of cases of suspected PID includes cervical specimens for detection of *N. gonorrhoeae* and *C. trachomatis*. One can increase the microbiologic yield by swabbing the urethra in addition to the cervix. To reduce costs, one may put the urethral and cervical swabs in the same transport medium. Cervical or vaginal cultures for anaerobic or facultative organisms or for *M. hominis* are of little value. These microorganisms are present in the lower genital tract of many healthy women, and the culture results do not reflect upper genital tract flora. Some investigators aspirate endometrial material for culture of facultative and anaerobic microorganisms in patients with suspected PID. To get endometrial specimens, the sampling device must be introduced through the cervix. This and other authors believe that cervical contamination is possible even with triple-lumen sampling devices. Only via the laparoscope can we get reliable culture specimens from the upper genital tract.

It is easy to aspirate peritoneal fluid in the physician's office by culdocentesis. Most patients with acute PID have WBCs in the peritoneal fluid. However, like most other signs associated with PID, WBCs in the peritoneal fluid are not specific for PID. Women with extragenital infections (e.g., appendicitis) may also have WBCs in the peritoneal fluid. Culdocentesis can still be a useful procedure in women with acute abdominal pain. Purulent fluid suggests PID or appendicitis; bloody, nonclotting fluid points to ectopic pregnancy or a ruptured luteal cyst.

By transvaginal ultrasound examination, thickened fluid-filled tubes, polycystic-like ovaries, and free pelvic fluid are criteria associated with plasma cell endometritis among women with lower abdominal pain. In obese women and in those with rigid abdomens because of peritonitis, ultrasound examination is useful to detect tuboovarian abscesses. Ultrasound examination is furthermore useful for following the regression of abscesses during treatment.

THERAPY

Treatment of PID must not be delayed. A prospective study based on 443 cases of acute salpingitis verified by laparoscopy showed that women who delayed seeking care for PID were three times more likely to experience infertility or ectopic pregnancy than women who sought care promptly. An additional "doctor's delay" might not improve on the fertility of these patients. Antibiotic therapy is the mainstay of PID treatment. A large number of studies of antibiotic therapy for PID are available. However, most studies are not comparable because investigators have used different criteria for enrollment and outcome. Many studies include unconfirmed cases of PID. Most studies have followed the patients until clinical cure only and therefore provide no information about infertility. The CDC together with experts from around the nation has come up with treatment recommendations for acute PID. The recommendations take available literature and knowledge of the most common microbial agents causing PID into account. The antibiotic combinations recommended for ambulatory therapy aim at eradicating *C. trachomatis*, *N. goriorrhoeae*, gram-negative facultative bacteria, anaerobes, and streptococci.

No single therapeutic regimen has been established for women with PID. Doxycycline and the oxychinolone ofloxacin are effective drugs against *C. trachomatis*. Other drugs active against *C. trachomatis* are erythromycin, azitromycin, and clindamycin. Clindamycin might be an excellent alternative to doxycycline because this drug is active against anaerobic microorganisms in addition to *M. hominis* and *C. trachomatis*.

Doxycycline eradicates most gonococci, but an increasing number of gonococcal strains are resistant to tetracyclines. One should therefore not rely on doxycycline alone in the treatment of PID. To lessen the chance of undertreating gonococci, one should add a β-lactam antibiotic. Ampicillin and amoxicillin are no longer recommended for U.S. patients with acute PID because of the high percentage of β-lactamase–producing gonococci. Therefore the CDC recommends β-lactamase–resistant antibiotics, including cefoxitin, ceftriaxone, ceftizoxime, and cefotaxime, in combination with doxycycline for outpatient treatment of PID. This regimen does not offer good coverage for enterococci, but these organisms rarely cause PID (Table 12-4). Ofloxacin is active against *C. trachomatis*, *N. gonorrhoeae*, and gram-negative facultative organisms. A combination of ofloxacin and clindamycin or metronidazole is an alternative outpatient treatment regimen for PID.

Compliance with the prescribed oral antibiotic treatment might be a problem for many women with acute PID. According to one telephone survey of women discharged from a municipal emergency department with a diagnosis of PID and a 10-day prescription for doxycycline, only 31%

TABLE 12-4. Recommended regimens for ambulatory treatment of acute pelvic inflammatory disease

---

Cefoxitin (2.0 g intramuscularly) plus probenencid, 1 g orally in a single dose concurrently, or
Certriaxone (250 mg intramuscularly)
Plus
Doxycycline 100 mg orally two times a day for 14 days
Or
Ofloxacin 400 mg orally two times a day for 14 days
Plus
Clindamycin 450 mg orally four times a day, or
Metronidazole 500 mg orally two times a day for 14 days

Adapted from Centers for Disease Control: *MMWR* 42:79, 1993.

reported complete compliance, and 28% did not fill their prescriptions at all. This should be considered in the choice of antibiotic regimen and in cases of failed treatment. In fact, the CDC recommends inpatient treatment for women with PID who are probably not going to be compliant.

Treatment of sex partners is imperative to reduce the risk of recurrent disease. One should examine, culture, and treat all men with whom the patient has had intercourse during the previous 30 days. Male partners should be cultured for *C. trachomatis* and *N. gonorrhoeae* from the urethra. They should be treated even when no symptoms and signs of urethritis are present. The partner may have an infection with *C. trachomatis* or *N. gonorrhoeae* without having symptoms or even signs of the infection. Recommended treatment of partners is doxycycline 100 mg orally for 7 days or azithromycin 1 g orally in a single dose in combination with ofloxacin 400 mg, cefixime 400 mg, or ciprofloxacin 500 mg orally in a single dose or an injection with ceftriaxone (125 mg intramuscularly).

BIBLIOGRAPHY

Brookoff D: Compliance with doxycycline therapy for outpatient treatment of pelvic inflammatory disease, *South Med J* 87:1088, 1994.

Brunham RC, Paavonen J, Stevens C, et al: Mucopurulent cervicitis: the ignored counterpart in women of urethritis in men, *N Engl J Med* 311:1, 1984.

Cacciatore B, Leminen A, Ingman-Friberg S, et al: Transvaginal sonographic findings in ambulatory patients with suspected pelvic inflammatory disease, *Obstet Gynecol* 80:912, 1992.

Centers for Disease Control: 1993 sexually transmitted diseases treatment guidelines, *MMWR* 42:1, 1993.

Critchlow CW, Wølner-Hanssen P, Eschenbach DA: Determinants of cervical ectopy and cervicitis: age, oral contraception, specific cervical infection, smoking, and douching, *Am J Obstet Gynecol* 173:534, 1995.

Eschenbach DA, Buchanan RM, Pollock HM, et al: Polymicrobial etiology of acute pelvic inflammatory disease, *N Engl J Med* 293:166, 1975.

Eschenbach DA, Wølner-Hanssen P: Fitz-Hugh–Curtis syndrome. In Holmes KK, Mårdh PA, Sparling PF, et al, editors: *Sexually transmitted diseases*, ed 2, New York, 1989, McGraw-Hill.

Farley TM, Rosenberg MJ, Rowe PJ, et al: Intrauterine devices and pelvic inflammatory disease: an international perspective, *Lancet* 339:785, 1992.

Hillis SD, Joesoef R, Marschbanks PA, et al: Delayed care of pelvic inflammatory disease as a risk factor for impaired fertility, *Am J Obstet Gynecol* 168:1503, 1993.

Jacobson L, Weström L: Objectivized diagnosis of pelvic inflammatory disease, *Am J Obstet Gynecol* 105:1088, 1969.

Joesoef MR, Weström L, Reynolds G, et al: Recurrent ectopic pregnancy: the role of salpingitis, *Am J Obstet Gynecol* 165:46, 1991.

Jossens MO, Schachter J, Sweet RL: Risk factors associated with pelvic inflammatory disease of differing microbial etiologies, *Obstet Gynecol* 83:989, 1994.

Landers DV, Wølner-Hanssen P, Paavonen J, et al: Combination antimicrobial therapy in the treatment of acute pelvic inflammatory disease, *Obstet Gynecol* 164:849, 1991.

Moore DE, Spadoni LR, Foy HM, et al: Increased frequency of serum antibodies to *Chlamydia trachomatis* in infertility due to distal tubal disease, *Lancet* 2:574, 1982.

Rolfs RT, Galaid EI, Zaidi AA: Pelvic inflammatory disease: trends in hospitalizations and office visits, 1979 through 1988, *Am J Obstet Gynecol* 166:983, 1992.

Scholes D, Daling JR, Stergachis A, et al: Vaginal douching as a risk factor for acute pelvic inflammatory disease, *Obstet Gynecol* 81:601, 1993.

Wasserheit JD, Bell TA, Kiviat NB, et al: Microbial causes of proven pelvic inflammatory disease and efficacy of clindamycin and tobramycin, *Ann Intern Med* 104:187, 1986.

Weström L, Joesoef R, Reynolds G, et al: Pelvic inflammatory disease and fertility. A cohort study of 1844 women with laparoscopically verified disease and 657 control women with normal laparoscopic results, *Sex Transm Dis* 19: 185, 1992.

Wølner-Hanssen P: Silent pelvic inflammatory disease: is it overstated? *Obstet Gynecol* 1995, in press.

Wølner-Hanssen P, Eschenbach DA, Paavonen J, et al: Association between vaginal douching and pelvic inflammatory disease, *JAMA* 263:1936, 1990.

Wølner-Hanssen P, Eschenbach DA, Paavonen J, et al: Decreased risk of chlamydial pelvic inflammatory disease associated with oral contraceptive use, *JAMA* 263:54, 1990.

Wølner-Hanssen P, Mårdh PA, Svensson L, et al: Laparoscopy in women with chlamydial infection and pelvic pain: a comparison of patients with and without salpingitis, *Obstet Gynecol* 61:299, 1983.

CHAPTER 13

Management of the Abnormal or Atypical Papanicolaou Smear

HISHAM K. TAMIMI

Papanicolaou and Traut published their historic monograph in 1943 on cervicovaginal cytology. In their classic description of exfoliative cervical cytology, they noted that vaginal smears "contained atypical cells . . . so closely related to malignant cells." They suggested that these atypical cell changes might be incipient malignancy. Since 1943 cervicovaginal cytology

356

has played a major role in the screening for early detection of cervical cancer and its precursors.

In 1925 Hans Hensselman designed and coined the name of his instrument, the colposcope. His purpose was to detect the earliest possible stage of invasive cancer of the cervix. With experience it became clear that the procedure, colposcopy, had the potential of detecting certain epithelial changes that are consistent with pathologic findings of preinvasive cervical neoplasia. The widespread use of colposcopy in the United States was relatively recent, particularly in conjunction with cervicovaginal cytology. The current management and early detection of cervical neoplasia is the product of cytology and colposcopy. One modality complements the other, and current knowledge dictates the use of both modalities.

The mortality rate of cervical cancer has decreased in communities where Papanicolaou smear screening programs have been established. In communities where screening programs have not taken place, there has been an increase in mortality from cervical carcinoma. The reduction in the incidence of cervical cancer was also associated with the presence of screening programs. Furthermore, the ratio of stage I to stages II, III, and IV has increased significantly after the screening program. Several controversies are still unresolved as to the frequency of testing of Papanicolaou smears, the characterization of factors of high risk, more accurate methods of cytology reporting, and the role of education of adolescent women in prevention, early detection, and treatment of sexually transmitted diseases. Human papillomavirus (HPV) emerged as the most common cause of an atypical Papanicolaou smear. Gynecologists and cytopathologists are facing a relatively new disease entity in HPV infection because it might be strongly associated with malignancy in millions of women in the United States.

EPIDEMIOLOGIC STUDIES

The incidence of cervical cancer is significantly higher in married and widowed women than in those who have never been married and in nuns. Cervical cancer is also related to pregnancy at an early age and to early marriage (or both). Cervical cancer is associated with early coitus, and the age of the first intercourse has the same implications. Several authors have demonstrated the importance of multiple sexual partners as a risk factor for cervical cancer. The male factor and its important role in cervical cancer is clear yct complex in nature. Many decades ago, smegma was considered a carcinogenic agent in patients with penile cancer, and its low incidence was associated with circumcised men. Smegma was also considered a carcinogenic agent related to women with cervical cancer. Therefore sexual activity is considered the main association that explains the increased incidence of cervical cancer. Of the sexually transmitted diseases, herpes simplex virus type 2 (HSV-2) and HPV are possibly related to the cause of cervical cancer. HSV-2 in the last three decades was the subject of extensive epidemiologic and biologic studies. Retrospective serologic studies indicated that women with cervical cancer had higher serum levels of HSV-2 antibodies as compared with the control group. However, prospective study indicated that the frequency of elevated HSV-2 antibody levels in patients with cervical cancer were similar to matched controls. Such epidemiologic studies failed to confirm a positive role in the carcinogenicity of *human* cervical cancer for HSV-2.

In the late 1980s HPV infection emerged as the agent investigated with a potential role in carcinogenesis in cervical cancer. Recent advances in pathologic studies, deoxyribonucleic acid (DNA) hybridization, and Southern blot techniques identified several HPV types and linked them to cervical dysplasia and cervical cancer. More than 60 types of HPV were identified, and of these 13 to 14 types were recognized in the anogenital tract. Investigators are in the process of correlating the various HPV types and the gross morphologic and clinical appearances. Human papillomavirus type 11 is known to be associated with the condylomatous cauliflower-like lesions known to be benign and distributed over the lower portion of the vagina, vulva, perineum, and anogenital epithelia. Human papillomavirus type 16 is associated with a high degree of dysplasia or atypia of squamous epithelia of the lower genital tract. Human papillomavirus type 18 is associated with invasive cervical cancer, including the adenocarcinoma variety, and is thought to be responsible for the "aggressive" cervical cancer seen in young women and seen in patients with cervical adenocarcinoma. For more details of this subject the reader is referred to the chapter on vulvar disease in this book. The use of serotyping of HPV is not currently available.

PAPANICOLAOU SMEAR

The Papanicolaou smear is an extremely specific test for detecting invasive cancer and cervical intraepithelial neoplasia class 3 (CIN 3) that has few false-positive results. The Papanicolaou smear is somewhat less specific for low-grade squamous intraepithelial lesion (SIL). The Papanicolaou smear is not a sensitive enough test to detect invasive cervical cancer, and the rates of false-negative smears are thought to be in the range of 8% to 50%. The use of the cytobrush is superior, with higher detection of CIN.

The controversy of how frequently women should undergo cervical cytologic screening is still unsettled. It is important to maintain perspective, avoid rigid recommendations, and allow flexible policies to be periodically reviewed to involve most women in the screening program. Statistical evidence might prove that repeated Papanicolaou smears every 2 years are safe while every 3 years carries risks, yet the annual interval would seem more adapted to current medical practice in the U.S. patient's acceptance and because many women are at risk.

Additional benefits to having Papanicolaou smears are that they are done as part of the annual general examination (blood pressure, diabetes, cholesterol level, breast cancer, ovarian cancer, etc.), which yields several advantages. Some oncologists advocate annual screening for ovarian cancer for every woman at a certain age, yet cervical cancer and its precursors are more frequent than ovarian cancer. Financial considerations and cost containment efforts should be directed toward prevention through education and identifying groups at risk at the earliest time and grade.

CERVICAL CYTOLOGY

The Papanicolaou smear is not intended to establish a diagnosis because a diagnosis should be accomplished by histopathologic findings; it is intended to identify patients with an extreme risk of invasive cervical cancer by detecting its precursors. Cervicovaginal cytology is therefore a screening tool, and like many other medical tests and procedures it has its own limitations. The factors that influence these limitations are false-negative, false-positive, and inconclusive results. The factors that determine reliable smears depend on proper cell sampling, technical preparation in obtaining an evenly spread specimen, timely fixation, and cytologic interpretation. Other factors are related to local (cervical and vaginal) factors. Bleeding, severe cervicitis, and vaginitis might partially or completely obscure important cytologic details. The epithelium of postmenopausal patients without exogenous estrogen replacement tends to be thin and atrophic and has scanty cellularity as is seen in patients after pelvic irradiation. It is controversial that the absence of endocervical cells is an indicator of the adequacy of a Papanicolaou smear, particularly in postmenopausal women.

The original Papanicolaou smear classification was numerical and extended from 1 through 5. Class 1 was reserved for benign and normal findings, and class 5 was defined as positive and the abnormal cells were consistent with invasive cancer (Table 13-1). The use of numerical classification led to several modifications of the original classes. Some of the modifications became too extensive and now carry little resemblance to the original Papanicolaou classification. Table 13-2 demonstrates the various classification systems during the past 45 years following the original classification system. Several laboratories adhered to the numerical classes, but others introduced additional ones that resulted in confusion. It became evident that clinicians and cytopathologists were dissatisfied with the numerical classification. The implications of class 3,

TABLE 13-1.   Cytologic classification of cervical cytology smears

Class	Papanicolaou definition	Modern definition
I	Benign	Normal
II	Atypical benign	Atypical cells below the level of cervical neoplasia
III	Suspicious	Abnormal cells consistent with dysplasia
IV	Probably positive	Abnormal cells consistent with carcinoma in situ
V	Positive	Abnormal cells consistent with invasive carcinoma

TABLE 13-2.   Various systems for classification of cervicovaginal cytology

Papanicolaou class	Dysplasia	CIN*	Bethesda system
Class I			
Normal smear	Negative	Negative	Within normal limits
Class II			
Atypical cells, no dysplasia	Reactive atypia		Regeneration, repair
	Koilocytosis or HPV*	Koilocytosis or HPV	Inflammation
	Mild dysplasia	CIN 1	Low-grade squamous intraepithelial lesion
Class III			
Abnormal cells consistent with dysplasia	Moderate dysplasia	CIN 2	
Class IV			
Abnormal cells consistent with CIS*	Severe dysplasia, CIS	CIN 2 CIN 3	High-grade squamous intraepithelial lesion
Class V			
Abnormal cells consistent with invasive or squamous cell origin	Squamous cell carcinoma	Squamous cell carcinoma	Squamous cell carcinoma

*CIN, Cervical intraepithelial neoplasia; CIS, carcinoma in situ; HPV, human papillomavirus.

for example, in one laboratory carried a totally different meaning to that of another laboratory. Hence there was a need for improvement in cytologic reporting practices to enhance understanding and communication between clinicians and cytopathologists. A narrative description of the cytologic findings was introduced by several laboratories. The National Institutes of Health (NIH) consensus report on cytology reporting was

TABLE 13-3. Summary of the 1988 Bethesda system for reporting abnormal squamous cervicovaginal cytology

Atypical squamous cells
Squamous intraepithelial lesions (HPV*)
Low-grade
HPV
Mild dysplasia/CIN* I
High-grade
Moderate dysplasia/CIN 2
Carcinoma in situ/CIN 3
Squamous cell carcinoma

CIN, Cervical intraepithelial neoplasia; *HPV*, human papillomavirus.

published with the main goal of improvement in reporting cervical and vaginal cytologic diagnoses (Tables 13-3 and 13-4). The conclusion was that the descriptive diagnosis as a narrative statement should facilitate communication and eliminate sources of confusion. The 1988 Bethesda system recommendation is to abandon the Papanicolaou classification because "it does not reflect the current understanding of cervical and vaginal neoplasm." Papanicolaou classes have no equivalent in diagnosis to histopathologic terminology, and as a result of numerous modifications the specific Papanicolaou classes no longer reflect diagnostic interpretation uniformly. The Bethesda system was not accepted by the entire medical community, particularly the recommendation of considering cytology report a medical consultation. The recommendations for further evaluation and treatment that were issued by laboratory technicians and cytopathologists far removed from the clinical arena have several implications. The Bethesda system's terminology is somewhat confusing, particularly the consideration of HPV as a low-grade SIL.

The observation that patients with genital tract condylomas have a higher incidence of abnormal Papanicolaou smears has a significant impact on the current understanding of HPV. Further evaluation confirmed the direct effect of HPV infection on the histopathologic changes in patients with cervical intraepithelial neoplasia class 1 (CIN 1) and higher degrees of neoplasia. Additional confirmation was supported by the identification of HPV antigen and the detection of HPV DNA. A recent study indicated that 91% of patients with CIN and 89% of patients with squamous cell cervical cancer contained HPV DNA; perhaps the most convincing evidence is the presence of HPV DNA in positive pelvic and paraaortic lymph nodes in patients with invasive cervical cancer while similar patients with negative lymph nodes failed to demonstrate HPV DNA. It is also noted that the positive lymph node metastasis had the same HPV type as the primary invasive cervical cancer.

TABLE 13-4. The 1988 Bethesda system for reporting cervical/vaginal cytologic diagnosis

Statement on the specimen adequacy

Satisfactory for interpretation
Less than optimal
Unsatisfactory
Explanation for less than optimal or unsatisfactory specimen
  Scan cellularity
  Poor fixation or preservation
  Presence of foreign material (e.g., lubricant)
  Partially or completely obscuring inflammation
  Partially or completely obscuring blood
  Excessive cytolysis or autolysis
  No endocervical component in a premenopausal women who has a cervix
  Not representative of the anatomic site
  Other

General categorizaton

With normal limits
  Other
    See descriptive diagnosis
    Further action recommended

Descriptive diagnosis

Infection
  Fungal
    Fungal organisms morphologically consistent with *Candida* species
    Other
  Bacterial
    Microorganism morphologically consistent with *Gardnerella* species
    Microorganism morphologically consistent with *Actinomyces*
    Cellular changes suggestive of *Chlamydia* species infection, subject to confirmatory studies
    Other
  Protozoan
    Trichomonas vaginalis
    Other
  Viral
    Cellular changes associated with cytomegalovirus (CMV)
    Cellular changes associated with herpes simplex virus
    Cellular changes associated with human papillomavirus (HPV)
    Other
    (Note: for HPV refer to "Epithelial cell abnormalities, Squamous cell")
  Other
Reactive and reparative changes
  Inflammation
    Associated cellular changes
    Follicular cervicitis

TABLE 13-4. The 1988 Bethesda system for reporting cervical/vaginal cytologic diagnosis—cont'd

Miscellaneous (as related to patient history)
  Effects of therapy
  Ionizing radiation
  Chemotherapy
  Effects of mechanical devices (e.g., intrauterine device)
  Effect of nonsteroidal estrogen exposure (e.g., diethylstilbestrol)
  Other
Epithelial cell abnormalities

Squamous cell
  Atypical squamous cells of undetermined significance (recommended follow-up type of further investigation: specify)
  Squamous intraepithelial lesion (SIL) (comment to presence of cellular changes associated with HPV if applicable)
    Low-grade squamous intraepithelial lesions encompassing
      Cellular changes consistent with HPV
      Mild (slight) dysplasia/cervical intraepithelial neoplasia 1 (CIN 1)
    High-grade squamous intraepithelial lesion encompassing
      Moderate dysplasia/CIN 2
      Severe dysplasia/CIN 3
      Carcinoma in situ/CIN 3
  Squamous cell carcinoma
Glandular cell
  Presence of endometrial cells in one of the following circumstances:
    Out of phase in menstruating woman
    In postmenopausal woman
    No menstrual history available
  Atypical glandular cells of undetermined significance (recommend follow-up or the type of further investigation [specify]):
    Endometrial
    Endocervical
    Not otherwise specified
  Adenocarcinoma
    Specify probable site of origin: endocervical, endometrial, not otherwise specified
  Other epithelial malignant neoplasm (specify)
Nonepithelial malignant neoplasm (specify)
Hormonal evaluation (applied to vaginal smears only)
  Normal pattern compatible with age and history
  Hormonal pattern incompatible with age and history: specify
  Hormonal evaluation not possible
    Cervical specimen
    Inflammation
    Insufficient patient history

Other

Human Immunodeficiency Virus

The incidence of human immunodeficiency virus (HIV) infections in women is increasing, and infections in women represent 40% of all HIV cases. The close relationship of immunosuppression and lower genital dysplasia is well known in patients with kidney transplant and in patients with chronic prednisone exposure. The Centers for Disease Control and Prevention (CDC) has added to the definition of acquired immunodeficiency syndrome (AIDS) HIV-positive female patients with invasive squamous cell carcinoma of the cervix.

The incidence and prevalence of HIV infection varies according to the population group. Cervical cancer, preinvasive diseases, and invasive diseases may precede the clinical diagnosis of HIV infection. In high-prevalence areas, HIV screening and counseling programs are warranted. Women who are HIV-positive are known to have a higher incidence of abnormal vaginal cytology. The severity of atypia and neoplasia runs parallel to the severity of immunosuppression.

Women who are HIV-positive demonstrate a clinically extensive and aggressive form of CIN. The entire lower genital tract may be affected, and the cervical involvement may extend to the endocervical canal. The severity of the neoplasia is also associated with T-cell function. Furthermore, HIV-positive women with CIN are likely to encounter significant persistence and recurrence after conventional therapy.

Causes of Atypical Papanicolaou Smear

The causes of abnormal Papanicolaou smears are outlined in Table 13-5. The agents of atypical Papanicolaou smears caused by infections are fungi, bacteria, protozoans, and viruses (cytomegalovirus [CMV], HPV, herpes). *Candida* is a common example of the fungal group. Several bacterial agents are *Gardnerella, Chlamydia,* and *Actinomyces. Gardnerella* is the pathogen responsible for nonspecific vaginitis. *Chlamydia trachomatis* is a sexually transmitted intracellular obligatory parasite. Several studies have shown an association of chlamydial cervicitis with abnormal Papanicolaou smears. Treatment of chlamydial cervicitis reverses the abnormal cellular changes seen on a Papanicolaou smear. Follicular cervicitis is often associated with chlamydial cervicitis that can be detected on vaginal cytology. *Actinomyces* has been identified on the Papanicolaou smear of patients using intrauterine devices (IUD).

Trichomonas vaginalis is the agent that results in *Trichomonas* vaginitis, a sexually transmitted disease, and can be associated with an atypical Papanicolaou smear.

The three viral agents CMV, HSV-2, and HPV are detectable on Papanicolaou smears, and each one has a characteristic cytologic finding. The CMV inclusion body is pathognomonic for CMV infection. Multinucle-

TABLE 13-5. Causes of an atypical Papanicolaou smear

Infection

Fungal: *Candida*
Bacterial: *Gardnerella, Actinomyces, Chlamydia*
Protozoan: *Trichomonas vaginalis*
Viral: cytomegalovirus (CMV), herpes simplex virus, human papillomavirus (HPV)

Reactive and reparative

Effects of therapy
Radiation
Chemotherapy
Mechanical device (e.g., intrauterine device)
Follicular cervicitus

Neoplastic

Lower genital tract
  Cervical intraepithelial neoplasia
  Carcinoma in situ
  Invasive cervical or vaginal cancer, squamous cell, or adenocarcinoma
Upper genital tract
  Endometrial cancer and its precursors
  Tubal or ovarian cancer
Extragenital
  Bowel cancer
  Pancreatic cancer
  Gastric cancer

---

ated giant cells are cytologic evidence of HSV-2 infection on Papanicolaou smears. The atypical cells produced by HPV infection are currently designated as koilocytes. Cytologic features of these cells are characterized by an abnormal nucleus surrounded by a "halo," a ballooned, vacuolated cytoplasm. The evidence is overwhelming and indicates that koilocytes represent HPV infection. The presence of koilocytes is the most common reason for an abnormal Papanicolaou smear. Reactive and repair changes are seen with the inflammation of follicular cervicitis; the effects of therapy, chemotherapy, and radiation; and the effects of mechanical devices (e.g., IUDs).

Epithelial abnormalities caused by squamous cells are CIN of all grades or squamous cell carcinoma of the cervix or vagina. Epithelial abnormalities caused by glandular cells might be due to atypical glandular cervical cells, malignant endocervical cells, atypical endometrial cells, and adenocarcinoma of the endometrium. Upper genital tract lesions such as tubal or ovarian cancer rarely cause abnormal Papanicolaou smears. Extragenital sources may be detected on vaginal Papanicolaou smears.

Technique for Obtaining the Papanicolaou Smear

Information should be given to the patient before the office visit. The patient should avoid douching and sexual intercourse the day before the examination. Heavy menstrual bleeding obscures the cytologic findings of importance; therefore elective and routine Papanicolaou smears should be arranged to avoid heavy menstrual flow. Abnormal vaginal bleeding is not a *contraindication* for obtaining a Papanicolaou smear. A delay in cervical cancer diagnosis has anecdotally been attributed to the reluctance of obtaining a Papanicolaou smear in the presence of vaginal bleeding.

After a thorough inspection of the vulva and external genitalia and with an adequate light source, a moistened bivalve speculum should be inserted without lubricant to expose the vagina and cervix. Lubricating materials interfere with proper cytologic interpretation. Abnormalities should be recorded, particularly gross lesions, ulcerations, abnormal vascularity, and contact bleeding. Attention should then be paid to identification of the cervical os. A cytobrush or moistened cotton-tipped applicator is inserted into the cervix, and the endocervical canal is sampled by twisting the cytobrush applicator and withdrawing it toward the external os. Remove the applicator, and gently spread the collected material on a glass slide. It is important to avoid a thick specimen because it may fail to reveal important cytologic details. Once the smear is made, it should be immediately immersed in a fixative solution; a delay in fixation may lead to cell

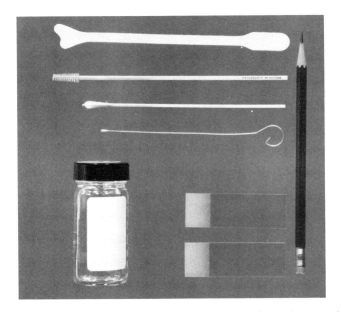

FIGURE 13-1. The supplies required for cervicovaginal cytology include a cytobrush, cotton-tipped swab, large swab, glass with a frosted end, 95% alcohol jar, and a pencil and label to be used for proper identification.

dehydration and to artifacts. The cytobrush improves the quality and accuracy of regular Papanicolaou smears. For postmenopausal patients and patients with cervical stenosis, the endocervical canal can be sampled by using a Calgi swab. A wooden or plastic spatula is then placed against the ectocervix, and the cervix should be gently yet firmly scraped (Fig. 13-1). The material should be transferred to another glass slide and rapidly transferred to the fixative. To avoid mishaps, a label (containing the patient's name and hospital number, etc.) should be placed on the fixed slide for identification. Close attention should be paid to the entire vaginal epithelium to exclude the possibility of vaginal dysplasia or warts. The presence of a gross lesion or lesions demands immediate biopsy. In the current method, the use of 95% alcohol remains the most effective fixative. Other practical methods, such as hair sprays containing alcohol as a fixative, are still in practice and are acceptable.

COLPOSCOPY

The colposcope is a binocular microscope with intense light and magnification. Its advantage is to localize the source and extent of atypical cells detected by a Papanicolaou smear. Colposcopy is not suitable for routine and screening measures.

The indications for colposcopic examination include an evaluation of patients with abnormal vaginal cytology results, an abnormal-looking cervix with or without gross lesions, patients with postcoital bleeding, patients with diethylstilbestrol (DES) exposure in utero, and management of atypical genital warts. Colposcopic examination of the vulva and vagina is of value in the management of precursors and squamous cell carcinoma of the vulva and vagina.

Colposcope

The colposcope is a low-power (6× to 10×) binocular microscope with a powerful source of illumination. The light source is also provided with a green filter for superior highlighting of vascular patterns. Most of the manufacturers provide several powers and focusing capabilities. The addition of a camera for photography either for prints or transparencies is an option available for most models. A teaching arm is also available for allowing more than one individual to view the colposcopic findings (Fig. 13-2).

Colposcopy Procedure

The patient should be well informed about the steps of the procedure and fully prepared before the procedure begins. A thorough pelvic examination is absolutely necessary before colposcopic examination. The pelvic examination should include inspection and palpation of the vulva and bimanual

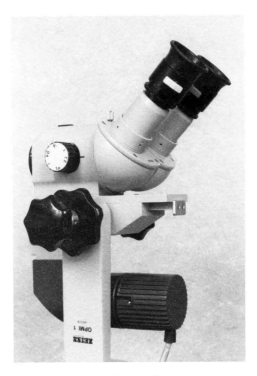

FIGURE 13-2. Colposcope.

examination. The selection of a speculum should be determined by known and suspected pathology, findings of bimanual examination, age, menopausal status, pregnancy, DES exposure, and so on.

The appropriate speculum should be selected and inserted to expose the cervix and upper fornices. A repeat Papanicolaou smear should be performed to compare with histologic findings. Vaginal discharge and cervical mucus should be removed. The colposcopic examination starts with systematic inspection of the entire cervix and upper portion of the vagina. Proper colposcopic examination is a time-consuming procedure. Acetic acid in a 3% solution should then be applied to dehydrate the cell cytoplasm and intensify nuclei. The findings should be recorded narratively and should diagrammatically depict abnormal findings, their location, and the sites of any biopsies performed (Fig. 13-3). Endocervical curettage (ECC) is considered an integral part of the colposcopic evaluation except in pregnancy (Fig. 13-4). Additional staining is probably not required, although some colposcopists use Lugol's solution, toluidine blue stains, or both. It is questionable whether these stains are of significant additive value except in the case of HPV infection, where Schiller iodine staining might distinguish benign from neoplastic epithelium. A thorough colposcopic evaluation is needed to eliminate unnecessary repeat examinations. The

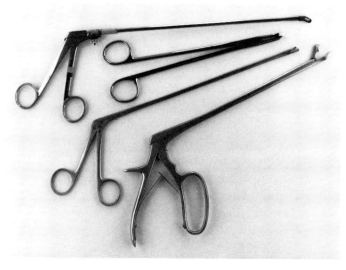

FIGURE 13-3. Various cervical biopsy instruments.

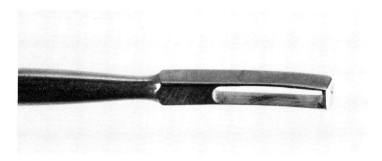

FIGURE 13-4. Endocervical curette (Kevorkian).

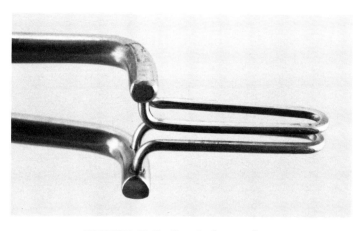

FIGURE 13-5. Cervical speculum.

examiner should try to avoid fixating on immediately evident abnormalities to the exclusion of a systematic colposcopic assessment. Proper colposcopic evaluation requires time to allow the visual adaptation needed. To avoid errors, careful colposcopic examination and the liberal use of multiple cervical biopsy specimens should be considered. The entire transitional zone may be seen in some cases with endocervical speculum use (Fig. 13-5).

Interpretation of Colposcopic Findings

There are many textbooks dedicated to the interpretation and teaching of colposcopy. The practical advantages of colposcopy are related to the early discovery of invasive or preinvasive cervical cancer and its precursors. The majority of diagnostic cone biopsy samples can be avoided, and precursors of cervical cancer can be managed on an outpatient basis with efficiency, safety, and cost-effectiveness.

The normal colposcopic pattern is characterized by a hairpin or network vascular appearance of capillaries. The columnar epithelium is easily identified after being exposed to 3% acetic acid and forms the grapelike appearance. Metaplastic epithelium may exhibit various degrees of maturity and exhibit a mild whitish coloration, in contrast to fully mature or native squamous epithelium, which demonstrates slightly gray gland openings. Smooth-appearing squamous epithelium directly adjacent to columnar epithelium is the pattern of the typical transformation zone. The diagnostic criteria used to determine colposcopic abnormalities are listed in Table 13-6.

Trichomonas infection exhibits a specific colposcopic appearance of double-looped capillaries and a poorly defined punctation-like picture. Colposcopic examination can be of value in evaluating a patient with HPV infection because it distinguishes clinically evident condylomas from noncondylomatous cervical warts described as flat condyloma. In the presence of HPV infection and with the application of 3% acetic acid the cervical epithelium may exhibit lesions of a whitish appearance. These acetowhite lesions are not limited to the transformation zone or to the squamocolumnar junction but involve the ectocervix and vaginal mucosa as well. Colposcopic examination of HPV and dysplasia might require an experienced colposcopist because the predictive value of colposcopy in such

TABLE 13-6.   Colposcopic diagnostic criteria of abnormal transformation zone

Vascular pattern (mosaic, punctation, and atypical vessels)
Intercapillary distance
Color tones and response to acetic acid
Surface contour
Character and sharpness of border between normal and abnormal epithelium

lesions is not always accurate. The use of Schiller's test is often helpful to identify high-grade neoplasia.

After cryotherapy (and less pronounced in laser therapy) colposcopic examination might demonstrate a unique vascular linear arrangement. Similar effects were seen after surgical cone biopsy.

For colposcopic examination to be considered adequate or satisfactory and to avoid diagnostic cone biopsy the following conditions must be met:
1. The squamocolumnar junction must be seen in its entirety.
2. The lesion must be seen completely.
3. There must be agreement between cytologic, colposcopic, and histologic impressions.

Cervicography

Cervicography was originally described by Dr. Adolf Stafl in 1981. He developed the technique of photographically depicting the cervix through the colposcope. These photographs can be sent to experts for interpretation and recommendation.

Cervicography is not a substitute for cytology, and the technique is associated with various degrees of false negative and false positive results. Furthermore, the expense associated with cervicography is prohibitive for its use as a routine screening method.

Management of Patients with Diethylstilbestrol Exposure In Utero

Diethylstilbestrol is a nonsteroidal estrogen synthesized in 1936. Between 1940 and 1971 the obstetric use of DES was for the management of high-risk pregnancy to prevent threatened abortion and help control diabetes mellitus and habitual abortion. None of these uses proved appropriate. Clear-cell carcinoma of the vagina, a previously extremely rare entity, was linked to DES exposure in utero as described in 1971 by Herbst, Ulfelder, and Postkanzer. The Registry for Clear-Cell Carcinoma was established and included patients with vaginal and cervical clear-cell carcinoma.

Screening programs were established to examine young women with a known history of DES exposure in utero. Several noncancerous lesions of the cervix and vagina were discovered. The cervical abnormalities were estimated to occur in nearly every patient investigated for in utero exposure to DES by speculum inspection, colposcopy, and cytology.

The benign cervical changes described in DES-exposed women include a wide transformation zone, cervical sulcus, recess of the endocervical epithelium to the vagina, and a pseudopolyp cockscomb or anterior cervical ridge. Vaginal adenosis is a benign vaginal change and presents in several ways, including adenosis, cystic adenosis, constricting vaginal membrane, cockscomblike vaginal membrane, fibrous vaginal band, apical vaginal narrowing, fornix obliteration, and vaginal septum.

Schiller's Test

Schiller's test uses the known quality that glycogenated squamous epithelium retains the stain of elemental iodine; therefore mature normal squamous epithelium stains a mahogany color, whereas the epithelium of immature squamous, dysplastic, and columnar epithelium fails to maintain the characteristic stain. Schiller's test is nonspecific and carries significant degrees of false-positive and false-negative findings. The main benefit of Schiller's test is the identification of surgical margins for resection of a cone biopsy specimen. Additional indications for Schiller's test are in patients with posthysterectomy dysplasia because it assists in selecting sites for vaginal biopsies in the presence of atypical vaginal cytology. It is also indicated for patients with HPV infection, as previously mentioned.

Cervical Biopsy

Before the era of colposcopic-directed biopsy, patients with atypical Papanicolaou smears were managed by random cervical biopsy of arbitrarily selected sites (e.g., 3, 6, 9, and 12 o'clock positions). Current practice indicates a need for colposcopic guidance in all patients with abnormal Papanicolaou smears. The use of random cervical biopsy specimens should be limited to patients with gross cervical lesions. The advantage is evident in pregnant women; confusion between ectopy and an abnormal cervix in these patients can be distinguished by colposcopic evaluation. Cervical biopsy is rarely required to resolve such cases.

Endocervical Curettage

The use of ECC is considered an integral part of evaluating a patient with an abnormal Papanicolaou smear. The rationale for its use is as follows: ECC might detect invasive cervical cancer, so cervical cone biopsy can be avoided, and ECC might detect endocervical in situ or invasive endocervical adenocarcinoma despite the appearance of adequate colposcopy.

DIAGNOSIS AND OFFICE MANAGEMENT OF CERVICAL INTRAEPITHELIAL NEOPLASIA

The Papanicolaou smear remains the most useful screening technique for the early detection of cervical neoplasia and cervical cancer. The recent clarification that CIN is a continuum has significant ramifications for management. The modern cytology reporting scheme includes a narrative portion that gives the clinician information beyond the original Papanicolaou smear classifications of 1 to 5. This is especially helpful in interpretation of the atypical smear. Recent attention to condylomatous changes as a potentially precancerous lesion has resulted in the early use of colposcopy in these clinical situations.

The options for treatment in patients with CIN are several, and before embarking on any specific treatment, it is of value to return the patient to the clinic to discuss these options. It is important to review the cytology, colposcopy, and pathology materials with the patient and members of the family to explain the details of each option of treatment, risks, possible complications, alternative methods of treatment, and future follow-up.

Nonsurgical methods for the management of CIN are available as investigational protocols at the present time. Several new modalities of therapy are available and include topical interferon, high-dose oral folic acid, and carotine.

Excision

The rationale for the use of simple local excision of a cervical lesion was based on the experience that a negative Papanicolaou smear continued long after excision of limited cervical lesions. The excision can be accomplished either by the use of cervical biopsy forceps (see Fig. 13-3) or a scalpel. Local excision carries significant failure rates of at least 40%. This method of treatment should be reserved for young women when adequate colposcopy shows a lesion limited to the ectocervix, single in focus, and no worse than CIN 1 or 2. Because of the high failure rate of local excision, most lesions should be eradicated with a modality that encompasses the entire transformation zone and squamocolumnar junction.

Cryotherapy

The era of current application of cryotherapy in the management of CIN was heralded by Crisp and others in 1967. The instrument uses the well-known effect of Joule-Thompson. Compressed gas, when allowed to escape through a small orifice under pressure, causes a significant drop in surface temperature. Various gases were used as refrigerants, including nitrogen, carbon dioxide, freon, and nitrous oxide. The latter is the most commonly used for gynecologic procedures. Probes are applied directly to the surface to be treated. The ice ball formation is the result of lowering the temperature of the probe. The ice ball should extend beyond the abnormal cervical epithelium. Mechanisms postulated to explain the effect of cryotherapy are dehydration and toxic concentrations of electrolytes, crystallization with rupture of cell membrane, denaturation of protein molecules within the cell membrane, thermal shock, and vascular stasis.

Cryotherapy is one of the most suitable methods for the treatment of early CIN in young women. The procedure is performed on an outpatient basis without anesthesia, and it has minimal morbidity and an excellent success rate. Proper selection of patients depends on meticulous colposcopic investigation, histologic diagnosis confirmed by multiple cervical biopsies, and an ECC to avoid the risk of occult invasive cancer. The pretreatment evaluation and not the method of treatment is the most important factor in treating patients with CIN managed by conservative methods. After several years of experience, the following are prerequisites to be met before performing cryotherapy:

1. Cervical biopsy specimens confirm CIN. Microinvasive or invasive carcinoma is excluded.
2. Negative ECC.
3. Satisfactory colposcopy. The squamocolumnar junction and the entire lesion are visible.
4. Results of cytology are in agreement with cervical biopsy samples.
5. Glandular cell abnormalities are excluded by cervical biopsies, cytology, or both.
6. Long-term follow-up is ensured.

Some investigators limit cryotherapy to young patients with the diagnosis of CIN 1 or CIN 2 and consider CIN 3 and endocervical extension a relative contraindication.

Several cryosurgery instruments are available on the market. The selection of suitable ones depends on size, portability, expense, and the refrigerant to be used. The handheld cryosurgical probe with a pistol grip (Fig. 13-6) and interchangeable probe tips (Fig. 13-7) remains the most popular one for gynecologic practice. Nitrous oxide remains the preferable refrigerant, although freon and CO_2 are available.

Cryotherapy is performed as an office procedure and without anesthesia. The patient should be informed of the details of the procedure, such as discomfort, the rare event of vasomotor reaction, and the expectations of excessive vaginal discharge. The timing of the cryotherapy should coincide with the follicular phase of the menstrual cycle to avoid freezing the cervix during pregnancy. Pregnancy tests should be used in questionable cases to rule out pregnancy. The selection of a large speculum is necessary to retract the vaginal epithelium away from the cryotherapy probe and to fully expose

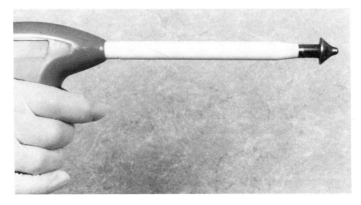

FIGURE 13-6. Cryosurgery unit.

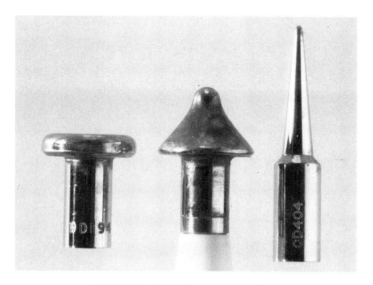

FIGURE 13-7. Cryosurgery tips.

the entire cervix. Colposcopy should be reevaluated to determine the extent, size, and configuration of the lesion to select the proper probe that covers the lesion best. A thin layer of lubricant is applied to the probe to enhance thermal transfer, and the probe is applied against the cervix and an ice ball raised. The size of the ice ball should exceed the lesion by 4 to 5 mm. The duration of freezing is perhaps of less importance than the size of the ice ball and close contact to the probe. Once defrosting is performed, colposcopic examination should be repeated to ensure proper application. We prefer a double-freeze technique with a 3-minute exposure in each freeze and at least 3 minutes between the freezing cycles. Large lesions might require several applications of cryotherapy with attention to overlap of the ice balls to avoid undertreatment.

Excessive vaginal discharge is the major complaint of patients treated by cryotherapy. Drainage continues 2 to 4 weeks after treatment, and discharge gradually subsides. Patients are instructed to avoid the use of tampons, and coitus is discouraged during the period of watery vaginal discharge. The patient should be instructed to return in 3 to 4 months for a Papanicolaou smear and for inspection of the cervix. Cervical stenosis should be managed by repeated cervical dilation. Significant stenosis can be managed by inserting a small *Laminaria* tent for 12 to 24 hours.

Frequent and periodic cytologic examination is essential to detect early failure of therapy. Routine ECC is probably not indicated, although a careful Papanicolaou smear that includes adequate sampling of the cervical canal is warranted. The transformation zone migrates upward toward the internal os after cryotherapy.

The treatment failures of cryotherapy are closely related to the following features:

1. Increasing histologic severity, particularly carcinoma in situ (CIS)
2. Increasing age
3. Endocervical involvement
4. Large lesions
5. Inadequate colposcopy
6. Technical applications (type and shape of the probe, shape of the cervical os, freeze time)

The failure rate can be reduced to a significant degree by proper selection of cryotherapy candidates based on the prerequisites described earlier.

Laser

Laser therapy is becoming a frequent method of treatment of several gynecologic conditions. The first use of lasers in gynecologic practice was for the treatment of cervical erosion (ectopy): CO_2 laser vaporization by Kaplan in 1973. Several types of laser therapy are currently available, with each having certain advantages and characteristics (Table 13-7). The types common for gynecologic practice include CO_2, KTP (potassium titanyl phosphate), Nd:YAG (neodymium: yttrium-aluminum-garnet), and argon. The carbon dioxide laser is the most frequently used in the management of CIN of the cervix and vulvar neoplasia. Vaporization is an outpatient or office procedure with minimal patient discomfort. Laser conization requires an operating room setting and anesthetic.

Major advantages of CO_2 laser therapy include the following:

1. High clinical efficacy
2. Bloodless field
3. Microscopic precision
4. Sparing of normal tissue
5. Rapid healing with minimal scar formation
6. Small number of complications
7. Outpatient procedure

Special precautions should be followed to protect patients, staff, and personnel from laser injury. Eye protection for patients is performed by

TABLE 13-7.   Characteristics of various lasers

Laser	Watt	Wavelength (μm)	Visible beam	Coagulation	Cutting	Plume	Flexible fibers	Water cooling
CO_2	100	10.6	No	+	+ + +	+ + +	No	No
KTP	20	0.532	Yes	+ +	+ +	+ +	Yes	Yes
YAG	20	1064	No	+ + +	+	+	Yes	Yes
Argon	20	0.48-0.515	Yes	+ +	+ +	+ +	Yes	Yes

applying eyeglasses; for patients under anesthesia, moist gauze applied to both eyes is secure protection. Staff and personnel eye protection is accomplished by the use of eyeglasses.

Protection against fire is maintained through a rigorous program of avoiding the use of inflammable paper drapes and anesthetic agents. It is also important to avoid operating the laser on tissues cleaned with flammable solutions (e.g., alcohol or ether). The use of nonreflective instruments is essential to the safety of laser therapy.

Prerequisites for laser vaporization are similar to the ones applied for cryotherapy. Cervical biopsy specimens confirm the worst part of the lesion on colposcopic examination. The pathologic material confirms the presence of CIN without a suspicion of microinvasion of the invasive process. Colposcopic assessment identifies the entire extent of the lesion by showing the ectocervical and endocervical margins. Before the vaporization, adequate assurance of future follow-up and informed consent should be obtained from the patient.

It is preferable to vaporize the cervix during the proliferative phase of the menstrual cycle so that the endocervical canal is spared, the healing process is enhanced, and the risk of cervical stenosis is minimized.

The laser machine should be calibrated by measuring the spot size on a tongue blade at a power density greater than 1000 W/cm^2. Rapid beam movement reduces thermal tissue conductivity, minimizes potential scarring, and reduces heat buildup in the cervical tissue with a reduction in uterine cramping and discomfort. The end result is rapid healing and minimal scarring. The laser beam is moved in multiple directions diagonally, horizontally, and vertically to prevent furrowing. The surface area to be lasered is divided into smaller segments, and one segment should be completed at a time. To assess the depth of vaporization a microruler is used to confirm the depth of vaporization. Vaporization should extend to a depth of 5 to 7 mm and 3 mm of peripheral margin. A power density below 350 W/cm^2 is not recommended because of increased time required for vaporization. A spot size of 1.5 to 2 mm is mandatory for vaporization. A power density greater than 1000 W/cm^2 is considered appropriate.

Healing is usually complete in 3 weeks. The new squamocolumnar junction is almost always located at the level of the external os. This renders future follow-up colposcopy and cytology satisfactory. The entire transformation zone should be vaporized.

Laser Cone Biopsy

The indications for diagnostic conization are endocervical extension, previously failed laser vaporization, disparity between cytologic and histologic findings (assumed negative colposcopic examination of the vagina), and inadequate colposcopy.

Electrocautery

Outpatient electrocautery is a well-known procedure used by many gynecologists for the management of benign cervical, vaginal, and vulvar lesions. With the advent of cryotherapy, electrocautery gradually became less popular in general and particularly for CIN.

There is a resurgence of the use of electrocautery, and several manufacturers produce several units for various applications. The idea is to transform electric energy to heat by passing an electric current through a wire with high resistance. The newer units use electrodiathermy.

The indications and prerequisites for electrocautery should be similar to the various methods of management of patients with CIN. Adequate colposcopy, negative ECC findings, and agreement of colposcopic and cytologic criteria are all necessary. Disadvantages of electrocautery include discomfort, cervical stenosis, and vaginal discharge.

Channen and Hollyock used electrocautery under anesthesia with comparable results to cryotherapy. The requirement of general anesthesia to destroy the endocervical cleft is a significant disadvantage in the current practice of cost containment. Channen and Rome reported on their extensive experience without significant side effects: that one method of treatment is better than another in an individual case is based on the patient's age, availability of the technology to be used, financial considerations, and personal preference. Postpartum cautery of the cervix was considered effective in preventing cervical cancer. Channen's experience with electrocautery for CIN produced results that are comparable to cryotherapy and laser therapy. The precautions and prerequisites for electrocautery should be identical to laser therapy.

Loop Electrosurgical Excision Procedure

Loop electrosurgical excision procedure (LEEP) uses a fine wire loop to excise a portion of the cervix or the entire transformation zone in the management of patients with various degrees of CIN. New concepts of management are emerging, with the aim of treatment at the initial evaluation. Such concepts advocate LEEP at the same time as colposcopic diagnosis. This procedure has the advantage of being performed in the physician's office under local anesthesia. It is perhaps safer for the inexperienced practitioner to adopt two visits, the first one for diagnosis and the second visit for treatment. Some European centers have advocated one visit for the management of atypical Papanicolaou smear. The treatment consists of colposcopic examination followed by LEEP with the aim of dual benefits: diagnosis and therapy accomplished in one visit. An additional potential benefit is a reduction in the incidence of cone biopsy.

Outpatient and office management is frequently successful in patients with squamous CIS. However, LEEP is not an appropriate management for adenocarcinoma in situ.

As with other procedures, the prerequisites that should be present before considering LEEP are the presence of significant atypia of Papanicolaou smear (CIN 2 or 3), colposcopically defined cervical lesions without suspicion of invasive disease, and persistent low-grade SIL.

Large loop excision of the transformation zone (LLETZ) is the natural extension of LEEP and involves the removal of the entire transformation zone. The disadvantage of LEEP and LLETZ is the thermal damage at the margins of resection, which might interfere with the histologic interpretation of extent of surgical margins and the presence of early invasion.

Summary of Office Management

It is important to individualize each patient based on the review of the entire record and findings of cytology, colposcopy, cervical biopsy, ECC, and previous treatment. Table 13-8 lists various factors that influence failure of CIN office and outpatient therapy. The physician should have a strong conviction of the importance of the prerequisites described for each modality. The presence of inadequate colposcopy or CIN material on ECC demands further evaluation before selecting any treatment plan in order to avoid inappropriate treatment of patients with invasive cervical cancer. Cryotherapy, laser therapy, and electrocautery result in tissue destruction without the benefit of pathology assessment. It is probably true that the method of treatment is less important than pretreatment evaluation, such as the extent of disease, size of the lesion, and presence of glandular and cervical canal involvement. Pregnant women with CIN rarely require any treatment during pregnancy, and once the risk of invasion is excluded, postpartum therapy is recommended.

Regardless of the method of treatment, close follow-up is essential. A surveillance program of frequent cytologic examination every 3 to 4 months for 2 years and annually thereafter is appropriate for the patient with posttherapy negative cytologic findings. Attempts should be made to reduce the chance of recurrence by adhering to the previously described guidelines for Papanicolaou smear frequency.

The diagnosis of invasive squamous cell carcinoma of the cervix based on cervical biopsy demands pathologic evaluation to determine the degree of invasion, lymphatic or vascular permeation, and confluence. The entity of microinvasive cervical cancer remains an ambiguous definition. In

TABLE 13-8. Reasons for failure of cervical intraepithelial neoplasia

Failure to completely evaluate the area at risk
Failure to obtain histologic conformation
Failure to follow up after therapy
Failure to perform endocervical curettage
Failure to recognize adenocarcinoma of the cervix

TABLE 13-9. Cervical cancer: FIGO Staging System, 1989

Stage I	The carcinoma is strictly confined to the cervix (extension to the corpus should be disregarded).
Stage Ia	Preclinical carcinomas of the cervix, that is, those diagnosed only by microscopy.
Stage Ia1	Minimal microscopically evident stromal invasion.
Stage Ia2	Lesions detected microscopically *that can be measured.* The upper limit of the measurement should not show a depth of invasion of more than 5 mm taken from the base of the epithelium, either surface or glandular, from which it originates, and a second dimension, the horizontal spread, must not exceed 7 mm. Larger lesions should be staged as Ib.
Stage Ib	Lesions of greater dimensions than stage Ia2, whether seen clinically or not. Preformed space involvement should not alter the staging but should be specifically recorded so as to determine whether it should affect treatment decisions in the future.
Stage II	Extension beyond the cervix, but not on to the pelvic wall. The carcinoma involves the vagina, but not the lower third.
Stage IIa	The carcinoma involves the vagina, but not the lower third. No obvious extension to the parametrium.
Stage IIb	The carcinoma involves the vagina, but not the lower third. Obvious extension to the parametrium, but not onto the pelvic wall.
Stage III	The carcinoma has extended to the pelvic wall. On rectal examination, there is no cancer-free space between the tumor and the pelvic wall. The tumor involves the lower third of the vagina.
Stage IIIa	No extension onto the pelvic wall.
Stage IIIb	Extension onto the pelvic wall.
Stage IV	The carcinoma has extended beyond the true pelvis or has involved the mucosa of the bladder or rectum. A bullous edema as such does not permit allotment of a case to stage IV.

January 1974, the Society of Gynecologic Oncologists (SGO) accepted the following statements on microinvasion in cancer of the cervix: (1) Cases of intraepithelial carcinoma with questionable invasion should be regarded as intraepithelial carcinoma and invasive. (2) A microinvasive lesion should be defined as one in which neoplastic epithelium invades the stroma in one or more places to a depth of 3 mm or less below the base of the epithelium and in which lymphatic or vascular involvement is not demonstrated. The depth of invasion is accepted by the majority of gynecologic oncologists according to the statement by the SGO and without evidence of lymphatic or vascular involvement and without confluence. In 1989 the International Federation of Gynecologists and Obstetricians (FIGO) presented the most recent modifications of the staging system for cervical cancer (Table 13-9).

Microinvasive squamous cell carcinoma of the cervix can be managed by a nonradical surgical approach. Hysterectomy is considered the treatment of choice, particularly if further reproductive function is no longer desirable. If pathologic findings indicate that the disease is beyond the confines of a microinvasive process, radical therapy is required. Treatment options include radical radiation therapy or radical hysterectomy with bilateral pelvic lymphadenectomy.

The diagnosis of adenocarcinoma in situ of the cervix should be based on cone biopsy evaluation. Some pathologists are introducing the new pathologic entity of microinvasive adenocarcinoma. Definitions and criteria for such an entity are lacking. Published data on the subject are sparse and mainly based on retrospective reviews. The entire canal of the cervix is at risk of being involved with adenocarcinoma of the cervix, whereas CIN's risk is confined to the squamocolumnar junction. Therefore hysterectomy is the preferable therapy in the management of women with so-called adenocarcinoma in situ.

SPECIAL PROBLEMS
Atrophy

Postmenopause and postirradiation changes pose a special difficulty in managing a patient with cervicovaginal cytologic findings. Atrophy is a form of atypia. It is not unusual that the degree of atypia might obscure the diagnosis of dysplasia or malignancy. The use of topical estrogen can be of help in determining the nature and extent of the atypia. Caution should be exercised in patients after they have undergone irradiation. Performing multiple and overzealous biopsies should be avoided because vesicovaginal fistulas have resulted after such procedures. Atrophic vaginitis might be associated with an infectious process. Topical antibiotics might be indicated to clear an intense inflammatory reaction associated with inflammatory atypia.

There is no reason to exclude women over 65 years of age from screening for cancer of the cervix. The postmenopause period presents special and often difficult clinical management problems. In these situations, the cervix is small, does not protrude, and is flush to the vaginal vault. The cervical os is often stenotic or even nonvisible, and the vaginal fornices are often not present. Cone biopsy is not infrequently associated with technical difficulties that might preclude obtaining an optimal specimen.

Papanicolaou Smear during Pregnancy

The management of a patient with an atypical Papanicolaou smear during pregnancy is greatly influenced by several factors, including the degree of atypia, the duration of pregnancy, the desire to maintain the pregnancy, and the availability of an experienced colposcopist. Before the advent of colposcopy, patients with atypical Papanicolaou smears during pregnancy were managed by diagnostic cone biopsy because random cervical biopsy specimens are inadequate to rule out invasive cervical cancer. The need for diagnostic cone biopsy was significantly reduced as a result of colposcopy. The main objective of the use of cervical cytology during pregnancy is to detect invasive cervical cancer, so the mere detection or recovery of atypical cells is not an indication to perform a cervical cone biopsy unless the atypia is advanced and worrisome enough to reflect or suggest an invasive process. Therefore the diagnosis of CIN detected during pregnancy does not require prenatal treatment because the final management can be performed in the postpartum period.

The physiologic changes during pregnancy give an adequate colposcopic view of the cervix because of cervical eversion, even in the early stages of pregnancy. The squamocolumnar junction is often visible; therefore ECC is rarely required.

The initial management of patients with abnormal Papanicolaou smears during pregnancy should include a thorough evaluation of the past history of neoplasia, previous treatments and type, and cytologic and pathologic degrees of abnormalities. A thorough colposcopic evaluation by an experienced colposcopist should be performed. Cervical biopsy might be required to clarify a cytologic and colposcopic discrepancy or for any suggestion of an invasive or microinvasive process. Patients with adequate colposcopy and low-grade CIN can be managed by repeat colposcopy and cytologic tests every 2 to 3 months until delivery. Severe colposcopic abnormalities require cervical biopsy or conization, depending on the severity and extent of cervical involvement. Cervical wedge resection is often satisfactory to establish the histologic diagnosis. Several investigators have confirmed the safety of such a program, and it is acceptable in the hands of experienced colposcopists. Once invasive or microinvasive processes are excluded, the patient should be managed according to what the obstetric condition dictates.

Papanicolaou Smear of the Vaginal Vault

Patients with a previous history of cervical or vulvar carcinoma, neoplasia, or invasive carcinoma are at a higher risk of developing vaginal neoplasm, and they perhaps share the same etiology, epidemiology, and pathogens. Vaginal cytology remains necessary and should be performed for routine surveillance, particularly in the high-risk group identified earlier.

Vaginal carcinoma in situ is asymptomatic and is detected by vaginal cytology or when seen in conjunction with lesions associated with HPV. Colposcopy should be performed to determine the location and number of lesions. The vaginal vault is the most common location, and young women tend to have multifocal lesions that may be associated with concomitant HPV or a past history of HPV. Vaginal biopsy is essential in establishing a diagnosis. The use of Schiller's test in selecting sites to obtain vaginal biopsy specimens is based on the retention of iodine staining and might be of value for preoperative mapping of the abnormal vaginal epithelium before excision or laser therapy. Because some patients with vaginal neoplasia are in the postmenopausal period, the vaginal mucosa might be atrophic and prove difficult to diagnose and treat. (See the section on atrophy.) Hence there is an advantage for the use of estrogen, topical or systemic. Vaginal biopsy may be carried out with a punch biopsy forceps. It might be necessary to resort to the use of a skin hook to grasp and elevate the vaginal mucosa to adequately perform a vaginal vault biopsy.

The treatment of vaginal intraepithelial neoplasia should be individualized according to the following factors: patient age, previous history of lower genital neoplasia, previous history of irradiation, previous therapy and its response, and the extent of the disease.

Local excision of a limited lesion can be satisfactorily performed. However, limited upper vaginectomy might be required, when the disease is limited to the upper vaginal vault and is of a unifocal nature.

The use of intravaginal fluorouracil (5-FU), 5% cream (Efudex), was used with success, particularly in patients with vaginal intraepithelial neoplasia after pelvic irradiation for cervical cancer. Multifocal lesions when associated with HPV are amenable to the use of intravaginal 5-FU cream.

Laser therapy is a tool to be considered in the treatment of vaginal neoplasia. It is clear that laser therapy is an effective method of treatment if properly selected, performed by an experienced surgeon, and performed on patients known to adhere to close follow-up. The use of vaginal cryotherapy has been declining since the introduction of laser therapy. Cryotherapy lacks the precision that laser therapy maintains and can have serious (particularly intestinal) complications.

Under certain circumstances, vaginal irradiation by using a vaginal cylinder is used in the treatment of vaginal carcinoma in situ and with success.

Papanicolaou Smear in the Presence of Atypical Glandular Cells

The presence of atypical glandular cells is worrisome and requires further evaluation. The assessment approach should be slightly different from the one used in patients with abnormal squamous cells. The sources of these abnormal glandular cells might be from the cervix, endometrium, tube, ovary, gastrointestinal tract, or breast.

Adenocarcinoma of the cervix has been noted to have a higher relative incidence in the past 30 to 40 years. The reason for this phenomenon is unknown. It is possible that the active cytology screening programs and the effective measures to eradicate cervical cancer precursors have resulted in a relative increase in adenocarcinoma. A thorough pelvic examination, colposcopic evaluation, ECC, and endometrial sampling provide the primary assessment. The detection of cervical adenocarcinoma or endometrial cancer should be managed according to the stage of the cancer. Persistent abnormal glandular cells with negative evaluation of the cervix and endometrium might require laparoscopy. The presence of an adnexal mass should promptly lead to laparotomy, and further management depends on the operative findings. It is suggested that annual Papanicolaou smears may hasten the detection of extravaginal primary carcinomas, and Papanicolaou smears in one study were more often indicative of noncervical than cervical malignancies.

BIBLIOGRAPHY

Baggish MS: Management of cervical intraepithelial neoplasia by carbon dioxide laser, *Obstet Gynecol* 60:379, 1982.

Baggish MS, editor: *Basic and advanced laser surgery in gynecology*, Norwalk, Conn, 1985, Appleton-Century-Crofts.

Baggish MS, Dorsey JH: The laser combination cone, *Am J Obstet Gynecol* 151:23, 1985.

Channen W, Hollyock VE: Colposcope and the conservative management of cervical dysplasia and carcinoma in situ, *Obstet Gynecol* 43:527, 1974.

Charles EH, Savage EW: Cryosurgical treatment of cervical intraepithelial neoplasia, *Obstet Gynecol* 35:539, 1980.

Coppelson M, Pixley E, Reid B: *Colposcopy*, Springfield, Ill, 1971, Charles C Thomas.

Crisp WE: Cryosurgical treatment of neoplasia of the uterine cervix, *Obstet Gynecol* 39:495, 1972.

Day NE: Effect of cervical cancer screening in Scandinavia, *Obstet Gynecol* 63:714, 1984.

Ferenczy A: Comparison of cryo- and carbon dioxide laser therapy of cervical intraepithelial neoplasia, *Obstet Gynecol* 66:793, 1985.

Figge DC, Creasman WT: Cryotherapy in the treatment of cervical intraepithelial neoplasia, *Obstet Gynecol* 62:353, 1983.

Fruchter RG, Maiman M, Sillmen FH, et al: Characteristics of cervical intraepithelial neoplasia in women infected with human immunodeficiency virus, *Am J Obstet Gynecol* 171:531, 1994.

Herbst AL, Ulfelder H, Postkanzer DC: Adenocarcinoma of the vagina: association of maternal stilbestrol therapy with tumor appearance in young women, *N Engl J Med* 284:878, 1971.

Kaplan I, Goldman J, Ger R: The treatment of erosion of the uterine cervix by means of carbon dioxide laser, *Obstet Gynecol* 41:795, 1973.

Kaufman RH, Irwin LF: The cryosurgical therapy of cervical neoplasia, *Am J Obstet Gynecol* 131:381, 1978.

Kolstad P, Stafl A: *Atlas of colposcopy*, Baltimore, 1972, University Park Press.

Krumholz BA, Knapp RC: Colposcopic selection of biopsy sites, *Obstet Gynecol* 39:22, 1972.

Kurman RJ, Schiffman MH, Lancerster WD, et al: Analysis of individual human papillomavirus types in cervical neoplasia, *Am J Obstet Gynecol* 159:295, 1988.

National Cancer Institute Workshop: The 1988 Bethesda system for reporting cervical/vaginal diagnoses, *JAMA* 252:931, 1988.

Ostergard DR, Gondos B: Outpatient therapy of pre-invasive cervical neoplasia: selection of patients with the use of colposcopy, *Am J Obstet Gynecol* 89:223, 1964.

Papanicolaou GN, Traut HE: *Diagnosis of uterine cancer by vaginal smear,* New York, 1943, Commonwealth Fund.

Prendiville W, Cullimore J, Normal S: Large loop excision of the transformation zone (LLETZ): new method of management of women with cervical intraepithelial neoplasia, *Br J Obstet Gynaecol* 96:1054, 1989.

Richart RM: Natural history of cervical intraepithelial neoplasia, *Clin Obstet Gynecol* 10:749, 1967.

Shy K, Chu J, Mandelson M, et al: Papanicolaou smear screening interval and risk of cervical cancer, *Obstet Gynecol* 74:838, 1989.

Stafl A, Mattingly RF: Colposcopic diagnosis of cervical neoplasia, *Obstet Gynecol* 41:168, 1973.

Urcuyo R, Rome R, Nelson JH: Some observation on the value of endocervical curettage performed as an integral part of colposcopic examination of patients with abnormal cervical cytology, *Am J Obstet Gynecol* 128:787, 1977.

Vonka V, Kanka J, Kirsch I, et al: Prospective study on the relationship between cervical neoplasia and herpes simplex type-2 virus. Herpes simplex type-2 antibody presence in sera taken at enrollment, *Int J Cancer* 33:61, 1984.

Wright TC, Gagnon S, Richart RM, Ferenczy A: Treatment of cervical intraepithelial neoplasia using the loop electrosurgical excision procedure, *Obstet Gynecol* 79:173, 1992.

Wright VC, Davies E, Rioplle MA: Laser surgery for cervical intraepithelial neoplasia: principles and results, *Am J Obstet Gynecol* 145:181, 1983.

CHAPTER **14**

Primary and Secondary Amenorrhea and Hirsutism

MICHAEL R. SOULES

The simplest definition of amenorrhea is the absence of menses at an age when menstrual function should be present. The age range for menstrual function is broad. The average age of menarche and menopause is 13 and 50 years, respectively. If one includes the accepted extremes of these averages, menstrual function can occur between the ages of 10 and 58 years and still be considered normal. For most women, it takes several years for regular menstrual cycles to develop after the initial menstrual period (menarche), and menstrual periods generally become irregular for 3 to 5 years before the last menstrual period (menopause). Therefore the age range in which we expect to find *regular* menstrual cycles is essentially 15 to 45 years. Women in this age range should have regular menstrual periods that occur every 21 to 35 days on average.

Amenorrhea (absence of menstruation) has classically been divided into primary and secondary. The definition of primary amenorrhea is the lack of a spontaneous menstrual period by 16 years of age. To have secondary amenorrhea, a woman must have had at least one spontaneous menstrual period. Once a woman has established regular cycles, if she fails to have regular menstrual periods for a disputed period of time, she is considered to have secondary amenorrhea.

There is no established definition for secondary amenorrhea. Some authors have claimed that the lack of menses for 3 months is sufficient for the diagnosis of secondary amenorrhea, and other experts have stuck to the more classic definition of 12 months without menses. Others have used 6 months as the critical diagnostic interval. This controversy regarding the length of time sufficient to meet the diagnosis should simply be recognized and should not be a cause for concern. Rather than be stymied over this lack of consensus, the clinician should use a commonsense approach to decide which patients should be evaluated for secondary amenorrhea. Examples of a commonsense approach would be the following:

1. A young woman 14 years old whose menarche occurred 18 months ago does not need to be evaluated if her menstrual periods are occurring every 4 months.
2. A 24-year-old woman who has always had 28-day cycles and now has experienced 4 months of amenorrhea should be evaluated.

There are several general clinical caveats that apply to the evaluation of amenorrhea. An important point to remember is that amenorrhea is a *symptom*, not a final diagnosis. There is a long list of disease states that can lead to primary or secondary amenorrhea. It is important for the clinician to focus his or her attention on the potential disease states that led to the symptom (amenorrhea). The second general point to remember is that the evaluation of amenorrhea is rarely an emergency situation. The diseases that lead to amenorrhea can often be complex and diverse. The diagnostic challenge can be formidable, but there is rarely a legitimate reason to press for a quick diagnosis that precludes a focused workup. The only emergency situation that applies to the diagnosis of amenorrhea is ectopic pregnancy. If ectopic pregnancy is a possible diagnosis, based on the history and physical examination, a serum human chorionic gonadotropin (HCG) level can be obtained. If the HCG level is negative, the practitioner can proceed with a stepwise evaluation. Clinically, it is not ''bad form'' to initiate a workup for amenorrhea and then take the necessary time to think over the findings and do some directed reading.

This chapter will be divided into three sections devoted to primary amenorrhea, secondary amenorrhea, and hirsutism, respectively. In each section, a diagnostic method will be presented. Each diagnostic method seeks to compartmentalize the malfunction and identify the source. Once the level of the defect has been identified, the reader can focus on the diseases that are known to occur in that compartment.

PHYSIOLOGY OF NORMAL MENSTRUAL FUNCTION

The hypothalamic-pituitary-ovarian-uterine axis must function in a co-ordinated manner to achieve normal menstrual function. Withdrawal menstrual flow is the end result of a series of orchestrated events. If one part of the system is malfunctioning, withdrawal menses do not occur, and amenorrhea is the symptom. Normal female reproductive function depends on the arcuate nucleus in the medial basal hypothalamus.

The arcuate nucleus must release the decapeptide gonadotropin-releasing hormone (GnRH) in an intermittent (pulsatile) fashion. The GnRH is secreted into the portal blood system approximately every 90 minutes in the first half of a normal cycle. In the second half of a normal cycle (luteal phase), GnRH is secreted intermittently every 4 to 6 hours. The principal pituitary hormones that control reproduction—luteinizing hormone (LH) and follicle-stimulating hormone (FSH)—are secreted intermittently in response to the GnRH pulses. In this manner, the medial basal hypothalamus controls the pituitary secretion of gonadotropins. If GnRH is not secreted or is released in an irregular manner, normal physiologic gonadotropin levels are not realized. The FSH is secreted by the pituitary at a relatively higher level during the late luteal and early follicular cycle phases (the intercycle FSH rise). This transient elevation of FSH levels is the basis for follicular recruitment within the ovary. Once follicular recruitment has occurred and there is a selected and dominant follicle, FSH secretion is suppressed secondary to the negative feedback signal of estradiol (and possibly inhibin).

In a classic 28-day menstrual cycle, a follicle has been selected and is dominant by cycle day 7 (Fig. 14-1). The dominant follicle is the principal source of estradiol during the remainder of the follicular phase. The oocyte matures within the dominant follicle as it approaches ovulation. Estradiol is also a major part of the feedback signal to the hypothalamus/pituitary that triggers a bolus release of gonadotropin—the LH/FSH surge. The LH surge leads to final follicular maturation events, the resumption of meiosis in the oocyte, and ovulation. Ovulation occurs 36 to 48 hours after initiation of the LH surge.

After ovulation, the follicle undergoes a rapid metamorphosis into a corpus luteum. The principal secretory product of the corpus luteum is progesterone. Progesterone feeds back on the arcuate nucleus and modifies the secretion of GnRH into the infrequent pattern that is appropriate for the

OVARIAN FOLLICULAR DEVELOPMENT

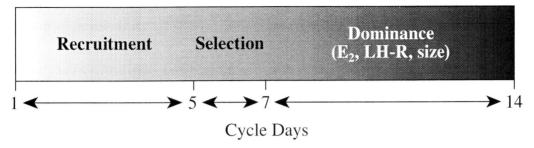

FIGURE 14-1. The ovarian follicle that is destined to ovulate undergoes recruitment and selection during the first 7 days of the menstrual cycle. Cycle days 7 to 14 the selected dominant follicle undergoes maturation before ovulation.

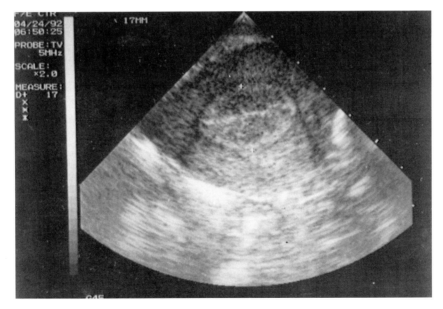

FIGURE 14-2. Transvaginal ultrasound of uterus. Uterine cavity is in the center of the image and appears as a trilaminar image. The center of the three stripes is the endometrial cavity and the outer two stripes are the basalis myometrial junctions.

luteal phase. This luteal secretion pattern of GnRH causes less frequent but relatively larger LH pulses from the pituitary that, in turn, stimulate progesterone secretion from the corpus luteum. With the demise of the corpus luteum, the arcuate nucleus returns to a rapid follicular-phase GnRH secretion pattern, the intercycle FSH rise occurs, and a new cycle begins.

While the hypothalamus-pituitary-ovary system is interacting in this complex loop of stimulus-response-feedback, the endometrium is receiving its own set of signals from the ovary. In the follicular phase, estradiol causes a profound growth response in the uterine lining (Fig. 14-2). Through concentrated mitotic activity, the residual endometrium of the basalis layer grows several millimeters thick. With the advent of progesterone secretion in the second half of the cycle, the endometrium undergoes maturational changes preparing for potential implantation. The endometrial glands (apocrine) become tortuous and convoluted and secrete glycogen. The stroma at first becomes edematous and then undergoes a decidual reaction. If no implantation occurs, estradiol and progesterone levels fall, and this "overripe" uterine lining sloughs. The sloughing of the endometrium (menses) is actually the beginning of the next menstrual cycle. This steroid hormone–induced withdrawal flow is self-limited because the uterus has intrinsic hemostatic mechanisms and the stimulus of estradiol during the next cycle also leads to a rapid repair response.

PRIMARY AMENORRHEA
General Principles and Common Causes

There are several simple etiologic clues readily available on first encountering a patient with primary amenorrhea. These are physical clues that are apparent even before a complete physical examination. For instance, mature breast development (Tanner stages 4 or 5, Fig. 14-3) requires an intact hypothalamic-pituitary-gonadal axis and a normal chromosome complement. Therefore the presence of normal breast development in primary amenorrhea points to a probable uterine-vaginal problem as the most likely cause. The contrary is also helpful; a lack of mature breast development leads one to suspect hypothalamic/pituitary or gonadal disease as the likely cause of the patient's primary amenorrhea. A second etiologic clue is obtained by noting the patient's stature. If she is of short stature (less than 5 feet tall) and past the age of 14 years, one can reasonably expect to find a sex chromosome anomaly or hypopituitarism as the cause of her delayed menarche. It is also important to realize that ordinarily adrenarche and the early stages of thelarche occur secondary to only adrenal hormone secretion. Therefore small amounts (stage 2 or 3 of breast or pubic hair development, Figs. 14-3 and 14-4) of secondary sexual development are

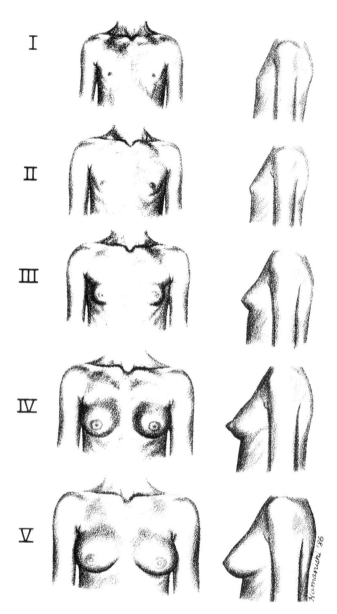

FIGURE 14-3. The Tanner stages of breast development (I through V) are illustrated.

(Redrawn from Marshall WA, Tanner JM: *Arch Dis Child* 44:291, 1969.)

I   II   III

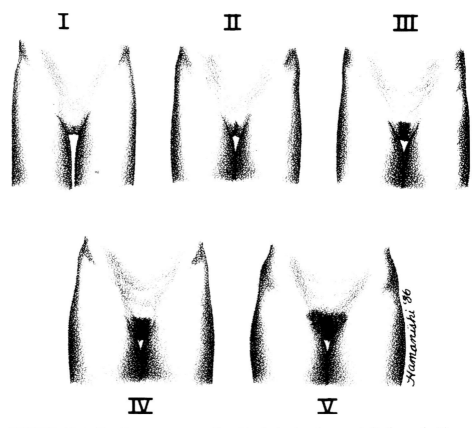

IV   V

FIGURE 14-4. The Tanner stages of pubic hair development (I through V) are illustrated.

(Redrawn from Marshall WA, Tanner JM: *Arch Dis Child* 44:291, 1969.)

usually found in most primary amenorrhea patients even if they have gonadal failure.

It is helpful to consider which diagnoses are most common among patients with primary amenorrhea. Gonadal dysgenesis (and all its variant forms with many possible sex chromosome aberrations) is the single most common cause of primary amenorrhea. Müllerian (uterovaginal) anomalies are the next most frequent group. Hypothalamic/pituitary causes (which vary from congenital central nervous system defects to isolated gonadotropin deficiency) are individually rare but as a group are relatively common. The next most common is constitutional delay, where primary amenorrhea results from an immature hypothalamic-pituitary axis. Constitutional delay is the most common of the hypothalamic-pituitary etiologies. It is a "rule-out" diagnosis that is present when all other known causes for

TABLE 14-1. Common causes of primary amenorrhea

Cause	Frequency (%)
Gonadal dysgenesis	33
Müllerian anomalies	20
Hypothalamic/pituitary	15
Constitutional delay	10
Other	22

hypothalamic-pituitary disease have been excluded. Table 14-1 lists these common causes with approximate percentages indicated.

Table 14-2 lists most of the known causes of primary amenorrhea. This outline is divided into six main divisions (subheadings) that group together similar diseases. The disease states that can result in primary amenorrhea are generally one of two types. The first type includes those diseases that occur early in life, are intrinsic diseases of the reproductive system, and usually cause primary amenorrhea. Examples of this first type of disease would be congenital hypopituitarism, gonadal dysgenesis, and müllerian agenesis. The second type consists of those diseases that can occur at any time in one's life span, can involve the reproductive system, and may cause primary amenorrhea if they happen to affect the individual before her menarche. Examples of the second type of disease would be pituitary adenomas, onset of a debilitating systemic disease, and anorexia nervosa. Obviously, this second category of diseases includes most of the maladies known to cause secondary amenorrhea.

Evaluation

A complete history and physical examination are extremely important elements in the evaluation of a young woman with primary amenorrhea. It is crucial to obtain a good history of growth and development. A well-kept pediatric growth chart is invaluable here. Even if a growth chart is not available, historical clues about the growth spurt are available: Over a span of about 1 year, did the child outgrow all of her clothes? Obviously, it is important to ask questions about puberty. Has breast and pubic hair development begun? If so, how far has it advanced? As part of the physical examination, it is important to accurately record the height, weight, and arm span. Remember to check for the common anomalies associated with gonadal dysgenesis: neck folds, setting of the ears and hairline, chest configuration, whether the fourth metacarpal is short, and cubitis valgus. For both breast and pubic hair development, grade the degree of development according to the Marshall-Tanner stages. For reference, these are indicated in Figs. 14-3 and 14-4.

TABLE 14-2. Etiology of primary amenorrhea

Central nervous system (general)

Infection
  Encephalitis
  Meningitis
Neoplasm
  Craniopharyngioma
  Glioma
  Pineal tumor
Congenital anomalies
  Hydrocephaly
  Sellar malformation

Hypothalamic

Infection
  Tuberculosis (granuloma)
  Syphilis (gumma)
Inflammatory
  Sarcoidosis (granuloma)
Neoplasm
  Craniopharyngioma
  Midline teratoma
Syndromes
  Kallman's syndrome
  Fröhlich's syndrome
  Bardet-Biedl syndrome
Tumor
  Hamartoma
  Hand-Schüller-Christian disease
Congenital anomaly
  Idiopathic hypogonadotropic hypogonadism
Constitutional delay
Hypothalamic hyperprolactinemia

Pituitary

Neoplasm
  Adenoma
    Lactotrophic
    Cushing's disease
    Acromegaly
    Chromophobe
  Idiopathic (congenital) hypopituitarism—partial or complete
Space-occupying lesion
  Arterial aneurysm
  Empty sella
Inflammatory
  Sarcoidosis
Infiltrative
  Hemachromatosis
    Idiopathic
    Congenital anemia (e.g., thalassemia)
Trauma

TABLE 14-2. Etiology of primary amenorrhea—cont'd

Gonadal

Gonadal dysgenesis
  Turner's syndrome
  Pure gonadal dysgenesis
  Mixed gonadal dysgenesis
  XX gonadal dysgenesis
  XY gonadal dysgenesis (Swyer's syndrome)
Insensitive ovary
  Resistant ovary—Savage's syndrome
  Afollicular ovary
    Idiopathic—premature aging
    Injury (e.g., radiation, chemotherapy)
    Autoimmune disease
    Infection (e.g., mumps oophoritis)
    Infiltrative—mucopolysaccharidosis
Gonadal agenesis
  Anorchia (early, late)
  Ovarian agenesis
    Idiopathic
    Surgical
Ovarian tumor
  Androgen-producing
True hermaphroditism

Uterine-vaginal

Müllerian agenesis (Rokitansky's syndrome)
Vaginal agenesis—isolated
Cervical agenesis—isolated
Vaginal septum—transverse
Imperforate hymen
Asherman's syndrome—infectious

General conditions

Endocrinopathy
Thyroid disease
  Hypothyroidism
  Hyperthyroidism
Adrenal disease
  Cushing's syndrome
  Congenital adrenal hyperplasia
  Adrenal androgen tumor
Androgen excess syndrome
  Polycystic ovarian disease
  Exogenous androgen therapy
Male pseudohermaphroditism
  Androgen insensitivity syndromes
  Androgen biosynthetic defects
Estrogen biosynthetic defects

Continued.

TABLE 14-2.   Etiology of primary amenorrhea—cont'd

Systemic disease (severe)

Examples
  Crohn's disease
  Hepatic failure
  Glomerulonephritis
  Systemic lupus erythematosus

Nutritional problem

Generalized malnutrition (moderate to severe)
Weight fluctuations—acute

Psychiatric disease

Anorexia nervosa
Psychosis

Miscellaneous conditions

Exercise induced
Stress-related

The pelvic examination should be gentle but thorough. It is most important to determine whether a vagina and uterus are present and whether there are any adnexal masses. The presence of a cervix at the end of the vaginal canal is sufficient evidence for the presence of a uterus. Vaginal mucosa that has not been exposed to estrogen is somewhat erythematous because estrogen causes thickening of the skin and vaginal rugation. If clear cervical mucus is present in the cervical os, that is a good indication for the presence of estrogen. Sometimes, in the office setting, it is feasible to perform a rectal examination only if the young woman is particularly squeamish about a pelvic examination. A rectal examination is fully capable of ascertaining the presence and size of a uterus. Remember to check the sense of smell as part of the physical examination. Common, easily recognized odors are recommended (e.g., tobacco, ground coffee, soap flakes). First cranial nerve function directly relates to the diagnosis of congenital hypothalamic GnRH deficiency (Kallman's syndrome).

There is a myriad of possible diagnostic tests when it comes to the laboratory evaluation of amenorrhea. One approach that is sometimes taken (but is not recommended) is the "shotgun" approach. Clinicians who practice in this manner order a wide number and spectrum of laboratory tests in the hope of finding one or several that are abnormal. This approach not only wastes time and money, but more often than not, it leads to confusion. The recommended approach is to order a select number of laboratory tests based on the impression formed from the history and physical examination. Once these focused tests have been ordered and

TABLE 14-3. Diagnostic tests for amenorrhea

Hypothalamic-pituitary compartment

Serum hormone levels: LH, FSH, TSH, prolactin, growth hormone, AM and PM cortisol
Dynamic tests: GnRH, TRH, and CRH challenge tests; insulin tolerance test; water deprivation test
Imaging: lateral skull film, CT scan or MRI of the pituitary and sella

Ovarian compartment

Serum hormone levels: LH, FSH, estradiol, progesterone
Diagnostic tests: progestin challenge
Imaging: pelvic ultrasound, dual-photon absorptiometry or DEXA, bone age (hand/wrist)
Other: karyotype (banded), ovarian antibody panel, ovarian biopsy, basal body temperature chart

Uterine-vaginal compartment

Serum hormone levels: human chorionic gonadotropin
Dynamic tests: estrogen plus progestin challenge test
Imaging: pelvic ultrasound, hysterosalpingogram, MRI
Other: endometrial biopsy

Additional tests of other organ systems

Serum hormone levels: testosterone, DHEAS, 3α-androstanediol glucuronide, 17-OH progesterone, thyroxine, T_3 uptake, carotene, insulin, glucose tolerance test
Dynamic tests: ACTH stimulation test, dexamethasone suppression test, TRH stimulation test
Imaging: adrenal CT scan, iodocholesterol scan, thyroid scan
Other: selective venous catheterization

ACTH, Adrenocorticotropic hormone; *CRH,* corticotropin-releasing hormone; *CT,* computed tomography; *DEXA,* dual-energy x-ray absorptiometry; *DHEAS,* dehydroepiandrosterone sulfate; *FSH,* follicle-stimulating hormone; *GnRH,* gonadotropin-releasing hormone; *LH,* luteinizing hormone; *MRI,* magnetic resonance imaging; *TRH,* thyrotropin-releasing hormone; *TSH,* thyroid-stimulating hormone.

---

interpreted, the diagnosis is usually apparent. If the diagnosis is not clear at that time, the patient could be referred to a subspecialist (reproductive endocrinologist). It sometimes takes several clinic visits and several series of tests to finally diagnose the cause of a given patient's amenorrhea. However, in most primary amenorrhea cases, only one set of laboratory tests is required for an accurate diagnosis.

Table 14-3 lists most of the possible laboratory tests that are used for making a diagnosis of amenorrhea. In most cases it is necessary to perform only a select few. The list divides the tests according to the different anatomic compartments, the function of which they are designed to assess. Some of the tests are simple and readily available; other tests are complex and available only through subspecialists at major medical centers. Because some of the tests will not be familiar to every reader, a brief explanation of some of them follows.

Low gonadotropin levels (FSH and LH < 5 mIU/ml) indicate that the hypothalamic/pituitary compartment is nonfunctional; high levels (>40 mIU/ml) indicate that there is gonadal failure when they are elevated into the menopausal range. Therefore gonadotropin levels are helpful in isolating the problem to these two different compartments. When assessing anterior pituitary hormone function by serum levels, there generally is not a readily available radioimmunoassay for adrenocorticotropic hormone (ACTH). Therefore when it is pertinent to assess ACTH function cortisol levels are usually obtained at 7:00 AM and 7:00 PM to check for normal diurnal variation in ACTH secretion. Pituitary dynamic tests are usually performed when initial tests indicate that the patient may have complete or partial hypopituitarism. These tests are complex and usually performed under the direction of a reproductive endocrinologist as an inpatient procedure. Computed tomography (CT) and magnetic resonance imaging (MRI) of the pituitary and sella are essentially equal tests to diagnose pituitary microadenoma, and a plain lateral sella film can be used in selected cases to rule out a macroadenoma (which will invariably enlarge the sella turcica).

In the ovarian compartment, a progesterone challenge test is a basic and helpful test. Either oral medroxyprogesterone acetate (10 mg/day for 5 days) or progesterone in oil (100 mg intramuscular) can be administered, with the onset of menses expected within 1 week of the last dose. When this progesterone challenge test is positive, it indicates that there is sufficient hypothalamic pituitary and ovarian function to promote sufficient estradiol secretion to stimulate the endometrial lining to a proliferative level. A positive progesterone challenge test finding indicates that there is only partial suppression of the system and less severe amenorrhea is present. When a patient is hypoestrogenic with a negative progesterone challenge finding, it is often important to assess bone density to check for osteoporosis. Bone density can be best assessed by dual-energy x-ray absorptiometry (DEXA) or a quantitative CT scan of the spine. The newer DEXA machines are quick (3 to 5 minutes), and the total radiation exposure is about 10 mREM (one tenth the dose of a chest x-ray). The best place to look initially for osteoporosis is the trabecular bone of the lumbar spine. A banded karyotype is an expensive but key laboratory test for the diagnosis of primary amenorrhea.

The uterine/vaginal compartment can be easily and economically tested by a 30-day exposure to estrogen (conjugated estrogen, 1.25 mg/day or equivalent) combined with progestin (medroxyprogesterone acetate, 10 mg/day) for the last 10 to 14 days. If the endometrial lining is capable of responding, the patient will have some degree of uterine withdrawal bleeding after this challenge. The most straightforward test to assess the endometrial cavity other than the hormone challenge test is a hysterosalpingogram.

In the evaluation of amenorrhea, it is often necessary to test other endocrine systems. The most common tests in this area are for androgen excess. A serum testosterone level assesses both the ovary and the adrenal, and a serum dehydroepiandrosterone sulfate (DHEAS) level gives a strong indication of the level of testosterone secretion from only the adrenal gland. A 3α-androstanediol-glucuronide (3α-diol-G), serum level (a metabolite of dihydrotestosterone) gives a good indication of the level of androgen activity at the pilosebaceous end organ in the skin. A 17-hydroxyprogesterone serum level will assess for mild forms of congenital adrenal hyperplasia that usually do not become apparent until after puberty.

Some diagnoses of primary amenorrhea are evident at the end of the history and physical examination; usually, however, the diagnosis is not evident at this point, and selected laboratory tests or imaging studies are necessary in order to move from a clinical impression to a diagnosis. The clinician must form a logical laboratory evaluation plan at this time based on the clinical impression. The basis for the formulation of this plan is the degree of breast development and the presence or absence of müllerian structures. This proven clinical method for the diagnosis of primary amenorrhea based on the degree of breast development and the presence of müllerian structures enables a practitioner to focus his or her diagnostic tests. For the purpose of this system, if breast development is indicated as a plus sign it refers to stage 4 or 5 development. (This degree of development is present only when there has been a functioning gonad.) When the müllerian structures are indicated with a plus sign, this indicates that a uterus/vagina was present on pelvic examination. The clinical usefulness of this system will be illustrated here by reviewing a series of cases.

Breast development negative, uterus/vagina positive. Patients with findings of minimal breast development and the presence of a uterus/vagina (Fig. 14-5) tend to have little (if any) secondary sexual development. They may have breast budding (stage 2 or 3) and some pubic hair, but sexual development is not advanced. On pelvic examination they clearly have a uterus and a vagina, but these young women demonstrate no estrogen effects; the uterus is hypoplastic, and the vaginal epithelium is thin and not rugated. In this situation such patients have had little (if any) gonadal function. Either there is a central nervous system defect wherein the gonads are not being stimulated (hypogonadotropic – case A), or the gonads are not present or nonfunctional (hypergonadotropic – case B). Therefore determination of a serum level of LH and FSH indicates whether the hypoestrogenism is either gonadal or hypothalamic/pituitary in etiology.

When the LH and FSH levels are low (hypogonadotropism), the cause of the primary amenorrhea is whatever disease or condition is suppressing the hypothalamic/pituitary axis. It is not necessary in the hypogonadotropic group to obtain a karyotype; if determined, it would be 46XX. A wide variety

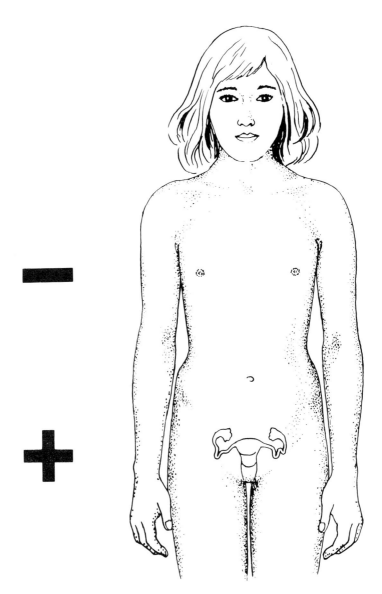

FIGURE 14-5. A drawing of a young woman that illustrates minimal breast development (stages 1 or 2); a vagina and uterus are present on pelvic examination.

of tests are available to evaluate the central nervous system (see Table 14-3). While testing the hypothalamic/pituitary unit it is also important to determine whether any level of gonadal function is present. This is most easily determined by a progesterone challenge test, a bone age test, and a serum estradiol level test.

Case A. Table 14-4 illustrates the use of this diagnostic scheme for a young woman with minimal breast development who has an immature

TABLE 14-4. Primary amenorrhea, case A: diagnostic tests

First visit

Bone age (left hand and wrist): 15 years
Estradiol: 24 pg/ml
   Normal values: follicular phase, 20=100 pg/ml
LH: 3 mIU/ml; FSH: 2 mIU/ml
   Normal values: LH, 5-20 mIU/ml; FSH, 4-16 mIU/ml
Progesterone challenge test: no withdrawal flow

Second visit

Lateral skull x-ray: normal anatomy of sella turcica
Growth hormone: 6 ng/ml
   Normal values: 0.5-13.0 ng/ml
Cortisol: 14 μg/dl
   Normal values: 0700-0900 hr, 9-24 μg/dl; 1600-1800 hr, 2-14
   μg/dl
Prolactin: 5 ng/ml
   Normal values: 0-20 ng/ml
TSH: 5 μIU/ml
   Normal values: 0.4-5.0 μIU/ml

LH, Luteinizing hormone; *FSH,* follicle-stimulating hormone; *TSH,* thyroid-stimulating hormone.

uterus/vagina. This 18-year-old woman with primary amenorrhea had a bone age immature for her age (Fig. 14-6), a low estradiol level, and no withdrawal bleeding to 100 mg progesterone-in-oil administered intramuscularly. Her gonadotropin levels were low as well. These tests all indicate that she did not have gonadal function secondary to a lack of ovarian stimulation by the hypothalamic/pituitary unit. The other baseline pituitary hormone levels, other than the gonadotropins, were normal as indicated. The patient was then given a GnRH challenge test of 100 μg of subcutaneous GnRH with essentially no change in her LH and FSH levels over a period of 2 hours after this injection. She was then "primed" with GnRH by using an intermittent pump that administered intravenous GnRH at a dose of 2.5 μg every 90 minutes for 7 days. At the end of that 7-day period of time, she was given a second 100-μg subcutaneous GnRH challenge test. There still was no response of serum LH and FSH over a period of 120 minutes (Fig. 14-7). Therefore this patient had isolated hypogonadotropic hypogonadism or partial hypopituitarism involving the gonadotropic axis only. She requires cyclic estrogen-progestin replacement therapy until she wishes to conceive, at which time she will require exogenous gonadotropin treatment.

    The second group of patients in this category (minimal breast development, uterus/vagina present, see Fig. 14-5) with hypergonadotropism (elevated LH and FSH serum levels) have gonadal failure. A banded karyotype is necessary to further delineate their problem. Often, the karyotype will reveal an X-chromosome abnormality. With an X-chromosome abnormality, the patients have gonadal dysgenesis, the gonads are streaks, and no opera-

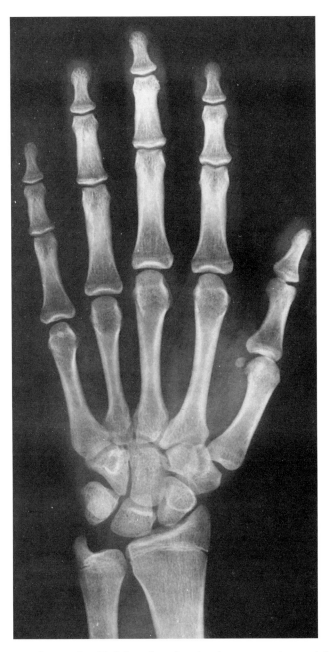

FIGURE 14-6. Radiograph of left hand and wrist demonstrating epiphyseal fusion as found in a normal 15-year-old girl.

tive procedure is necessary. In any patient with gonadal dysgenesis, it is important to perform special tests (e.g., chest x-ray, electrocardiogram [ECG], intravenous pyelogram, thyroid functions) in search of problems in other organ systems commonly associated with this diagnosis. When the hypergonadotropic patient has a 46XY karyotype, an operative procedure

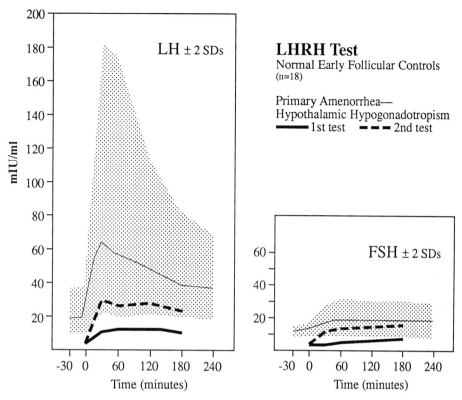

FIGURE 14-7. Gonadotropin-releasing hormone (luteinizing hormone–releasing hormone) stimulation test in an 18-year-old woman with primary amenorrhea. She received 100 μg GnRH subcutaneously with essentially no response at the time of her first test. A week later she received a second 100-μg GnRH test dose after undergoing intermittent priming with GnRH and still had essentially no response of LH or FSH.

with gonadal extirpation is necessary. When there is a normal 46XX karyotype, it is necessary to perform an operative procedure, visualize the gonads, and perhaps perform a biopsy if the gonad is any larger than a classic streak. This biopsy is usually best performed through a small laparotomy incision to ensure adequate tissue for diagnosis. The histologic determination will check for the presence of follicles and leukocytic or other types of infiltration. However, the most likely finding on ovarian biopsy is ovarian stroma with no primordial follicles.

Case B. A case example of an evaluation in a 17-year-old woman with minimal breast development, a uterus and vagina present, and elevated levels of LH and FSH is illustrated in Table 14-5. The karyotype in this patient was 46XY, but the testosterone level was in the low female range. The presence of a functional uterus was confirmed by the estrogen-progestin challenge test. At the time of laparoscopy and exploratory laparotomy, there was no gonad present in the inguinal canal or the abdominal cavity. This

TABLE 14-5.   Primary amenorrhea, case B: diagnostic tests

First visit

Bone age: 13-14 years
LH: 37 mIU/ml; FSH: 81 mIU/ml
  Normal values: LH, 5-20 mIU/ml; FSH, 4-16 mIU/ml
Progesterone challenge test: no withdrawal flow

Second visit

Estradiol: <20 pg/ml
  Normal values: follicular phase, 20-100 pg/ml
Karyotype: 46XY
Testosterone: 38 ng/dl
  Normal values: 20-70 ng/dl
Estrogen and progestin challenge test: normal withdrawal flow

---

LH, Luteinizing hormone; *FSH*, follicle-stimulating hormone.

was a case example of anorchia, or the "vanishing testes" syndrome. The fact that a uterus and vagina were present indicates that the testes vanished before 9 weeks of gestation. (It is at approximately 9 weeks that müllerian inhibitory factor (MIF) is secreted.) There would be no uterus/vagina if MIF had been secreted. This woman needed no reconstructive surgery but will need lifelong estrogen and progestin replacement.

Breast development positive, uterus/vagina positive. Patients with breast development (stage 4 to 5) and a uterus would be expected to achieve menarche (see Fig. 14-8). That is, they have the müllerian tissue to respond to estrogen, and the degree of breast development documents a moderate amount of gonadal function. The types of medical problems that lead to primary amenorrhea in this group are generally those disorders that have occurred once puberty is well advanced. Several laboratory tests are helpful to sort out the disorders in this group. A karyotype will pick up the milder forms of gonadal dysgenesis that will rarely allow some gonadal function and mature breast development. A bone age determination is used to further determine the extent of estrogen exposure. The determination of LH and FSH levels does not establish a diagnosis for any of the diseases in this group, but it will help support many of the diagnoses. For instance, women with stress or weight loss amenorrhea, if severe, would have low gonadotropin levels. The androgen-excess states with elevated testosterone or increased levels of other androgens belong in this group (e.g., polycystic ovarian disease). These patients usually (but not always) demonstrate hirsutism or other signs of androgen excess. If the patient has an onset of hyperprolactinemia later in puberty, she will be in this group as well (although she may not have galactorrhea). The elevated prolactin concentration could be secondary to any of the known causes of hyperprolactinemia.

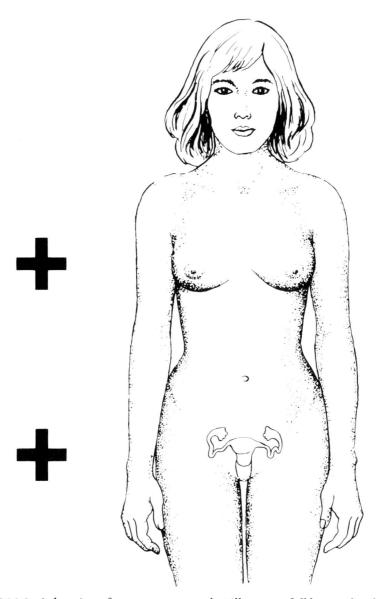

FIGURE 14-8. A drawing of a young woman that illustrates full breast development (stages 4 or 5); a vagina and uterus are present on pelvic examination.

Once these five tests have been obtained, the diagnosis is usually apparent.

Case C. An example of a clinical case in this category is presented in Table 14-6. A 19-year-old student had primary amenorrhea. Over the past several years she had purposely dieted for fear of excess weight gain. She was a compulsive individual who had an outstanding scholastic record and was involved in many social activities. She achieved full adult breast development at approximately 14 years of age but never had a menstrual

TABLE 14-6. Primary amenorrhea, case C: diagnostic tests

First visit
Bone age: 15 years
LH: <2 mIU/ml; FSH: 3 mIU/ml
Normal values: LH, 5-20 mIU/ml; FSH, 4-16 mIU/ml
Prolactin: 6 ng/ml
Normal values: 0-20 ng/ml
Progesterone challenge test: no withdrawal flow
Second visit
Cortisol: 19 μg/dl
Normal values: 0700-0900 hr, 9-24 μg/dl; 1600-1800 hr 2-14 μg/dl
Growth hormone: 12 ng/ml
Normal values: 0.5-13.0 ng/ml
Estradiol: <20 pg/ml
Normal values: follicular phase, 20-100 pg/ml
Estrogen-progestin challenge test: positive withdrawal flow
Lateral skull x-ray: normal sella turcica anatomy

LH, Luteinizing hormone; *FSH*, follicle-stimulating hormone.

period. Her weight loss began about the same time. On physical examination, she was 66 in. tall and weighed 103 lb (her ideal body weight is 124 lb). She had a small hypoplastic uterus on pelvic examination. Her bone age was immature. Her LH and FSH levels were low, and therefore no karyotype was necessary because she did not have ovarian failure. She failed to withdraw to progesterone-in-oil (100 mg intramuscularly), but did have a menstrual period when given a full month of oral estrogen with progestin added the last 2 weeks. Interestingly enough, the referring physician had obtained serum levels of cortisol and growth hormone, both of which were elevated. This patient has psychogenic weight loss amenorrhea (she was 17% below her ideal body weight and therefore does not meet the criteria of 25% weight loss for the diagnosis of anorexia nervosa). The psychopathology intervened about the time of her expected menarche. Her hypothalamic-pituitary-ovarian/müllerian axis was anatomically normal. She simply had a disease state that occurred during her puberty that led to primary amenorrhea. Primary therapy in this case would be psychiatric, but estrogen plus progestin cyclic therapy would be appropriate during the interim.

Breast development positive, uterus/vagina negative. Patients with normal breast development but no uterus or vagina (Fig. 14-9), have a completely normal puberty until they fail to achieve a menarche. On pelvic examination, the vaginal depth is rarely more than 1 to 2 cm. There are two diagnostic possibilities with this presentation: müllerian agenesis (Roki-

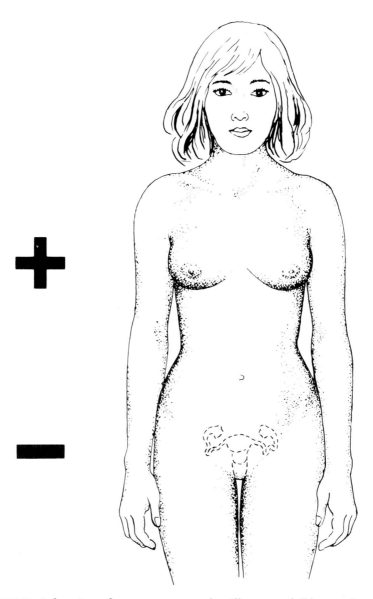

FIGURE 14-9. A drawing of a young woman that illustrates full breast development (stages 4 or 5); absence of vagina and uterus on pelvic examination.

tansky's syndrome) or androgen insensitivity (testicular feminization syndrome). A testosterone level and a karyotype determination distinguish these two entities. In androgen insensitivity, the karyotype is 46XY, and the testosterone level is in the male range (300 to 1200 ng/dl). Patients with androgen insensitivity syndrome have some unique and obvious features: large breasts with immature nipples, no axillary or pubic hair, and possibly gonads in the inguinal canal. The karyotype in müllerian agenesis is 46XX,

TABLE 14-7.   Primary amenorrhea, case D: diagnostic tests

First visit

Testosterone: 64 ng/dl
  Normal values: 20-70 ng/dl
Estradiol: 183 pg/ml
  Normal values: follicular phase, 20-100 pg/ml
Karyotype: 46XX

Second visit

Intravenous pyelogram: unilateral renal agenesis

and the testosterone is in the normal female range (20 to 70 ng/dl). Women with müllerian agenesis have normal pubic hair and mature nipples.

Case D. Table 14-7 illustrates a case in this category. This 17-year-old woman had primary amenorrhea. She was of normal stature (66 in., 133 lb). Her thelarche began at 9 years of age and adrenarche at age 10. She achieved complete breast and pubic hair development by 14 years of age. When her family physician was consulted because she had no menstrual periods at 15 years of age, she was given only tacit reassurance. At 16 years of age she was given medroxyprogesterone acetate (10 mg orally for 5 days) without withdrawal menses. She had never had more than a cursory pelvic examination. At the current visit she was noted to have normal female external genitalia except for the vagina, which was only a 2-cm blind pouch. On rectal examination no uterine or müllerian structures could be palpated. Her testosterone was in the famale range, her karyotype was normal, and the estradiol level definitely indicated ovarian function. She had müllerian agenesis (Rokitansky-Kuster-Hauser-Mayer syndrome). An intravenous pyelogram noted that she had a hypertophied left kidney and an absent right kidney (associated renal anomalies occur in 40% to 50% of women with müllerian agenesis) (Fig. 14-10). At the appropriate time, therapy would consist of progressive vaginal dilation or a McIndoe vaginoplasty that incorporates a split-thickness skin graft as a neovagina.

Breast development negative, uterus/vagina negative. This combination of physical findings (lack of both breast development and uterus/vagina, see Fig. 14-11) in patients with primary amenorrhea is rare. The lack of breast development indicates gonadal failure, and the lack of müllerian structures would indicate MIF activity from testes. Both diseases in this category are associated with elevated gonadotropin levels and gonadal failure in 46XY males. (LH and FSH levels and a karyotype are the recommended diagnostic tests.) The first possible disease entity is anorchia (loss of the testes after MIF activity but before testosterone production). At laparotomy no gonad would be present. The second possible disease entity is a

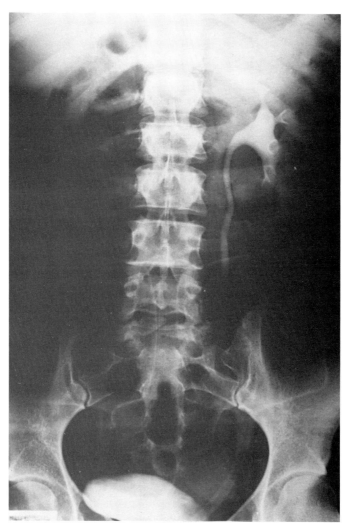

FIGURE 14-10. A radiograph of an intravenous pyelogram demonstrating hypertrophied left kidney and absence of right kidney in a woman with müllerian agenesis.

testosterone biosynthetic defect in which there is an enzyme block early in the steroid biosynthetic pathway and the testes are present but located in the abdominal cavity.

Breast development positive, uterus/vagina? Young women in this category have clearly normal secondary sexual development, but there is confusion after completion of the pelvic examination as to whether müllerian tissue is present (see Fig. 14-12). The normal breast development indicates a normally functioning gonad but not necessarily an ovary. At this point it is best to document the chromosomal sex (karyotype) of such a patient. In addition, this is the time to incorporate selected radiographic,

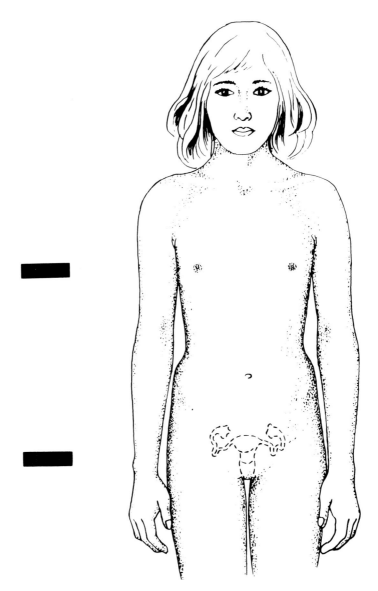

FIGURE 14-11. A drawing of a young woman that illustrates minimal breast development (stages 1 or 2); absence of vagina and uterus on pelvic examination.

endoscopic, and operative procedures that are collectively capable of sorting out the existence and extent of müllerian structures. The disease states that fall into this category are imperforate hymen, complete transverse vaginal septum, partial vaginal agenesis, cervical aplasia, and true hermaphroditism. Generally, these patients require operative treatment by a gynecologic surgeon. These disease entities usually have active

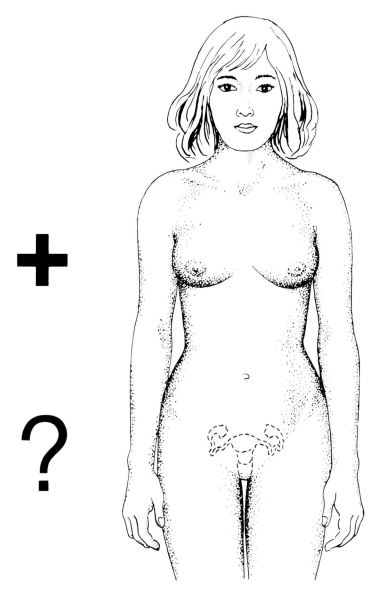

FIGURE 14-12. A drawing of a young woman that illustrates full breast development (stages 4 or 5); on pelvic examination it is unclear whether a vagina and/or uterus is present.

endometrium and outflow obstruction, so the patient is at risk for the development of endometriosis.

Case E. Table 14-8 illustrates such a case. This young woman was evaluated at 14 years of age (earlier than the usual age cutoff recommended for a primary amenorrhea evaluation) because of pelvic pain. The pelvic examination noted a tender adnexal mass that was determined to be cystic

TABLE 14-8.   Primary amenorrhea, case E: diagnostic tests

First visit

Karyotype: 46XX

Ultrasound: 3 × 4–cm cystic mass in the right ovary with diffuse internal echoes

Second visit

Ca-125: 77 U/ml
  Normal values: 0-35 U/ml

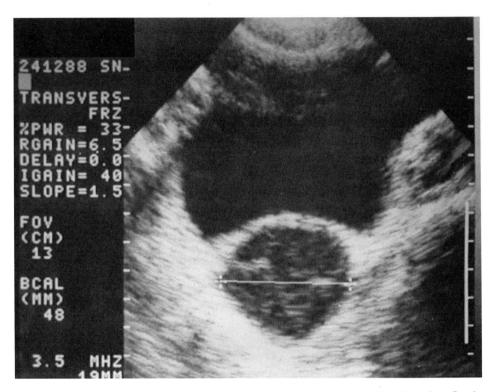

FIGURE 14-13. Transabdominal ultrasound revealing a round unilocular fluid-filled mass with central echoes in the vicinity of the cervix. This woman had partial vaginal agenesis, and the mass was a distal hematocolpos.

with internal echoes on ultrasound examination (Fig. 14-13). The CA-125 (an ovarian carcinoma tumor antigen) level was compatible with endometriosis. The diagnosis was not completely established until laparotomy, at which time the mass was determined to be a distal hematocolpos, and the patient was found to have partial vaginal agenesis.

SECONDARY AMENORRHEA
History

It cannot be emphasized enough that the medical history is extremely important to the diagnosis of secondary amenorrhea. The ages at which the patient realized her pubertal milestones should be noted (e.g., Did she achieve her menarche at a normal age?) Once menstrual function was established, what was her cycle regularity? Regular menstrual cycles are those that occur between 21 and 35 days. There is no established normal duration of menstrual flow, but it should be generally constant month to month. The presence of cycle regularity leads to a strong presumption of ovulation. Symptoms that indicate probable ovulation are brief episodes of unilateral midcycle pain (mittelschmerz) and a potpourri of subjective premenstrual symptoms (e.g., bloating) that indicate the imminent onset of menses. It is important to ascertain when and how the patient deviated from her prior menstrual cyclicity. Did the cycles cease abruptly, or did she experience cycle irregularity for a period of time leading up to the cessation of menses? It should be established whether or not the patient has ever been pregnant, as well as what the outcome was of any gestations. Does she currently or did she in the past use any contraception? Has she ever tested her fertility? Could she currently be pregnant? If any pregnancy events are historically close to the onset of her amenorrhea, it is pertinent to obtain further history in regard to delivery, the absence or presence of postpartum hemorrhage, and lactation.

It is important to seek information regarding the patient's general medical condition. Has she ever been admitted to a hospital or had any operations? Does she have any chronic disease (e.g., diabetes)? Is she currently taking any medications? Other questions should determine whether the patient has experienced the growth of cxccss body hair on the face, chest, abdomen, or upper portion of the back. Hirsutism (androgen excess) is a common cause of secondary amenorrhea and is usually associated with increased sebaceous activity of the skin (acne). Another important set of questions has to do with the presence or absence of breast milk (galactorrhea). Slight, even unilateral, galactorrhea is significant if it is persistent. If there is a question of whether breast fluid is actually milk or some other secretion, a Sudan stain can be performed by mixing a drop of stain with a drop of the breast fluid and examining this mixture under low power. The presence of fat droplets indicates milk. The potential for thyroid disease is also important to cover in the history. (Note: most thyroid diseases are more common in women.) Questions regarding weight changes, skin texture, energy level, bowel habits, and temperature tolerance are pertinent for potential thyroid symptomatology. Also, remember to inquire about a family history of thyroid disease. A general family history of secondary amenorrhea is relevant but not of primary importance.

Social habits are pertinent to the diagnosis of secondary amenorrhea. The patient's habits in regard to exercise and eating are extremely relevant. Amenorrhea is common (about 40%) in female athletes. The prevalence of amenorrhea increases with the intensity and duration of exercise. Eating habits and weight changes can affect menstrual function. Being underweight or overweight is detrimental to normal menstrual function. An acute weight change in either direction can suppress the menstrual cycle even if the patient remains in her normal weight range. Psychosocial stress is another known cause of secondary amenorrhea that can be secondary to occupation, lifestyle, extrinsic life events, and so on. Therefore never skip the social habits section of the medical history in patients with amenorrhea.

Physical Examination

The vital signs are extremely important in the physical examination of a woman with amenorrhea. Her height and weight should be noted and related to either a table that indicates normal averages (e.g., Metropolitan Life Tables) or a calculated ideal body weight (IBW) (IBW [lb; cb = 100 + 4 [height in inches − 60]). The resting pulse should be noted as well because it will be either slow in patients with hypothyroidism or fast in patients with hyperthyroidism. The blood pressure (BP) should be carefully noted because this can be an indication of certain androgen excess states and other endocrinopathies (e.g., Cushing's syndrome). The skin should be carefully examined for acne and hirsutism. If hirsutism is noted, it should be scored according to an objective rating system (Fig. 14-14). Another important aspect in regard to the skin is the pigmentation. Women who ingest a large amount of vitamin A and have elevated levels of serum carotene will have an orange tinge to their skin that also involves the palms and soles. Elevated serum carotene levels are usually associated with being underweight and with peculiar dietary habits. A careful examination of the thyroid gland is important; determine the overall size and the presence or absence of nodularity. The degree of breast development should be noted because this indicates the completeness of puberty. The presence or absence of galactorrhea should always be noted. The abdominal examination is more important in terms of surface findings (e.g., the presence of a male pattern to the hair growth or striae). Of course, the pelvic examination is beneficial to the physical diagnosis of amenorrhea. The presence and degree of vaginal rugation (which is an indication of estrogen effect) should be noted on pelvic examination. A good indication of overall estrogen status is the cervical mucus—the

Hirsutism Classification

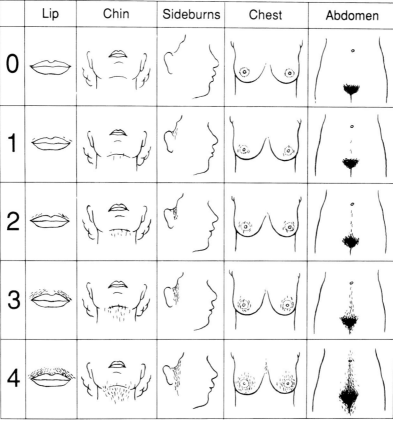

Adapted from Thomas and Ferriman, 1957

FIGURE 14-14. A scoring system for midline body hair that is useful in the clinic setting. The lip, chin, sideburns, chest, and abdomen are scored on a scale of 0 to 4 for the degree of hair growth. A score of 6 or more is abnormal and indicates the presence of hirsutism.

amount, stretchability (spinnbarkeit), and whether it will form a fern pattern when dried on a glass slide (Fig. 14-15). Estrogenized cervical mucus indicates some degree of ovarian activity, and the clinician can reasonably expect the patient to withdraw to a progesterone challenge. There are not many uterine causes of secondary amenorrhea that are apparent on pelvic examination. The only exception is a common but sometimes overlooked situation—pregnancy, wherein the uterus is soft and enlarged. The adnexal areas of the pelvis are often revealing in patients with amenorrhea. A unilateral ovarian enlargement can mean a virilizing or steroid hormone–producing tumor. Symmetrically enlarged ovaries usually indicate that the patient has polycystic ovarian disease, which can be a cause of amenorrhea, although most women with polycystic ovaries have oligomenorrhea. The deep tendon reflexes (DTRs) are pertinent to the diagnosis of amenorrhea. The patient's thyroid status can be ascertained by the briskness of the DTRs, with special attention given to the speed of the relaxation phase.

The proven clinical method for the diagnosis of secondary amenorrhea relies on a good history and physical examination with focused diagnostic tests that seek to compartmentalize the defect. As discussed previously, it is helpful to isolate the disease to the hypothalamic/pituitary, ovarian, or uterine/vaginal compartment. Once the etiology of a patient's amenorrhea has been isolated to a particular compartment, then the clinician can do some selective reading of the particular diagnosis if it is not already obvious. This diagnostic method will be illustrated with a series of case examples.

Hypothalamic/pituitary compartment

Case F. A 27-year-old G3, para (P)3 white female had a 5-year history of secondary amenorrhea. Her menarche was at age 14, and through high school her menstrual periods were every 28 to 30 days with 4 days of regular flow. She experienced menstrual irregularity her first 2 years of college with menstrual flow every 2 to 3 months; her last 2 years of college, she took oral contraceptives for contraceptive reasons and thereby resumed regular menstrual cycles. She discontinued oral contraceptive usage at 22 years of age and has had no further spontaneous menstrual periods. She has not experienced hot flashes but does have vaginal irritation with intercourse. She was using a diaphragm for contraception at that time. She consulted a physician for her amenorrhea problem on two occasions in the preceding 5 years; both times she received oral medroxyprogesterone acetate as a progesterone challenge, to which she had no withdrawal menses. There was no further workup. The remainder of her medical history is noncontributory. She was working 40 to 60 hours per week as a sales representative at the time of examination. She had lost 15 lb gradually over the previous 4 years. She had regular eating habits, denied bulimia, and followed no particular dietary pattern. She exercised daily, which consisted primarily of running 5 to 7 miles per day. On physical examination she was noted to be a thin, white female. She was 5 ft 5 in. tall and weighed 103 lb (IBW = 120 lb). Her skin was clear, and there was no hirsutism. Her thyroid was noted to be normal size with no nodularity present. Her breasts were stage 5 development without masses or galactorrhea. On pelvic examination the vagina had normal rugation and no cervical mucus. The uterus was nulliparous in size, and there were no adnexal masses. Her DTRs were brisk with a normal relaxation phase.

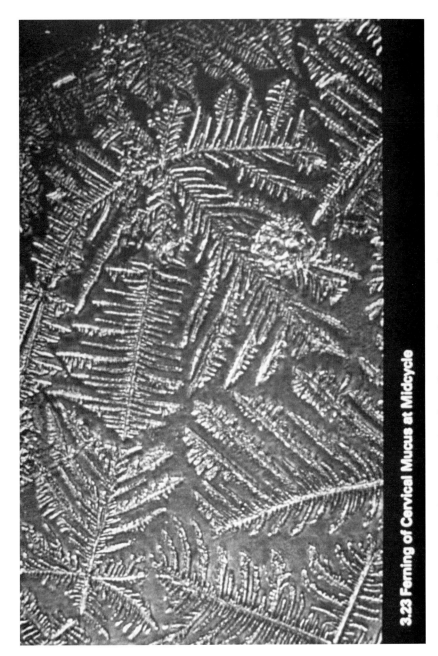

3.23 Ferning of Cervical Mucus at Midcycle

FIGURE 14-15. Cervical mucus under the influence of unopposed estrogen dries in a fernlike pattern on a microscope slide.

TABLE 14-9. Secondary amenorrhea, case F: diagnostic tests

First visit

LH: 4 mIU/ml; FSH: 3 mIU/ml
 Normal values: LH, 5-20 mIU/ml; FSH, 4-16 mIU/ml
Prolactin: 7 ng/ml
 Normal values: 0-20 ng/ml
Progestin challenge: no withdrawal flow
TSH: 2 μIU/ml; T_4: 8.1 μg/dl; T_3 uptake: 33%
 Normal values: TSH, 0.4-5.0 μIU/ml; T_4: 4.8-10.8 μg/dl; T_3: 33%-45%

Second visit

Estradiol: <20 pg/ml
 Normal values: follicular phase, 20-100 pg/ml
DEXA: bone density 3 SD below normal for age
Estrogen and progestin challenge: withdrawal flow

DEXA, Dual-energy x-ray absorptiometry; *FSH*, follicle-stimulating hormone; *LH*, luteinizing hormone; *SD*, standard deviation; *TSH*, thyroid-stimulating hormone.

The diagnostic tests ordered and laboratory results for Case F are given in Table 14-9. The gonadotropin levels obtained at her first visit were noted to be low. Her prolactin level was low normal. She did not have withdrawal flow to a progesterone challenge test, which indicated minimal endogenous estrogen compatible with her lack of cervical mucus. These test results taken together isolated her amenorrhea problem to the hypothalamic-pituitary compartment. Her thyroid function tests were normal, and hyperthyroidism was thereby eliminated as a potential cause for her low weight. On her second visit, hypoestrogenism was confirmed by a serum estradiol level in the menopausal range. It was determined that her uterus could respond to appropriate steroid hormones when she had a positive withdrawal flow to an estrogen/progestin challenge test. The DEXA scan indicates that she had significant osteoporosis that was compatible with 5 years of hypoestrogenism (Fig. 14-16). Therefore this patient's final diagnosis was hypothalamic secondary amenorrhea. Her low weight, the stress of her job, and her heavy exercise pattern were the presumptive causes for her low gonadotropin levels and lack of ovarian stimulation. Appropriate treatment would be estrogen replacement therapy in consideration of her osteoporosis. She should be encouraged to undergo changes in her lifestyle (weight, occupational stress, and exercise pattern).

Case G. This patient is a 24-year-old, gravida (G)3 P3 single Asian female who had postpartum secondary amenorrhea. She delivered at term 13 months ago, after appearing in the emergency room in labor with no prior

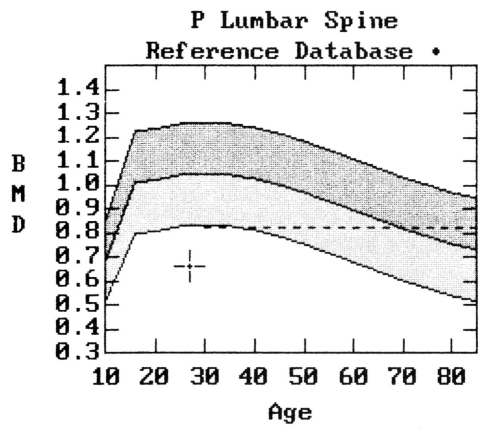

FIGURE 14-16. The average bone mineral density of the lumbar spine is approximately 3 standard deviations below the expected value for this 27-year-old woman.

prenatal care. At that time her profuse vaginal bleeding, uterine tenderness, and intrauterine fetal demise were all compatible with the diagnosis of abruptio placentae. She delivered 2 hours after admission and proceeded to have a postpartum hemorrhage secondary to uterine atony. Her estimated blood loss was 12 units, and she received, over the course of that admission, an 8-unit transfusion. Despite the transfusion, her postpartum hematocrit stabilized at only 24%. She required no suppression of lactation. She took oral contraceptives for 4 months and had regular withdrawal periods but has not experienced any spontaneous menses since discontinuing their use. She had a 23-lb weight gain during the pregnancy and has gained another 20 lb since delivery. She complained of chronic fatigue and malaise and had a decreased appetite. She was chronically cold, and her skin was dry and scaly. Her past medical history was noncontributory for significant prior illnesses. She was a single parent who worked part-time and did not participate in regular exercise. On physical examination, her BP was noted to be 92/60, with a pulse of 64 and regular. Her height was 5 ft 2 in. and she weighed 151 lb (IBW = 108 lb). Her skin was noted to be dry and without hirsutism. The thyroid gland was small and without nodularity. Her breasts were stage 5 development and without masses or galactorrhea. On pelvic examination, she was noted to have vaginal rugation and a small amount of clear cervical mucus in her cervical os. The uterus was multiparous in size, and there were no adnexal masses. Her DTRs were sluggish, with a slow relaxation phase.

The diagnostic tests for case G are presented in Table 14-10. On the first series of tests the patient was noted to have a small amount of endogenous estrogen by the fact that she had some withdrawal bleeding to progesterone challenge and her estradiol was in the early follicular-phase range. Baseline anterior pituitary hormone tests were low (hypogonadotropic with a low thyroid-stimulating hormone [TSH] level). Although the cortisol was in the normal range, it was drawn at 0900 hours, a time when it should be higher in accordance with normal diurnal variation. Overall, the results of the tests at the end of this first visit isolated the problem to the hypothalamic/pituitary compartment. On the second visit, the results of an estrogen-progestin challenge test indicated that her uterus had the ability to respond. The working diagnosis at this point was hypopituitarism, and she was admitted for 2 days of dynamic pituitary testing. (All these tests are sophisticated, somewhat difficult to interpret, and are best performed by a subspecialist in the hospital setting.) These tests indicated that she did not have diabetes insipidus because the antidiuretic hormone function of her posterior pituitary was normal. However, her anterior pituitary function test results were all abnormal, with sluggish responses recorded for growth hormone, cortisol, prolactin, TSH, and gonadotropins. Altogether, this patient had a very low level of anterior pituitary function and no pituitary reserve when challenged. Her final diagnosis was secondary amenorrhea caused by complete hypopituitarism resulting from postpartum hemorrhage, which was severe enough to lead to infarction of the anterior pituitary (Sheehan's syndrome). Her secondary amenorrhea was the direct result of low gonadotropin levels, but her hypothyroid status and Addison's disease were also contributory. Her therapy calls for estrogen/progestin replacement therapy and thyroid and glucocorticoid replacement.

Ovarian Compartment

Case H. A 31-year-old G1, P1 married black female had an 8-month history of secondary amenorrhea. Her menarche was at 12 years of age, and her menstrual periods were always regular every 28 days until age 29. For the past 2 years, her menstrual periods had been every 30 to 60 days without

TABLE 14-10. Secondary amenorrhea, case G: diagnostic tests

First visit

LH: 4 mIU/ml; FSH: 3 mIU/ml
  Normal values: LH, 5-20 mIU/ml; FSH, 4-16 mIU/ml
Estradiol: 45 pg/ml
  Normal values: follicular phase, 20-100 pg/ml
Prolactin: 3 ng/ml
  Normal values: 0-20 ng/ml
TSH: 0.5 μIU/ml; T_4: 2.0 μg/dl; T_3 uptake: 41%
  Normal values: TSH, 0.4-5.0 μIU/ml; T_4, 4.8-10.8 μg/dl; T_3 uptake: 33%-45%
Cortisol: 6 μg/dl
  Normal values: 0700-0900 hr, 9-24 μg/dl; 1600-1800 hr, 2-14 μg/dl
Growth hormone: 1.2 ng/ml
  Normal values: 0.5-13.0 ng/ml
  Progesterone challenge: spotting for 1 day

Second visit

Estrogen and progestin challenge: withdrawal flow

Third visit

Hospital admission for pituitary dynamic testing
Overnight H_2O deprivation test: urine specific gravity was 1.023 with urine osmolality of 70 mOsm
  Normal values: 100-1000 mOsm
Insulin tolerance test
  Growth hormone: baseline, 4 ng/ml; peak, 6.6 ng/ml
    Normal values: stimulated should be >10 ng/ml
  Cortisol: baseline, 8 μg/dl; peak, 12 μg/dl
    Normal values: stimulated should at least be double baseline value
TRH stimulation test
  Prolactin: baseline, 4 ng/ml; peak, 13 ng/ml
    Normal values: stimulated should be >30 ng/ml
  TSH: baseline, 1.2 μIU/ml; peak, 4.7 μIU/ml
    Normal values: stimulated should be >12 μIU/ml
GnRH stimulation test
  LH: baseline, 3 mIU/ml; peak, 7 mIU/ml
    Normal values: stimulated should be >20 mIU/ml

FSH, Follicle-stimulating hormone; *GnRH*, gonadotropin-releasing hormone; *LH*, luteinizing hormone; *TRH*, thyrotropin-releasing hormone; *TSH*, thyroid-stimulating hormone.

her prior premenstrual symptoms. She conceived easily and had an uncomplicated term pregnancy at 26 years of age. Besides concerns about her lack of menstrual periods, she also wanted to conceive again in the near future. Her history was notable for frequent hot flashes that occurred two to three times per day and often disturbed her sleep. She also complained of vaginal dryness. Among first-degree family relatives, her family history was negative for any menstrual dysfunction. Her medical history was negative. She denied any weight changes, thyroid symptomatology, galactorrhea, and hirsutism. She was a homemaker and did not exercise heavily. On physical examination, she was noted to be 5 ft 7 in. tall and weigh 129 lb (IBW = 128 lb). Her BP was 114/72, with a pulse of 72 and regular. Her skin was clear, and she had no hirsutism. Her thyroid was normal in size and without nodularity. Her breasts showed stage 5 development without masses or galactorrhea. On pelvic examination she was noted to have normal vaginal rugation with a multiparous cervix and no cervical mucus. The uterus was multiparous size, and there were no adnexal masses. Her DTRs were brisk, with a normal relaxation phase.

The series of diagnostic tests performed on case H are illustrated in Table 14-11. Based on the results of her first visit, she was noted to be hypergonadotropic, euprolactinemic, and hypoestrogenic because she did not respond to a progesterone challenge. The elevated gonadotropin levels isolate the problem to the ovarian compartment. A series of focused laboratory tests were done at the second visit to evaluate her premature gonadal failure. The normal karyotype indicates that she did not have a mild form of gonadal dysgenesis. The serum estradiol level confirmed that her estrogen was in the menopausal range. Although most cases of premature ovarian failure are idiopathic in etiology, it is pertinent to look for polyglandular autoimmunity as a potential cause. The associated endocrine glands that can be involved in polyglandular autoimmunity are the thyroid, parathyroid, adrenal cortex, and the islet cells of the pancreas. Other associated findings with this autoimmune syndrome can be alopecia, pernicious anemia, and vitiligo. The laboratory tests performed to look for autoimmunity on her second visit were suspicious for incipient Addison's disease with the relatively low 24-hour urinary free cortisol level. (Note: tests for adrenal and ovarian antibodies are available from only a few laboratories.) The presence of antithyroid antibodies and the elevated TSH level indicated that there was impending thyroid failure. Her thyroid was functioning normally at that time (as indicated by the thyroxin level). She did not have any diabetes mellitus, parathyroid disease, or anemia. On her third visit, the ACTH stimulation test indicated that her adrenal reserve was low, and she was at risk to develop Addison's disease. Therefore this patient had premature ovarian failure presumably secondary to ovarian autoimmunity. The ovarian antibody tests currently available are not sensitive, and this assumption of ovarian autoimmunity was based on the fact that she had definite signs of impending adrenal and thyroid failure. She requires estrogen replacement therapy to prevent osteoporosis and suppress the hot flashes. Her thyroid and adrenal status will be followed closely over the years, and when the levels dip below normal, appropriate replacement should be instituted.

TABLE 14-11.   Secondary amenorrhea, case H: diagnostic tests

---

First visit

LH: 87 mIU/ml; FSH: 119 mIU/ml
  Normal values: LH, 5-20 mIU/ml; FSH, 4-16 mIU/ml
Prolactin: 4 ng/ml
  Normal values: 0-20 ng/ml
Progestin challenge: no withdrawal flow

Second visit

Estradiol: <20 pg/ml
  Normal values: follicular phase, 20-100 pg/ml
Karyotype: 46XX
Ovarian and adrenal antibodies: negative
24-hour urine-free cortisol: 21 ng/24 hr
  Normal values: 0-96 ng/24 hr
Hermatocrit: 39%
  Normal values: 36%-45%
TSH: 8 μIU/ml; T_4: 6.8 μg/dl; T_3 uptake: 38%
  Normal values: TSH, 0.4-5.0 μIU/ml; T_4, 4.8-10.8 μg/dl; T_3 uptake: 33%-45%
Thyroid antibodies: antimicrosomal, positive; antithyroglobin, positive
ANA: negative
Serum calcium: 9.4 mg/dl
  Normal values: 8.9-10.2 mg/dl
Serum phosphorus: 3.1 mg/dl
  Normal values: 3.0-4.5 mg/dl
Glucose: 87 mg/dl
  Normal values: 70-100 mg/dl

Third visit

ACTH stimulation test
  Cortisol: baseline, 4 μg/dl; peak (60 min), 4.5 μg/ml
  Normal values: stimulates should be 2× baseline value

ACTH, Adrenocorticotropic hormone; *ANA*, antinuclear antibodies; *FSH*, follicle-stimulating hormone; *LH*, luteinizing hormone; *TSH*, thyroid-stimulating hormone.

Uterine/vaginal compartment

Case I. This patient is a 31-year-old, G2, P2 white female who had 14 months of secondary amenorrhea. The patient's menarche was at 11 years of age, and she always had regular monthly menstrual periods. She conceived with her second pregnancy approximately 2 years ago after discontinuing use of a diaphragm, and she had an uncomplicated full-term vaginal delivery 14 months ago. Two weeks after delivery, she entered the emergency room at her local hospital with profuse vaginal bleeding. It was necessary for her to be taken to the operating room, and a dilation and curettage (D & C) was performed in which a retained placental cotyledon was found. Following the D & C, she required oral antibiotics for low-grade endometritis and a 2-unit transfusion. She breast-fed for 5 months and then went back on barrier contraception. Ten months postpartum she went to her obstetrician because of a lack of menstrual periods. She denied significant weight changes, galactorrhea, thyroid symptoms, hirsutism, and change in lifestyle. She was in otherwise good health. On physical examination, her vital signs were height 5 ft 6 in., weight 137 lb (IBW = 124 lb), and BP 116/74 with a regular pulse of 72. Her skin was clear and without hirsutism. Her thyroid was normal and without nodularity. Her breasts were stage 5 development without masses, and there was 1+ bilateral galactorrhea. On pelvic examination, the vagina had normal rugation, the cervix was multiparous, and there was a 3+ quantity of clear cervical mucus that was fern-positive. The uterus was multiparous in size, and there were no adnexal masses. The DTRs were brisk, with a normal relaxation phase. The remainder of the physical examination was normal.

The diagnostic tests for case I are presented in Table 14-12. The laboratory results from the first visit indicated that the serum gonadotropin levels were normal. The patient demonstrated a moderate amount of ovarian activity based on the level of her serum estradiol. With that level of estradiol and clear cervical mucus, a withdrawal flow to a progesterone challenge would have been expected. The patient was placed on a basal body temperature (BBT) chart for 1 month, and there was a 2-week segment during which she had a definite temperature elevation. The results of the tests at this first visit placed the disorder in the uterine/vaginal compartment. This was confirmed with the estrogen-progestin challenge test, which did not result in any withdrawal flow. Next, a hysterosalpingogram was performed that documented intrauterine synechiae acting as a mechanical block to endometrial stimulation and

TABLE 14-12. Secondary amenorrhea, case I: diagnostic tests

First visit
LH: 12 mIU/ml; FSH: 9 mIU/ml
  Normal values: LH, 5-20 mIU/ml; FSH, 4-16 mIU/ml
Prolactin: 11 ng/ml
  Normal values: 0-20 ng/ml
Progesterone challenge test: no withdrawal flow
Estradiol: 129 pg/ml
  Normal values: follicular phase, 20-100 pg/ml
BBT chart: biphasic response

Second visit
  Estrogen and progestin challenge test: no withdrawal flow

Third visit
Hysterosalpingogram: filling defects encompassing 90% of the endometrial cavity

BBT, Basal body temperature; FSH, follicle-stimulating hormone; LH, luteinizing hormone.

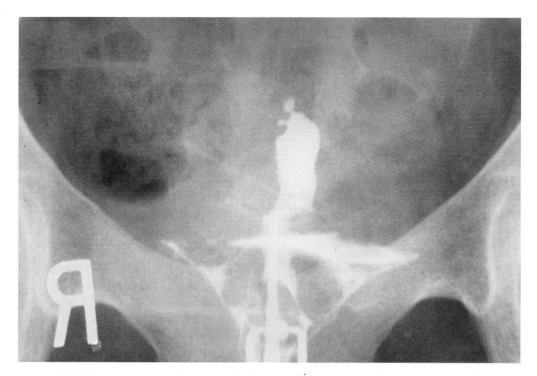

FIGURE 14-17. A radiograph of a hysterosalpingogram demonstrating infusion of radiopaque medium into the cervical canal. The medium progresses to the level of the internal cervical os and does not progress further. This woman has complete Asherman's syndrome.

withdrawal bleeding (Fig. 14-17). The diagnosis in this patient was Asherman's syndrome secondary to her postpartum hemorrhage and endometritis. She required hysteroscopic lysis of adhesions as a primary treatment.

HIRSUTISM

Female androgen excess can present some of the most difficult diagnostic problems in reproductive medicine. First, the physician should pay close attention to the degree of symptomatology. The first and lowest level of androgen excess symptoms is acne and hirsutism, The next level is menstrual dysfunction, and the third level is frank virilization. The prevailing androgen (testosterone) levels are correspondingly higher according to the degree of symptomatology (Fig. 14-18). Therefore the history in a woman with hirsutism should pay special attention to menstrual function and signs of virilization. When virilization is present, all of the possible symptoms are not necessarily present (e.g., a patient can have deepening of her voice without clitoromegaly). In regard to hirsutism, it

Female Hyperandrogenism

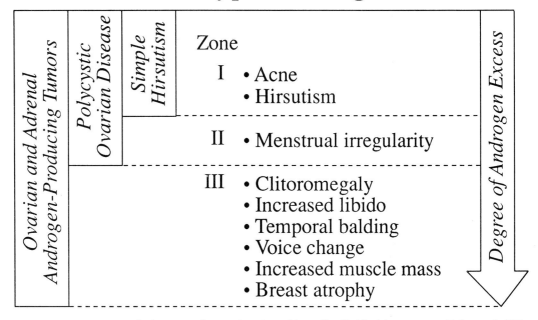

FIGURE 14-18. Female hyperandrogenism is arbitrarily divided into zones I through III. Zone I has mild androgen elevations and is exemplified by the diagnosis of simple hirsutism. Zone II has moderate elevations of androgen levels and is exemplified by polycystic ovarian disease. Zone III has severe elevations of androgen levels and is exemplified by a virilizing tumor.

should be noted that we are discussing midline body hair. If a patient has excessive hair growth on her extremities, this is referred to as hypertrichosis, which is genetic and is not mediated by androgenic hormones. The amount of midline body hair for a nonhirsute normal woman depends on her familial and ethnic background. The clinician must be familiar with the expected amount of body hair for a particular ethnic background. Extreme examples of this would be the minimal midline body hair of Asians versus the relatively heavy midline body hair of women of Mediterranean descent. Remember that hirsutism and acne should usually be present simultaneously because both segments of the pilosebaceous unit should be equally responsive to excess androgens. The following cases illustrate the evaluation of women with hirsutism.

Case J. This 19-year-old, G0, P0, single, white female had 2½ years of secondary amenorrhea and an associated complaint of hirsutism. Her menarche was at 12 years of age, and her menstrual periods were somewhat regular, every 30 to 40 days until age 14. From 14 to 16 years of age her menstrual periods occurred every 3 to 4 months and have been absent for the past 2½ years. Although she always had a tendency toward being

TABLE 14-13. Secondary amenorrhea, case J: diagnostic tests

First visit

LH: 7 mIU/ml; FSH: 8 m IU/ml
   Normal values: LH, 5-20mIU/ml; FSH, 4-16 mIU/ml
Total testosterone: 106 ng/dl
   Normal values: 20-70 ng/dl
Free testosterone: 5.2 pg/ml
   Normal values: 0.6-3.2 pg/ml
DHEAS: 412 µg/dl
   Normal values: 81-256 µg/dl
Progesterone challenge test: positive withdrawal flow

Second visit

Blood samples obtained in fasting state at 0800 hr
Insulin: 81 µU/ml
   Normal values: 0-20 µU/ml
Glucose: 108 mg/dl
   Normal values: 70-100 mg/dl
17-OH-progesterone: 180 ng/dl
   Normal values: <300 ng/dl

DHEAS, Dehydroepiandrosterone sulfate; *FSH*, follicle-stimulating hormones; *LH*, luteinizing hormone.

overweight, her weight problem had exacerbated over the past 5 years. At age 12, she weighed 120 lb; at age 16 she weighed 178 lb and currently is 243 lb. For the previous several years, she had noted intermittent bouts of moderate to severe acne and a gradual increase in facial and abdominal hair. She was not sexually active and used no contraception. She had not experienced hot flashes or vaginal dryness. Her energy level was adequate. She had normal temperature tolerance and no family history of thyroid disease. She denied galactorrhea. The remainder of her family medical history was noncontributory. On physical examination her vital signs were height 5 ft 3 in., weight 243 lb (IBW= 112 lb), pulse 84 and regular, and BP 140/84. Examination of her skin noted moderate facial acne, and she had severe hirsutism involving the sideburns, lip, chin, chest, and lower portion of the abdomen (score of 19—see Fig. 14-14). She also had white striae on the lower part of her abdomen. The patient demonstrated hyperpigmented, verrucous velvety skin along the neck folds and the axilla and in the inguinal region. Her thyroid and breast examinations were normal. On pelvic examination, vaginal rugation was normal. The cervix was nulliparous, with a 2+ quantity, clear cervical mucus that was fern-positive. The uterus was small and nulliparous in size, with normal ovaries and no adnexal masses. The DTRs were brisk, with a normal relaxation phase.

The diagnostic tests for case J are illustrated in Table 14-13. The serum androgen profile noted definite elevations in total and free testosterone levels with an adrenal component demonstrated by the elevated DHEAS level. As expected, based on her cervical mucus, she had positive withdrawal flow to a progesterone challenge. This indicated some level of ovarian activity. Her LH/FSH ratio was not elevated, and her gonadotropin levels were normal. On the basis of these initial tests, the patient's problem was classified as androgen excess in origin. (This is an example of disease in other organ systems that can affect the hypothalamic-pituitary-gonadal axis.) At her second visit, more focused blood tests were ordered to find the specific cause of her androgen excess. In the fasting state her serum insulin level was noted to be greatly elevated, with a normal glucose level. She did not demonstrate cryptic (adult-onset) congenital adrenal hyperplasia because her 17-hydroxyprogesterone level was normal. This patient's diagnosis is the so-called "HAIR-AN" syndrome (hyperandrogenemia, insulin resistance, and acanthosis nigricans). The elevated levels of insulin (secondary to an insulin receptor defect) are known to contribute to excess androgen secretion by the ovaries. Many of these women are erroneously diagnosed as having polycystic ovarian disease, which includes a milder form of insulin resistance. The minimum treatment is to induce regular progestin withdrawal bleeding, but most patients request suppression of the hyperandrogenemia. This can be accomplished with oral contraceptives or spironolactone. She should be strongly encouraged to lose weight because the insulin resistance is a major part of the pathophysiology.

Case K. This 27-year-old, G1, P1, married, white female had a history of chronic, persistent hirsutism. Her menarche was at age 13, and her menstrual cycles have always been every 28 days, with nondebilitating premenstrual symptomatology without dysmenorrhea. She conceived without difficulty at age 21 and had a full-term vaginal delivery without complications. She was using a barrier method for contraception at the time of examination. Her weight had been stable, her energy was good, there was no family history of thyroid disease, and she was not taking any regular medications. Her ethnic background was of mixed middle-European descent (German, Scottish, French). In regard to the hirsutism she had noted a gradual increase in hair growth on her lip, chin, chest, and lower abdomen. This hair growth had been present for years but was gradually becoming more thick and noticeable. She either plucked or shaved the hair 2 to 3 times per week. During her late teenage years, she had problems with facial acne. On examination her complexion was blemish-free except she used special soaps to manage her chronic oily skin texture.

On physical examination, the presence and pattern of her abnormal hair growth was noted using a scoring system with a maximum of 5 points per location. Her sideburns were 2; lip, 3; neck, 3; chest, 2; and abdomen, 3, for a total score of 13, which is moderate hirsutism (see Fig. 14-14). There was

TABLE 14-14. Androgen excess, case K

> Progesterone: 7.3 ng/ml
>   Normal values: 0.5-18 ng/ml
> Testosterone (total): 67 ng/dl
>   Normal values: 20-70 ng/dl
> Testosterone (free): 2.9 pg/ml
>   Normal values: 0.6-3.2 pg/ml
> DHEAS: 241 μg/dl
>   Normal values: 81-256 μg/dl
> 3-α-androstanediol glucuronide: 338 ng/dl
>   Normal values: 60-300 ng/dl

DHEAS, Dehydroepiandrosterone sulfate.

no visible acne. The remainder of her physical and pelvic examination was normal.

The patient had moderate hirsutism without menstrual dysfunction or virilization (level 1 androgen excess). She had hirsutism, not hypertrichosis, and the entire pilosebaceous unit was involved as attested to by her oily complexion. The following laboratory tests were ordered with the results presented in Table 14-14: total and free testosterone, DHEAS, and 3-alpha-androstanediol glucuronide (3-α-diol G). The progesterone level confirms that her regular cycles were ovulatory. The DHEAS level represents a good indication of total androgen secretion from the adrenal gland. Therefore if the DHEAS level is elevated, it can be assumed that the adrenal is also secreting excess quantities of more potent androgens (e.g., testosterone). The testosterone levels give an indication of the overall degree of androgen excess but do not distinguish between an ovarian and an adrenal source. The level of free testosterone is a reflection of the sex-binding protein levels, which decrease as a chronic response to elevated circulating levels of androgens. It is a significant clinical finding if either total or free testosterone is elevated. In this case total testosterone, free testosterone, and DHEAS were not elevated, indicating a lack of evidence for elevated androgen secretion. The 3-α-diol G level was elevated, indicative of increased conversion of testosterone to dihydrotestosterone at the end organ (hair follicle). In the past, patients with this set of findings would have been given the diagnosis of idiopathic hirsutism. This diagnosis was used when there was no evidence for increased levels of circulating androgens. With the more recent ability to assess androgen activity at the level of the pilosebaceous unit, most of these former diagnoses of idiopathic hirsutism would be more properly classified as end-organ hyperactivity cases. (In this case the enzyme 5α reductase is hyperactive.) One term that has been applied to women with this set of findings is *simple hirsutism*. In women with simple hirsutism, the best therapy is partial androgen receptor blockade with spironolactone (100 to 200 mg/day).

CONCLUSION

The intent of this chapter was to present diagnostic methods for establishing the etiology of primary and secondary amenorrhea and hirsutism. It should be remembered that amenorrhea and hirsutism are symptoms and not diseases. Once a clinician is presented with either of these symptoms, a focused evaluation is necessary. Once this evaluation is undertaken and the symptom has been isolated to a particular compartment, the clinician can do some directed reading regarding specific diseases that affect the particular compartment in question; additional, more directed tests can then be performed. Once the diagnosis has been clearly established, a treatment plan can be designed.

BIBLIOGRAPHY

Biller BMK, Baum HBA, Rosenthal DI, et al: Progressive trabecular osteopenia in women with hyperprolactinemic amenorrhea, *J Clin Endocrinol Metab* 75:692, 1992.

Boyar RM: Endocrine changes in anorexia nervosa, *Med Clin North Am* 62:297, 1978.

Cowan BD, Morrison JC: Management of abnormal genital bleeding in girls and women, *N Engl J Med* 324:1710, 1991.

Crosby PDA, Rittmaster RS: Predictors of clinical response in hirsute women treated with spironolactone, *Fertil Steril* 55:1076, 1991.

Drinkwater BL, Nilson K, Chestnut CH III, et al: Bone mineral content of amenorrheic and eumenorrheic athletes, *N Engl J Med* 311:277, 1984.

Fritz MA, Speroff L: The endocrinology of the menstrual cycle: the interaction of folliculogenesis and neuroendocrine mechanisms, *Fertil Steril* 38:509, 1982.

Fujimoto VY, Clifton DK, Cohen NL, Soules MR: Variability of serum prolactin and progesterone levels in normal women: the relevance of single hormone measurements in the clinical setting, *Obstet Gynecol* 76:71, 1990.

Griffin JE: Androgen resistance: the clinical and molecular spectrum, *N Engl J Med* 326:611, 1992.

Griffin JE, Edwards C, Madden JD, et al: Congenital absence of the vagina. The Mayer-Rokitansky-Kuster-Hauser syndrome, *Ann Intern Med* 85:224, 1976.

Jacobs HS, Knuth UA, Hull MG, et al: Post-"pill" amenorrhea—cause or coincidence? *Br Med J* 2:940, 1977.

Jialal I, Naidoo C, Norman RJ, et al: Pituitary function in Sheehan's syndrome, *Obstet Gynecol* 63:15, 1984.

Kallmann FJ, Schoenfeld WA, Barrera SE: The genetic aspects of primary eunuchoidism, *Am J Ment Defic* 48:203, 1944.

Kletzky OA, Davajan V: Hyperprolactinemia: diagnosis and treatment, in Mishell DR Jr, Davajan V, Lobo RA (eds): *Infertility, contraception and reproductive endocrinology*, ed 3. Boston; Blackwell Scientific Publications, 1991, 396-421.

Kohler PO: Thyroid function and reproduction. In Riddick DH, editor: *Reproductive physiology in clinical practice*, New York, 1987, Thieme Medical.

Marshall WA, Tanner JM: Variation in pattern of pubertal changes in girls, *Arch Dis Child* 44:291, 1969.

Nader S: Polycystic ovary syndrome and the androgen-insulin connection, *Am J Obstet Gynecol* 165:346, 1991.

Portuondo JA, Barral A, Melchor JC, et al: Chromosomal complements in primary gonadal failure, *Obstet Gynecol* 64:757, 1984.

Rarick LD, Shangold MM, Ahmed SW: Cervical mucus and serum estradiol as predictors of response to progestin challenge, *Fertil Steril* 54:353, 1990.

Reame N, Sauder SE, Kelch RP, Marshall JC: Pulsatile gonadotropin secretion during the human menstrual cycle: evidence for altered frequency of gonadotropin-releasing hormone secretion, *J Clin Endocrinol Metab* 59: 328, 1984.

Rebar RW: Practical evaluation of hormonal status. In Yen SSC, Jaffe RB, editors: *Reproductive endocrinology: physiology, pathophysiology and clinical management*, ed 3, Philadelphia, 1991, Saunders.

Rebar RW, Connolly HV: Clinical features of young women with hypergonadotropic amenorrhea, *Fertil Steril* 53:804, 1990.

Reindollar RH, Byrd JR, Mcdonough PG: Delayed sexual development: a study of 252 patients, *Am J Obstet Gynecol* 140:371, 1981.

Schlecte J, Dolan K, Sherman B, et al: The natural history of untreated hyperprolactinemia: a prospective analysis, *J Clin Endocrinol Metab* 68:412, 1989.

Sluijmer AV, Lappöhn RE: Clinical history and outcome of 59 patients with idiopathic hyperprolactinemia, *Fertil Steril* 58:72, 1992.

Snyder PJ, Rudenstein RS, Gardner DF, et al: Repetitive infusion of LHRH distinguishes hypothalamic from pituitary hypogonadism, *J Clin Endocrinol Metab* 48:864, 1979.

Stein AL, Levenick MN, Kletzky OA: Computed tomography versus magnetic resonance imaging for the evaluation of suspected pituitary adnomas, *Obstet Gynecol* 73:996, 1989.

Styne DM, Grumbach MM: Disorders of puberty in the male and female. In Yen SSC, Jaffe RB, editors: *Reproductive endocrinology: physiology, pathophysiology and clinical management*, ed 3, Philadelphia, 1991, Saunders.

Warren M: The effects of exercise on pubertal progression and reproduction function in girls, *J Clin Endocrinol Metab* 51:1150, 1980.

CHAPTER **15**

Abnormal Vaginal Bleeding

DEBORAH J. DOTTERS
WILLIAM DROEGEMUELLER

    Abnormal bleeding is one of the most common gynecologic problems. As many as 15% of outpatient visits and 25% of gynecologic surgeries are directly related to the symptoms of abnormal bleeding. Although this symptom is common, it is difficult to rigidly define. This is because every patient defines abnormal bleeding as bleeding that is different from what she is used to experiencing. Thus abnormal bleeding may have an infinite variety of presentations, from scant to profuse, from every day to every few months. In the office setting we are dealing with the patient's definition of abnormality rather than that of the textbooks. Regular periodic flow is a sign of normality. Irregular, unusual, or heavy bleeding produces anxiety. Thus when the patient has abnormal uterine bleeding, education is as important as diagnosis and correction in the treatment plan.

This chapter will review normal menses and its physiology, timing, and duration. The differential diagnosis of abnormal bleeding will be discussed. The diagnostic evaluation of this symptom complex will be presented in four sections: history, physical examination, laboratory and imaging tests, and endometrial sampling. Office and outpatient treatment modalities will then be presented. In the final section we will provide brief case histories and discuss their workup and treatment.

NORMAL BLEEDING

Although abnormal bleeding is different for each woman, physiologic norms and definitions have been established empirically over the past four decades (Table 15-1). Normal menstrual bleeding, representing regular ovulation, occurs every 28 days with a normal range of 21 to 35 days. The duration of flow is 4½ days with a normal range of 2 to 7 days. Thus a woman with bleeding every 21 days for 7 days would be within the boundary of the physiologic norms. Several studies have shown that normal blood loss at menses is 35 ml, with a range of 20 to 80 ml. Menstrual bleeding of greater than 80 ml or greater than 7 days in duration is defined as menorrhagia, also called hypermenorrhea. About 10% to 20% of all women lose more than 80 ml of blood per cycle. Bleeding that occurs in intervals greater than 5 weeks (35 days) is defined as oligomenorrhea.

Regular menstrual bleeding is a function of cyclic hormonal stimulation by both estrogen and progesterone of the uterine lining. Abnormalities in any step of this process (excess estrogen, inadequate progesterone, distortion of endometrial architecture, disease of platelets or thrombin, or an increase in fibrinolysis) may lead to abnormal bleeding patterns.

Early in the cycle estradiol, secreted by the growing ovarian follicle, stimulates growth of the superficial layers of the endometrium. Small spiral arterioles and glandular elements expand through the loose stroma. The lining of the endometrium at this stage consists of simple columnar cells in continuity with the endometrial glands. After the appropriately timed luteinizing hormone (LH) surge from the pituitary gland, ovulation occurs, and the reorganized follicular structure, the corpus luteum, secretes progesterone as well as estrogen. Progesterone acts directly on the endometrium to induce cell differentiation and secretions from the glandular elements, to inhibit endometrial growth by inhibition and down-regulation of estrogen receptors, and to initiate cellular changes in

TABLE 15-1.   Normal bleeding

1. 28-day intervals: range, 21-35 days
2. 4½ days of flow cycle; range, 2-7 days
3. 35 ml normal blood loss: range, 20-80 ml

the stromal matrix and spiral arterioles that allow for uniform sloughing of the endometrium when the corpus luteum degenerates and estrogen and progesterone levels decline.

The withdrawal of hormonal support of the endometrium leads to waves of vasoconstriction within the spiral arterioles. The outer endometrial layers degenerate because of the resulting ischemia. The tissue integrity of the superficial blood vessels and glandular elements is lost. In the first 24 hours of menses, thrombin and platelet plugs in the small vessels control bleeding as superficial tissue is sloughed. The vast majority of blood loss is within this first 72 hours. Over the next 2 days a new ovarian follicle begins to grow and secrete estrogen. The epithelial lining regenerates from deep glands and from endometrium of the isthmus and cornu to restore the integrity of the endometrium. During this time hemostasis is primarily from proximal vascular spasm.

DIFFERENTIAL DIAGNOSIS

The differential diagnosis of abnormal bleeding is affected by the patient's age, medications, past medical history, and past social history. In general there are two categories of pathophysiology from which a patient's differential may be developed: abnormal hormonal signals (such as bleeding secondary to anovulation) and abnormal local factors (such as bleeding from a polyp). At the most fundamental level, for bleeding to begin and also to stop at the appropriate time and with a normal amount, a woman must have an anatomically normal endometrium, intact coagulation system, and regular and appropriate progression of ovarian hormonal secretion. It is important to note that most etiologies of abnormal bleeding disrupt more than one aspect of the normal physiology.

Congenital or acquired deficiencies in the coagulation pathways may lead to abnormal bleeding. Platelet and fibrin plugs are the immediate mechanism for menstrual hemostasis in the first 24 to 48 hours. In one series up to 20% of severe menorrhagia in adolescents was found to be due to clotting deficiencies, primarily von Willebrand's disease, Glanzmann's disease, and thrombocytopenia. Acquired deficiencies that may lead to excessive menstrual bleeding include leukemia and immune thrombocytopenic purpura. Several medications may interfere with the coagulation pathways, the most common being warfarin (coumadin) therapy.

In contrast to a deficiency in the clotting pathways, inappropriate activation of the fibrinolytic system may also lead to abnormal bleeding. Plasminogen activator levels have been found to be elevated in the menstrual efflux of women with abnormal bleeding. Inflammation and infection, which may activate the fibrinolytic system, are well-established causes of abnormal uterine bleeding. Prostaglandins are involved at several important points in the control and timing of normal menstrual bleeding.

The myometrium contains high levels of prostaglandin $F_{2\alpha}$ ($PGF_{2\alpha}$), a potent vasoconstrictor. Many investigators believe that $PGF_{2\alpha}$ may induce the endometrial vasospasm and vasoconstriction that initiate menses. The endometrium in some women with excessive bleeding has been found to have less-than-normal levels of $PGF_{2\alpha}$. Prostaglandin E_2 (PGE_2) and prostacyclin are vasodilators. Increased levels of PGE_2 receptors have been found in the myometrium of menorrhagic women. The PGE_2 may act to redistribute blood flow from the myometrium to the endometrium, thus also allowing for increased menstrual flow. Increased levels of PGE_2 and prostacyclin have also been found in the endometrium of women with abnormal bleeding. Increased levels of PGE_2 metabolites have been found in the menstrual efflux of menorrhagic women. In another study of endometrial biopsy specimens of menorrhagic women, an increased ratio of prostacyclin to thromboxane metabolites was found. Hormonal irregularities such an anovulation may cause bleeding partially through altered levels of prostaglandins.

Women with anovulation or abnormal ovulation often have atypical estrogen and progesterone levels. If there is too much estrogen, the endometrial lining continues to grow and develop and becomes structurally unstable. Prolonged estrogen stimulation results in small sections of the endometrium sloughing off with resultant irregular bleeding. Anovulation, causing increased estrogen levels without progesterone, is one of the most common causes of abnormal bleeding. Adolescents are particularly susceptible to this cause of abnormal bleeding. If there are inadequate progesterone levels or an increased estrogen-to-progesterone ratio, the stimulus for synchronous vasospasm in the endometrial vessels may be altered. Although a secretory pattern may be seen on endometrial biopsy, the patient may still experience menorrhagia. Between 50% and 60% of premenopausal women with abnormal bleeding and menorrhagia have a secretory endometrium found on endometrial biopsy samples. Investigators have found similar levels of LH, follicle-stimulating hormone (FSH), estradiol, and progesterone in women with menorrhagia as compared with controls.

For menstrual bleeding to stop, neoformation of the surface endometrial epithelium must occur. The old endometrial lining must be cleanly sloughed, and tissue repair must be unimpeded. Only a basal level of estrogen is needed for this to occur. Incomplete sloughing of the endometrium with hormonal irregularities may cause excessive bleeding.

One of the most common causes of abnormal bleeding is pregnancy. The discussion of the physiology and pathophysiology of pregnancy bleeding is beyond the scope of this chapter. However, it is necessary for the clinician to keep this diagnosis in mind in any menstrual-age patient.

The following outline provides a differential diagnosis of abnormal uterine bleeding.

I. Pregnancy related
  A. Intrauterine pregnancy
    1. Threatened abortion
    2. Incomplete abortion
    3. Missed abortion
    4. Septic abortion
  B. Ectopic pregnancy
  C. Gestational trophoblastic neoplasm
    1. Hydatidiform mole
    2. Placental site trophoblastic tumor
    3. Choriocarcinoma
II. Infections-endometritis
  A. Ascending infection and sexually transmitted diseases
  B. Systemic hematogenously derived infections (tuberculosis)
  C. Infection related to use of intrauterine device (IUD)
  D. Endometritis related to degenerating or prolapsed leiomyomas
  E. Postinstrumentation infection
III. Endocrine causes
  A. Anovulation
    1. Hypothalamic
    2. Polycystic ovarian syndrome
    3. Follicle depletion (perimenopausal)
  B. Hypothyroidism and hyperthyroidism
  C. Prolactin-secreting tumors
IV. Neoplasia
  A. Benign polyps
  B. Myomas
  C. Endometrial hyperplasia
  D. Malignancy
    1. Endometrial carcinoma
    2. Cervical or endocervical carcinoma
    3. Ovarian (granulosa cell, metastatic)
    4. Tubal carcinoma
V. Coagulation disorders
  A. Inherited (e.g., von Willebrand's, hemophilia)
  B. Acquired (e.g., idiopathic thrombocytopenic purpura [ITP], leukemia)
  C. Drug induced—coumadin, heparin, aspirin
VI. Systemic disease
  A. Renal failure
  B. Severe liver disease with secondary coagulopathy
VII. Endometrial atrophy

   VIII. Factitious bleeding (not from the uterine cavity)
      A. Gastrointestinal tract origin
      B. Urinary tract origin
      C. Cervical/vaginal bleeding
   IX. Unexplained bleeding

The differential diagnosis of abnormal bleeding is confounded by numerous clinical and not-so-clinical classifications. The most common classifications of abnormal bleeding are pregnancy, organic bleeding, and dysfunctional bleeding. Organic bleeding includes diagnoses such as neoplasm or infections, with dysfunctional bleeding defined by exclusion when all other diagnoses are ruled out. Some authors have defined dysfunctional bleeding as anovulatory bleeding in the absence of uterine neoplasia. In general we do not like to use the term *dysfunctional bleeding* because ovulation does occur in the majority of women without infection, neoplasms, or coagulopathies. In other words, dysfunctional uterine bleeding does not connote anovulation. In addition, dysfunctional uterine bleeding is a pejorative term to patients and a confusing term to clinicians.

EVALUATION OF ABNORMAL BLEEDING

The evaluation of abnormal bleeding is based on two questions: Is the blood loss too excessive, and thus a danger to the woman's health? Is the bleeding caused by an underlying malignancy? The first question is answered through patient history, physical examination, and simple laboratory procedures. The issue of malignancy is also approached through patient history, and management is guided by the patient's age and duration of symptoms.

In evaluating and treating abnormal bleeding, it is important to assess the relationship between the patient's symptoms, her feelings about the symptoms of abnormal bleeding, and whether or not there is excessive blood loss. Excessive bleeding over a prolonged period obviously may lead to anemia. Bleeding may be abnormal not only in a temporal sense (when it is the wrong time of the cycle [metrorrhagia]), but may also be abnormal when the menses lasts too long. When bleeding is abnormal in a quantitative sense (when there is too much bleeding) the symptom is called menorrhagia.

Objective means of assessing blood loss are impractical in the clinical setting because they involve saving all the pads and tampons a woman uses and then measuring blood loss, usually with the alkaline hematin method. Thus it is our practice to assess the symptomatology as a deviation from the patient's normal and usual amount of bleeding.

Studies that have measured the relationship between perceived and actual blood loss have found a poor correlation between symptomatology and blood passage. In a classic study from Oxford of women with menorrhagia but regular menses, there was no correlation between a patient's perception of menses and her measured blood loss. The patient's assessment of whether the periods were light, moderate, or heavy did not relate to the loss of quantified hemoglobin. In addition, there was no correlation with the patient's impression of whether her periods were light, moderate, or heavy; the number of tampons or pads that she used; or her duration of flow. In another study of blood loss and patient's perceptions, 40% of women with menorrhagia, defined as greater than 80 ml of blood loss, considered their flow scant or moderate. In a group of women with extreme menorrhagia, greater than 200 ml per cycle, there was also no correlation between the patient's perceptions, the amount of blood loss, and the duration of menses. When women have been asked to quantify flow from spotting to heavy, the range of what women consider spotting is 0.1 to 16 ml with a mean of 2.5 ml. Women have considered heavy bleeding to range from 1.4 ml to 216 ml per day, with a mean of 22 ml. Tampon and pad use does not correlate with whether bleeding is heavy but is based more on individual habit. In addition, different brands of pads and tampons absorb different amounts of menstrual flow. Thus clinicians should not try to quantify blood loss from questions such as "How many pads did you use?" Investigations of perceived blood loss have also shown that 90% of blood loss occurs in the first 3 days regardless of whether menorrhagia or normal flow is occurring.

The discrepancy of a woman's perception of her menstruation and measured blood loss is affected by the constituents of menstrual efflux. The mean hematocrit of menstrual flow is 36%; however, the range is from 2% to 80%. The major component of menstrual efflux is endometrial tissue, not blood. Secretions (vaginal and cervical) make up little of the efflux. It is likely that variable etiologies of abnormal bleeding may influence the ratio of blood to endometrial tissue in menstrual efflux. For example, in one study, women with a menorrhagia caused by IUDs had a higher ratio of blood to tissue than did non-IUD users. Perceptions of amount of bleeding are not the only highly subjective factor; assessment of timing is also to some extent subjective. Some women may count 28-day cycles as regular, whereas some consider wide fluctuations as acceptable if they occur once a calendar month. The clinical corollary of the patient's individual evaluation of both timing and quantity of blood make the review of a menstrual diary, an ongoing patient-kept calendar, extremely helpful to the clinician.

In summary, although the standard for assessing the "heaviness" of abnormal bleeding is the measurement of the patient's hematocrit, the patient's hematocrit may not reflect the severity of the symptom complex to the patient. A woman may have a hematocrit of 39% and have bleeding 15 out of 30 days of the month. As clinicians we must treat the patient's problem, not just the laboratory value.

HISTORY

A glance at the differential diagnosis of abnormal bleeding indicates that the causes of bleeding are myriad and often systemic; therefore they require perceptive clinical acumen and a good history.

Abnormal bleeding should be defined by both timing and amount. It is valuable to know when bleeding begins, whether it is spotting or heavy, how long the bleeding lasts, whether or not it is daily spotting, and how heavy the heavy days are. Many women keep menstrual calendars and will offer them if asked. The timing of bleeding and the relationship to previous cycles and previous years is also valuable information. For example, daily spotting is more indicative of a polyp or low-grade infection, whereas heavy flow tapering to spotting, then to no bleeding for a few days, and then to a heavy flow again is more characteristic of anovulatory bleeding.

The patient should be asked whether she has seen a physician for these symptoms before and what the outcome was. Inquiring about contraceptive use and sexual history is essential. The history of the chief complaint should include information about premenstrual symptoms, such as bloating, breast tenderness, or anxiety. The presence of molimina usually indicates ovulation. Pain with intercourse, defecation, or urination or pelvic heaviness in association with abnormal bleeding may indicate a persistent corpus luteum cyst, endometriosis, or myomas. The presence or absence of clots is not particularly helpful.

Other aspects of the history should include questions about drugs and medications, many of which may affect bleeding or ovulation. A history of fever, chills, or respiratory symptoms may indicate a chronic infection. Recent changes in the patient's weight, in her life, or in her activity or exercise patterns should be discussed. These factors may affect ovulation at the hypothalamic level. Dietary fads may also affect bleeding; for example, ginseng cream or tea has a mild estrogenic effect and can alter normal hormonal patterns. Changes in body hair, body habitus, or spontaneous milk production may indicate endocrinologic pathology. A history of other bleeding and bruising should also be sought. Changes in bowel or bladder function should also be questioned. Patients may have bleeding from the rectum or the urethra and confuse this symptom with uterine bleeding.

The patient should also be asked about other systemic diseases with open-ended questions such as "Are you seeing or have you recently seen a physician for any other problems?" Open-ended questions are helpful because a patient frightened by her bleeding often regresses to concrete thinking and may answer questions literally. A separate question about psychiatric medications such as antidepressants should also be made. When patients feel embarrassed about the use of such medications, they may not admit to their prescriptions under the generic question, "Are you taking any medications?"

A final helpful question at the end of the history is "Are there other symptoms or problems that seem worrisome to you?" The "last clue" is often valuable, from "I was almost transfused after dental work" to "I may have left a tampon inside me."

PHYSICAL EXAMINATION

The physical examination should include vital signs, particularly pulse. Abnormalities in the pulse rate may reflect thyroid disease or anemia. Thyroid size and abdominal masses merit special attention in the physical examination. The pelvic examination must ensure that bleeding is uterine; thus urethral inspection and stool guaic are helpful parts of the workup. Cervical bleeding from erosion, polyps, or cervicitis is extremely common. If the vaginal vault does not contain blood, inspection of the vaginal discharge is helpful. Cervicitis from *Chlamydia* may also cause endometritis and abnormal bleeding. *Gardnerella* endometritis is an uncommon (but not rare) cause of abnormal bleeding. Bleeding from inflammation is usually a daily occurrence. Changes in the cervical mucus can also be helpful in assessing ovulation. If ovulation has occurred, the cervical mucus changes from thin and stringy to thick and tenacious. Air-dried slides of cervical mucus show a ferning pattern in an estrogen-dominant situation. Ferning in the second half of the cycle indicates anovulation. The uterus should also be evaluated for tenderness, size, and shape. Careful assessment of the adnexa is mandatory.

LABORATORY AND IMAGING TESTS

In most patients the history and physical examination either strongly suggests or eliminates most etiologies of abnormal bleeding. However, some laboratory tests are helpful. A sensitive pregnancy test is the most important. It must be emphasized that regardless of the sexual history, there is no lower age limit for pregnancy in a menstruating teenager. The positive pregnancy test result does not indicate whether the gestation is viable or whether it is extrauterine or intrauterine.

A complete blood count is also helpful in establishing hemoglobin and hematocrit levels, red blood cell indices, and the platelet count. If anovulation is suspected, a prolactin, a thyroid panel, and a thyroid-stimulating hormone (TSH) screen are also useful tests. Determination of creatinine levels may also be appropriate if renal disease is suspected. A urinalysis is also important to look for evidence of nonspecific urethritis, as well as blood in the urine. Coagulation studies (prothrombin time, partial activated thromboplastin time, and bleeding time) are useful in adolescents. Women with bruising or other suspicious histories of bleeding diathesis should have a coagulation profile. From the history, physical examination, and limited laboratory tests, a working diagnosis may be established in over 90% of patients.

ENDOMETRIAL SAMPLING

After the history is taken and a physical examination is performed, further diagnostic testing may be unnecessary. If a cause for bleeding is uncovered, appropriate laboratory tests should be obtained. However, often a specific diagnosis is not apparent. In these cases we use the patient's age and duration of symptoms to guide subsequent management. If the woman is over 40 or has a history suggestive of chronic annovulation, we suggest endometrial sampling to rule out hyperplasia or malignancy. If she is younger than 40 and symptoms are acute or of only short duration, we usually proceed directly to a trial of hormonal therapy. The rationale for endometrial sampling is to diagnose a neoplastic or refractory cause for bleeding. As stated, endometrial sampling is indicated in women over 40 years of age, women with chronic anovulation, or women of any age without a diagnosis who have failed empiric hormonal therapy (Table 15-2). Endometrial sampling should be performed whenever there is anticipation of the possible diagnosis of endometrial hyperplasia or neoplasia.

For many years there was debate regarding endometrial sampling in the office versus dilation and curettage (D & C). Office endometrial sampling is preferable to outpatient D & C for the diagnosis of abnormal bleeding for several reasons. Office endometrial biopsies are in practice as effective as outpatient D & Cs in establishing a diagnosis of abnormal bleeding and are considerably less expensive. In addition, D & C is only temporarily effective for correction of refractory bleeding. About 65% of women treated with a D & C have resumption of their abnormal bleeding within three cycles. Except for the temporary emergency control of refractory bleeding, office endometrial biopsy is preferable to D & C.

If infection is suspected, antibiotic treatment should be initiated empirically after appropriate cervical cultures are performed. Complications of endometrial sampling are extremely rare (1 to 2 per 1000). The

TABLE 15-2. Indications for endometrial sampling

Women over 40 years of age
Chronic anovulation
Suspicion of chronic infection
Women with persistent symptoms despite hormonal therapy

major complications of endometrial sampling are perforation and infection. Perforation may be managed conservatively. However, postinstrumentation infection usually requires parenteral broad-spectrum antibiotics.

Endometrial sampling detects endometrial polyps in 1% to 2% of cases in women under the age of 40 years. Another 1% to 2% of women have hyperplasia without cellular atypia. Atypical hyperplasia is found in fewer than 1% of women and endometrial carcinoma in fewer than 1%. A significant percentage of women under the age of 40 years (in some series as high as 60%) is found to have secretory endometrium. In perimenopausal women between the ages of 41 and menopause, abnormal hyperplasia and malignancy are found in an increasing percentage of cases as age increases; however, this percentage is still under 10%. Up to 20% of postmenopausal women who are not taking hormone medication have malignancy.

Atypical endometrial hyperplasia may be found in another 10% to 15%. Atrophic endometrium is the single largest cause of abnormal uterine bleeding in the postmenopausal age group. In the presence of atrophic endometrium, endometrial sampling of specimens often returns with a histologic diagnosis of insufficient tissue. If the endometrial thickness is 5 mm or greater, repeat sampling is indicated. If abnormal bleeding continues despite a normal endometrial biopsy, further diagnostic studies, such as sonohysterography or hysteroscopy, are indicated.

Endometrial biopsy may be performed without analgesia in the majority of subjects. Some clinicians prefer a paracervical block with 1% lidocaine. Alternatively, the use of intracervical viscous lidocaine, applied liberally with a cotton-tipped applicator, provides inexpensive and rapid analgesia. Many clinicians pretreat patients 30 minutes before the procedure with an oral prostaglandin synthetase inhibitor such as ibuprofen or naproxen. Paracervical block is particularly useful for the woman with a stenotic cervical os and for the woman with a predilection for vasovagal episodes. The plastic cannulas are small enough and flexible enough to pass through almost all cervical canals, with elderly, nulliparous patients being the most common exception.

An endometrial biopsy is best performed late in the menstrual cycle (days 20 to 28). If ovulation has occurred, a secretory pattern can be seen in the endometrium. Endometrial biopsy greater than 14 days after conception may disrupt a pregnancy. Light bleeding is not a contraindication to endometrial biopsy. If mucopurulent cervicitis is present, a culture should be taken and the infection treated with doxycycline (100 mg twice daily for 10 days) before endometrial sampling. Antibiotic prophylaxis for subacute bacterial endocarditis (SBE) is no longer recommended for patients undergoing D & C or endometrial biopsy in the absence of infection.

There are multiple instruments available for endometrial sampling. The older hollow metal curette devices (the Randall and Novak curettes) have few indications in current office practice. They are more painful than the newer instruments and do not obtain a more accurate sample. The flexible, thin, plastic endometrial cannulas include the Vabra aspirator and soft plastic devices such as the Pipelle and the Z-sampler (Fig. 15-1). These devices have equal efficacy in obtaining tissue samples and often do not require the use of a cervical tenaculum. They are currently the instruments of choice for endometrial biopsy.

Before endometrial sampling the cervix may be cleaned with povidone-iodine (betadine) or an alternative antiseptic solution. A bimanual pelvic examination should be performed to assess the uterine position. The endometrial biopsy is performed by inserting the instrument gently up to the fundus. Suction is then obtained, and the flexible curette is moved up and down in the endometrial cavity while rotating it throughout the inner circumference of the uterus (Fig. 15-2). We recommend obtaining samples from all four walls of the uterus.

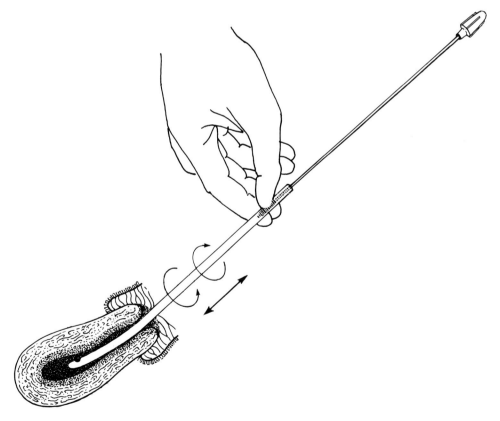

FIGURE 15-1. Endometrial biopsy being performed with the Pipelle (Unimar). Suction is maintained by sliding and extending the inner plastic stem.

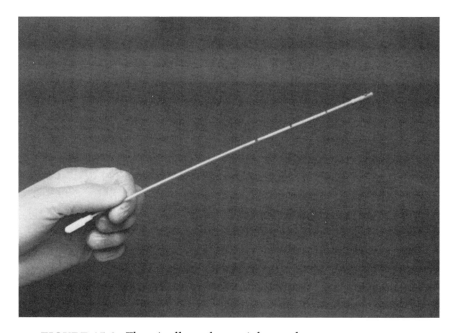

FIGURE 15-2. The pipelle endometrial sampler.

From Herbst AL, et al: *Comprehensive gynecology*, ed 2, St Louis, 1992, Mosby.

Suction may be obtained by a syringe, an intrinsic device, or a self-contained pump. Light bleeding may persist for 1 to 2 days after endometrial sampling. Cramps are usually mild and end within 10 to 15 minutes.

ULTRASOUND

Another tool for diagnostic evaluation of abnormal bleeding is endovaginal ultrasound. Endovaginal ultrasound has developed rapidly in the past several years. Common uses of endovaginal ultrasound in patients with abnormal bleeding include ruling out ectopic pregnancy, assessment of myomas and abnormal uterine size, measurement of endometrial thickness, and with saline installation sonohysterography—evaluation of the endometrial cavity. Endometrial polyps and submucous myomas may also be seen. Studies in postmenopausal women not taking hormones indicate that endometrial thickness should not exceed 4 mm. If an endometrial thickness greater than 4 mm is seen, histologic diagnosis by endometrial sampling is indicated. Sonohysterography is an extremely valuable technique in which saline is instilled into the uterine cavity, distending the cavity and outlining such structures as polyps, submucous myomas, and adhesions (Fig. 15-3). Sonohyster-

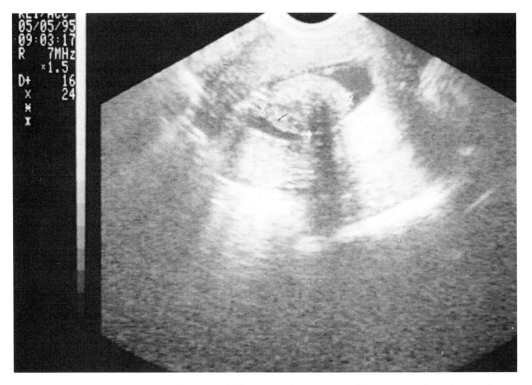

FIGURE 15-3. An endovaginal ultrasound using sonohysterography of an endometrial polyp. The patient was perimenopausal and had abnormal bleeding. The endometrial biopsy had shown secretory endometrium.

ography may also be used when an endometrial biopsy does not provide an explanation for bleeding and when the patient has a poor response to hormonal therapy.

HYSTEROSCOPY

An additional procedure besides ultrasound for the evaluation of abnormal bleeding is hysteroscopy. The hysteroscope may be used whenever persistent bleeding occurs despite hormonal treatment, when endometrial samples return as insufficient tissue, or when intrauterine pathology is suspected. Some investigators have suggested that hysteroscopy should be performed at all times rather than just for biopsy. However, availability, patient acceptance, and cost limit this technique as a first-approach standard of care at this time. The hysteroscope may be used for complex operative procedures such as ablation of the endometrium with electrocautery or laser, myomectomy, and intrauterine surgery for congenital uterine anomalies or the synechiae of Asherman's syndrome. Complex operative hysteroscopy is best performed in an operative suite. Diagnostic hysteroscopy for visualization and simple biopsy or for removal of small polyps or IUDs may be performed in the office setting.

Anesthesia similar to that for endometrial biopsy is usually all that is necessary for a simple imaging hysteroscopic examination. Because the procedure takes longer and the distention of the uterus frequently causes mild to moderate cramping, many patients may benefit from mild sedation with diazepam (Valium) or fentanyl (Sublimaze).

Hysteroscopes are used with a distending medium, such as CO_2, saline, or Hyskon. The latter is not miscible with blood and thus is the distending medium of choice in the woman who is bleeding heavily. Diagnostic hysteroscopes have small calibers of 4 to 6 mm. Predilation of the cervix is usually not necessary and may even prohibit successful observation by causing increased bleeding or by allowing the distending medium to leak out.

Hysteroscopy, although simple, should be performed by experienced physicians. The infusion medium must be monitored carefully. Hyskon has been noted to cause anaphylaxis. Both Hyskon and saline solutions may cause intravascular volume overload and pulmonary edema when given excessively. Carbon dioxide instillation under excess pressure has been associated with cardiac arrest. Other complications are rare and include infection, perforation, and bleeding. It is appropriate to perform a sensitive urine pregnancy test before hysteroscopy. If visual inspection of the vaginal vault or pelvic examination suggests acute infection, treatment of infection should precede hysteroscopy.

As helpful as office hysteroscopy is, most clinicians have found sonohysterography much easier and much less expensive. In most practices, sonohysterography is replacing hysteroscopy as the initial diagnostic technique of choice for refractory abnormal bleeding. It is rarely necessary to need more complicated imaging techniques such as magnetic resonance imaging (MRI), computed tomography (CT), or hysterosalpingogram in the diagnosis of abnormal bleeding. Studies have confirmed the accuracy of endovaginal ultrasound in these settings compared with CT or MRI.

TREATMENT OF ENDOMETRIAL BLEEDING

Treatment of endometrial bleeding depends on the severity of the bleeding, the acuteness of the symptoms, and the etiology. For women who are not hemorrhaging or hypovolemic, treatment may be performed on an outpatient basis. For women who are hemorrhaging, treatment should be under direct observation in the hospital with parenteral medication or D & C. If malignancy is suspected, D & C is usually most definitive.

The foundation of treatment for abnormal bleeding is the correction of any underlying pathology. For example, if hypothyroid disease is diagnosed, correction with thyroid hormone adjusts the abnormal menses. However, if no obvious etiology is apparent and the woman is younger than the age of 40 years without a history suggestive of chronic anovulation, treatment may be empiric. If abnormal bleeding does not fall into these categories, endometrial sampling should be performed before treatment.

There are two primary medical therapies for a woman who has heavy bleeding (Table 15-3). The first is the use of conjugated estrogens with progestins; the second is oral contraceptives. Both therapies use estrogens to restore endometrial integrity and progestins to induce endometrial differentiation and a controlled sloughing of the endometrial lining.

In the first type of therapy, 5 mg of oral conjugated estrogen (such as Premarin) are prescribed for 10 days. For the same 10 days, 10 mg of medroxyprogesterone acetate (Provera) are prescribed. If bleeding is light and more a pattern of continued spotting, progesterone may be used alone in the dose of 10 mg daily for 10 days.

Estrogens are necessary in situations where significant amounts of the endometrium have been sloughed and stabilization of the endometrial lining is necessary before inducing progesterone changes. A full 10 days of progesterone is used because this is the minimum time needed to produce the cellular changes for a physiologic sloughing of the endometrial lining. The advantage of using estrogen and progesterone is that treatment induces a relatively physiologic endometrium.

When the patient has finished with the estrogen-progesterone protocol, bleeding ensues within 1 to 7 days in the majority of women. The patient should be warned that these menses may be heavier than normal. The subsequent two menstrual cycles are best treated with 10 mg of medroxyprogesterone on days 16 to 25 of the cycle. If intermenstrual bleeding or spotting occurs, endometrial biopsy or hysteroscopy should be performed to exclude the presence of intrauterine pathology. The occurrence of continued spotting with abnormal bleeding may suggest chronic infection.

TABLE 15-3.   Oral hormonal regimens for abnormal bleeding

1. Conjugated estrogen 5 mg/day for 10 days
   Provera 10 mg/day for 10 days
   Taken simultaneously for the same 10 days
2. Oral contraceptives: 35 µg monophasic estrogen pill taken twice daily for 1 week, followed by a 35-µg pill taken daily for 2 months, days 1-21

Many clinicians prefer to use oral contraceptives to control abnormal bleeding. A 35-μg estrogen monophasic pill is taken twice a day for a week. This method arrests acute bleeding in the majority of women within 48 hours. The ensuing period is slightly heavier than normal. The next two cycles are also treated with 35 μg birth control pills taken one per day. If bleeding persists during this regimen, sonohysterography, hysteroscopy, or an endometrial sampling is indicated. Advantages of using oral contraceptives are low cost, good success, ease of explanation, and good compliance on the part of patients. The disadvantage of the use of oral contraceptives for abnormal bleeding is that they produce a relatively nonphysiologic endometrium. There is also fear in many patients of oral contraceptives and their side effects. In patients who have an atrophic endometrium or areas of sloughed endometrium, the excess progestogen may not completely control bleeding.

When patients have severe bleeding, parenteral treatment is indicated. Conjugated estrogens, 25 mg, are given intravenously (IV). This dose may be repeated every 2 to 6 hours for three times. If bleeding continues despite IV estrogen, D & C is indicated.

Once bleeding has stopped and the patient has stabilized, she should be treated with a combination of oral estrogen and oral progesterone for 10 days. If the patient is an adolescent, coagulation profiles should be obtained. Several recent studies in patients with severe renal disease and uremia have shown that the administration of IV estrogen leads to a decrease in bleeding time within 3 to 4 days. The mechanism for this effect is unclear. If either IV or high-dose estrogen is given to arrest severe bleeding, the progestogen treatment should not be started until bleeding has ceased or declined to staining or spotting. The success rate of parenteral estrogen and then oral estrogen and progestin is 90%. In the rare case of the woman who continues to have heavy bleeding that is refractory to both hormonal therapy and D & C, a large-bore Foley catheter with a 30-cc bulb may be used to tamponade the uterine cavity. The tip is cut off to allow flow if necessary. The bladder is drained, and the Foley catheter is inserted into the uterus. The large bulb is blown up, and uterine tamponade is effected. The catheter is left in place for 24 hours. A recent report on the use of this technique found that it was initially successful in 17 of 20 cases and partially successful in two.

Rarely, when severe bleeding cannot be stopped, selective embolization of abnormal vessels may be considered. Selective embolization may be used with plastic coils, Gelfoam, or both. The procedure is performed in an angiography suite by a skilled vascular radiologist. Although this technique has been used successfully in obstetric and postoperative patients, little has been published about it in women with severe menorrhagia. A final treatment is hysterectomy.

After successful hormonal therapy, a long-term plan should be established with the patient. If this is the first episode of bleeding, 3 months of treatment with an oral contraceptive is usually sufficient. If this is the second or third episode and no etiology has been found, the patient may be treated with the addition of progesterone at the end of every other cycle, a progesterone-containing IUD, or the addition of nonsteroidal antiinflammatory drugs (NSAIDs) during menses. Studies have shown that naproxen, mefenamic acid, ibuprofen, and indomethacin are all useful in reducing the amount of menstrual blood flow. The use of progestogens at the end of the luteal phase and NSAIDs is more effective than either therapy alone. As discussed, prostaglandins play an essential role in the initiation of menstrual bleeding. Prostaglandin synthetase inhibitors, by decreasing prostacyclin and PGE_2, may work to effect a more normal menstrual sloughing. It is notable that the prostaglandin synthase inhibitors do not decrease menstrual blood loss in patients with submucous myomas or endometrial polyps. If heavy bleeding continues in the face of the use of NSAIDs, hysteroscopy is suggested.

The prostaglandin synthetase inhibitors may be given in standard dosages. The agents should be taken with the onset of menstrual bleeding and continue until bleeding is finished. The reduction of blood loss varies between 30% and 50% when compared with the patient's previous periods. Prostaglandin synthetase inhibitors are also excellent in treatment of excess bleeding with an IUD. Long-term effects from the use of prostaglandin synthetase inhibitors include potential renal toxicity. Evidence of compromised renal function would preclude the use of these agents.

After bleeding has been stabilized in the patient who is a poor surgical candidate or wants to preserve her uterus, ablation of the endometrium may be performed through the hysteroscope. Many patients have light bleeding after endometrial ablation. It is essential that endometrial sampling be performed before the use of definitive surgical hysteroscopic therapy to rule out a carcinoma. Endometrial ablation by either electrocautery or laser is successful in stopping menses in half of patients, and the remaining 50% have substantially decreased bleeding.

Other less common medical treatments to prevent abnormal bleeding from recurring have included the use of danazol or gonadotropin-releasing hormone (GnRH) agonists. Although these treatments are usually successful when intrauterine pathology has been ruled out, both are costly and are associated with significant side effects. Studies have shown that 200 mg of danazol per day is the ideal dose. In one series the blood loss was noted to be 183 ml per day before danazol treatment and reduced to 38 and 26 ml in the next two cycles. Because the endometrium is so atrophied by the use of danazol, the effect usually lasts for a month or two after discontinuation of the drug; however, beyond that point abnormal bleeding may return. It is important to remember that because danazol is not effective as birth control in low doses and because it can be teratogenic, the woman should use other contraception. The use of a GnRH agonist is only a temporary stopgap measure.

Many patients who prefer not to bleed at all but who do not wish surgical therapy may benefit from the use of intramuscular (IM) medroxyprogesterone acetate (Depo-Provera). The use of 150 mg IM every 3 months produces amenorrhea in a significant proportion of patients. The advantages of this technique are that it is necessary to give only every few months, it is available for patients who may not take estrogens, and it may also reduce uterine size.

Several studies in the late 1980s investigated the use of antifibrinolytic agents. Large doses of these agents are needed, and most have appreciable side effects. E-Aminocaproic acid may be given in doses of 20 to 25 g per day. Other antifibrinolytic agents have been used successfully, such as tranexamic acid in doses of 4 g per day. Side effects of nausea, headache, and dizziness occur in 80% of patients. In addition, the possibilities of intravascular coagulation are serious and not insignificant. Intracranial arterial thrombosis has been reported in patients taking these agents.

THEORETIC CASES
Case 1

The patient is a 14-year-old gravida (G)0 who denies sexual activity. She began her menarche at 11 years of age and has a history of menstrual periods every 6 to 10 weeks. She has had heavy vaginal bleeding, two to three pads per hour, for the past 6 hours. She has had no problems with intermenstrual bleeding. She has no bleeding problems with dental work. She has normal body habitus and normal vital signs. She is anxious and frightened, as is her mother, because of the heavy bleeding. She has not had episodes of severe bleeding over the past 3 years other than this bleed.

This patient's bleeding most likely represents an anovulatory cycle. Because of the absence of a history of severe bleeding, initial therapy with estrogen and progestins may be prescribed. We would recommend the use of Premarin, 5 mg daily for 10 days, with the addition of Provera, 10 mg per day. If bleeding does not stop within 24 hours IV Premarin should be used. We would then offer the patient oral contraceptives for 3 months.

An alternative therapy is a progestational agent such as medroxypro-gesterone acetate (10 mg) for 10 days of the month for 3 months. After 3 months she could stop medication to see if regular and lighter bleeding develops.

Case 2

A 25-year-old G2, para (P)1, presents with periods every 10 days. One period is 3 to 4 days of light spotting, and the other period lasts 5 days, beginning with 2 days of heavy bleeding and then tapering to 3 days of spotting. She has no other bleeding. She is not sexually active. She takes no medication. Her vital signs are stable, and her hematocrit is 37%.

This patient's pattern of abnormal bleeding is most likely consistent with a small estrogen withdrawal bleed at the time of ovulation. If she wishes, oral contraceptives may be prescribed at this time. An alternative therapy would be the addition of a slight amount of estrogen, 0.625 mg for 3 to 4 days starting on day 13 of the cycle.

Case 3

The patient is a thin 34-year-old G3, P2, status post–tubal ligation with her last child 6 years old, and with no other contributory past medical history. Her chief complaint is 2 to 3 days of spotting before the beginning of her menses. Her menses are regular and are preceded by molimina. Because of the age of this patient endometrial sampling is probably unnecessary, although she may have a myoma or endometrial polyp. We would begin treatment with 10 mg of Provera on days 16 to 25 for two cycles. If she continues to spot while taking the Provera, a hysteroscopy or sonohyster-ography should be used to visualize the endometrial cavity. This patient most likely has an early progesterone withdrawal bleed and may represent a variant of corpus luteum dysfunction. Thyroid studies are indicated in this patient if initial hormonal therapy is unsuccessful.

Case 4

This patient is a 26-year-old female who has been bleeding intermittently for the past 6 weeks. She starts with a few days of spotting and then passes heavy clots without warning, with enough bleeding to make her seek bed rest. Then she has 2 to 3 days of spotting followed by 2 to 3 days without bleeding. This patient is best managed with Premarin and progesterone after a urine pregnancy test. We would begin the Premarin at 5 mg per day and the Provera at 10 mg per day. This patient may also be treated with oral contraceptives, three per day for 1 week. If the bleeding is still heavy, the dose of estrogen must be increased. If the bleeding reoccurs within the next year, endometrial sampling or hysteroscopy is indicated.

Case 5

This is a 30-year-old G0, P0, with acute leukemia and corresponding thrombocytopenia. She has heavy bleeding. The optimum management of this patient is the suppression of ovarian function and subsequent endometrial bleeding. Norethindrone (Aygestin), 10 to 40 mg, may be given daily. This progestin suppresses ovarian function and leads to atrophy of the endometrial lining. Advantages include easy compliance and once-a-day use. An alternative would be a GnRH agonist, although this regimen is more expensive, and would cause menopausal symptoms.

BIBLIOGRAPHY

Adelantado JM, Rees MCP, Bernal AL, et al: Increased uterine prostaglandin E receptors in menorrhagic women, *Br J Obstet Gynaecol* 95:162, 1988.

Ambriz F, Pizzuto J, Morales M, et al: Therapeutic effect of danazol on metrorrhagia in patients with idiopathic thrombocytopenic purpura (ITP), *Hematology* 28:275, 1986.

Andersson JK, Rybo G: Levonorgestrel-releasing intrauterine device in the treatment of menorrhagia, *Br J Obstet Gynaecol* 97:690, 1990.

Brooks PG, Serden SP: Hysteroscopic findings after unsuccessful dilatation and curettage for abnormal uterine bleeding, *Am J Obstet Gynecol* 158:1354, 1988.

Chimbira TH, Anderson ABM, Naish C, et al: Reduction of menstrual blood loss by danazol in unexplained menorrhagia: lack of effect of placebo, *Br J Obstet Gynaecol* 87:1152, 1980.

Chimbira TH, Anderson ABM, Turnbull AC: Relation between menstrual blood loss and patient's subjective assessment of loss, duration of bleeding, number of sanitary towels used, uterine weight and endometrial surface area, *Br J Obstet Gynaecol* 87:603, 1980.

Choo YC, Mak KC, Hsu C, et al: Postmenopausal uterine bleeding of nonorganic cause, *Obstet Gynecol* 66:225, 1985.

Claessens EA, Cowell CA: Acute adolescent menorrhagia, *Am J Obstet Gynecol* 139:277, 1981.

DeVore GR, Owens O, Kase N: Use of intravenous Premarin in the treatment of dysfunctional uterine bleeding—a double-blind randomized control study, *Obstet Gynecol* 59:285, 1982.

Dockeray CJ, Sheppard BL, Bonnar J: Comparison between mefenamic acid and danazol in the treatment of established menorrhagia, *Br J Obstet Gynaecol* 96:840, 1989.

Eldred JM, Thomas EJ: Pituitary and ovarian hormone levels in unexplained menorrhagia, *Obstet Gynecol* 84:775, 1994.

Emanuel MH, Verdel MJ, Wamsteker K, et al: A prospective comparison of transvaginal ultrasonography and diagnostic hysteroscopy in the evaluation of patients with abnormal uterine bleeding: clinical implications, *Am J Obstet Gynecol* 172:547, 1995.

Falcone T, Desjardins C, Bourque J, et al: Dysfunctional uterine bleeding in adolescents, *J Reprod Med* 39:761, 1994.

Feldman S, Shapter A, Welch, et al: Two year follow-up of 263 patients with post/perimenopausal vaginal bleeding and negative initial biopsy, *Gynecol Oncol* 55:56, 1994.

Ferenczy A: Studies on the cytodynamics of human endometrial regeneration, *Am J Obstet Gynecol* 124:64, 1976.

Ferenczy A, Bertrand G, Gelfand MM: Studies on the cytodynamics of human endometrial regeneration, *Am J Obstet Gynecol* 134:297, 1979.

Finikiotis G: Hysteroscopy: a review, *Obstet Gynecol Surv* 49:273, 1994.

Fraser IS: Menorrhagia due to myometrial hypertrophy: treatment with tamoxifin, *Obstet Gynecol* 70:505, 1987.

Fraser IS, McCarron G, Markham R: A preliminary study of factors influencing perception of menstrual blood loss volume, *Am J Obstet Gynecol* 149:788, 1984.

Fraser IS, McCarron G, Markham R, et al: Long-term treatment of menorrhagia with mefenamic acid, *Obstet Gynecol* 61:109, 1983.

Fraser IS, McCarron G, Markham R, et al: Blood and total fluid content of menstrual discharge, *Obstet Gynecol* 61:194, 1985.

Gimpelson RJ, Rappold HO: A comparative study between panoramic hysteroscopy with directed biopsies and dilatation and curettage, *Am J Obstet Gynecol* 158:489, 1988.

Goldrath MH: Uterine tamponade for the control of acute uterine bleeding, *Am J Obstet Gynecol* 147:869, 1983.

Goldstein SR: *Contemporary Ob Gyn* 80:9, 1995.

Hammond RH, Oppenheimer LW, Saunders PG: Diagnostic role of dilatation and curettage in the management of abnormal premenopausal bleeding, *Br J Obstet Gynaecol* 96:496, 1989.

Herbst AL, Mishell D, Stenchever M, et al: *Comprehensive gynecology*, ed 2, St Louis, 1992, Mosby.

Hill NCW, Oppenheimer LW, Morton KE: The aetiology of vaginal bleeding in children. A 20-year review, *Br J Obstet Gynaecol* 96:467, 1989.

Hopkins MP, Androff L, Benninghoff AS: Ginseng face cream and unexplained vaginal bleeding, *Am J Obstet Gynecol* 159:1121, 1988.

Kaminski PF, Stevens CW: The value of endometrial sampling in abnormal uterine bleeding, *Am J Gynecol Health* 2:130, 1988.

Karlsson B, Granberg S, Wikland M: Transvaginal ultrasonography of the endometrium in women with postmenopausal bleeding—a nordic multicenter study, *Am J Obstet Gynecol* 172:1488, 1995.

Lavin RJ, Wagner G: Absorption of menstrual discharge by tampons inserted during menstruation: quantitative assessment of blood and total fluid content, *Br J Obstet Gynaecol* 93:765, 1986.

Lidor A, Ismajovich B, Confino E, et al: Histopathological findings in 226 women with postmenopausal uterine bleeding, *Acta Obstet Gynecol Scand* 65:41, 1986.

Loffer FD: Hysteroscopy with selective endometrial sampling compared with D&C for abnormal uterine bleeding: the value of a negative hysteroscopic view, *Obstet Gynecol* 73:16, 1989.

Macdonald R: Modern treatment of menorrhagia, *Br J Obstet Gynaecol* 97:3, 1990.

Makarainen L, Ylikorkala O: Ibuprofen prevents IUCD-induced increase in menstrual blood loss, *Br J Obstet Gynaecol* 93:285, 1986.

Mencaglia L, Perino A, Hamou J: Hysteroscopy in perimenopausal and postmenopausal women with abnormal uterine bleeding, *J Reprod Med* 32:577, 1987.

Odell WD, Meikle AW: Menometrorrhagia, infertility, elevated serum estradiol, and hyperprolactinemia resulting from increased aromatase activity (MIEHA syndrome), *Fertil Steril* 46:321, 1986.

Parmer J: Long-term suppression of hypermenorrhea by progesterone intrauterine contraceptive devices, *Am J Obstet Gynecol* 149:578, 1984.

Pellerito JS, McCarthy SM, Doyle MB, et al: Diagnosis of uterine anomalies: relative accuracy of MR imaging, endovaginal sonography, and hysterosalpingography, *Radiology* 83:795, 1992.

Rees MCP, Dederholm-Williams SA, Turnbull AC: Coagulation factors and fibrinolytic proteins in menstrual fluid collected from normal and menorrhagic women, *Br J Obstet Gynaecol* 92:1164, 1985.

Rees MCP, Demers LM, Anderson ABM, et al: A functional study of platelets in menstrual fluid, *Br J Obstet Gynaecol* 91:662, 1984.

Rees MCP, Dunnill MS, Anderson ABM, et al: Quantitative uterine histology during the menstrual cycle in relation to measured menstrual blood loss, *Br J Obstet Gynaecol* 91:662, 1984.

Rosenfield RL, Barnes RB: Menstrual disorders in adolescence, *Endocrinol Metab Clin North Am* 22:491, 1993.

Rosenthal DM, Colapinto R: Angiographic arterial embolization in the management of postoperative vaginal hemorrhage, *Am J Obstet Gynecol* 151:227, 1985.

Schweiger U, Schwingenschloegel M, Laessle R, et al: Diet-induced menstrual irregularities: effects of age and weight loss, *Fertil Steril* 48:746, 1987.

Smiley RK, Tittley P, Rock G: Studies on the prolonged bleeding time in von Willebrand's disease, *Thromb Res* 53:417, 1989.

Smith SK, Kelly RW, Abel MH, et al: A role for prostacyclin (PGI$_2$) in excessive menstrual bleeding, *Lancet* 1:552, 1981.

Turksoy RN, Safaii HS: Immediate effect of prostaglandin F$_{2\alpha}$ during the luteal phase of the menstrual cycle, *Fertil Steril* 26:634, 1975.

Valle RF: Hysteroscopic evaluation of patients with abnormal uterine bleed-ing, *Surg Gynecol Obstet* 153:521, 1981.

Vancaillie Thierry G: Electrocoagulation of the endometrium with the ball-end resectoscope, *Obstet Gynecol* 74:425, 1989.

Van Den Bosch T, Vandendael A, Van Schoubroeck D, et al: Combining vaginal ultrasonography and office endometrial sampling in the diagnosis of endometrial disease in postmenopausal women, *Obstet Gynecol* 85:349, 1995.

Van Eijkeren MA, Christiaens GCML, Sixma JJ, et al: Menorrhagia: a review, *Obstet Gynecol Surv* 44:421, 1989.

Wilansky DL, Greisman B: Early hypothyroidism in patients with menorrhagia, *Am J Obstet Gynecol* 160:673, 1989.

Wortman M, Daggett A: Hysteroscopic endomyometrial resection: a new technique for the treatment of menorrhagia, *Obstet Gynecol* 83:295, 1994.

Ylikorkala O, Pekonen F: Naproxen reduces idiopathic but not fibromyoma-induced menorrhagia, *Obstet Gynecol* 68:10, 1986.

Zupi E, Luciano AA, Valli E, et al: The use of topical anesthesia in diagnostic hysteroscopy and endometrial biopsy, *Fertil Steril* 63:414, 1995.

CHAPTER 16

Office Management of Endometriosis

KAMRAN S. MOGHISSI

Endometriosis is a common and disabling disease of women of reproductive age and is defined by the presence of tissue that is biologically and morphologically similar to normal endometrium in locations other than the endometrial cavity and myometrium. It affects approximately 7% to 10% of premenopausal women. Among infertile women the incidence is believed to be as high as 30% to 60%. The etiology of endometriosis has not been clearly established and may include retrograde menstruation, vascular or lymphatic dissemination, direct implantation, and metaplasia. Other factors, such as genetic predisposition and immunologic disturbances, may play a role. Contrary to previous opinion, black women, particularly those in higher socioeconomic classes, and adolescents may also be affected.

Clinical manifestations of endometriosis consist of pelvic pain associated with menses, dyspareunia, dysmenorrhea, and abnormal uterine bleeding. The condition is commonly associated with infertility. In the presence of advanced lesions, anatomic distortion of pelvic structure, or adhesions caused by endometriosis, infertility may be readily explained; however, no satisfactory hypothesis has been advanced to explain the association of mild endometriosis with infertility.

The clinical presentation and severity of symptoms of endometriosis to some degree relate to the anatomic location and the extent of the disease; however, on occasion, severe endometriosis may be asymptomatic, and minimal disease may be associated with severe and disabling symptoms. Deep implants are usually found in patients with pain, whereas superficial implants are most frequently associated with infertility. Endometriotic lesions are usually confined to the pelvis, although they can occur at distant sites and even outside of the abdomen. The most common sites of involvement are the ovaries, pelvic peritoneum, cul-de-sac, and uterosacral ligaments. Adjacent bowels, bladder, and ureters may also be affected. Extraabdominal foci can occur in almost any organ of the body, including the umbilicus, rectal sheath, cervix, vagina, vulva, rectovaginal septum, liver, diaphragm, and lungs.

DIAGNOSIS

Endometriosis is suspected when pain or other characteristic symptoms and signs of the disease are present. Unfortunately, the symptoms may be highly variable from one subject to another, and the severity of symptoms may not correlate with the extent of the disease. Detection of posterior cul-de-sac nodularity, a tender fixed-retroverted uterus, and an adnexal mass is helpful in establishing the diagnosis; however, these signs are frequently absent in early disease. In all patients suspected of having endometriosis, laparoscopy is indicated and establishes the definitive diagnosis. This procedure should also be performed in all women with unexplained infertility, persistent pelvic pain, and those showing abnormal pelvic findings by other diagnostic procedures such as hysterosalpingography or ultrasonography.

Diagnostic laparoscopy should be performed by the two-puncture technique, and pelvic and abdominal structures should be systematically visualized. The classic appearance of endometriosis is that of puckered black-and-blue lesions, which are also called powder burns or blueberries. Scarred white endometriosis lesions are more difficult to visualize and may be confused with fibrotic tissue from previous inflammatory disease. Strawberry-like reddish lesions are the most active lesions. Finally, clear vesicular lesions often found in younger women are the most difficult to visualize. Experience is necessary to recognize different types of endometriosis, as well as unrelated lesions. Documentation of the site of endometriotic implants and the extent of disease is most important. All patients should be staged by using one of the existing staging systems, such as the American Society for Reproductive Medicine (ASRM) revised classification (Fig. 16-1). Photographs may be taken through the laparoscope to document the findings for future reference and compare treatment modalities. Videotape recording is performed by many physicians and is also helpful. In lesions appearing to be similar to typical endometriosis, histologic evaluation has revealed hemangioma, carbon, old suture material, trophoblastic tissue, necrotic ectopic pregnancies, psammoma bodies, and other pathologic entities. Thus biopsy of suspected lesions should be performed when the diagnosis is in doubt. Biopsies obtained from normal-appearing peritoneum in the vicinity of endometrial implants have also shown endometriotic lesions that were not readily identified through the laparoscope. The diagnosis of extrapelvic endometriosis should always be considered when symptoms of pain or a palpable mass or lesion occur in a cyclic sequence with menses.

WHEN TO TREAT ENDOMETRIOSIS

Major indications for the treatment of endometriosis consist of the presence of pelvic pain, dysmenorrhea, or dyspareunia; pelvic pathology such as ovarian cysts, endometrioma, and adhesions; and infertility. Prophylactic treatment of endometriosis should also be considered to prevent future pelvic disorders associated with advanced stages of the disease (stage III and IV ASRM). More controversial is the need for therapy in cases of stage I and II (ASRM) endometriosis that are merely associated with infertility or asymptomatic disease that is detected in the course of unrelated laparoscopy (e.g., for tubal ligation).

HOW TO TREAT ENDOMETRIOSIS

Several treatment modalities of endometriosis have evolved in the past few decades. The presence of advanced lesions, anatomic distortion of pelvic structure, or adhesions requires surgical therapy.

When minimal to moderate disease is associated with clinical symptoms of pain or infertility, hormonal treatment, laser vaporization, and fulguration with low-voltage electrocautery through the laparoscope are preferred. The advantage of fulguration or vaporization is the immediate result, particularly when infertility is the major complaint. There is, however, considerable evidence suggesting that all endometrial implants are not readily visible or recognized during endoscopic procedures. Thus medical treatment, because of its generalized suppressive or pharmacologic effect, may be more effective (Table 16-1).

Occasionally, combined medical and surgical therapy may be preferred. A short course of medical treatment may be attempted before surgical management of advanced disease to facilitate surgical excision of large

458 Office Gynecology

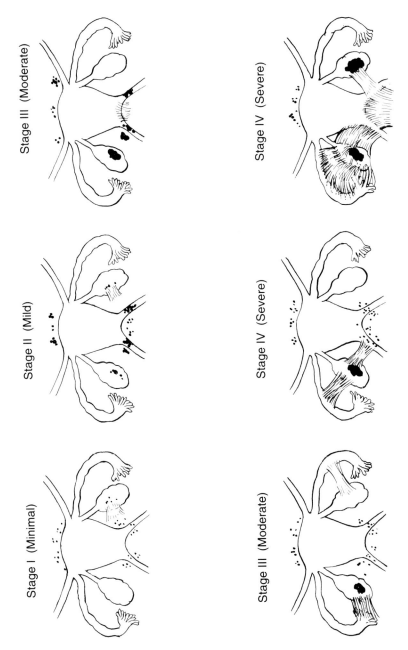

FIGURE 16-1. The American Society for Reproductive Medicine revised classification of endometriosis.

TABLE 16-1. Modalities of treatment available for the management of endometriosis

MEDICAL TREATMENT
Estrogen-progestogen combination
Progestogens: injectable, oral
Danazol
Gonadotropin-releasing hormone agonists
SURGICAL
Laser ablation
Fulguration
Surgical excision
COMBINATION OF MEDICAL AND SURGICAL THERAPY
Preoperative medical treatment (6-12 wk)
Postoperative medical treatment (6-24 wk)

endometrioma associated with severe adhesive disease. Similarly, postoperative medical therapy may be necessary after surgical management of advanced endometriosis associated with severe symptomatology to eradicate potential residual lesions.

Endometriosis may persist during the entire reproductive life of a woman and for as long as functioning ovarian tissues are present. It is therefore essential that a concerned physician and informed patient develop a long-term management plan combining or alternating various surgical and medical treatment modalities and taking into consideration the patient's desire for fertility, family size, and marital and professional obligations.

PSEUDOPREGNANCY

It has long been recognized that estrogen and progesterone are the major regulators of endometrial growth and function and that symptomatic and objective findings of endometriosis ameliorate during pregnancy. Endometriotic lesions contain specific binding sites for estrogen, progesterone, and androgen, and their distribution is similar to that found in the endometrium from the same subject. These findings suggest that endometriotic implants respond to all three classes of steroid hormones. Based on the assumption that a combination of estrogen and progestin may simulate the beneficial effects of pregnancy, Kistner introduced the pseudopregnancy regimen for the treatment of endometriosis. This regimen results in an anovulatory acyclic hormone environment and is presumed to bring about a resolution of endometrial implants.

High-dose oral contraceptives were used initially in an increasing dosage schedule to mimic the pregnancy state. With increased experience, however, it was recognized that the continuous use of low-dose oral contraceptives, which were associated with fewer side effects, has similar beneficial results.

Almost all estrogen-progestin combinations result in anovulation, amenorrhea and progressive decidualization, and ultimate necrobiosis and resorption of ectopic endometrial tissue.

Current technique involves the use of low-dose (30 to 35 μg ethinyl estradiol) oral contraceptives continuously for 6 to 9 months. The treatment is usually begun with 1 tablet daily and increased to 2 or more tablets per day only if breakthrough bleeding occurs. The lowest dose of hormone that produces amenorrhea is then maintained during the course of therapy. The decidual reaction and necrobiosis produced by low-dose formulations are just as extensive as noted in previously used high-dose regimens.

During the initial 2 to 3 months of treatment, most patients are beset with worsening symptoms referable to the endometriosis, in addition to those specifically related to the estrogen-progestogen combination. The latter side effects are frequent, numerous, and sometimes severe. They range from abdominal swelling, depression, breast pain and tenderness, increased appetite, weight gain, and edema (seen in almost all patients) to break-through bleeding, nausea, and breast secretion. Superficial-vein varicosities may occasionally appear, and there is an increased risk of deep-vein thrombosis. Ovulation and menstruation usually resume within 4 to 6 weeks after therapy has been discontinued.

The estrogen-progestogen regimen has been used extensively in the past for the treatment of endometriosis. Symptomatic relief of the disease has been reported in 75% to 100% of cases. Pregnancy rates in women who complained of infertility in addition to endometriosis have ranged from 10% to 58%. Several studies have shown that both danazol and surgical therapies result in greater symptomatic improvement and pregnancy rates as compared with pseudopregnancy regimens alone or in combination with surgery.

The diversity in pregnancy rates among published reports undoubtedly reflects differences in patient selection for this modality of treatment and the extent to which other contributing infertility factors were evaluated and treated. Also, the majority of reports published during this period were hampered by the lack of adequately designed and prospective controlled studies, the wide variety of drugs and dosages employed, the absence of a standard classification system, appropriate statistical analysis, and the frequency with which pseudopregnancy was combined with other forms of therapy, including surgery. Nonetheless, pseudopregnancy represented the most effective medical therapy of its time; however, because of troublesome side effects, which many patients and physicians were unable to tolerate, other modalities of treatment were explored.

Today, estrogen and progestin in combination are not used as a first line of treatment and should be considered only if other therapeutic regimens are contraindicated or cannot be employed. There is evidence that women who have used oral contraceptives are less likely to develop endometriosis. Also, the use of oral contraceptives in the usual cyclic fashion may delay the recurrence of the disease.

PROGESTOGENS

Progestogens alone have been used for the medical management of endometriosis for over two decades. These agents produce a hypoestrogenic acyclic hormonal environment by suppressing gonadotropin, inhibiting ovulation, and producing amenorrhea. In addition, progestogens have a variety of effects on endometriotic tissue. Progestational agents have the theoretic advantage of being better tolerated and avoid the complications of estrogen therapy. Because of the increased rate of breakthrough bleeding, these agents have not been as enthusiastically received or adequately evaluated as danazol for suppression of endometrial implants. Recently there has been a resurgence of interest in the use of progestogens, partly because of the side effects and intolerance of other therapeutic agents by some women.

Medroxyprogesterone Acetate

Medroxyprogesterone acetate (MPA), an extremely potent progestational agent, has proved to be an effective inhibitor of gonadotropic function in the human female when given intramuscularly. An injection of 50 mg of MPA produces secretory changes in the proliferative endometrium within 6 or 7 days.

The use of this progestogen was advocated by Kistner, who recommended it for patients who demonstrated unusual or excessive side effects to the estrogenic component of oral contraceptive (pseudopregnancy) regimens. The regimen used consisted of 100 mg of depot MPA every 2 weeks for four doses, followed by 200 mg monthly for 4 months. When breakthrough bleeding occurred, ethinyl estradiol, 0.02 mg daily for 25 days of each month, was added. A significant drawback to the use of depot MPA is the prolonged interval to resumption of ovulation after cessation of therapy. Because of this complication, the drug should not be used in women desirous of immediate pregnancy.

Adequate data to document the effectiveness of parenteral MPA either for suppression of endometriosis or to enhance fertility among infertile women with endometriosis are not available.

Parenteral administration of MPA in doses of 150 mg intramuscularly every 2 weeks decreases the high-density lipoprotein (HDL) concentration in a dose-dependent way and in the same direction as other progestins. The HDL reduction is confined to the HDL_2 subfraction, which is decreased by

58% after 24 weeks of treatment. Low-density lipoprotein (LDL) levels are not affected.

The use of oral MPA in doses of 30 mg per day continuously for a period of 90 days was first reported by Moghissi and Boyce. In a pilot study of 35 patients with mild to moderate endometriosis documented by laparoscopy, subjective and objective improvement was observed in all patients. Repeat laparoscopy generally showed a decrease in the size or disappearance of endometrial implants.

Histologic examination of endometrial biopsy specimens or endometriomas removed during subsequent laparoscopy or laparotomy showed marked glandular atrophy and decidual reaction. Serial monitoring of serum progesterone levels was consistent with ovulation in the pretreatment cycle. Serum progesterone suppression indicative of anovulation was observed throughout therapy. By day 22 of the posttreatment cycle, a significant rise in serum progesterone levels consistent with ovulation occurred.

The first posttreatment cycle was occasionally prolonged by approximately 7 days, and the first ovulation usually occurred 2 to 3 weeks after the termination of MPA therapy.

In a small group of 10 women who had no other infertility problem, 9 achieved pregnancy (90%) within 8 months after therapy. Patients normally remained amenorrheic throughout MPA therapy and tolerated the treatment well. The most prominent side effects consisted of spotting in 26% and breakthrough bleeding in 23% of patients. Other side effects included depression, weight gain, and bloating. Improvement or remission was observed even in those with breakthrough bleeding. Patients treated with MPA and then subjected to surgery demonstrated significant softening of the endometrial lesions that facilitated operation.

Larger doses of oral MPA do not seem to be more effective or associated with a lower rate of breakthrough bleeding.

The effectiveness of oral MPA has also been compared with that of danazol in the management of stages I and II endometriosis associated with infertility. At a 30-month follow-up, there were no significant differences in pregnancy rates between patients receiving MPA and those treated with danazol.

Other Progestogens

Several other progestogens have been used to treat endometriosis. Lynestrenol in doses of 10 mg has yielded fair results.

More recently another progestogen, gestrinone (R2323), an unsaturated 19-norsteroid, has been studied in several European countries. Gestrinone is a weak progestin that usually forms a relatively unstable interaction with the progesterone receptor. It has minimal estrogenic activity but behaves as an antiestrogen in vivo, and it has no uterotropic activity.

Centrally, gestrinone acts on the hypothalamic-pituitary system to suppress midcycle surges of luteinizing hormone (LH) and follicle-stimulating hormone (FSH) and folliculogenesis, thus diminishing estrogen synthesis. Randomized clinical trials comparing the effectiveness of gestrinone with that of danazol have been reported from several centers. In these studies the patients received 2.5 mg gestrinone either two or three times a week for 6 months. Amenorrhea and symptomatic relief was established in 85% to 90% of the women within 2 months. Side effects were moderate, transient, and primarily related to androgenic and anabolic activity of the drug. Among treated women with no other infertility factor, pregnancy rates of approximately 60% have been reported.

Megestrol acetate, another progestational agent with antiandrogenic effect and suppressive action on gonadotropins, also has been used for the treatment of endometriosis. In doses of 40 mg per day for up to 24 weeks it has been found to relieve the symptoms of endometriosis in 86% of treated subjects.

DANAZOL

Danazol is an isoxazole derivative of the synthetic steroid 17α-ethinyl testosterone. It is well absorbed by the gastrointestinal tract and is rapidly metabolized by the liver. A major metabolite of danazol is 17α-ethinyl testosterone, which is known to be both a progestogen and a weak androgen. Danazol binds to intracellular receptors, sex hormone-binding globulin, and corticosteroid-binding globulin. Thus danazol may be considered biologically to be an androgen and glucocorticoid agonist. Danazol also binds to intranuclear progesterone receptors and appears to have a mixed agonist-antagonist activity with respect to the progesterone and estrogen receptors, but it has no estrogenic activity. In women, danazol has a mild suppressive effect on gonadotropin secretion, abolishes LH surge, and has an inhibitory effect on the growth of normal and ectopic endometrium. Thus the drug creates an anovulatory amenorrheic, high-androgen, low-estrogen milieu that is extremely hostile to the growth of endometriotic implants.

Clinical Application

When initially introduced, the standard regimen of danazol consisted of a dosage of 800 mg daily in divided doses for a period of 6 months or longer. Subsequently it was shown that lower dosages of 400 to 800 mg per day were equally effective. At lower doses, however, the rate of breakthrough bleeding increases. For this reason, a dosage of 600 mg/day for 6 months is recommended and appears to be effective in relieving symptoms and suppressing the endometriotic lesions. In practice, the dosage of danazol should be individualized and adjusted to the need of the patient, extent of the disease, and severity of side effects. The medication should be started after the completion of a normal menstruation. Danazol should not be administered to pregnant women because it may cause virilization of the external genitalia of the female fetus. Thus in patients with irregular or abnormal menstrual cycles the presence of an early pregnancy should be excluded by a sensitive pregnancy test before this medication is given. A barrier contraceptive should be used by patients using danazol, particularly those using less than 400-mg daily dosages.

The therapy interval also should be individualized. For preoperative and postoperative drug adjuvant therapy a period of 12 weeks of treatment may be adequate, whereas primary medical treatment necessitates a period of 6 months or longer.

Therapeutic Results

Danazol is highly effective in the treatment of dysmenorrhea but less effective in the management of chronic pelvic pain. Various studies have indicated symptomatic relief in 60% to 100% of cases. On the average, over 90% of patients experience improvement or resolution of dysmenorrhea, and over 80% note relief when dyspareunia or chronic pelvic pain is the predominant symptom.

The effect of danazol on endometriotic lesions has been assessed at second-look laparoscopy in several studies. Resolution of endometriotic implants occurs in almost 100% of minimal to mild cases (ASRM stages I and II) and in 50% to 70% of cases of more advanced lesions. Endometriomas greater than 1 cm in diameter, particularly those located in the ovary, respond poorly to danazol.

Pregnancy rates after danazol usage vary greatly with patient population, severity of disease, presence or absence of other infertility factors, and length of follow-up.

Collectively, current data indicate that danazol in doses of 600 to 800 mg per day for a period of 6 months is highly effective in alleviating the symptoms of endometriosis, particularly in early stages of the disease. Large endometriomas and advanced lesions are less likely to respond to this medication. Danazol may be used in combination with surgery in extensive endometrioses. The ability of danazol to enhance fertility in early stages of endometriosis has not been documented.

Side Effects

Danazol is an androgenic steroid, and its use results in side effects associated with a hyperandrogen state. These include weight gain, acne, hirsutism, oily skin, and a decrease in breast size. Other troubling side effects include muscle cramps, flushing, mood changes, depression, and edema. Patients receiving danazol are usually amenorrheic; however, breakthrough bleeding may occur when doses of 400 mg or less are given. Danazol has some adverse effect on lipid metabolism. It decreases HDL and increases LDL levels, but very low-density lipoprotein (VLDL) levels are unchanged. Fortunately, these changes are reversible within 3 to 5 months after therapy. Hepatic dysfunction, as evidenced by reversible elevated serum enzyme or jaundice, has also been reported in patients receiving a daily dosage of danazol of 400 mg or more. Thus the drug should be used cautiously in patients with hyperlipidemia or impaired liver function, and prolonged and repeated courses of the drug should be avoided. Inadvertent exposure to danazol during pregnancy may cause deformities of the external genitalia in the female fetus. Therefore patients receiving danazol therapy should use a barrier contraceptive during the entire course of treatment.

GONADOTROPIN-RELEASING HORMONE AGONISTS

Gonadotropin-releasing hormone (GnRH) is produced and released in pulsatile fashion from the arcuate nucleus and preoptic anterior hypothalamic area. It reaches the anterior pituitary through the portal system and is believed to bind to specific receptors in the anterior pituitary, where it stimulates the synthesis and secretion of LH and FSH in both males and females. Follicle-stimulating hormone and LH in turn are essential for gonadal function. Gonadotropin-releasing hormone is a decapeptide with an identical structure in all mammals, including humans. Like several other brain peptides, GnRH is synthesized as part of a much larger precursor peptide. When administered to women or men, GnRH stimulates a prompt and large release of LH and a smaller secretion of FSH.

Gonadotropin-releasing hormone is rapidly degraded by peptidase and cleared by glomerular filtration. Its half-life in peripheral circulation is only 2 to 4 minutes. To increase the potency and duration of action of GnRH, analogues with agonistic or antagonistic properties have been synthesized. Substitution of an amino acid at the 6 or 10 position results in analogues with agonistic activity. Administration of GnRH agonists (GnRH-a) produces an initial stimulation of pituitary gonadotropes that results in secretion of FSH and LH and the expected gonadal response. However, continuous or repeated administration of an agonist at nonphysiologic doses produces an inhibition of the pituitary-gonadal axis. Functional changes resulting from this inhibition include pituitary GnRH receptor down-regulation, gonadal gonadotropin receptor down-regulation, attenuated gonadotropin secretion, and decreased steroidogenesis. The inhibitory effects of analogues are fully reversible. Gonadotropin-releasing hormone receptor messenger RNA is also expressed in granulosa-lutein cells of human ovary across different functional stages, suggesting that the administration of GnRH analogs may have a direct action on the human ovary.

Gonadotropin-releasing hormone agonists are potent therapeutic agents with considerable advantages for clinical use. They cannot be administered orally because they are readily destroyed by the digestive process, but they may be given parenterally, by nasal spray, or in vaginal pessaries. Implants containing GnRH analogues and capable of slow drug release have been developed and are currently available. The biologic efficacy of GnRH-a administered by a nasal formulation is only 2% to 5% of the subcutaneous route. Gonadotropin-releasing hormone agonists are well tolerated, and their side effects are minimal.

The ability of GnRH-a to produce amenorrhea and anovulation has provided the basis for their use in the management of endometriosis (Table 16-2). A large number of clinical studies in the United States and European countries have demonstrated the efficacy of GnRH-a in the management of endometriosis.

Nafarelin (Synarel), a GnRH superagonist, was the first analogue introduced in the United States for the management of endometriosis. In a parallel double-blind study design, 204 patients with endometriosis were randomly treated with danazol or with 400 µg or 800 µg doses of nafarelin for 6 months. In another randomized clinical trial, 104 patients received nafarelin, 400 µg per day, and 63 were given danazol, 600 µg per day. A similar degree of relief of symptoms and regression of endometrial implants was observed in all groups. During the course of therapy there was an initial rise of gonadotropin and estradiol levels followed by sustained hypoestrogenism, amenorrhea, and anovulation. In another major multicenter clinical trial 315 patients with stage I-IV endometriosis (revised ASRM classification) were treated with goserelin acetate (Zoladex, 3.6 mg every 28 days by subcutaneous injection) or danazol (800 mg daily for 24 weeks). The

TABLE 16-2. Gonadotropin-releasing hormone agonists studied for management of endometriosis

Generic name	Route of administration	Dosage
Buserelin	Subcutaneous	200 µg/day
	Intranasal	300-344 µg × 4/days
Decapeptyl	Intramuscular depot	3 mg/mo
Goserelin	Subcutaneous implant*	3.6 mg/mo
Histerelin	Subcutaneous injection	100 µg/day
Leuprolide	Subcutaneous injection*	500-1000 µg/day
	Intranasal	400 µg × 4/day
	Intramuscular depot*	3.75-7.5 mg/mo
Nafarelin	Intranasal*	200 µg × 2/day
	Intramuscular depot	3 mg/mo
Tryptorelin	Intramuscular depot	2-4 mg/mo

*Available in the United States.

women were randomized in a 2:1 ratio (208 Zoladex:107 danazol). Both treatments significantly reduced mean subjective signs and symptoms of the disease during and after treatment. The mean percent reduction in the endometrial implant scores after 24 weeks of treatment was 56% for goserelin and 46% for danazol. Changes in serum gonadotropins and estradiol level were similar to those observed with nafarelin. Leuprolide acetate depot, yet another GnRH agonist administered intramuscularly, has also been shown to be efficacious in the management of symptomatic endometriosis in several multicenter clinical trials.

Adverse reactions associated with GnRH agonists were limited to those attributable to hypoestrogenism, including hot flashes, vaginal dryness, and some largely reversible loss of vertebral trabecular bone. The anabolic and androgenic properties of danazol were reflected in a high incidence of such side effects as weight gain, edema, acne, reduced breast size, and seborrhea. Myalgia, emotional lability, and headaches were also reported more frequently by patients receiving danazol. In addition, danazol treatment was associated with increases in hepatic enzyme levels and adverse changes in the serum lipid profile.

Other agonists have similar suppressive effects on endometriosis. Several reports have documented the beneficial effect of buserelin given in a dose of 0.2 mg subcutaneously per day or 1.2 mg intranasally per day for 6 months or longer.

Pregnancy rates among infertile patients receiving GnRH agonist therapy appear to be comparable to those treated with danazol or progestins, and recurrence rates are also similar.

Prolonged treatment with GnRH agonists has a significant impact on bone metabolism. The extent to which bone loss occurs depends on the potency and dosage of the GnRH, duration of use, and ultimately the degree of hypoestrogenism resulting from such therapy. Bone resorption is most pronounced in sites with a high trabecular bone content. Usually the effects of the analogues on bone metabolism are reversible and may return to pretreatment levels within 6 months after the cessation of therapy. However, up to 12 months after treatment, a significant residual loss of trabecular bone mineral content persists. There is therefore some concern regarding the effect of repeated courses of GnRH agonist treatment on bone mineral content. Because of this concern, prolonged or repeated cycles of GnRH agonists have not been sanctioned by the Food and Drug Administration (FDA). GnRH agonists currently approved by the FDA in the United States for the management of endometriosis are nafarelin, which is recommended in doses of 400 µg daily, leuprolide acetate, which is administered in doses of 3.75 mg every 4 weeks, and goserelin, which is given subcutaneously in doses of 3.6 mg every 4 weeks for 6 months.

To obviate the undesirable effect of hypoestrogenism on bone metabolism and vasomotor system, concomitant administration of a progestational agent, alone or in conjunction with estrogen, along with a GnRH agonist has been proposed. The rationale for such an approach is the notion that there may be a differential threshold of serum estradiol (E_2) level to suppress endometriosis and to maintain normal bone metabolism and calcium turnover. The optimal E_2 target to achieve this goal remains to be defined, but preliminary evidence suggests that an E_2 target in the range of 30 pg/ml may be as clinically effective as an E_2 target of 15 pg/ml for the treatment of pelvic pain caused by endometriosis. Strategies for achieving an E_2 target of 30 pg/ml might include the combination of GnRH-a plus E_2 add back or adjustment of GnRH-a dose to achieve the desired E_2 target. In a preliminary clinical trial, Friedman and Hornstein administered a combination of leuprolide acetate depot (3.75 mg/m every 4 weeks for 24 months) plus oral conjugated estrogen 0.625 mg per day and MPA 2.5 mg per day taken from treatment months 3 through 24 to six women with symptomatic endometriosis. There was significant improvement in hypoestrogenic symptoms and no change of bone density measurement of lumbar spine with this regimen. Several other small studies have confirmed these results. Progestogens are known to be beneficial for the management of menopausal vasomotor symptoms, bone loss, and treatment of endometriosis. However, the addition of daily doses of 20 to 30 mg of MPA to GnRH-a regimen failed to affect pain or suppression of endometriosis, although it decreased the hypoestrogenic effect of GnRH-a therapy alone.

In another study the combination of norethinedrone (0.35 mg or more daily) with GnRH agonists caused significant relief of pain, vasomotor symptoms, and endometriosis. Bone mineral density of the distal portion of the radius was not reduced during therapy, although lumbar spine bone density assessed by quantitative computed tomography was minimally but reversibly reduced. These preliminary data indicate that the combination of norethindrone or estrogen and progestogen with a GnRH-a is a well-tolerated and effective means of treating symptomatic endometriosis and may prevent undesirable side effects of GnRH-a therapy. However, properly controlled large-scale clinical trials are required to resolve this issue. A barrier contraceptive should be used during treatment with GnRH-a to prevent inadvertant exposure of a conceptus to the potential teratogenic effect of these drugs.

ANTIPROGESTINS

Antiprogestins are a group of steroid compounds that bind to progesterone receptors and exert antiprogesterone and antiglucocorticoid activities. Although many antiprogestins are being evaluated by pharmaceutic companies for various therapeutic purposes, only one (mifesterone [RU-486]) has been extensively studied in human beings. The drug has been widely used and is marketed in several European countries for termination of early pregnancy. Preliminary reports indicate that RU-486 may be effective in a variety of other conditions.

Because ectopic endometrial tissue contains both estrogen and progesterone receptors and is sensitive to hormonal agents that affect these receptors, it has been suggested that RU-486 could be beneficial in women with symptomatic endometriosis. In preliminary studies Kettel, Murphy, Mortola, and others have reported that RU-486 at a dose of 100 mg per day for 3 months in women with laparoscopically diagnosed pelvic endometriosis induced amenorrhea and brought about an improvement of pelvic pain. Serum estradiol and estrone (E_1), testosterone, androstenedione, serum FSH, thyroid-stimulating hormone, and prolactin remained unchanged throughout treatment course, whereas 24-hour mean serum cortisol and adrenocorticotropic hormone (ACTH) concentrations were increased after RU-486 treatment. The rise of cortisol and ACTH was most apparent during the early morning hours. These findings indicated that RU-486 at 100-mg daily dose induced an antiglucocorticoid effect. Side effects of this drug included atypical flushes, anorexia, and fatigue. Long-term treatment of endometriosis with RU-486 at a lower dose of 50 mg daily for 6 months has also been reported. Once again, all patients became anovulatory and amenorrheic. All subjects reported a significant decrease in pelvic pain that lasted throughout therapy. Laparoscopic assessment of endometriotic implants showed a decrease in eight of nine subjects. Bone mineral density of the lumbar spine and femur remained constant throughout therapy. The 24-hour mean serum cortisol was unchanged and the normal circadian rhythm was preserved.

These preliminary studies demonstrate the effectiveness of long-term low-dose RU-486 in achieving a condition of ovarian acyclicity and improving both pain and extent of pelvic endometriosis. Thus RU-486 may provide a safe and well-tolerated alternative for the medical management of endometriosis if these results are confirmed by larger clinical trials.

RELATIONSHIP OF ENDOMETRIOSIS AND INFERTILITY

A critical question is whether mild endometriosis actually causes infertility and whether treatment of endometriosis per se improves fertility. A large body of evidence indicates that considerable hormonal, biochemical, and immunologic alterations are related to or result from the presence of ectopic endometrial implants, including

1. Ovulatory defects, estimated to range from 17% to 27% of patients, that include abnormal gonadotropin secretion, abnormalities in follicular growth, and luteal phase defect
2. Alteration in the systemic immune response characterized by changes in humoral immunity (appearance of antiendometrial autoantibodies and

antiphospholipids in the serum), cell-mediated immune response, and altered peritoneal fluid local immune response

3. Direct toxic effect of prostaglandins or other cellular products of peritoneal fluid on the gametes or embryo
4. Possible increase in early pregnancy loss.

Thus, as suggested by Halme and Surrey, the cause of infertility in patients with endometriosis appears to be multifactorial. Central and local factors may affect normal ovulatory function in some patients. However, chronic inflammatory changes secondary to activation of local immune mechanisms, including macrophages and lymphocytes, play an important role in the impairment of the reproductive process. It is also possible that endometriosis affects each subject differently. Some women experience only a slight or no decrease in fecundity, whereas a more profound impairment takes place in others. A cyclic variability in the degree of impairment is also conceivable.

Theoretically, the role of any therapy for endometriosis is to suppress the hypothalamic-pituitary axis, prevent estrogen-mediated proliferation of endometrial implants, and produce necrobiosis and atrophy of existing implants. Additionally, such treatment should inhibit humoral and cell-mediated immune alterations and abolish cytotoxic and embryotoxic effects of factors observed in the presence of endometriosis. Many drugs used for the management of endometriosis meet some or all of these criteria. Do they, however, improve fertility? Until a few years ago, based on uncontrolled studies, it was generally thought that they do. Since 1982, seven controlled studies have appeared that cast doubt on this premise. Four of these studies used a randomized, untreated group of infertility patients and compared them with those treated with either danazol or a progestogen (MPA or gestrinone). All four reports indicated no significant differences between the treated and the untreated or placebo-treated group of patients. Another controlled but not randomized study compared the effectiveness of danazol, MPA, and no treatment in 144 patients with stage I and II endometriosis associated with infertility. Cumulative pregnancy rates as determined by life table analysis were 55% for controls, 71% for MPA-treated patients, and 46% for danazol-treated patients. There were no significant differences in these rates. In these studies, associated infertility factors were either excluded or, if present, treated. Another important factor is that the fecundity rate (the rate at which a couple achieves pregnancy in a given month) is reduced even with mild endometriosis.

These results may be interpreted in two ways. First, it may be concluded that mild endometriosis does not play a role in the etiology of infertility. This interpretation is probably too simplistic. Second, it may be argued that in some infertile women the presence of endometriosis is coincidental and the lesions exert little or no influence on fecundity, whereas in other subjects it can induce some or all of the biochemical and immunologic changes listed previously. Unfortunately, at present our diagnostic tools are too crude and our ability to adequately recognize affected patients too limited to enable us to differentiate between those who may benefit from therapeutic measures and those who will not.

Until we understand more precisely why endometriosis is so frequently (four to six times more) associated with infertility and identify the factor or factors that contribute to this relationship, prudence dictates that medical management of endometriosis be used in selected infertility patients.

We therefore suggest that in asymptomatic patients with stage I and II endometriosis, approximately 6 to 12 months of expectant management along with correction of other infertility factors is warranted before medical therapy is contemplated.

SURGICAL MANAGEMENT OF ENDOMETRIOSIS

Several modalities of surgical therapy may be used for conservative management of endometriosis. These include endoscopic surgery using either fulguration with thermal cautery or ablation with laser and surgical resection and removal by laparotomy.

Laparoscopic treatment of endometriosis has several advantages. The disease can be accurately diagnosed, staged, and immediately resected or ablated all in the course of one procedure. Additionally, adhesions can be lysed and endometriomas drained or excised when indicated and possible.

Electrocoagulation may be performed by using either a unipolar or bipolar source of electrical energy. Thermal damage to peritoneum, bowel, or other adjacent structures may occasionally occur when unipolar cauterization is performed. When bipolar electrical systems are used, the current passes from the generator across the jaws of the instrument back to the generator. Consequently, the heat generated is restricted to the tissue between the jaws of the insulated instrument. Bipolar systems are safer than unipolar, but accidents are still possible.

Ablation of endometriosis is achieved with the CO_2 laser. The CO_2 laser beam is precise and causes minimal damage to adjacent tissue. The immediate and near-total tissue absorption of the CO_2 laser beam limits thermal damage to surrounding tissue. Tissue coagulation is also accomplished when using other types of laser, such as argon or KTP (potassium tantanyl phosphate) lasers. These lasers destroy the tissue primarily by photocoagulation rather than vaporization.

Studies comparing the effectiveness of thermocoagulation or laser ablation with conservative surgery or medical therapy are not available. In a randomized study of 123 infertile patients, 60.8% of those whose endometriotic implants were fulgurated conceived within 8 months after laparoscopy, whereas only 18.5% of women whose endometriotic implants were not coagulated achieved a pregnancy. Numerous publications have appeared on the results achieved with laser therapy for endometriosis. Generally, these indicate a pregnancy rate of 50% to 60% in patients treated with CO_2 laser and somewhat higher when endometriosis was the only infertility factor identified. Unfortunately, the majority of these studies are uncontrolled and thus difficult to evaluate. Furthermore, while providing some data on pregnancy, as an end point they lack information relative to the relief of symptoms such as pain and recurrence. A review of the few studies containing such information indicates the following:

1. The percentage of patients obtaining relief of dysmenorrhea, dyspareunia, and pelvic pain with endoscopic surgery is similar to that reported for other therapeutic modalities, including laparotomy.
2. Using newer techniques and instrumentations the majority of cases of mild and moderate pelvic endometriosis may be managed by laparoscopic approach. Laser laparoscopy is a safe and effective treatment in alleviating pain symptoms with stages I to III (ASRM) endometriosis.

Surgical Excision

Removal of endometrial implants during laparoscopy is an alternative to fulguration and laser ablation. However, because of complications such as bleeding and adhesion development, as well as difficulties in removing lesions located in sites such as the bowel or ureter, laser ablation is preferred. For extensive endometriosis, conservative surgery by laparotomy is the method of choice. Laser or thermocoagulation may be used during these operations to ablate or fulgurate implants or lyse adhesions. Preoperative or postoperative medical treatment is commonly combined with conservative surgery for advanced diseases. For practical purposes, mild and moderate endometriosis may be treated by a laparoscopic approach or medical therapy, whereas extensive endometriosis, particularly lesions involving bowel or urinary tract, require surgical therapy, usually through a laparotomy.

Hysterectomy with removal of ovaries should be considered in patients who have severe symptomatic disease and are no longer interested in future pregnancies.

RECURRENCE OF ENDOMETRIOSIS

Endometriosis has the potential of recurring any time during the reproductive age. Only menopause or hysterectomy with bilateral oophorectomy may produce a cure. Thus the disease may reappear after all medical or conservative surgical modalities of treatment. The recurrence rate of endometriosis varies in different women and probably depends on the invasiveness of the disease, host resistance, and possibly intervening pregnancies. In some patients, a single course of medical treatment or surgical intervention may be followed by a prolonged period of relief, whereas in others, recurrences occur within a few months after termination of treatment. After a course of danazol therapy, for example, the recurrence of symptoms and lesions is approximately 5% to 20% per year. A second course of medical therapy may be provided if, in fact, the initial course resulted in a remission of disease.

BIBLIOGRAPHY

American Fertility Society: Revised classification of endometriosis, *Fertil Steril* 43:351, 1985.

Andrews WE, Larson GD: Endometriosis: treatment with hormonal pseudopregnancy and/or operation, *Am J Obstet Gynecol* 118:643, 1974.

Azadian-Boulanger G, Secchi J, Tournemine C, et al: Hormonal activity profile of drugs for endometriosis therapy. In Raynaud JP, et al, editors: *Medical management of endometriosis*, New York, 1984, Raven Press.

Barbieri RL, Hornstein MD: Medical therapy of endometriosis. In Wilson EA, editor: *Endometriosis*, New York, 1987, Alan R Liss.

Barbieri RL, Gordon AC: Hormonal therapy of endometriosis. The estradiol target, *Fertil Steril* 56:820, 1991.

Bayer SR, Seibel MM: Medical treatment: danazol. In Schenken RS, editor: *Endometriosis: contemporary concepts in clinical management*, Philadelphia, 1989, Lippincott.

Bayer SR, Seibel MM, Saffan DS, et al: Effect of danazol treatment for minimal endometriosis in infertile women. A prospective randomized study, *J Reprod Med* 33:179, 1988.

Bergqvist A, Carlstrom K, Jepson S, et al: Histochemical localization of specific estrogen and progesterone binding in human endometrium and endometriotic tissue, *Acta Obstet Gynecol Scand* 123(suppl):15, 1984.

Berguist C: Effects of nafarelin versus danazol on lipids and calcium metabolism, *Am J Obstet Gynecol* 162:589, 1990.

Cedars MI, Lu JKH, Meldrum DR, et al: Treatment of endometriosis with a long acting gonadotropin releasing hormone agonist plus medroxyprogesterone acetate, *Obstet Gynecol* 75:641, 1990.

Claesson B, Bergquist C: Clinical experience treating endometriosis with nafarelin, *J Reprod Med* 34:1025, 1989.

Corbin A, Frederick J, Jones B, et al: Comparison of LHRH agonists and antagonists anti-fertility and therapeutic developments. In Labrie F, Belanger A, editors: *LHRH and its analogs*, New York, 1984, Elsevier Science Publishers.

Cornillie FJ, Oosterlynck D, Lauweryns JM, et al: Deeply infiltrating pelvic endometriosis: histology and clinical significance, *Fertil Steril* 53:978, 1990.

Dawood MY, Spellacy WN, Dmowski WP, et al: A comparison of the efficacy and safety of buserelin vs danazol in the treatment of endometriosis. In Chadha DR, Buttram VC Jr, editors: *Current concepts in endometriosis*, New York, 1990, Alan R Liss.

Dawood Y, Lewis V, Ramos J: Cortical and trabelcular bone mineral content in women with endometriosis: effect of gonadotropin releasing hormone agonist and danazol, *Fertil Steril* 52:21, 1989.

Dmowski WP, Radwanska E, Binor Z, et al: Ovarian suppression induced with buserelin or danazol in the management of endometriosis: a randomized comparative study, *Fertil Steril* 51:395, 1989.

Fahraeus L, Sydsjo A, Wallentin L: Lipoprotein changes during treatment of pelvic endometriosis with medroxyprogesterone acetate, *Fertil Steril* 45:503, 1986.

Friedman AJ, Hornstein MD: Gonadotropin releasing hormone agonist plus estrogen-progestin "add back" therapy for endometriosis related pelvic pain, *Fertil Steril* 60:236, 1993.

Halme J, Surrey ES: Endometriosis and infertility: the mechanisms involved. In Chadha DR, Buttram VC Jr, editors: *Current concepts in endometriosis*, New York, 1990, Alan R Liss.

Hammond CB: Conservative treatment of endometriosis, *Fertil Steril* 30:497, 1978.

Hammond CB, Rock JA, Parker RT: Conservative treatment of endometriosis. The effects of limited surgery and hormonal pseudopregnancy, *Fertil Steril* 27:756, 1976.

Henzl M, Corson S, Moghissi K, et al: Administration of nasal nafarelin versus oral danazol for endometriosis. A multicenter double-blind comparative clinical trial, *N Engl J Med* 318:485, 1988.

Henzl MR, Long K: Efficacy and safety of nafarelin in the treatment of endometriosis, *Am J Obstet Gynecol* 162:570, 1990.

Hughes EG, Federkow DM, Collins JA: A quantitative overview of controlled trials in endometriosis associated infertility, *Fertil Steril* 59:963, 1993.

Hull ME, Moghissi KS, Magyar DM, et al: Comparison of different treatment modalities of endometriosis in infertile women, *Fertil Steril* 47:40, 1987.

Johanson JS, Rus BJ, Hassager C, et al: The effect of a gonadotropin-releasing hormone agonist analog (nafarelin) on bone metabolism, *J Clin Endocrinol Metab* 67:701, 1988.

Kettel LM, Murphy AA, Mortola JF, et al: Endocrine responses to long term administration of the antiprogesterone RU-486 in patients with pelvic endometriosis, *Fertil Steril* 56:402, 1991.

Kistner RW: The use of newer progestins in the treatment of endometriosis, *Clin Obstet Gynecol* 9:271, 1958.

Kistner RW: Management of endometriosis in infertile patient, *Fertil Steril* 26:1151, 1975.

Knobil E: The neuroendocrine control of the menstrual cycle, *Recent Prog Horm Res* 36:53, 1980.

Martin DC, Diamond MP: Operative laparoscopy. Comparison of laser with other techniques, *Curr Probl Obstet Gynecol Fertil* 9:564, 1986.

McArthur JW, Ulfelder H: The effect of pregnancy upon endometriosis, *Obstet Gynecol Surv* 20:709, 1965.

Minartzis D, Jakubowski M, Mortola JF, et al: Gonadotropin-releasing hormone receptor gene expression in human ovary and granulosa lutein cells, *J Clin Endocrinol Metab* 8:430, 1995.

Moghissi KS, Boyce CR: Management of endometriosis with oral medroxyprogesterone acetate, *Obstet Gynecol* 47:265, 1976.

Noble AD, Letchworth AT: Medical treatment of endometriosis. A comparative trial, *Postgrad Med* 5(suppl):37, 1979.

Nowroozi K, Chase JS, Check JH, et al: The importance of laparoscopic coagulation of mild endometriosis in infertile women, *Int J Fertil* 32:422, 1987.

Rock JA, Markham SM: Extrapelvic endometriosis. In Wilson EA, editor: *Endometriosis*, New York, 1987, Alan R Liss.

Rock JA, Truglia JA, Caplan RJ, et al: Zoladex (Goserelin acetate implant) in the treatment of endometriosis: a randomized comparison with danazol, *Obstet Gynecol* 82:198, 1993.

Schlaff WD, Dugoff L, Damewood MD, et al: Magestrol acetate for treatment of endometriosis, *Obstet Gynecol* 75:646, 1990.

Shaw RW: Female pseudohermaphroditism associated with danazol exposure in utero. Case report, *Br J Obstet Gynaecol* 91:386, 1984.

Shaw RW: Goserelin-depot preparation of LHRH analogues used in the treatment of endometriosis. In Chadha DR, Buttram VC Jr, editor: *Current concepts in endometriosis*, New York, 1990, Alan R Liss.

Surrey ES, Gambone JC, Lu JKH, et al: The effect of combining norethindrone with a gonadotropin-releasing hormone agonist with treatment of symptomatic endometriosis, *Fertil Steril* 53: 620, 1990.

Sutton CJG, Ewen SP, Whitelaw N, et al: Prospective, randomized, double blind controlled trial of laser laparoscopy in the treatment of pelvic pain associated with minimal, mild and moderate endometriosis, *Fertil Steril* 62:696, 1994.

Telimaa S: Danazol and medroxyprogesterone acetate inefficacies in the treatment modalities of endometriosis in infertile women, *Fertil Steril* 47:40, 1987.

Thomas EJ, Cook ID: Successful treatment of asymptomatic endometriosis: does it benefit infertile women, *Br Med J* 294:1117, 1987.

Tummon IS, Pepping M, Binor Z, et al: A randomized, prospective comparison of endocrine changes induced with intranasal leuprolide or danazol for treatment of endometriosis, *Fertil Steril* 51:390, 1989.

Waibel-Treber S, Minne HW, Scharla SH, et al: Reversible bone loss in women treated with GnRH agonists for endometriosis and uterine leiomyoma, *Hum Reprod* 4:384, 1989.

Wheeler JM, Kettle JD, Miller JD: Depot leuprolide acetate versus danazol in the treatment of women with symptomatic endometriosis: a multicenter double blind randomized clinical trial. II. Assessment of safety, *Am J Obstet Gynecol* 169:26, 1993.

Yeu SSC: Use of antiprogestins in the management of endometriosis and leiomyoma. In Donaldson MS, Dorflinger L, Brown SS, et al, editors: *Clinical application of mifepristone (RU-486)*, Washington, DC, 1993, National Academy Press.

CHAPTER 17

Pelvic Mass: Detection, Diagnosis, and Management

JOANNA M. CAIN

The need to accurately diagnose the etiology of a pelvic mass is based on the need to plan further management carefully. The oldest route for detection of pelvic abnormalities, a careful pelvic examination, remains the safest and cheapest method as well as one that is critical in decisions about further evaluation. Understanding the workup and management of pelvic masses detected by any means may help prevent unnecessary, costly, and delaying workups. This chapter will focus on detection, workup, and appropriate management patterns for pelvic masses.

SCREENING PELVIC EXAMINATIONS, ULTRASOUND, AND TUMOR MARKERS

The need to improve on the initial detection of pelvic masses is a product of concern about the presence of a pelvic malignancy. Because of the continuing difficulty in curing epithelial ovarian cancer, the potential of early detection of these malignancies has given birth to a number of screening formats for detection of pelvic masses and for assessing the potential for malignancy. Whether or not these formats hold any cost-effective chance of improving our early detection of these cancers, they do hold some clues about the potential utility of screening forms such as ultrasound and serum tumor markers. This desire for early detection of asymptomatic pelvic malignancies, primarily ovarian, has led to a number of trials, some of which are outlined in Table 17-1. These trials are hampered by the fact that the incidence of these malignancies is relatively low (1.7% risk per patient) and the number needed to evaluate screening is large. These trials are reporting on already present ovarian enlargements over short periods of time rather than the development or detection of such masses in a population over longer periods. Follow-up over a number of years is difficult because of poor patient compliance. At present, we have no evidence that such screening patterns will detect ovarian cancers earlier or prove cost-effective for the general population.

There is a group of patients at risk for ovarian cancer, however, who may benefit from such screening solely because the incidence of ovarian cancer is much higher for the group. These are the patients who have a familial history of ovarian cancer. Unfortunately, the main national registry is dependent on referral of patients and families to their database. Therefore, although we use the material from this group, the information from this

TABLE 17-1. Screening trials for ovarian cancer

Trial	Method	Number of patients	Comments
Andolf et al	Ultrasound	801	Population: 40-70 yr and increased risk. No correlation found.
Bhan et al	Ultrasound	5479	Population: self-selected ongoing trial with numerous papers on this group. No conclusion regarding screening. Five malignancies found.
Bourne et al	Transvaginal (TV) color ultrasound	50	Population: previous abnormal TV ultrasound. Seven malignancies. Identifies characteristics of malignant masses.
Jacobs et al	Ca-125 + exam, then ultrasound	1010	Highest specificity when all three were combined.
van Nagell et al	Transvaginal ultrasound	1000	Population: >40 yr asymptomatic. One malignant tumor found.
Grover et al	Pelvic exam	2623	Population 25-92. High specificity.
Schutter et al	Ca-125 + exam, then ultrasound	228	Highest specificity when all three combined.

database cannot represent a true population-based study. In these families, a proposed inheritable autosomal dominant pattern is identified by the presence of two or more first-degree relatives with ovarian cancer or a family tree with many second-degree relatives with ovarian cancer. The risk may approach 50% for those with two first-degree relatives, particularly if they occur at ages less than 50. For this reason, the registry recommends screening every 6 months with Ca-125, pelvic examinations, and pelvic ultrasound. Again, data documenting a clear increase in early detection and increased survival benefit from such screening are not available; however, the increased incidence in these select families may lend itself to an increase in detection by such screening methods. Genetic screening for the small group of women with hereditary syndromes may be appropriate in the future as clarification of appropriate genetic markers continues (BRCA1). Women who are members of high-risk families have expressed a high rate of interest in such screening.

HISTORY

Once a pelvic mass is detected, the workup should proceed with the fewest unnecessary tests to the diagnosis. This is not simple. Because the pelvis contains not only reproductive organs but also major components of the gastrointestinal (GI) tract, the urinary tract, and the pelvic vascular system, the potential origins of a pelvic mass (Table 17-2) can cause great confusion. The first elements to identify are the history associated with the mass and a careful identification of the location by physical examination before further evaluation proceeds. Although none of these is conclusive, combined they can identify the extent of further evaluation required.

History taking assumes paramount importance with the evaluation of a pelvic mass. Because of the numerous potential sites of origin the history cannot be limited to gynecologic history only. If a systems approach is used, information in the following areas should be elicited:

Past history: History of stroke, diabetes, medications, previous malignancies.
Ob/Gyn history: Any pelvic surgery; pelvic infections; gravidity/parity; details of obstetric history; present menstrual status, especially detailing abnormal bleeding and chance of present pregnancy; previous Papanicolaou history.
Urinary history: Frequency, hematuria, incontinence, onset and inciting factors, voiding patterns.
Gastrointestinal: Increased girth, nausea, bowel dysfunction, tarry stools, blood in stools, diarrhea/constipation, pressure/nausea.
Developmental history: Any known congenital anomalies, neurologic motor problems.

TABLE 17-2. Partial listing of potential sources of pelvic masses

CENTRAL NERVOUS SYSTEM

Meningocele

URINARY TRACT

Pelvic kidney
Bladder malignancy

VASCULAR/LYMPHATIC

Hemangioma
Aneurysm
Lymph node enlargement

GASTROINTESTINAL

Appendicocele abscess
Diverticular abscess
Gastrointestinal malignancy

REPRODUCTIVE ORGANS

Pregnancy—in or out of uterus
Congenital anomalies
Cervical mass—benign and malignant
Uterine mass—benign and malignant
Parametrial mass—benign and malignant
Adnexal mass—benign and malignant

RETROPERITONEAL/PERITONEAL MASSES

Peritoneal inclusion cyst
Retroperitoneal mass—fibrosarcoma, desmoid tumor
Endometriosis implants

Vascular:	Known aneurysms or hemangioma elsewhere, assessment of vascular supply to legs.
Infection:	Fever, chills; when/how long?
Medication:	Clomid and others.

Positive findings in one of these areas should lead to further detailed questioning.

PHYSICAL EXAMINATION

The importance of a thorough physical examination cannot be overstated. Without it, for example, how are we to know that the pelvic mass might be a metastatic focus from a palpable breast mass? We will delete the details of a full examination, however, to concentrate on valuable elements of the abdominal and pelvic examination. Often the physical examination *alone* is adequate to plan surgery without future evaluation as in the case of a postmenopausal woman who has a large pelvic mass with palpable metastatic disease and ascites.

Abdomen: Hepatic size, epigastric mass, splenic size, fluid wave, palpable mass, rebound, guarding, tenderness, trauma, or scars.

Pelvis: Identify cervix position (if present), uterine contour and position, and central or lateral position of mass and mass attachments; rectovaginal and rectal examination with stool guaiac test should be done for all patients. The access to a full sacral, cul-de-sac, and rectal mucosal evaluation with the rectal examination is important.

If, at this time, the site and potential for malignancy are identified, the workup appropriate for that area should proceed.

TRIAGE OF WORKUP

Differentiating between a central or lateral location can serve to triage lesions. A definite site of origin can often be easily identified (ovary or uterus, for example) from the history and physical examination. The ambiguous mass presents the most challenging problems. Clues from location of the mass and the history may help diagnose even such rare conditions as the following:

Neurogenic bladder: History of stroke, diabetes, dribbling, or incontinence may all be clues. A red rubber catheter may produce complete resolution of the mass.

Meningocele or retroperitoneal mass: Uterus seems pushed anterior only. Rectal examination suggests a mass posterior to the rectum or a rectum displaced to the side, not ballotable, and no space from anterior part of the sacrum.

Specifically, masses that are localized solely in the lateral area or on the sidewall might be as follows:

Right: Gastrointestinal; a cecal or appendicocoele mass will often be found higher than the ovarian position, although the mass can extend down to parametria.

Left: Rectosigmoid mass.

Either: Ovarian or paraovarian; if on the pelvic sidewall and not connected to reproductive structures, consider lymph node enlargement or pelvic aneurysm. Is there a transmitted pulse with the mass?

Both: Bilateral ovarian masses are of concern because bilaterality may double the risk of malignancy.

The majority of masses, unfortunately, fall into areas involving both midline and lateral areas. Further workup is warranted at this point based on identification or an inability to define the primary site (Fig. 17-1).

GENERAL WORKUP
Use of Ultrasound Evaluation of the Pelvis

When the site cannot be identified, ultrasound, transabdominal or transvaginal, can be a rapid, low-risk approach to site evaluation. It can

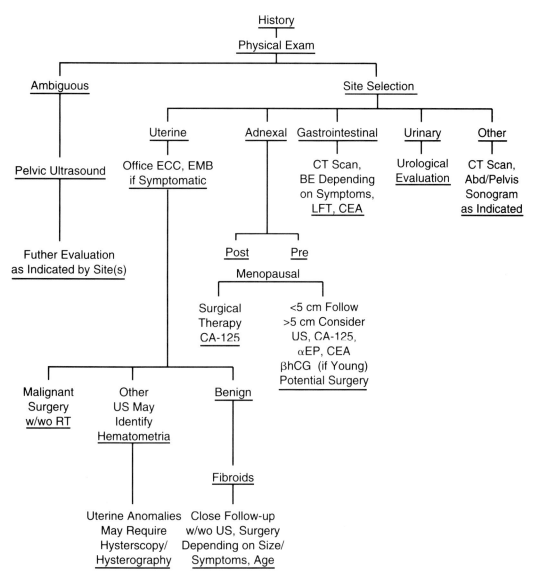

FIGURE 17-1. Evaluation of a pelvic mass.

potentially identify all the lesions listed in Table 17-2. The office use of vaginal ultrasound has expanded the availability of such screening of ambiguous pelvic masses and appears to have little variability between well-trained observers. Certain technological developments such as color flow imaging may help define the characteristics of a mass that suggest malignancy. Furthermore, combining other evaluations such as Ca-125 with ultrasound findings may increase the likelihood of identifying patients more likely to have malignant ovarian masses and thereby direct them to early oncologic management to facilitate their overall treatment.

The question must be, however, whether this examination changes the proposed therapy. If the patient is postmenopausal with a large pelvic or abdominal mass, performance of ultrasound evaluation does not change the need for surgical exploration. A metastatic workup based on the history would be more valuable because it would add to presurgical assessment of potential surgical problems and indicate origin and possible reasons to forego surgery (such as liver function tests, creatinine, barium enema if colonic obstruction or colon primary is suspected, bone scan if there is a history of breast cancer, etc.).

Fine-needle biopsy or aspiration of a new pelvic mass is generally discouraged because of the potential to export or extend a primary malignancy. However, confirmation of recurrence of a known primary such as a pelvic mass may be aided by fine-needle biopsy, which would allow patients with some malignancies to avoid surgical exploration.

Magnetic Resonance Imaging/Computed Tomography

Magnetic resonance imaging (MRI) and computed tomography are costly procedures that should be limited to patients for whom specific questions must be answered. They may be of special help when a congenital anomaly is suspected (uterine, pelvic kidney, meningocele) or concerns about a GI malignancy are present, especially in the evaluation of metastatic disease (hepatic lesions, for example). In one study by Gore, Cooke, Wiltshaw, and others, management of patients with suspected ovarian cancer was not significantly altered by these evaluations even when they disagreed with the clinical presentation. Considering their cost, they should not be a part of routine evaluation for a suspected ovarian neoplasm.

Angiography

Vascular anomalies can often be identified first by ultrasound Doppler examinations; however, definitive evaluation and potential embolization or sclerosis will require experienced angiographic skills.

Laboratory Evaluation: Ca-125

Tumor markers, primarily Ca-125, have come to hold an increasing position in preoperative decision making about the management of pelvic masses and the potential referral of a patient to a tertiary-care center or subspecialist. In that context, it is important to recognize the limits of such testing. According to Bast, Klug, St. John, and associates, the original intent of the Ca-125 test was to monitor the course of epithelial ovarian cancers, still the most frequent use of this tumor marker. The initial choice of greater than 35 units/ml as abnormal was arbitrary. At this level 1.4% of apparently healthy women controls, 6.3% of patients with benign diseases, and 28.5% of patients with nongynecologic cancers had elevated levels, while 82% of known epithelial malignancies had elevated levels. It is obvious from this that a negative Ca-125 result does not rule out malignancy. Other studies extending the use of Ca-125 into preoperative evaluation of pelvic masses suggest that the sensitivity of the test for pelvic malignancy (including endometrial cancer, nonepithelial or ovarian cancer, etc.) may be as high as 95%. Still other studies show a differentiation in sensitivity based on menopausal status, with a greater specificity and sensitivity in postmenopausal patients where benign conditions such as active endometriosis can confuse the findings. Panels of serum markers are being evaluated for increasing the accuracy of preoperative diagnosis, but the Ca-125 test remains the most available.

The primary use of Ca-125, however, remains as a marker to follow the treatment of epithelial ovarian cancers. Therefore when ovarian cancer is the presumed diagnosis on physical examination alone, a Ca-125 reference level should be obtained before any treatment.

SPECIFIC SITES
Ovarian Neoplasms

At present, the most accurate preoperative evaluations of ovarian masses are those that combine physical examination, history of menopausal status and age, and Ca-125 and ultrasound findings.

Grave physical findings include any or all of the following: pulmonary effusion, cul-de-sac nodularity, an upper abdominal mass suggestive of an omental cake, ascites, and bilaterality of the masses. Menopausal status has an impact on the likelihood that an ovarian neoplasm is malignant: It raises the risk for ages 60 to 69 years to twelvefold greater than ages 20 to 29. In premenopausal women the risk that any ovarian neoplasm is malignant is about 13%, but this increases to about 45% in postmenopausal women.

Ultrasound findings taken by themselves can present the most confusing picture. Sonography has been noted, quite frankly, to be misleading in up to 15% of patients, where it has misrepresented the benign or malignant nature of the lesion. The positive predictive value for diagnosing malignancy in one study was only 73%. Even characteristics associated with benign diagnoses such as clear cysts without septa at larger than 5 cm have been reported by various authors to have up to a 29% incidence of neoplastic changes and a 9% incidence of malignancy in postmenopausal patients. However, cysts less than 5 cm without septa, even in postmenopausal patients, did not demonstrate malignancy in most studies except for a patient with papillate formations present on the wall. Not surprisingly, characteristics such as larger size, multiple septa, solid parts, or papillate growths on a wall increased the likelihood of a malignancy being present.

Compiling these data with a general framework for management of clinically palpable ovarian masses can give some guidelines:

1. Reevaluation with physical examination alone after ovarian suppression or the completion of the next menstrual cycle is appropriate for premenopausal (or younger than 40-year-old) patients with unilateral, clinically nonsuspicious masses less than 5 cm. If persistent, ultrasound evaluation may be of benefit.

2. Baseline transvaginal or transabdominal ultrasound evaluation may be helpful in management decisions for patients with clinically nonsuspicious masses who are postmenopausal or those of any age who have masses larger than 5 cm or bilateral masses.

3. Patients with multiple grave physical findings require surgical evaluation, and a baseline Ca-125 value should be obtained and the patient referred for oncologic care. Needle aspiration of the mass is discouraged.

4. Patients with abnormal ultrasound findings should have appropriate tumor markers drawn and the potential referral to oncologic care for surgery based on the levels of these and the ultrasound abnormalities. For example, a patient with an elevated Ca-125 value and papillate formations visible on ultrasound has a high likelihood of malignancy.

5. Patients with symptoms, examination findings consistent with endometriosis, and a suspected endometrioma often have elevated Ca-125 value as well. These can present a confusing picture, and at least a diagnostic laparoscopy should be planned to confirm the diagnosis before conservative therapy is carried out for endometriosis.

6. In women younger than 35 years of age, a primarily solid mass on ultrasound can also indicate a primary germ cell malignancy of the ovary. The serum markers for these tumors include primarily β–human chorionic gonadotropin (βHCG) and α-fetoprotein (αFP), lactic dehydrogenase (LDH), and carcinoembryonic antigen (CEA). Besides their assistance in diagnosis, these markers are critical in evaluating the response to postoperative therapy.

Uterine Masses

In premenopausal women, pregnancy and uterine leiomyomas are common sources of a pelvic mass. Pregnancy lends itself to rapid diagnosis with physical examination and measurement of HCG. If a hydatidiform mole is suspected because of unusual bleeding, passage of tissue, size and date lack of correlation, or a failure to find fetal heart tones, serum measurement of βHCG and an ultrasound should be obtained.

If uterine leiomyomas are suspected on physical examination, further workup might include pelvic ultrasound if the ovaries cannot be clearly palpated separately. If there are associated symptoms, particularly abnormal uterine bleeding, further evaluation is required. An endocervical scraping and endometrial biopsy specimen will help rule out the possibility of malignancy or hyperplasia. Hysterograms and hysteroscopy may be of value when the bleeding or discharge is suspected to arise from a submucous fibroid or a prolapsing fibroid. Resection of smaller submucous fibroids can also be accomplished through the hysteroscope in many cases. Documentation of the size of the fibroids and the impact of increased bleeding on the hemoglobin and hematocrit are important in patient management.

Rapidly enlarging fibroids present a particular problem in patient management for both premenopausal and postmenopausal patients. Rapid growth most commonly represents infarction or bleeding in a fibroid but raises the specter of uterine sarcomas in the clinician's mind. The frequency of sarcomatous changes in leiomyomas is unknown because the base population of fibroids is unknown but may be around 1.5%. The majority of patients with sarcomas also have associated abnormal uterine bleeding, and an endometrial biopsy or curettage may diagnose the condition. Ultrasound and MRI may be of value when rapid growth occurs if areas of hemorrhage or characteristics of malignancy can be identified. Laparoscopy is not generally of help because the external uterine surface may have minimal if any abnormalities even with sarcoma present. For patients in whom real concern exists and the diagnostic tests are not definitive, removal of the supposed myoma or the uterus may be the only definitive test.

Other conditions leading to uterine enlargement are numerous. Adenomyosis, rare tumors of the uterus, and congenital anomalies such as enlargement of a blind uterine horn after menarche are some examples. The differential diagnosis follows the pattern of careful physical examination with endometrial sampling for symptoms and ultrasound or MRI for ambiguous findings.

Conservative management of any pelvic mass can be based only on the most careful pelvic, laboratory, and for some circumstances ultrasound or radiographic demonstration of the diagnosis. Further management of specific diagnoses are well covered elsewhere.

BIBLIOGRAPHY

Andolf E, Jorgensen C: Cystic lesions in elderly women diagnosed by ultrasound, *Br J Obstet Gynaecol* 96:1076, 1989.

Andolf E, Jorgensen C, Astedt B: Ultrasound examination for detection of ovarian carcinoma in risk groups, *Obstet Gynecol* 75:106, 1990.

Bast RC, Klug TL, St John E, et al: A radioimmunoassay using a monoclonal antibody to monitor the course of epithelial ovarian cancer, *N Engl J Med* 309:883, 1983.

Bernacerrif BR, Finkler NJ, Wojciechowski C, et al: Sonographic accuracy in the diagnosis of ovarian masses, *J Reprod Med* 35: 49, 1990.

Bhan V, Amso N, Whitehead MI, et al: Characteristics of persistent ovarian masses in asymptomatic women, *Br J Obstet Gynaecol* 96:1382, 1989.

Bourne T, Campbell S, Steer C, et al: Transvaginal color flow imaging: a possible new screening technique for ovarian cancer, *Br Med J* 229:1367, 1989.

Campbell S, Royston P, Bhan V, et al: Novel screening strategies for early ovarian cancer by transabdominal ultrasonography, *Br J Obstet Gynaecol* 97:304, 1990.

Einhorn N, Bast RC, Knapp RC, et al: Preoperative evaluation of serum Ca 125 levels in patients with primary epithelial ovarian cancer, *Obstet Gynecol* 67:414, 1986.

Finkler NJ, Benacerraf B, Lavin PT, et al: Comparison of serum Ca 125 clinical impression, and ultrasound in preoperative evaluation of ovarian masses, *Obstet Gynecol* 72:659, 1988.

Fleischer AC, McKee MS, Gordon AN, et al: Transvaginal sonography of postmenopausal ovaries with pathologic correlation, *J Ultrasound Med* 9:637, 1990.

Gore ME, Cooke JC, Wiltshaw E, et al: The impact of computed sonography and ultrasonography on the management of patients with carcinoma of the ovary, *Br J Cancer* 60:751, 1989.

Granberg S, Wikland M, Jansson I: Macroscopic characterization of ovarian tumors and the relation to the histologic diagnosis: criteria to be used for ultrasound evaluation, *Gynecol Oncol* 35:139, 1989.

Greggi S, Genuardi M, Benedetti-Panci P, et al: Analysis of 138 consecutive ovarian cancer patients: incidence and characteristics of familial cases, *Gynecol Oncol* 39:300, 1990.

Grover S, Quinn MA, Weideman P: Patterns of inheritance of ovarian cancer: an analysis from an ovarian cancer screening program, *Cancer* 72:526, 1993.

Higgins RV, van Nagell JR, Woods CH, et al: Interobserver variation in ovarian measurements using transvaginal sonography, *Gynecol Oncol* 39:69, 1990.

Hurwitz A, Yagel S, Zion I, et al: The management of persistent clear pelvic cysts diagnosed by ultrasound, *Obstet Gynecol* 72:320, 1988.

Iwamari A, Miyakoa J, Dati Y, et al: Differential diagnosis of ovarian cancer, benign ovarian tumor, and endometriosis by a combination assay of serum sialyl SSEA-1 antigen and Ca-125 levels, *Gynecol Obstet Invest* 29: 71, 1990.

Jacobs I, Stabile I, Bridges J, et al: Multimodal approach to screening for ovarian cancer, *Lancet* 1:268, 1988.

Koonings PP, Grimes PA, Campbell K, et al: Bilateral ovarian neoplasms and the risk of malignancy, *Am J Obstet Gynecol* 162:167, 1990.

Maggino T, Gadducci A, D'Addario V, et al: Prospective multicenter study on CA 125 in postmenopausal pelvic masses, *Gynecol Oncol* 54:117, 1994.

Montague ACW, Swartz DP, et al: Sarcoma arising in a leiomyoma of the uterus, *Am J Obstet Gynecol* 92:421, 1965.

Neuwirth RS: Hysteroscopic management of symptomatic submuceous fibroids, *Obstet Gynecol* 62:509, 1983.

O'Connell GJ, Ryan E, Murphy KJ, et al: Predictive value of Ca 125 for ovarian carcinoma in patients presenting with pelvic masses, *Obstet Gynecol* 70:930, 1987.

Schutter EM, Kenemans P, Sohn C, et al: Diagnostic value of pelvic examination, ultrasound, and serum CA 125 in postmenopausal women with a pelvic mass. An international multicenter study, *Cancer* 74:1398, 1994.

Tholander B, Taube A, Lindgren A, et al: Pretreatment serum levels of Ca 125, carcinoembryonic antigen, tissue polypeptide antigen, and placental alkaline phosphalaise in patients with ovarian carcinoma, borderline tu mors, or benign adnexal masses: relevance for differential diagnosis, *Gynecol Oncol* 39:16, 1990.

Trimbos JB, Hacker NF: The case against aspirating ovarian cysts, *Cancer* 72:828, 1993.

van Dink T, Woodruff JP: Leiomyosarcoma of the uterus, *Am J Obstet Gynecol* 144:817, 1982.

Van Nagell JR Jr, Higgins RV, Donaldson ES, et al: Transvaginal sonography as a screening method for ovarian cancer, *Cancer* 1:573, 1990.

Weinreb JC, Barkoff ND, Megibow A, et al: The value of MR imaging in distinguishing leiomyomas from other solid pelvic masses when sonography is indeterminate, *Am J Roentgenol* 154:295, 1990.

Zanetta G, Brenna A, Pittelli M, et al: Transvaginal ultrasound-guided fine needle sampling of deep cancer recurrences in the pelvis: usefulness and limitations, *Gynecol Oncol* 54:59, 1994.

CHAPTER 18

Evaluation of the Infertile Couple

PAUL W. ZARUTSKIE

In the Western world, the inability to bear a child is a serious medical problem associated with significant emotional stress. Over the past two decades there has been a dramatic change in the number of couples seeking medical consultation for infertility. In the United States 600,000 visits for infertility evaluation were reported in 1968, and over a 6-year period (1982 to 1988) some 15 years later, services increased 25% (1.1 million to 1.35 million). At that time it was estimated that approximately 53 million women in the United States were in their reproductive years (15 to 44 years old) and that 8.5% of these women were infertile; however, the true scope of the problem is much greater in that these total population figures include unmarried women, women who are surgically sterile, and those who have not wanted to become pregnant. Also, most studies focus on female infertility, and there are few data available on male factor infertility. A more realistic estimate is that approximately 17.3 million couples desire children and approximately 2.4 million couples (13.9%) have a problem with conception. In terms of the number of individuals affected by a disease or handicap in the United States, this number is similar to the 3 million patients with diabetes.

DEFINITIONS

Infertility is generally defined as the inability of a couple to conceive within 12 months of unprotected intercourse. In contrast to sterility, which implies an inability to conceive under any circumstances, infertility is a state of subfecundity in which the time of achieving a pregnancy or the time between conceptions is abnormally lengthy. A woman who has never achieved a pregnancy or a man who has never initiated a pregnancy is classified as having *primary infertility*. The term *secondary infertility* is applied when a previous pregnancy has been achieved, in either the current relationship or in a previous relationship.

In clinical situations, the distinction between infertility and sterility is becoming less relevant because current technologies and social mores are making it possible for couples in which one member was previously categorized as sterile to achieve a pregnancy through in vitro fertilization (IVF), surrogacy, or donor gametes. It is also clinically practical to expand the definition of infertility to include those individuals who experience difficulty in carrying a pregnancy, although data on these patients are generally included in obstetric records as "pregnancy wastage."

As our technologies increase the number of treatment options more attention is being paid to defining outcomes. Fecundity is the ability to achieve a live birth from one menstrual cycle or attempt per treatment. Fecundability on the other hand is the probability (0.20 to 0.25, or 20% to 25% in a fertile couple) of achieving a pregnancy per cycle attempted.

EPIDEMIOLOGY

Over the past 200 years in the United States there has been a dramatic decline in the birth rate (from 8 to 1.8 births per woman). Societally, we have changed—marriages are deferred, womens' roles and aspirations have changed, and delays in childbearing are possible because of availability of contraception. The majority (85%) of the decline in the total fertility rate is due to these factors leading to avoidance of pregnancy in the early years of marriage. In the middle of this century (post–World War II) total fertility rates reached a modern-day peak of 3.8 births per woman; thus a greater number of men and women have delayed marriage and pregnancy plans than in any other time in history. This demographic change has led to the problems seen in achieving a pregnancy and being pregnant with advanced maternal age. The proportion of births attributed to this older age group will increase 72% by the turn of the century. Therefore the practitioner will see these couples who feel pressed for time and have a heightened desire to get pregnant in a shortened time frame. With this urgency come emotional, financial, personal, and medical management conflicts—for which the couple can benefit from the consultation services provided by a reproductive endocrinologist.

RISK FACTORS

The literature reporting causes of infertility and associated risk factors often cites findings associated with female infertility rather than male or couple infertility. For example, estimates from the National Survey of Family Growth involved surveys of women only. Similar data do not exist for men. A profile of infertility when treating couples would assume female pelvic factors (including ovulatory dysfunction, tubal disease, and endometriosis) to account for 30% to 40% of the cases, male factor infertility (primarily defined in the past as defects in sperm production) to account for an additional 30% to 40% of cases, with 10% to 15% combined male and female factors, and the remaining 5% to 10% with no known etiology.

Age

Infertility increases with age. A woman over the age of 35 is twice as likely to experience infertility as a woman 25 years of age. For women who delay childbearing, the probability of conception is reduced not only by the number of months available but by the risk of decreased fertility. Males at 25 years are three times more likely to initiate a pregnancy than are males at 40 years of age. These figures are not corrected for reduced frequency of intercourse that is commonly reported by older couples.

For women over 40 years old fecundity is decreased not only by an increased inability to conceive, but also by an associated increase in spontaneous abortion rate. In other words, once a pregnancy is achieved in this population the chance of a successful delivery is compromised by the increased risk of a miscarriage. This is reflected by the increasing incidence of both normal (euploid) and abnormal (aneuploid) abortuses with advancing maternal age. The spontaneous abortion rate for women over 40 years old is nearly 2.25 times that of women less than 20 years old (26% versus 12%). Using assisted reproductive technology (ART) data from the U.S. Registry for woman over 40 years of age, 34.4% of pregnancies (30.2% spontaneous, 4.2% induced) from in vitro fertilization resulted in a pregnancy loss, and 43.4% (41.2% spontaneous, 2.2% induced) from gamete intrafallopian transfer technology resulted in pregnancy loss. The cause for this increase in spontaneous abortion rate can be thought of as something wrong with either the resulting embryo (sperm or oocyte) or the implantation site (uterus or hormone milieu). Assisted reproductive technology data demonstrate that the defect is due to the aging oocyte and not the implantation site. Using oocytes donated from women less than 35 years of age there appears to be no decline in success rates (30% per cycle) for recipient women between the ages of 40 and 50 years. The spontaneous abortion rate in these recipient women increased as the age of the donor increased (14% with donors 20 to 24 years old versus 44.5% with donors older than 35), further suggesting that the increased risk of spontaneous abortion and the appearance of genetic defects associated with aging are due primarily to the aging oocyte.

Aging in the male is a less-studied but equally important area of knowledge. It appears that the quality of sperm does decrease with age. Advanced paternal age is correlated with increased frequency of male gene mutations with the appearance of new autosomal disease and increased nondisjunction resulting in an increased incidence of trisomies. It is less clear whether this decline in the quality of sperm seen in aging is correlated with fecundability.

Sexually Transmitted Diseases

One of the most important risk factors for both male and female infertility in the United States is sexually transmitted diseases. Over the past 20 years, the incidence of pelvic inflammatory disease (PID) has continued to rise to an estimate of 1 million cases per year. Subsequent damage to the fallopian tubes and ovaries results in tubal infertility in approximately 10% of these patients, with an increasing risk for infertility associated with each successive episode of PID. The same organisms responsible for PID in women cause male infertility. Changes in semen quality are seen when a gonococcal infection is present. Infection by *Neisseria gonorrhoeae* or *Chlamydia* can obstruct the vas deferens, seminal vesicles, or epididymis.

Sexually transmitted diseases are often asymptomatic or have subtle symptoms. In the male, infections are rarely reported unless there is acute orchitis or epididymitis. Similarly in women, approximately half of patients with tubal infertility have no history suggestive of PID. *Chlamydia trachomatis* is thought to be responsible for over 50% of the cases of acute epididymitis and may be a major causative factor in silent pelvic infections, partly because the symptoms are more subtle than those of gonorrhea.

Environmental and Lifestyle Factors

Multiple studies of animals and epidemiologic case-control studies in humans have suggested that women who smoke have an increased risk of impaired fertility, spontaneous abortion, ectopic pregnancy, earlier onset of menopause, poorer pregnancy outcomes, and cervical cancer. This increased risk could be secondary in part to the effect that smoking has on the menstrual cycle pattern, oocyte production, tubal function, and cervical mucus production. In addition the incidence of spontaneous abortion increases in proportion to the amount of smoking. Continuing to smoke at the time of treatment with IVF has been associated with delay in embryo cleavage and a reduced availability to transfer four or more embryos, suggesting a direct effect at the cellular level.

The data on the effects of nicotine on sperm production and function are less conclusive. Decreases in sperm count and motility, alterations in sperm morphology, and disruptions in hormone levels have been reported. Even passive exposure to tobacco smoke shows measurable levels of nicotine/cotinine in seminal plasma.

Alcohol consumption, caffeine ingestion, and the use of social drugs (e.g., marijuana, cocaine) have been demonstrated to have various effects on the reproductive process. These lifestyle factors have been particularly difficult to evaluate in an epidemiologic manner because exposure to one factor usually cannot be isolated from other variables, including sexually transmitted diseases, and from their effects. Using fecundability rates adjusted for risk factors known at the time of conception, researchers initially did not show any evidence for an adverse effect of caffeine; however, recent studies are reporting association between caffeine intake and delay in conception. A significant increase (relative risk greater than 1.5) in infertility resulting from an increased risk of tubal infertility and endometriosis has been suggested when a woman ingests as little as 7 g of caffeine per month, or two cups of caffeinated beverage per day. Therefore as the correlation between these factors and fertility becomes clearer and in the interest of good health in general, patients should be encouraged to diminish their exposure to all such agents. All parties should keep in mind that complete cessation can be extremely difficult, possibly diminishing the couple's well-being, increasing mental stress, and requiring counseling.

Another increasingly important risk factor is exposure to environmental chemicals, often in association with the patient's occupation. This is also a difficult area to document because exposure may have taken place many years before treatment for infertility, and the individuals may have been exposed to more than one hazardous substance. Sperm production has been noted to decrease with exposure to heat, vibration, ionizing radiation, and pesticides (such as dibromochloropropane). Oligospermia and azoospermia have been demonstrated with the glycoethers found in paints and varnishes. A twofold to sixfold increase in female infertility risk has been associated with noise, dry-cleaning chemicals, mercury, cadmium, and textile dyes.

Patients assessing their fertility are likely to be aware of additional risk factors that have surfaced in the lay press, specifically, the use of tight-fitting briefs by men, hot tub exposure, douching with various alkaline or acid preparations, and sexual positions. The issue for men is increased scrotal temperature, which has been shown to affect semen quality. Thus the use of noncotton material for underwear or exposure to hot tubs or saunas on a regular basis may have a major effect on men whose semen quality is already borderline for fertility. For women, unless a vaginal infection is present, the natural vaginal and cervical secretions are optimal for sperm survival in the middle of the menstrual cycle (days 12 to 14). Douching can change this natural environment and render it less favorable for sperm survival and function. Similarly, ejaculation into the vaginal vault bathes the cervix in sperm regardless of the woman's position, but liquefaction of sperm requires approximately 20 minutes. Thus remaining reclined for a short time after intercourse might be favorable, but positioning of the hips and other such ideas have not been shown to increase pregnancy success.

ASSESSMENT OF THE INFERTILE COUPLE

Infertility may be attributed to male factors, to female factors, to biologic and physiologic interaction between the members of the couple, or to a combination of independent male and female factors; therefore treatment for infertility requires evaluation of both partners and cooperation of both in the subsequent diagnostic and treatment process. To expedite this, a couple scheduling an office visit should be informed that a complete history and physical examination will be done on both partners.

It is preferable that the couple work with one primary health care provider who can coordinate the necessary services of specialists and laboratories to provide a complete assessment of the infertile couple (Table 18-1). In 1988 the Office for Technology Assistance (OTA) reported that almost half (45%) of the clinicians working with couples for infertility were clinicians in an obstetric-gynecologic (ob-gyn) practice. The next largest group was family practitioners (38%), and only 13.7% were urologists. Since 1988 these numbers have probably changed.

At the time of the OTA report there were approximately 200 centers in the United States offering assisted reproductive technologies. At the last report there were 267 centers reporting their data to the National Registry. With an increase in the availability of assisted reproductive technologies, more patients are being referred to such centers earlier in their diagnostic and therapeutic management. Also, with the continued growth of managed care in the United States and changes in insurance coverage for infertility services, fewer clinicians are working with infertile couples.

Most of a routine infertility evaluation of a couple can be conducted competently by a clinician in general practice or by an ob-gyn specialist.

TABLE 18-1.   Assessment of the infertile couple

Provides diagnostic/therapeutic options
Educational opportunity to explain basic reproductive physiology
Medical opportunity to provide preventive health care

However, when infertility is of unknown etiology and an in-depth evaluation of each partner is necessary or when complicated treatment or surgery is needed, referral to a reproductive endocrinologist is appropriate. Evaluating and treating infertile couples requires that clinicians extend their expertise beyond the primary focus of their training and interact effectively with other professionals, particularly those who are qualified to interpret sophisticated laboratory analyses. Failure to do this could result in incomplete workups, dependence on a limited number of diagnostic and therapeutic modalities, or continuation of a course of treatment beyond its probable period of efficacy.

The sequence in which a physician evaluates a couple's infertility can vary based on the particular personal and financial needs of the couple; however, the workup should be completed expeditiously and in an organized manner that provides the couple the greatest amount of information in the shortest amount of time. Within a 2- to 3-month period of time, the workup can cover a complete history and physical for both partners, semen analyses or sperm function testing on the male, basal body temperature (BBT) charts and urinary luteinizing hormone (LH) testing for the female, and a postcoital test. If indicated, an endometrial biopsy, serum progesterone, and a hysterosalpingogram (HSG) can be done within this time period. These studies should be sufficient to diagnose approximately 60% of couples undergoing infertility studies.

In assessing the infertile couple it should be the goal of the practitioner not just to achieve a pregnancy for all couples but to accelerate the workup in such a manner as to shorten the time period required to achieve that pregnancy. If a pregnancy has not been achieved within 1 year of the development of a management plan for a woman less than 35 years of age or within 6 months for a woman over 35 years old, the couple should be referred to a specialty center for further evaluation.

Patient History

A complete patient history should be obtained from each partner, including information on medical, surgical, cultural, and sexual backgrounds.

Detailed information often complements subsequent examinations and laboratory tests and supports recommendations for a course of treatment. Although a complete history often seems to include information about specific environmental, occupational, or personal factors for which there is no clearly established connection with infertility, it is important to collect these data to assist in determining the impact of factors such as caffeine, nicotine, and dietary and exercise habits on reproductive health. As a part of the environmental exposure history, lifestyle factors should be recorded to obtain specific data profiles for the patient so that appropriate counseling can be provided.

A complete sexual history is extremely important because it produces information that relates directly to infertility. It is necessary, however, to develop a strategy for obtaining personal information. Frequency of intercourse, the presence of dyspareunia, a history of sexually transmitted diseases, pregnancies achieved with prior partners, and specific sexual habits such as use of vaginal lubricants or douches can quickly identify specific factors that have an impact on the couple's fertility; however, attempting to obtain responses to these questions when a couple is together is likely to result in incomplete or biased responses. Delaying part or all of the sexual history taking until the time of the physical examination allows the individual an opportunity to provide specific information in a setting of physician-patient rapport. It also allows the physician to obtain individual histories and to compare any differences in the couple's psychosexual status.

For instance, if there is a major discrepancy in the frequency of intercourse reported by the two partners, this will lead the physician to attempt to clarify such discrepancies with the couple. This can be done in a nonconfrontational manner that allows the physician opportunity to educate the couple about how their habits and actions affect fertility. In an educational framework the information is not specifically directed toward one partner but is used as a springboard to future data collection.

At the time the history is obtained from both partners, the clinician should explore whether there are religious or cultural mandates that affect the couple's reproductive behaviors. This is also an excellent opportunity to educate the couple on basic reproductive physiology. Explaining the menstrual cycle to both husband and wife prepares the couple to understand the procedures and tests that will be carried out to evaluate ovulation, tubal patency, and other related fertility factors. Similarly, a discussion of male reproductive physiology is an important tool in determining the couple's working knowledge regarding the interpretation of semen analysis, sperm penetration assays (SPAs), and future information that might be required should the discussion of assisted technologies arises.

Female history. The female history should include the onset of the patient's menses; symptoms such as weight gain, hirsutism and acne (particularly of perimenstrual onset, which can be indicative of an androgen-excess syndrome), changes in menstrual flow, cycle length, and related symptomatologies; breast tenderness; and fluid retention or mood changes to assist in finding normal versus abnormal ovulation. Characteristics and occurrences of pelvic pain can assist in directing an evaluation for endometriosis.

The history of exposure to tuberculosis and prior surgical history are important information to obtain concerning possible tubal obstruction as the etiology for infertility. A history of prior gynecologic procedures (e.g., cauterization, conization, dilation and curettage) is helpful in evaluating cervical factors as possible etiologies of infertility. A history of intrauterine exposure to diethylstilbestrol (DES) has been implicated in a history of spontaneous habitual abortions and infertility.

Male history. Traditionally, males are more likely than females to have been exposed to environmental or occupational toxins that may have an impact on reproductive health, and the history should cover this possibility. The genital/urologic history should also be directed toward identifying men with symptoms but no prior diagnosis of chronic prostatitis, including specific questions addressing postvoid dribbling, burning urination, and nocturia.

Because sperm production may be affected by the presence of a varicocele, cryptorchidism, testicular failure secondary to viral infection, or various endocrinopathies, a careful history should be obtained for these parameters. For a history of varicocele, a man should be asked about prior surgery, prior trauma to the scrotal area, and the presence of a fullness in the scrotal area. A man should be asked whether he has ever examined his genital area and, if so, whether he has noted asymmetry in the size of the testes or fullness in the scrotal area. Although rare, adrenal genital syndrome, pituitary dysfunction, and hypothyroidism are endocrinopathies that can cause infertility: fatigue, dry skin, weight gain, and a decrease in activity could possibly lead to a diagnosis of hypothyroidism; persistent headaches, visual disturbances, or a decrease in sexual activity could mean a pituitary lesion; and acne, weight gain, oily skin, and blood pressure abnormalities could suggest an adrenal genital syndrome.

A childhood history is important to determine when the man noted descent of testes. It is essential that the testes descend by the age of 6 years. If the man is unable to give an exact history, it would be important to determine whether or not any surgeries were performed as a child for such a disorder. The presence of either viral or bacterial infections either in the past or present can have an effect on semen production. The classic history of exposure to mumps virus in puberty leading to mumps orchitis and sterility is well known. However, exposure to various other viruses and their results on infertility are unclear. Acute viral or bacterial infection can lead to a stress pattern with an observed decrease in semen parameters.

Examination

A thorough and complete physical examination of both partners is essential, not only as a tool to assist in providing evidence of a physiologic or anatomic basis for infertility, but also to provide an opportunity for preventive health care instruction.

Examination of the female. As part of the preventive health maintenance evaluation, blood pressure, height, and weight should be recorded. In the case of the female this should include examination of the breasts with education on routine self-examination. It should also include an annual Papanicolaou smear of the cervix and a pelvic/rectal examination. The external genitalia should be observed for any evidence of prior infection, the appearance of condylomata acuminata, and any evidence of herpes genitalis. The vagina should be examined carefully and evidence of estrogenation (rugation) should be observed. The presence of any vaginal discharges should be identified, and a wet-slide preparation should be made, along with a potassium hydroxide (KOH) preparation. The cervix should be observed for any lesions or malformations consistent with DES exposure.

The presence of cervical mucus should be recorded, and if mucus is observed, a specimen should be obtained for microscopic examination. In this initial specimen, mucus quality can be observed along with possible sperm survival based on where the patient is in her cycle and the time of last intercourse (Figs. 18-1 and 18-2). By indirectly observing the estrogen effects on the cervical glands, such as observing the characteristic changes

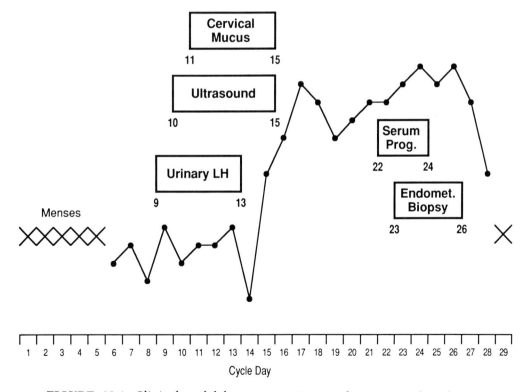

FIGURE 18-1. Clinical and laboratory testing in the menstrual cycle requires testing both around the time of the preovulatory event (cervical mucus, luteinizing hormone, ultrasound) and in the luteal phase (progesterone, endometrial biopsy).

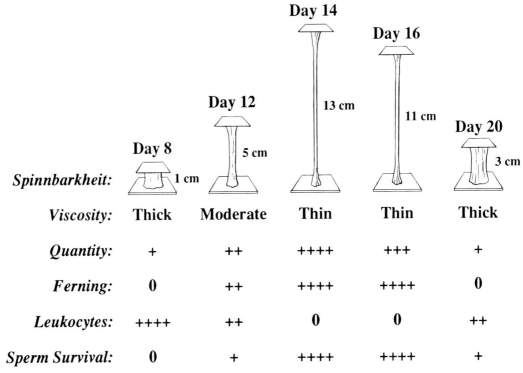

Spinnbarkheit:	Day 8 1 cm	Day 12 5 cm	Day 14 13 cm	Day 16 11 cm	Day 20 3 cm
Viscosity:	Thick	Moderate	Thin	Thin	Thick
Quantity:	+	++	++++	+++	+
Ferning:	0	++	++++	++++	0
Leukocytes:	++++	++	0	0	++
Sperm Survival:	0	+	++++	++++	+

FIGURE 18-2. The characteristics of the cervical mucus demonstrate maximal ferning, peak spinnbarkeit, and relative acellularity at the time of the ovulatory event. This change in mucus characteristics allows for optimal sperm survival and penetration of cervical mucus.

(Fig. 18-2), the postcoital test provides the practitioner insight into the patient's menstrual cycle. The test should be performed around the time of the midcycle LH surge (Fig. 18-1), thus necessitating accurate establishment of this event by various tests (Fig. 18-2). The role of the postcoital test in the basic infertility evaluation should not be extrapolated to become the definitive test for fertility. In fact in recent years it is becoming clearer that the postcoital test lacks validity, standardization of methodology, and definition of normality. Other investigators similarly have shown little value in using the postcoital test to predict pregnancy.

A bimanual examination should assess uterine size, shape, and contour. The pelvis should be examined and evaluated for masses, fixation of adnexal structures consistent with pelvic scarring from PID, and any evidence of tenderness. A rectal examination should also be performed to complete assessment of the posterior portion of the pelvis, with emphasis on obtaining evidence of endometriosis and evaluating the uterosacral ligaments. A stool guaiac test should be performed to screen for a possible gastrointestinal bleeding source (cancer, ulcers, colitis).

Physical findings associated with secondary sex characteristics are helpful in assessment of adrenal and gonadal hormone secretions and the systemic response to these hormones.

Examination of the male. Men in a fertility evaluation often report having their last physical examination either for a high school sports program or for the military, and they are extremely apprehensive about both the examination and possible findings. Therefore the clinician should offer the patient a routine physical examination, beginning with the standard measurements of blood pressure, height, and weight and a cardiopulmonary examination, and should emphasize health maintenance. Instruction and demonstration of self-examination of the scrotal contents emphasizes to the male the importance of his health maintenance and helps educate him as to his role in the couple's fertility.

A guaiac test for stool hemoglobin should be completed, and the prostate should be examined carefully, completing the procedure with a prostate massage. The prostatic discharge should be evaluated microscopically to look for the presence of white cells, prostatic crystals, and the presence of white cell cast. This examination can confirm historical data suggesting findings of chronic prostatitis.

The fertility evaluation should focus on determining the adequacy of the reproductive tract, with particular emphasis on identifying evidence of chronic infection, hernia, varicocele, or hypospadia. Testicle size should be recorded because testicular atrophy is directly correlated to sperm production.

Analysis of Fertility

Within the past decade, changes in the technologies available for diagnosis have led to expanded focus of fertility evaluations from determining sperm and oocyte production and identifying structural defects within the reproductive tract that prevent the union of the sperm and egg to studying the quality of the oocytes and function of sperm as related to fertilization.

Technologic advances greatly enhance the probability of a successful outcome for infertile couples, but the processes involved can have a profound effect on both the personal and professional lives of the couple. For the male, collection of semen by masturbation may be embarrassing or associated with inhibitions, or he may feel threatened having his sperm counted and his fertilization capacity scored. Because additional studies are required for the wife, many of which are invasive in nature, the male may feel helpless in having his partner go through the studies and guilty that such invasive procedures are not required of him. It is not uncommon for the woman to report that she feels manipulated and invaded and that she is being probed to excess. Multiple visits to her physician's office may have a significant impact on her personal and professional life. The demands and the nature of the diagnostic procedures may make coitus unpleasant for the couple. Midcycle patterns of impotence and sexual dysfunction can disrupt the timing sequences for diagnosing testing.

Not all tests are indicated in all diagnostic workups (Table 18-2). The workup should not be overly complex or lengthy because this may result in discouragement and failure to complete the recommended program. Nor should the workup be halted once an abnormality is identified because each procedure normally evaluates only a specific physiologic or anatomic aspect of reproductive function. However, it is important to complete the workup of the couple and simultaneously treat all identifiable abnormalities rather than initiate sequential therapies over several months (Table 18-3). This allows for a short but intense evaluation interval of only a few months, with early introduction of interventions necessary to achieve a pregnancy.

In most cases, critical tests should be repeated because physiologic parameters vary with time. For example, it is estimated that sperm maturation in the human takes approximately 10 weeks (72 days). Therefore the success of any corrective action that was undertaken to improve sperm quality would not be apparent for several months.

Male fertility. Historically, fertility evaluation of males has been hampered by our poor understanding of the male physiology. For many years, male fertility studies have examined the appearance of the sperm (morphology), the movement potential (motility), and the numbers (concentration) by using basic techniques such as seminal fluid analysis and the postcoital test. Male fertility is much more complex, however, than measurements of sperm morphology, motility, and concentration, and a major fertility or endocrinology center can now study the sequence of biochemical events that occur as sperm acquire the capacity to fertilize an oocyte. To understand the usefulness of these tests and to interpret the results, clinicians must understand capacitation and acrosome reactions, which are explained later in this chapter.

TABLE 18-2.   Fertility evaluation

Female	Male
Basal body temperature	Semen analysis
Urinary measurement of luteinizing hormone	Standard sperm penetration assay
Serum measurements of estradiol, progesterone	Postcoital test
Endometrial biopsy	
Follicular dynamics	
Hysteroscopy	
Laparoscopy	
Hysterosalpingogram	
Postcoital test	

TABLE 18-3. Fertility workup

INITIAL VISIT

Clinical
  History/physical for both partners
Laboratory
  Testing to assess specific medical findings
  Assess for sexually transmitted diseases
  Papanicolaou smear
  Semen analysis
Education
  Health maintenance (breast, scrotal self-examination)
  Ovulation monitoring

SECOND VISIT (SCHEDULE IN MIDCYCLE, I.E., PERIOVULATORY PORTION OF CYCLE)

Clinical
  Postcoital test
Laboratory
  Schedule midluteal progesterone/prolactin
  Sperm penetration assay
Educational
  Review ovulation monitoring data and laboratory findings
  Schedule midluteal endometrial biopsy

THIRD VISIT (SCHEDULE IN MIDLUTEAL PORTION OF CYCLE)

Clinical
  Endometrial biopsy
Laboratory
  Prolactin, progesterone
Educational
  Discuss need to assess tubal/uterine integrity (i.e., hysterosalpingogram vs.
    laparoscopy/hysterectomy)

FOURTH VISIT

Clinical
  Follow-up examination to assess efficacy of medical therapies
Laboratory
  Follow-up to assess efficacy of therapies
Educational
  Outline biochemical/physiologic bases of couple's infertility
  Outline management plans
  Discuss referrals for possible assisted reproductive technologies

Semen composition. A complete semen analysis should include the volume, pH, viscosity of seminal fluid, sperm count, motility, morphology, and presence of lymphocytes/leukocytes, all of which give a profile of the basic characteristics of sperm and seminal fluid. Because semen characteristics fluctuate considerably over a period of time, two or preferably three semen analyses over at least a 2- to 3-month period are recommended.

TABLE 18-4. World Health Organization standards for semen analysis

Parameter	Standard
Sperm concentration	$\geq 20 \times 10^6$/ml
Total motile count	$\geq 40 \times 10^6$/ejaculate
Sperm motility	$\geq 50\%$ progression or $\geq 25\%$ rapid progression
Sperm morphology	$\geq 30\%$ normal
Viability	$\geq 75\%$ alive
White blood cells	$< 1 \times 10^6$/ml
Immunobead test	$< 20\%$ spermatozoa with adherent particles

Standards for semen, as established by the World Health Organization (WHO) in 1992, are presented in Table 18-4. These standards do not imply that infertility would necessarily result if one of the parameters were abnormal. For example, a sperm count of 50 to 60 million per ml is usually thought to be necessary for fertilization. However, a count as low as 20 million sperm per ml is considered to be within normal limits, and counts lower than this do not preclude fertility.

The measurements of motility provided by the current computer-assisted semen analysis tests are greatly improved over the previous analytic methods (Table 18-5). However, assessment methods have not been standardized, and interpretation of these data requires consultation with an andrologist and laboratory staff versed in the testing procedures. With computer technologies, subtle measurements of sperm velocity, linearity, and the lateral deflection of the sperm head are gaining clinical relevance as they define male factor infertility more functionally.

The semen analysis can also be an adjunct to the history and physical examination in diagnosing prostate disease. The signs are the presence of bad odor, yellowish or reddish discoloration of the semen sample, high- or low-volume ejaculates, large fluctuations in pH, and poor liquefaction. Laboratory data associated with the semen analysis should be correlated to the physical examination and in particular the prostatic examination and prostate massage.

Sperm function. Until the last decade, the standard test for sperm function when assessing male fertility was the postcoital (or cervical mucus) test, which measures the ability of sperm to migrate through cervical mucus. This is a subjective measure of sperm vitality; one simply looks at the number of sperm present in cervical mucus a fixed number of hours after intercourse (usually either 4 to 6 hours or 8 to 12 hours) and their relative activity as measured by forward progression. In vivo human fertilization requires that the sperm not only swim through cervical mucus but also be transported through the female reproductive tract to the fallopian tube, capacitate, migrate through the cumulus matrix, recognize

TABLE 18-5. Computer-aided sperm motility analysis

DEFINITIONS

Velocity
Curvilinear (VCL)
  Sum of the lines joining sequential positions of the sperm read along its track per second
  Two-dimensional representation of the true three-dimensional path
  Highly dependent on the frame rate (Hz) of the camera
Straight line (VSL)
  Straight line distance between the start and end of the sperm track per second
  Straight line, i.e., progressive velocity
Linearity (LIN)
  LIN = VSL/VCL
    Measure of "straightness" of path
    Straight line, LIN = 100
    Perfect circle, LIN = 0
Amplitude of lateral head (ALH) deflection
  Distance between the recorded curvilinear path and the calculated smoothed (average) path
  Measure of flexing at the sperm's neck

ADVANTAGES OVER MANUAL ANALYSIS

Measures are more objective and reproducible
New measures not available manually
Comparisons before and after treatment or between treatments are made with greater accuracy

CLINICAL RELEVANCE

More precise classification of sperm into different motility categories (e.g., WHO classifications)
Progressively motile sperm population is biologically relevant; clinically significant
High ALH, VCL, LIN positively correlated with normal sperm penetration in sperm penetration assay (SPA)
Good VSL, high ALH necessary for normal cervical mucus penetration
High ALH, positively correlated with normal in vitro fertilization rates

---

and bind to the zona pellucida, undergo acrosome reaction in conjunction with the zona, penetrate the zona, bind and fuse with the oocyte plasma membrane, activate the egg to prevent polyspermia, enter the egg cytoplasm, decondense and form a pronucleus, and fuse with the female pronucleus to form a zygote. Thus over the past decade attention has been focused on establishing more objective tests of sperm function.

No single test has been devised to predict the ability of sperm to carry out its specific physiologic functions; however, the SPA accurately reflects several key steps, including capacitation (the ability of sperm to shed the protein coating) and acrosome reaction (the ability of the sperm to release enzymes), both of which are essential to fertilization of the ovum. Definitions, parameters, and assessment guidelines for this test are listed in

TABLE 18-6. Sperm penetration assay

DEFINITION OF SPERM FUNCTION

Capacitation
    Continuation of sperm differentiation
    Removal/modification of sperm surface proteins acquired during maturation
    Loss of cholesterol/cholesteryl esters increasing membrane fluidity
    Increased permeability to calcium
    Time correlated to the presence of fertilizable oocytes
Acrosome reaction
    Fusion of the plasma membrane with the outer acrosomal membrane
    Subsequent loss of the acrosomal cap

PARAMETERS AFFECTING THE ASSAY

Period of abstinence
Sperm-semen separation time
Medium (content, pH, osmolality)
Capacitation/acrosome reaction time
Concentration/type of protein supplement
Energy source supplement
Sperm/hamster ova exposure time

ASSESSMENT GUIDELINES

Definition of normal
Validity of the test as part of a sequence of tests
Standardization of test parameters
Independent, "blind" comparison with a standard used for diagnosis
Definition of patient characteristics and study setting
Reproducibility of test results (precision) and interpretation (observer variation)

Table 18-6. Only when the consulting andrology laboratory carefully standardizes the test parameters and the clinician follows specific assessment guidelines can the SPA be used clinically to define male infertility. The clinician should inquire about the timing used within the test because this has implications for the findings: A poor result on the SPA can result if the laboratory uses only one standardized capacitation time (20 to 22 hours) and the patient is atypical (e.g., has a shorter-than-normal capacitation time). When a shortened capacitation time is identified, the maximum gestation potential is at the time of ovulation rather than preceding it, and the couple can be offered ovulation timing advice. If this is ineffective, they are candidates for assisted techniques such as intrauterine insemination with pretreated sperm.

Although the clinical significance of the SPA (also known as the hamster ovum penetration assay) was controversial until recently, many clinical studies have now been carried out to demonstrate its applicability. In one major study of long-term infertility, in those cases in which no abnormalities could be found in the wife's workup, only 8% of the husbands had a normal

TABLE 18-7. Use of the sperm penetration assay

I. DEFINITION

Sensitivity: Ability to identify male *infertility*
Specificity: Ability to identify male *fertility*
Predictive value of an *abnormal* test: likelihood of a male with an abnormal sperm
    penetrating assay (SPA) being *infertile*
Predictive value of a *normal* test: likelihood of a male with an abnormal SPA
    being *fertile*

II. VALIDITY

Test	Sensitivity	Specificity	High score, "normal"	Low score, "abnormal"
Standard SPA	.82	.52	.90	.35
Follicular fluid SPA	.64	.97	.80	.93

SPA finding when using the hamster ovum penetration assay (versus 61% of husbands who demonstrated normal SPA results when the infertility was associated with an abnormality in the wife). Another study of infertile couples in which the woman tested normal showed that 68% of men with a normal or borderline penetration test successfully initiated a pregnancy within 1.5 years, as compared with only 19% with abnormal SPA results. Continued development in the testing systems have led to improved predictability of the SPA in defining male infertility. Defining the specificity and sensitivity of the assay is of critical importance in establishing the prognostic value of the SPA (Table 18-7).

When employing both the standard SPA and an enhanced assay (follicular fluid), our laboratory reports a sensitivity of 82% (versus 41% for seminal fluid analysis) and a specificity of 97% (compared with 90% for seminal fluid analysis). Thus the standard SPA is helpful (90% predictive value) in determining the likelihood of a male with abnormal SPA findings being fertile, and the follicular fluid SPA (FF-SPA) is predictive (93%) of the likelihood of a male with abnormal FF-SPA findings being infertile.

Immunologic disorders. Findings of agglutination in either semen analysis or cervical mucus have in the past warranted evaluation for possible immunologic disorders. In the absence of agglutination, tests measuring antibodies present on the sperm, in the seminal fluid, or in the female secretions may be useful in specific instances, but in general they correlate poorly with successful fertilization.

Endocrine evaluation. Normal sperm production requires a hormonal balance between the hypothalamus, pituitary, the testis, and other endocrine organs (e.g., adrenal and thyroid). Thus in a situation where sperm production appears compromised, evaluation of gonadotropins (LH and follicle-stimulating hormone [FSH]), prolactin, testosterone (free and total), and thyroid hormones is essential. In a case in which the hormone profile is normal, the physical examination (including testicular size) is normal, the semen analysis demonstrates no sperm in the ejaculate, and the presence of fructose in the ejaculate rules out the possibility of a congenital absence of the vas deferens and seminal vesicles, further operative evaluation must be done to determine whether there was an underlying defect in sperm production or a blockage of the sperm/ejaculatory system. A radiographic study injecting contrast dye into the vas deferens or the ejaculatory duct is valuable in identifying tubal obstruction. At the same time a testicular biopsy is often performed under local or general anesthesia to provide histologic evidence of sperm cell differentiation and Leydig's cell development.

Female fertility. Because routine infertility testing is often scheduled on the basis of specific events in the menstrual cycle, the cyclic events (hormonal, physiologic, and biochemical) must be clearly understood to officially complete the testing. Because of the rapid growth of over-the-counter products, infertile couples have become more informed than ever concerning basic diagnostic and treatment methods. In addition, the infertile couple often has initiated a workup in the past and is returning for either additional evaluation or follow-up. Thus the practitioner must determine what prior evaluation or therapies have been completed and appropriately choose the diagnostic technologies available to evaluate the infertile woman. In evaluating the female, ovulation must be documented, tubal patency demonstrated, and the absence of cervical/uterine factors demonstrated.

Ovulatory factors. Clinically, we have seen little change in the initial methods used to assess ovulation despite major development of laboratory (urine/serum) techniques. The two basic clinical tools remain BBT charting and assessing cervical mucus, although less importance is being assigned to these age-old clinical tools. Laboratory and ultrasound technologies are moving us out of the realm of using subjective interpretation of the whole-body response to objectively looking at ovarian hormone production and follicular development. Figure 18-1 outlines the time in the menstrual cycle when the various clinical laboratory parameters are used to assess the ovulatory event.

BASAL BODY TEMPERATURE. The BBT is a time-tested, popular, and cost-effective predictor of ovulation. The temperature-regulating centers in the hypothalamus are in part controlled by the production of progesterone. When ovulation occurs and the progesterone level rises, an upward shift of the BBT (greater than or equal to 0.5°F is often observed. Because resting (preovulatory) temperatures vary among individuals, it is the change in temperature rather than the absolute readings that correlate with ovulation. The observed increase in baseline temperature is not seen until a significant rise in peripheral progesterone (greater than 4 ng/ml) is recorded. This rise is seen approximately 2 days after the LH peak, and oocyte release occurs 1 day prior; thus the BBT should not be used exclusively as a tool to determine timing of coitus, but rather as a way to create a calendar of events for the menstrual cycle study.

In one out of five women, ovulation can occur in the face of a monophasic temperature recording, and biphasic recordings do not necessarily predict normal ovulation. If the BBT is used as a menstrual calendar, observation of a temperature rise of less than 11 days' duration has been correlated with a luteal-phase defect, as diagnosed by endometrial biopsy. Thus the BBT can be used as a menstrual calendar in which both the physician and couple can outline specific diagnostic steps in the workup and visually record for the couple the progress of the evaluation. Other ovulation-monitoring tests can be added to this calendar, which helps educate the patient on the specific role of other tests in the evaluation.

The BBT is a retrospective piece of data observing the overall effect of follicular hormone production on the hypothalamus. It does not reveal follicle growth or oocyte maturity, but rather the results of follicular luteinization, that is, progesterone production effect on the hypothalamic temperature regulatory system.

CERVICAL MUCUS. Changes in cervical mucus have long been used as a guide to contraception; however, observation of cervical mucus changes are also valuable for assessment of ovulation. In midcycle in conjunction with the ovulatory temperature rise, estrogen causes the cervical mucus to become thin, often causing a copious vaginal discharge. Evaluation of the characteristics of cervical mucus reveals specific patterns correlated to the midcycle ovulatory event (see Fig. 18-2). Increased osmolality can be seen as a fernlike pattern when cervical mucus is air-dried on a glass slide (ferning), and an increase in elasticity is demonstrated by the spinnbarkeit test. At the time of ovulation, the increased stretchability of cervical mucus may allow a span of 8 to 12 cm without breaking. When cervical mucus is clinically evaluated, a single drop of mucus placed on a slide with a coverslip should be observed for white cells, cellular debris, and pH.

More sophisticated testing of hormone-induced changes in cervical mucus is available through electronic devices to measure electrical resistance of saliva or vaginal mucus as a reflection of the hyperosmotic changes occurring midcycle. These devices are generally available and used by patients who, for various reasons, are unable to employ other monitoring techniques.

The BBT and cervical mucus tests provide retrospective evidence of the ovulatory event. To predict ovulation there are four laboratory procedures that can be initiated at midcycle and completed at the luteal phase of the menstrual cycle. These tests, which measure specific hormones and characterize ovulation, are packaged urinary LH tests, serum hormone tests, endometrial biopsy, and ultrasound monitoring.

URINARY LUTEINIZING HORMONE ASSAYS. In the past 10 years the rapid development of monoclonal antibodies has led to several ovulation prediction kits available over the counter. The majority of these kits employ specific antibody-LH reagent reactions that develop a characteristic color indicator when completed (Fig. 18-3). Thus an intense color develops when the LH level exceeds the kit's semiquantitative threshold level, and the quantitative color change can be compared with a reference indicator.

Because the midcycle LH surge precedes ovulation by an average of 24 to 28 hours, this kit can be used not only to document ovulation but also to time intercourse or insemination procedures as well. When using a specific LH surge kit, the practitioner should be familiar with the predictive accuracy of the kit and the testing schedule required for accurate prediction of the LH surge and should be prepared to counsel the couple on timing of intercourse.

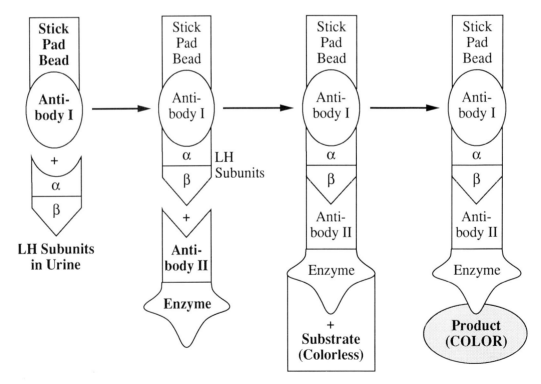

FIGURE 18-3. Step 1: add urine to the stick, pad, and bead. Step 2: add antibody/enzyme complex solution. Step 3: add substrate solution. Step 4: observe for color change resulting in the substrate undergoing enzymatic change to a colored product.

LABORATORY HORMONE TESTING. The initial evaluation of any historical or physical findings suggestive of an endocrinopathy (such as a thyroid, adrenal, or pituitary dysfunction) can be assessed by using specific hormone assays to measure thyroid hormones (thyroid-stimulating hormone [TSH]/ triiodothyronine [T_3], thyroxine [T_4]), adrenal hormones (dehydroepiandrosterone sulfate [DHEAS], serum cortisol, 24-hour urine total cortisol), pituitary hormones (gonadotropins, prolactin), and ovarian hormones (estrogen and progesterone).

To assess whether ovulation has occurred, progesterone is measured in the midluteal phase. A level greater than 10 ng/ml is considered an indication of adequate formation of corpus luteum and thus indirect evidence of adequate ovulation. A major drawback to assessing ovulation based on a single progesterone value is that, like the gonadotropins, secretion of these hormones into the bloodstream occurs in a pulsatile manner; thus a single midluteal serum progesterone value may not be a true indicator of "adequate" ovulation.

Ovulation (egg release) may be occurring, but poor formation of the corpus luteum may result in a syndrome known as the luteal-phase defect. Because of this clinical situation, it is often suggested that multiple progesterone levels be obtained and a profile of the luteal phase assessed in conjunction with an endometrial biopsy.

Measurement of estradiol, a secretory product of the granulosa cells, is not routinely used for diagnosis in the initial stages of a workup. However, in cases in which ovulation dysfunction is suspected and medication may be indicated to induce ovulation, it is extremely helpful in following follicular formation and assessing adequate oocyte maturation. The various, complex protocols employ a variety of gonadotropins and gonadotropin-releasing hormone agonists. Because of the possibility of ovarian hyperstimulation on such therapy, it is imperative that serum estradiol levels be monitored daily once medication is begun.

ENDOMETRIAL BIOPSY. The growth of the endometrium undergoes dramatic changes from the proliferative pattern observed in the follicular phase of the cycle to a secretory pattern observed in the luteal phase. Changes in the glands' structure and secretion, the supporting stroma, and the presence of perivascular decidualization have been used to date the endometrial lining in reference to the menstrual cycle days. Between days 22 and 25 of a 28-day menstrual cycle, an endometrial biopsy sample can be obtained. In the case of a patient with irregular menses (greater than or less than 28 days), the endometrial biopsy can be performed 7 to 9 days after documentation of ovulation by an LH surge. In conjunction with the endometrial biopsy, serum progesterone values can be obtained and correlated with the histologic findings determined after pathologic evaluation of the endometrium; an asynchrony between pathologic findings and the calendar day of

TABLE 18-8.　　Diagnostic use of pelvic ultrasound

UTERUS

Malformation (congenital, i.e., bicornuate, unicornuate)
Leiomyoma uteri
Gestational sac

OVIDUCT

Hydrosalpinx
Ectopic gestation

OVARY

Benign cyst (i.e., corpus luteum, follicle, functional cyst)
Polycystic (Stein-Leventhal syndrome)
Benign-malignant mass (cystic vs. solid)
Endometrioma

PERITONEUM

Endometriosis (mass, cystic/solid)
Malignancy (ascites, uterosacral nodules)

the menstrual cycle thus defines an out-of-phase biopsy. A greater than 2-day asynchrony must be observed in comparing the histologic findings to the menstrual dates in order to establish the biopsy as out of phase.

ULTRASONOGRAPHY. Use of pelvic ultrasound as an adjunct to the pelvic examination has increased the ability of the practitioner to assess the pelvis in cases where abnormal pathology is noted (Table 18-8). If the initial examination suggests an adnexal mass, pelvic nodularity, or uterine enlargement or irregularity, ultrasound can help discern the particular pathology. Of increasing importance is the use of ultrasound in assessing growth and development of the follicle, whether in natural cycles or during ovulation induction cycles (Fig. 18-4). In addition to growth and development of the follicles, follicular collapse and development of the corpus luteum can be documented by ultrasound techniques. In case of ovulation induction, ultrasound monitoring is often combined with other indicators of ovulation, such as BBT, estradiol, and cervical mucus evaluation.

Uterine and tubal factors. The fallopian tube is a dynamic structure, a highly sophisticated organ designed for ovum pickup, sperm transport, fertilization, early embryo development, and zygote transport. Its muscular and ciliary activities, in conjunction with specific secretory cell patterns of bicarbonate and protein production, render this organ a functional activity that has heretofore been ignored in diagnostic testing. Unfortunately, we lack the sophisticated biochemical/physiologic means to assess the function of the fallopian tube and thus have limited our evaluations to documentation of tubal form (patency versus nonpatency).

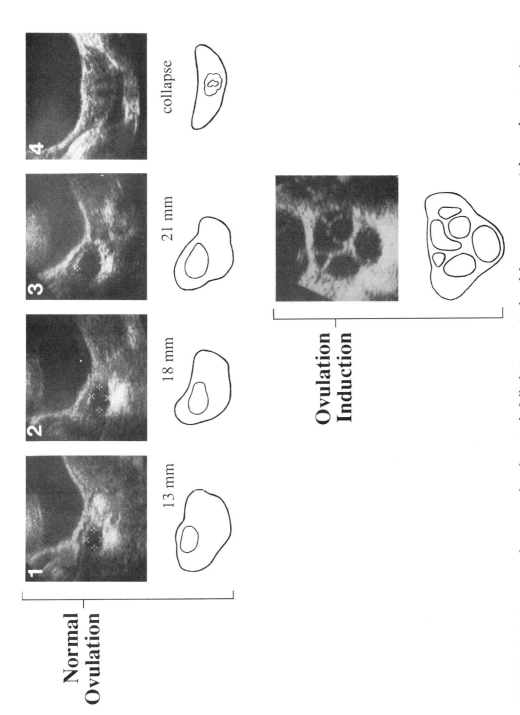

FIGURE 18-4. In a normal menstrual cycle a single follicle is recruited and demonstrates serial growth to a maximum diameter of 20 to 24 mm. Ovulation is confirmed by follicular collapse and subsequent corpus luteum development. Ovulation induction leads to the recruitment of several symmetrically sized follicles.

Over the past century, both operative and office procedures have been developed to assess tubal patency. Of historical note is the tubal insufflation test with carbon dioxide, described by Ruben in 1920, which involves the transcervical insufflation of carbon dioxide gas into the reproductive tract. The screening test is rarely used now because it provides no information on unilateral versus bilateral patency and correlates poorly with patencies demonstrated under direct visualization data in laparoscopy. Thus the procedure is not considered a part of current standard evaluation.

The most common outpatient procedure performed for evaluation of tubal patency is a radiologic procedure, the HSG (Fig. 18-5). Although it is a diagnostic test, in some cases it apparently has therapeutic value as well. It is critical that the test be performed in the first half of the menstrual cycle to minimize reflective endometrial tissue and decrease uterine spasms. This should also be considered a safety measure to avoid possible radiation exposure during an early gestation. Either an oil- or a water-based medium can be used, although the oil-based medium is slightly less irritating, and its delayed absorption can provide for a 24-hour delayed film of the pelvis to assess for loculated spillage and thus pelvic adhesions.

The evaluation should be performed under fluoroscopy to provide the operator direct visualization of the filling pattern observed in the contrast media. Slow and careful installation of contrast media is critical to interpretation because overly rapid administration can cause corneal spasms that block the fallopian tubes and air bubbles in the contrast medium can be mistaken for intrauterine polyps, fibroids, or other filling defects. The risk of embolism, reported in some of the older literature, essentially has been eliminated by halting the procedure immediately if lymphatic or intravascular extravasation is observed.

If corneal obstruction is observed or if the patient reports severe pain, the study is usually discontinued and rescheduled so that glucagon can be administered intravenously (IV) to minimize uterine spasms. If there is any suggestion of delayed tubal filling or spill, a delayed film should be obtained at 24 hours.

A patient with a recent positive *Chlamydia* titer should be given antibiotics (tetracycline, 250 mg twice daily [bid] or doxycycline, 100 mg bid) starting 1 day before HSG and continuing for 4 days. Such patients should be told to contact the physician after HSG if pain, fever, or increasing serosanguineous vaginal discharge is noted. Hysterosalpingogram should never be performed if there is tenderness or if pelvic masses are palpated during a pelvic examination before the HSG.

The HSG has limited value beyond assessing pathology directly related to uterine cavity shape, tubal patency, and peritubular adhesive disease because it fails to assess the presence of subtle pelvic pathology (e.g., intrauterine synechia, endometriosis, periovarian adhesions).

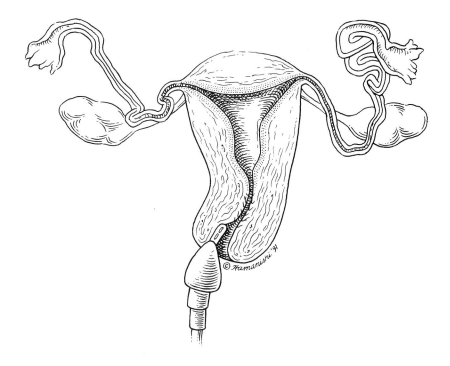

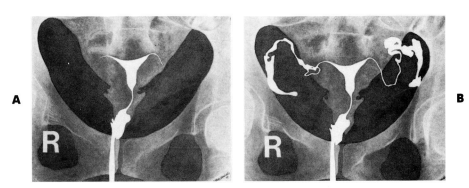

FIGURE 18-5. A normal hysterosalpingogram demonstrating uterine cavity and tubal patency. Anatomic tortuosity of the left tube is observed. **A,** Instillation of 1 to 2 ml of contrast medium to outline the uterine cavity and bilateral filling of the proximal fallopian tube. **B,** Instillation of an additional 3 to 5 ml of contrast medium to demonstrate bilateral tubal patency, tortuosity of the left tube, and peritoneal spillage.

Direct visualization of the reproductive tract is approached by employing various techniques. For direct visualization of the uterine cavity, a hysteroscope is passed through the cervix and the uterine cavity is expanded, if necessary, with either gas or liquid to look for polyps, septa, scar tissue, fibroids, or the presence of an imbedded intrauterine device. Similar operative techniques can often be employed to remove or correct such abnormalities. Recently, direct visualization of the fallopian tube has been reported by Kerin, Daykhovsky, Segalowitz, and others, who employed a falloposcope. Development of falloposcope technology will allow for not only the development of operative instruments to reestablish tubal patency, but also more precise diagnoses of tubal patency and assessment of tubal secretory activity.

The development of the laparoscope by obstetricians and gynecologists in the 1960s allowed for direct visualization of the female reproductive tract. After adequate insufflation of the abdominal cavity, the laparoscope can be introduced, and under direct visualization pelvic structures can be observed to screen for pelvic pathologies such as endometriosis, adhesions, PID, and pelvic masses. In addition, methylene blue dye can be installed transcervically to document tubal patency. Today the reproductive surgeon has an armament of operative procedures, tools, and technologies (such as laser dissection) that allow for completion of diagnostic and therapeutic procedures hitherto requiring exploratory laparotomy.

Cervical factors. The cervical mucus test, described in the section on male assessment, is often used to assess the physiologic characteristics of the female reproductive tract. Only during the preovulatory period when the cervical mucus is thin, watery, and hyperosmotic do sperm appear actively motile. Thus the widely held practice has been to evaluate the survival of sperm in cervical mucus in the preovulatory period. Test data from mucus studies correlate with sperm count and the number of motile sperm at the various levels but have failed to correlate with fertility.

Traditionally, a normal postcoital test is defined by the observation of greater than 10 motile sperm per high-power field with more than 50% showing good forward progression 2 hours after intercourse; however, even when few or no sperm have been observed in the cervical mucus, pregnancies have been reported, and laparoscopic studies have demonstrated motile sperm in the peritoneal cavity in many of such cases. Thus the postcoital test has value to ascertain cervical characteristics and determine sperm presence in cervical mucus, but it should not be considered definitive in assessment of sperm function and should not be used as a prognosticator of the ability of a given semen sample to result in a successful impregnation.

Because the mucus characteristics are dynamically controlled by the changing midcycle hormonal milieu, it is imperative that the preovulatory interval be defined by deploying methods such as urinary LH monitoring. With appropriate observation of an LH surge, intercourse can be arranged and a postcoital test performed. The time of observation after intercourse has traditionally been stated as 2 hours; however, many experts suggest that it should be performed 12 hours after intercourse to demonstrate active spermatozoa and demonstrate the function of the cervix as a reservoir for sperm.

PATIENT PROGNOSIS

At completion of the evaluation of the ovulatory function, semen function, tubal status, and cervical status, the couple should return for a consultation. The couple should be educated as to the particulars surrounding their reproductive capacity, and further testing that might be indicated should be outlined. If one or more conditions are identified for treatment or if there are several treatment options, these should be discussed with the couple, and further consultation visits should be scheduled at appropriate therapeutic landmarks. If, on the other hand, specific therapeutic options require the skills of a reproductive surgeon or endocrinologist or if all tests are within normal ranges, the couple should be referred to a specialist available at major fertility and endocrinology centers.

If all tests are within normal ranges and no pelvic or peritoneal pathology is identified, attention will most likely be directed to the fertilization potential of the sperm and the quality of the oocyte, which is the most rapidly developing field in reproductive endocrinology.

It is estimated that approximately 10% of couples completing a routine investigation will not have an established diagnosis. In the past this group was thought to have idiopathic or unexplained infertility. Assuming a routine workup has been completed, using this diagnosis is probably a misnomer for a fertilization failure. Failure to provide further diagnostic testing can rob the couple of appropriate treatment.

Empiric treatments for endometriosis, male factor, stress, and ovulatory irregularities have no effect on increasing the pregnancy rate in these couples. The average monthly fecundity in fertile couples is 25%, whereas the rate is 1.5% to 3.0% for couples with unexplained infertility. This rate increases 3 to 4 times from 9% per month fecundity with clomiphene therapy to 15% with combined gonadotropin and intrauterine insemination therapy. Assisted reproductive technologies can be used as a diagnostic as well as a therapeutic tool to assess the cause of a fertilization failure. Cumulative pregnancy rates in excess of 40% can be achieved using three treatment cycles of these technologies.

If a woman has failed to conceive within 2 years of an initial fertility evaluation, the probability of a successful unassisted pregnancy is extremely low (less than 4%), and it is estimated that as many as half the infertile couples seeking routine treatment will ultimately be unsuccessful in achieving pregnancy despite treatment. The decision on how long to continue conservative treatment and when to refer the couple should take into account the couple's age, motivation, and financial resources and the quality of professional care available locally. In general, if conception has not occurred during the first year of treatment or if the woman is over 39 years of age at the onset of evaluation, the couple is a candidate for referral to a major center specializing in ART.

ASSISTED REPRODUCTIVE TECHNOLOGIES (ART)

The birth of Louise Brown on July 25, 1978, the first baby conceived through IVF technology, marked the onset of the rapid use of ART to treat human infertility. Early treatment modalities were focused on coculturing sperm and oocytes to assist couples in cases where tubal pathology prevented conception. As knowledge of in vitro techniques increased, new treatments were developed to assist patients by using an expanding spectrum of diagnostic tools. Today ARTs consist of IVF, gamete intrafallopian transfer (GIFT), zygote intrafallopian transfer (ZIFT), cryopreserved embryo transfer (CPE), donor oocyte programs (DOP), and microoperative techniques such as intracytoplasmic sperm injection (ICSI). The availability of ART now offers patients with tubal disease, ovulatory dysfunction, male factor infertility, and advancing maternal age an opportunity hitherto unavailable to establish a pregnancy.

In 1989 the Society for Assisted Reproductive Technology established a voluntary registry to compile program activities. Today data reporting is mandatory for membership in the society and is subject to validation. Because of compelling public and governmental concerns surrounding both political and ethical issues as related to this area of medicine, almost all programs are reporting their data. As of 1993 (the last available published data as this book goes to press) 280 programs in the United States and Canada offer some sort of ART, and 267 programs submitted data to the Assisted Reproductive Technology Registry. These 267 programs reported initiation of a total of 43,975 cycles of ART treatment. As a result of all the procedures, a total of 8,741 deliveries was reported. This reflects nearly a doubling in activity since 1989 with 2.5 times the number of deliveries (4598 deliveries in 1989 versus 8741 deliveries in 1993) over this 4-year period. Increased availability of this technology and improvements in the technology itself have led to the success of this technology in treating infertile couples.

Clinical pregnancy rates vary based on the etiology of the couple's infertility and on the procedure performed (Table 18-9). Because of a variety of factors, approximately 12% to 14% of cycles initiated do not result in a procedure to retrieve oocytes. However, on a per retrieval basis the success of ART technologies is approaching and in some cases exceeding the estimated natural cycle success rate for human reproduction of 18% to 20%.

The dominant effects of the age of the female and male factor diagnosis continue to be reported (Table 18-10). A couple consisting of a younger woman and a man who has no identifiable problem with sperm parameters has the highest chance of achieving a pregnancy through the more commonly used technologies of IVF or GIFT. The age of 40 at the time of retrieval was arbitrarily selected for data collection, and in the next annual report data collection techniques will enable more precise determinations

TABLE 18-9.   Comparison of reported outcomes for all art procedures

Procedure	Number of retrievals	Number of pregnancies	Number of deliveries	Delivery rates (delivery/retrieval %)
In vitro fertilization	27,443	6,321	5,103	18.6
Gamete intrafallopian transfer	4,992	1,472	1,182	28.1
Zygote intrafallopian transfer	1,557	446	380	24.4
Cryopreserved embryo transfer	NA	984	791	NA
Donor oocyte program	2,368	895	716	30.2

From Society for Assisted Reproductive Technology (SART), American Society for Reproductive Medicine (ASRM): *Fertil Steril* 64:13, 1995.

TABLE 18-10.   Effects of age and diagnosis of male factor on assisted reproductive technology outcome*

Patient category		Number of retrievals	Cancellations†	Number of pregnancies	Number of deliveries‡	Delivery rate
Women <40, no	IVF§	17,847	12.4	4,703	3,833	21.5
male factor	GIFT§	2,804	13.0	1,106	903	32.2
Women ≥40, no	IVF	3,120	21.9	413	268	8.6
male factor	GIFT	635	27.5	136	54	11.8
Women <40,	IVF	5,198	11.6	1,076	864	16.6
male factor	GIFT	605	13.0	210	176	29.1
Women ≥40,	IVF	952	18.8	113	65	6.8
male factor	GIFT	157	20.3	20	14	8.9

From Society for Assisted Reproductive Technology (SART), American Society for Reproductive Medicine (ASRM); *Fertil Steril* 64:13, 1995.
*This table denotes information only on stimulated IVF cycles and included ($n = 9$) unstimulated GIFT cycles.
†Percent of stimulated cycles initiated that did not proceed to retrieval.
‡Deliveries with at least one liveborn infant.
§*GIFT*, Gamete intrafallopian transfer; *IVF*, in vitro fertilization.

of the probability of achieving a pregnancy for specific populations of women at each age. Similarly, data were not collected regarding sperm function, morphology, or antibodies; thus, in not using these characteristics, male factor is defined based only on sperm parameters of count and motility. Needless to say when a woman is 40 years old or older the presence of a concomitant male factor (as defined by count or motility) does little to suppress the already dramatically compromised delivery rate seen in this patient population (6.8% to 8.6% for IVF, 8.9% to 11.8% for GIFT). Yet using donor oocytes in this population yields a 30.2% delivery rate, equaling or exceeding rates for the younger population.

This success has in part come through increasing knowledge that allows us to enhance oocyte and sperm quality. In turn, these techniques can be applied to design specific infertility therapies to correct specific etiologic factors. New ovulation induction protocols employing gonadotropins in combination with gonadotropin-releasing hormone agonists were developed to improve oocyte number and quality; thus they have improved success rates for infertility patients who have failed prior attempts at ovulation induction with less aggressive therapies. Assisted reproductive technologies have also developed improvements in monitoring the ovulatory event, such as ultrasound monitoring of follicular development, urinary LH, and serum estradiol/progesterone, which in turn have improved oocyte quality and increased pregnancy rates on monitored cycles.

Similarly, sperm enhancement techniques are more available from increased knowledge of sperm physiology. Intrauterine inseminations can now be performed to mimic more closely the natural timing necessary to achieve fertilization. Sperm capacitation and the timing of the acrosome reaction can allow for preparation of a semen sample for intrauterine insemination to be placed at the optimal time for oocyte fertilization as determined by the ovulation monitoring techniques developed in ART. Assisted reproductive technology centers can now offer a combined nonsurgical procedure utilizing super ovulation, uterine replacement of sperm, capacitation of sperm, and enhancement of the timing of insemination (SOURCE). The major centers are reporting that the use of ovulation induction in combination with sperm enhancement has offered the couple with infertility of unknown etiology a cycle success rate near that of ART as a whole.

The future directions of ART are being determined by exciting findings from recent studies. The first area of investigation is to increase the success in transferring cryopreserved embryos to give a patient a higher per embryo success rate. This would translate into the couple having an increased pregnancy potential by undergoing embryo transfers more frequently using oocytes recovered from a single oocyte recovery procedure. When using oocytes from the intended recipient for these subsequent transfer cycles, the couple has an additional possibility (11.9%) of achieving a pregnancy and delivering.

The second area of study relates to establishing an optimal cultural environment that mimics normal tubal secretions. This need was suggested by the fact that higher pregnancy rates are seen with intrafallopian placement of either gametes or zygotes, which implies that the tubal environment may contribute something (a growth factor, a hormone milieu, a biochemical/physiologic environment) that is lacking in the IVF culture medium.

TABLE 18-11. Oocyte micromanipulation

Procedure	Number of retrievals	Number of pregnancies	Number of deliveries	Delivery rate (delivery/retrieval %)
Mixed transfer*	484	83	70	14.5
Exclusively micro-operative	888	94	75	8.4

From Society for Assisted Reproductive Technology (SART), American Society for Reproductive Medicine (ASRM); *Fertil Steril* 64:13, 1995.
*Includes both embryos generated by standard in vitro fertilization insemination and micromanipulation.

In the area of male factor infertility, developments are focused on both biochemical pretreatment of sperm, which enhances sperm capacitation and acrosome reaction, and on microsurgical techniques that range from dissection of the zona to direct ICSI. Reported oocyte micromanipulation data (Table 18-11) do not reflect specific technique but do show the outcome when this technology is employed in conjunction with routine IVF. In reviewing this data the reader should realize that candidates for oocyte micromanipulation would consist of couples with documented failed fertilizations in a prior ART procedure or demonstrated compromise in sperm function testing. Thus, using a redefinition of male factor infertility to include fertilization failures, microoperative treatments now available are able to yield pregnancies heretofore unachievable.

These early microoperative data are being eclipsed by the increased availability and exclusive use of ICSI, the most dramatic of the microoperative techniques. Reports of 25% per cycle pregnancy rates for this technology are not uncommon. This is remarkable in that men with severely compromised semen parameters of form, function, or both can achieve pregnancy rates equal to couples with non–male factor infertility.

Finally, with the development of embryo biopsy techniques, centers are now able to diagnose genetic disorders before implantation. This allows for preimplantation counseling for couples who might voluntarily be avoiding conception because of the risk of transmitting a gamete disorder to their newborn. Successful testing for cystic fibrosis, single-gene defects (Duchenne's muscular dystrophy, Tay-Sachs disease, Lesch-Nyhan syndrome, sickle cell disease), and X-linked disorders (hemophilia, X-linked mental retardation) are being reported. Use of preimplantation testing extends the role of ART even further by expanding the definition of infertility to include those individual clients who would like to have a child but have voluntarily become infertile.

In conclusion, the use of ART should not be reserved for therapeutic modalities but should be used as a diagnostic tool in cases of infertility of unknown etiology. One benefit of such a procedure for a specific couple is that placement of gametes, sperm, and eggs in a laboratory environment might allow for a better understanding of the issues of this problem. More and more frequently it is indicated that these couples have a problem related to the fertilization event, and with more sophisticated evaluation (i.e., enhanced SPA and zona-binding studies) improved therapies will be made available to infertile couples.

CONCLUSIONS

Treatment of infertility is a major challenge to health care providers in the United States. Particularly challenging are the couples who deferred childbearing until their midthirties, when reproductive capacity is normally decreased and the woman has a limited number of years in which to conceive children. The number of men and women who are infertile as a result of a history of sexually transmitted diseases continues to rise, as does the number who have been exposed to environmental risk factors and stress.

Concerns about infertility bring many people into the health care system who might not otherwise seek care. Therefore the clinician must use this entry to provide routine health care assessment and screening, with particular emphasis on Papanicolaou smear testing, breast examination, prostate and rectal screening, and patient education regarding lifestyle risk factors.

Practicing clinicians are well qualified to do the initial workup of the infertile couple, to provide patient education in reproductive physiology, and to provide treatment of observed defects. However, in many cases providing service to this client population requires collaboration with state-of-the-art laboratories and with reproductive systems specialists. The direction that reproductive infertility research has taken recently is to study the mechanisms of oocyte maturation and the physiologic processes of sperm function. Sophisticated studies are becoming available for those couples who fail to conceive even though they have completed a basic infertility workup that fails to identify an etiologic factor. In addition, ART is increasing the possibility for couples with identified reproductive failures to bear a child.

BIBLIOGRAPHY

Abdalla HI, Burton G, Kirkland A, et al: Age, pregnancy, and miscarriage: uterus versus ovarian factor, *Hum Reprod* 8:1512, 1993.

Armstrong BG, McDonald AD, Sloan M: Cigarette, alcohol, and caffeine consumption and spontaneous abortion, *Am J Public Health* 82:85, 1992.

Chlamydial infections, Washington, DC, 1987, American College of Obstetrics and Gynecology.

Collins JA, So Y, Wilson EH, et al: The post coital test as a predictor of pregnancy among 355 infertile couples, *Fertil Steril* 41:703, 1984.

Davajan V, Mishell DR Jr: Evaluation of the infertile couple. In Mishell DR Jr, Davajan V, editors: *Infertility, contraception and reproductive endocrinology*, ed 2, Oradel, NJ, 1986, Medical Economics Books.

Downs K, Gibson M: Basal body temperature graph and luteal phase defect, *Fertil Steril* 40:466, 1983.

Dubin Z, Amelar RD: Etiologic factors in 1294 consecutive cases of male infertility, *Fertil Steril* 22:469, 1971.

Dunihoo DR: Infertility. In *Fundamentals of Gynecology and Obstetrics*, Philadelphia, 1990, Lippincott.

Griffith CS, Grimes DA: The validity of the postcoital test, *Am J Obstet Gynecol* 162:615, 1990.

Grodstein F, Goldman MB, Ryan L, Cramer DW: Relation of female infertility to consumption of caffeinated beverages, *Am J Epidemiol* 137:1353, 1993.

Kerin J, Daykhovsky L, Segalowitz J, et al: Falloposcopy: a microendoscopic technique for visual exploration of the human fallopian tube from the uterotubal ostium to the fimbria using a transvaginal approach, *Fertil Steril* 54(suppl):390, 1990.

Luciano AA, Peluso J, Koch E, et al: Temporal relationship and reliability of the clinical, hormonal, and ultrasonographic indices of ovulation in infertile women, *Obstet Gynecol* 75:412, 1990.

Makler A: Evaluation and treatment of the infertile male. In DeCherney AH, editor: *Reproductive failure*, New York, 1986, Churchill Livingstone.

Mattison DR: The effects of smoking on fertility from gametogenesis to implantation, *Environ Res* 28:410, 1982.

Medical Research International, Society for Assisted Reproductive Technology, and the American Fertility Society: In vitro fertilization–embryo transfer (IVF-ET) in the United States: 1989 results from the IVF-ET Registry, *Fertil Steril* 55:14, 1991.

Megory E, Zuckerman H, Shoham (Schwartz) Z, et al: Infections and male fertility, *Obstet Gynecol Surv* 42:283, 1987.

Mosher WD, Pratt WF: The demography of infertility in the United States. In Asch RH, Studd JW, editors: *Annual progress in reproductive medicine*, Pearl River, NY, 1993, Parthenon.

Mueller BA, Daling JR: Epidemiology of infertility. In Soules MR, editor: *Controversies in reproductive endocrinology and infertility*, New York, 1989, Elsevier Science.

Muller CH, Zarutskie PW, Stenchever MA, et al: The sperm penetration assay, *Obstet Gynecol Rep* 2:412, 1990.

Pacifici R, Altieri F, Gardini L, et al: Environmental tobacco smoke: nicotine and cotinine concentrations in semen, *Environ Res* 68:69, 1995.

Phipps WR, Cramer DW, Schiff I: The association between smoking and female infertility as influenced by the cause of the infertility, *Fertil Steril* 488:377, 1987.

Rachootin P, Olsen J: The risk of infertility and delayed conception associated with exposures in the Danish workplace, *J Occup Med* 25:394, 1983.

Rosenfeld DL, Seidman SM, Bronson RA, et al: Unsuspected chronic pelvic inflammatory disease in the infertile female, *Fertil Steril* 39:44, 1983.

Sauer MV, Paulson RJ, Lobo RA: Reversing the natural decline in human fertility: an extended clinical trial of oocyte donation to women of advanced reproductive age, *JAMA* 268:1275, 1992.

Seibel MM: Work-up of the infertile couple. In Seibel MM, editor: *Infertility*, Norwalk, Conn, 1990, Appleton & Lange.

Shy KK, Stenchever MA, Muller CH: Sperm penetration assay and subsequent pregnancy: a prospective study of 74 infertile men, *Obstet Gynecol* 71:685, 1988.

Society for Assisted Reproductive Technology (SART), American Society for Reproductive Medicine (ASRM): Assisted reproductive technology in the United States and Canada: 1993 results generated from the American Society for Reproductive Medicine/ Society for Assisted Reproductive Technology Registry, *Fertil Steril* 64:13, 1995.

Spencer G: Projections of the population of the United States by age, sex, and race: 1983-2080, current population reports. In *Population estimates and projections*, U.S. Department of Commerce, May 1984, Series P-25, 952.

Stenchever MA, Spadoni LR, Smith WD, et al: Benefits of the sperm (hamster ova) penetration assay in the evaluation of the infertile couple, *Am J Obstet Gynecol* 143:91, 1982.

Stene J, Fischer G, Stene B, et al: Paternal age effect in Down's syndrome, *Ann Hum Genet* 40:299, 1977.

Svensson L, Westrom L, Ripa KT, et al: Differences in some clinical and laboratory parameters in acute salpingitis related to uterine and serologic findings, *Am J Obstet Gynecol* 138:1017, 1980.

U.S. Congress, Office of Technology Assessment: *Infertility: medical and social choices*, OTA-BA-358, vol 51, Washington, DC, 1988, U.S. Government Printing Office.

Weisberg E: Smoking and reproductive health, *Clin Reprod Fertil* 3:175, 1985.

Wentz AC: Cigarette smoking and infertility, *Fertil Steril* 46:365, 1986.

Westoff CF: Fertility in the United States, *Science* 234:554, 1986.

Wyrobek AJ, Gordon LA, Burkhart JG, et al: An evaluation of human sperm as indicators of chemically induced alterations of spermatogenic function, *Mutat Res* 115:73, 1983.

Yanagimachi R, Yanagimachi H, Rogers BJ: The use of zona-free animal ova as a test-system for assessment of the fertilizing capacity of human spermatozoa, *Biol Reprod* 15:471, 1976.

CHAPTER 19

Evaluation of Pelvic Relaxation: Nonoperative Management

MORTON A. STENCHEVER

Pelvic support structures in women may become weakened for a variety of reasons. These include congenital anatomic weakness, childbirth, physical injury, damage related to surgical intervention, and chronic stress such as that relating to straining or to chronic cough. With aging, the withdrawal of estrogen may further weaken the support structures both as a direct effect on the structures and as a reduction in their vascularity. This chapter will address the diagnosis and nonsurgical treatment of conditions related to the weakening of pelvic support structures.

ANATOMIC RELATIONSHIPS

Anatomic relationships involved in pelvic support are best understood by considering the relationships of the muscular and fascial supports of the pelvic floor. Perhaps the most important of these is the pelvic diaphragm, which consists primarily of two muscles, the coccygeus and the levator ani. These muscles, which evolved from the tail-wagging musculature of quadripeds and their fascial covering, completely close off the pelvic floor except for openings of the urethra, the vagina, and the rectum, which they encircle. The levator ani, which is the largest, has three components named for their origin and insertion: pubococcygeus, puborectalis, and iliococcygeus. The total muscle mass of the levator ani muscle extends from the pubic symphysis to the coccyx and between the two lateral pelvic sidewalls. The coccygeus is a triangular-shaped muscle that extends between both ischial spines and to the coccygeus as the apex of the triangle. The levator ani muscles play a major role in controlling urination, in the birth process, and in maintaining fecal continence, as well as supporting the abdominal and pelvic viscera (Fig. 19-1).

A second musculofascial diaphragm important in pelvic support is the more superficial urogenital diaphragm that extends from the pubic symphysis to a line between the two ischial tuberoscities. Its role is to support the anterior segment of the pelvic outlet, and it consists of three muscle bundles: the ischiocavernosus, which extends between the pubic symphysis and ischial tuberosities along the pubic ramus; the bulbocavernosus, which extends between the pubic symphysis and the perineal body surrounding the vaginal outlet; and the deep transverse perineal muscle, which extends from the ischial tuberosities to the perineal body. The transverse perineal muscles join with the external anal sphincter muscle surrounding the rectum. The urogenital diaphragm, in addition, supports

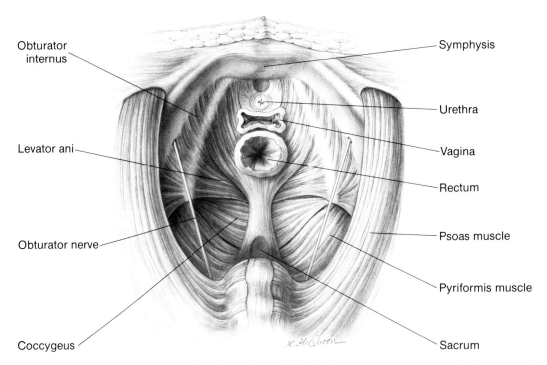

FIGURE 19-1. A superior view of the pelvic diaphragm demonstrates the levator ani and the coccygeus muscles.

Redrawn from Mattingly RF, Thompson JD: *Te Linde's operative gynecology*, ed 6, Philadelphia, 1985, Lippincott.

the external portion of the urethra and the introitus of the vagina. It contains pudendal blood vessels and nerves, the external sphincter of the urethra, and the dorsal nerve of the clitoris. It is important in maintaining the position of the bladder neck (Fig. 19-2). .

A number of so-called supporting ligaments also contribute to the support of the pelvic organs. Although these pelvic ligaments are called ligaments, they are really thickenings of endopelvic fascia. They tend to surround the vagina and the cervix as an endopelvic fascia. Anteriorly the portion that separates the vagina and cervix from the bladder is commonly called the pubocervical fascia. This helps support the bladder from herniating into the vagina. It blends laterally with the cardinal ligaments (Mackenrodt's ligaments), which extend from the lateral aspect of the upper portion of the vagina and cervix to the lateral pelvic wall bilaterally. The cardinal ligaments form the base of the broad ligament that is a tent of peritoneum draped across the round ligament in which are found the uterine artery and vein and the ureter. The ureter transverses the cardinal ligaments adjacent to the cervix. The posterior endopelvic investment fascia thickens into the uterosacral ligaments that join the cervix to the sacrum. Within these ligaments run nerve bundles that supply the uterus and cervix. The endopelvic fascia supports the pelvic structures that it invests and contributes (particularly via the uterosacral ligament) to the support of the cul-de-sac. The round ligament that extends from the fundus of the uterus into the inguinal canal offers little support but does help hold the uterus forward in an anteflexed position. It is part of the broad ligament.

PHYSIOLOGIC RELATIONSHIPS

Estrogen makes a major contribution toward the health and integrity of the pelvic support structures and improves the blood supply to these tissues. Loss of estrogen leads to atrophy of the epithelium of the vagina, bladder neck, and urethra and also weakens the elastic and collagen tissue of the endopelvic support fascia. These changes are reversible, and when estrogen is administered to a postmenopausal woman, improvement in the strength of these structures can be noted. Thus estrogen replacement therapy is an important component in the treatment of relaxation of pelvic supports.

PELVIC SUPPORT DEFECTS

When pelvic supports weaken, anatomic defects consisting of urethrocele, cystocele, rectocele, enterocele, and descensus of the uterus and cervix are possible. These conditions may occur singly or in combination in any given patient. Often the correction of these problems is surgical. Nonsurgical therapies are possible and may relieve the patient's symptoms appropriately. Therefore each anatomic defect will be considered from the standpoint of nonsurgical therapy for the purpose of this chapter.

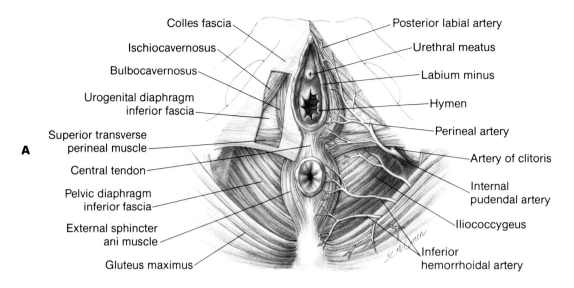

A

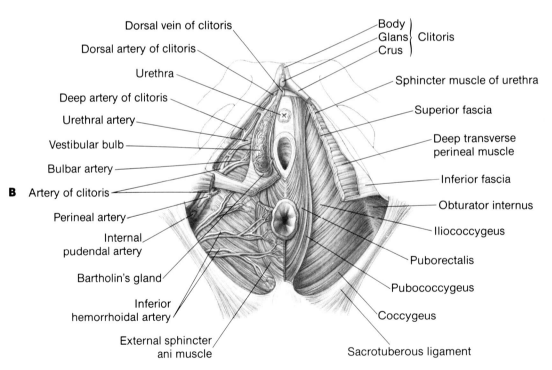

B

FIGURE 19-2. A, A schematic view of the perineum demonstrates the superficial structure of the urogenital diaphragm. **B,** A schematic view of the perineum demonstrates the superficial structures and deeper structures and shows the relationship of the levator ani and coccygeus muscles.

Redrawn from Pritchard JA, MacDonald PC, Gant NF: *Williams' obstetrics,* ed 17, New York, 1985, Appleton-Century-Crofts.

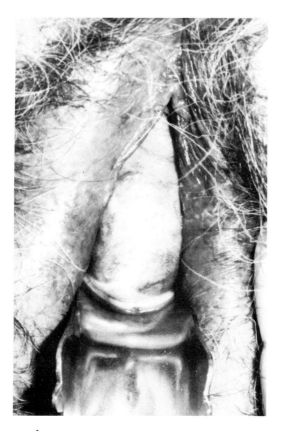

FIGURE 19-3. Cystocele.

From Stenchever MA: In Droegemueller W, Herbst AL, Mishell DR, et al, editors: *Comprehensive gynecology,* St Louis, 1987, Mosby. Used by permission.

Urethrocele and Cystocele

With weakening of the pubocervical fascia a herniation of the urethra (urethrocele) or the bladder neck or the bladder (cystocele) into the vagina is possible (Fig. 19-3). If the urethra and the bladder neck continue to be supported but a cystocele develops, the patient often does not suffer from stress urinary incontinence, but if the defect includes the urethra or the bladder neck, stress incontinence may be the presenting symptom. Women with wide subpubic arches such as those with a gynecoid pelvis may be at greater risk for damage to the pubocervical fascia during childbirth because of pressure of the fetal head directly against these structures. Women with narrower pelvic arches such as those with anthropoid or android pelvises may enjoy a degree of protection.

In addition to the symptoms of stress incontinence, patients with cystoceles often have a feeling of urgency or sensation of incomplete emptying after voiding. Also, such patients may complain of a heaviness in their pelvis, a sensation that a structure is falling out of the vagina, and if such is the case an awareness of a soft, bulging mass from the anterior wall of the vagina. Occasionally this mass must be replaced before the patient is able to void. With strain or cough the protrusion of the mass may be accentuated and may even occur outside the introitus. This mass may be apparent to the examining physician in either the lithotomy or standing position. Cystoceles are common, and patients with these may be completely asymptomatic. Although most patients are parous, cystoceles do occur in nulliparous women with congenitally or situationally weakened pelvic support structures.

The diagnosis of a cystocele is made with the patient in the lithotomy position and a posterior speculum blade placed into the vagina. The patient is then asked to bear down as the posterior blade is depressed, and the degree of the cystocele or urethrocele can be noted. At this point the physician should palpate the bladder neck and estimate its degree of support. If the bladder neck is well supported, the urethra will be as well, and it will be unlikely that the patient has stress incontinence. At this point in the examination it is appropriate to ask the patient to cough and note whether urine is lost. A repeat of this portion of the examination may be carried out with the patient in the standing position just to be sure that the specific circumstances of the cystocele or urethrocele are noted.

Urethroceles must be differentiated from other urethral and periurethral pathologic conditions such as inflammation and enlargement of Skene's glands and a urethral diverticulum. Occasionally bladder tumors or bladder diverticula may be mistaken for a cystocele. Inflamed Skene's glands are generally tender, and it may be possible to express pus from the urethra when they are palpated. Urethra diverticula generally feel different than a urethrocele in that the urethrocele is generally soft and pliable whereas the urethral diverticulum may offer resistance and if inflamed and infected may also be accompanied by the expression of pus through the urethra when palpated.

Nonoperative therapy for asymptomatic cystocele or urethrocele consists of estrogen replacement if the patient is postmenopausal, Kegel exercises to improve the tone of the pelvic diaphragm, and in some cases the use of a pessary.

Kegel exercises are isometric exercises first described by Kegel in 1956. At that time Kegel suggested that patients contract their pubococcygeal muscles five times on awakening, five times on arising, and five times every half hour throughout the day. These muscles can be demonstrated to the patient by asking her to contract the muscles that it takes to stop the urinary stream during urination. Once she knows which muscles to contract, Kegel exercises can be performed. Most patients, however, will not adhere to a rigorous schedule such as that laid down by Kegel. It probably suffices to ask them to exercise these muscles by contracting them 10 times to the count of 10 several times a day. Improving the muscular tone of the pelvic diaphragm may both improve the symptoms of stress incontinence and effect an apparent improvement in the strength of the pelvic support structures.

Other techniques have been used to attempt to improve the strength of pubococcygeal and levator ani muscles. Graduated vaginal weights, which the patient holds in place by contracting these muscles, have been used with some success. Devices have been designed that can be placed in the vagina and attached to a pressure device, allowing the patient to visually determine the strength of the contraction of these muscles. With this positive feedback, strength can be developed over time. Electric current can also be used to stimulate these muscles and to make them contract. Henalla, Hutchins, Robinson, and MacVicar studied 104 patients with stress incontinence divided into four groups. The first group ($n = 26$) was taught to perform pelvic floor exercises. The second group ($n = 25$) was treated with a course of 10 interferential (electric current) treatments over a 10-week period using one treatment per week. The third group ($n = 24$)) was given vaginal conjugated estrogen cream (2 g per night for 12 weeks, 1.25 mg conjugated estrogen/2-g dose). The fourth group ($N n = 25$) received no treatment at all and served as a control group. The groups were evaluated before and after therapy using a perineal pad weighing test and were evaluated by questionnaire 9 months after therapy. Sixty-five percent of the pelvic floor exercise group, 32% of the interferential group, 12% of the estrogen group, and none of the controls were found to either be completely relieved of their stress incontinence or greatly improved. In a separate report Henalla, Kerrwan, Castleden, and others, using a form of pelvic floor exercise under the direction of physical therapists at two different hospitals, demonstrated that 67% of patients had either completely achieved continence or were significantly improved of their symptoms.

The use of pessaries will be discussed later in this chapter.

Rectocele

Patients with rectoceles often complain of heaviness in the pelvis and a sensation that the rectum is falling out of the vagina. They may be constipated or may have a feeling of incomplete emptying of the rectum after a bowel movement and in extreme cases may need to splint the posterior wall of the vagina with their fingers to cause a bowel movement.

The rectocele is identified by retracting the anterior vaginal wall upward and having the patient strain. The rectum will then bulge into the vagina, and if the rectocele is large enough the bulge may protrude through the introitus (Fig. 19-4). The physician may make a specific diagnosis by placing

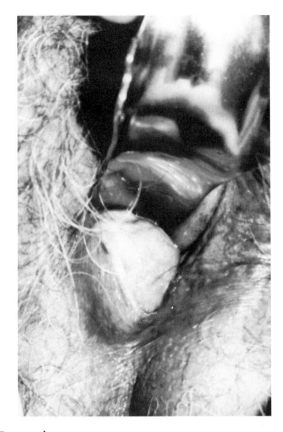

FIGURE 19-4. Rectocele.

From Stenchever MA: In Droegemueller W, Herbst AL, Mishell DR, et al, editors: *Comprehensive gynecology*, St Louis, 1987, Mosby. Used by permission.

one finger in the rectum and one in the vagina and palpating the herniation. The rectovaginal septum will appear paper thin, and the entire limits of the rectocele may be palpated. If an enterocele is present, with straining it may be possible to differentiate this sac from the rectocele. Small enteroceles may escape detection if the rectocele is large enough and may be found only at the time of surgical intervention.

Estrogen administration, Kegel exercises, and pessaries are also of value in treating the symptoms of rectocele nonoperatively. Definitive therapy relates to surgical correction.

Enterocele

An enterocele is a true hernia of the peritoneal cavity through the pouch of Douglas (cul-de-sac) between the uterosacral ligaments and into the rectovaginal septum (Fig. 19-5). Within the sac will be found the small bowel and frequently the omentum. The symptoms of an enterocele are heaviness in the pelvis and the detection of a bulge into the vagina or coming

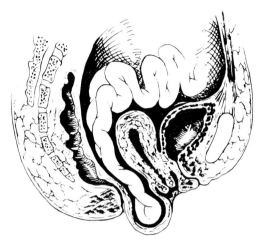

FIGURE 19-5. Enterocele and uterine prolapse.

From Symmonds RE: In Pernoll ML, editor: *Current obstetric and gynecologic diagnosis and treatment*, ed 7, Norwalk, Conn, 1991, Appleton & Lange. Used by permission.

through the introitus. Frequently it can be large. The enterocele is not always easy to differentiate from a rectocele, but it may be detected as a separate bulge on rectovaginal examination. If large enough it may be possible to transilluminate the sac and see the small-bowel shadows within it. It is often possible to reduce the hernia digitally, although of course it will not remain reduced without surgical intervention. Small enteroceles may be supported by a pessary, but when an enterocele is present, surgical intervention is usually necessary.

Uterine Prolapse (Descensus, Procidentia)

Prolapse of the uterus and cervix into the barrel of the vagina is often associated with injuries of the endopelvic fascia and injury to or relaxation of the pelvic floor muscles, particularly the levator ani muscles. Prolapse may occur during increased intraabdominal pressure such as may occur with ascites or a large pelvic or intraabdominal tumor superimposed on poor pelvic floor supports. In some cases, sacral nerve damage, particularly to sacral nerves S1 through S4, as may occur in tumors or in diabetic neuropathy, may be responsible. Chronic respiratory conditions, such as asthma, bronchitis, and bronchiectasis, or morbid obesity may also be associated. Young nulliparous women may develop a prolapse because of congenital abnormalities of the pelvic supports or relaxation of pelvic floor support because of trauma. Most patients with descensus, however, are multiparous, and the problem relates directly to childbirth trauma. It is unusual to have uterine prolapse without a cystocele or rectocele. Enteroceles are often present as well.

Descensus is graded in the following manner: a prolapse into the upper barrel of the vagina is defined as first degree; a prolapse through the barrel of the vagina to the region of the introitus is defined as second degree; and if the cervix and uterus prolapse through the introitus it is defined as a third-degree (or total) prolapse (Fig. 19-6). With total prolapse, the vagina everts around the uterus and cervix and is totally exteriorized. In such instances, particularly when estrogen replacement has not been given, dryness rapidly develops with thickening and chronic inflammation of the vaginal epithelium. Stasis ulcers, edema, and interference with the blood supply of the vaginal wall may occur. Although stasis ulcers are rarely cancerous, they should undergo biopsy to ensure that this is not the case.

Patients with descensus often complain of a feeling of heaviness or fullness and a feeling that something is falling out of the vagina. In second-degree prolapse, the cervix may be noted to be protruding at the introitus and give the patient the impression that a tumor is bulging out of her vagina. If total prolapse has occurred, the patient is aware of the mass. In addition, she may complain of symptoms of cystocele, rectocele, urinary incontinence, and vaginal bleeding. If infection of the vagina occurs, discharge may be present as well.

First-degree prolapse rarely requires any therapy. However, as the degree of prolapse increases and the cervix is displaced closer to the introitus, discomfort is usually more severe, and therapy either by pessary

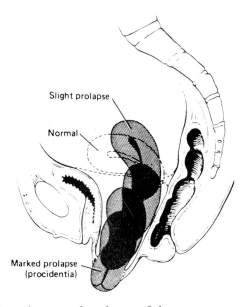

FIGURE 19-6. Various degrees of prolapse of the uterus.

From Symmonds RE: In Pernoll ML, editor: *Current obstetric and gynecologic diagnosis and treatment*, ed 7, Norwalk, Conn, 1991, Appleton & Lange. Used by permission.

or by surgical intervention is indicated. As with other pelvic relaxation problems, estrogen replacement is often helpful. In occasional cases, the prolapse may reduce itself partially or completely merely by having estrogen replaced.

Vaginal Vault Prolapse

Vaginal vault prolapse may occur in women who have previously had hysterectomies. Many of the reasons mentioned for total descensus of the uterus may be in play in such patients. Often, however, the prolapse occurs because the pelvic supports to the vaginal vault are weakened either through faulty operative technique or for other reasons that have occurred in the interim. The symptoms noted by the patient are similar to those for descensus of the uterus and include a feeling of heaviness and the prolapse of a structure through the introitus. Therapy is almost always surgical, but a trial of estrogen replacement and a pessary may be attempted. It is unusual to have only a vaginal vault prolapse, and often a cystocele, rectocele, or enterocele is also present.

Pessary Therapy

The goal of pessary therapy is to return the pelvic organs to their normal anatomic position and hold them there. A large number of different types of pessaries have been developed over the years, probably supporting the fact that no ideal pessary exists and that failure of pessary therapy is common. Nevertheless, in women who are poor surgical risks or who do not wish to have surgical therapy at a particular point in time, pessary therapy may have its place. Success often depends on the strength of the perineal body because the more gaping the introitus and the weaker the perineal body, the less likely it is that the patient can hold a pessary in place.

For the woman with descensus of the uterus, a doughnut or Smith-Hodge pessary may be appropriate and should probably be tried first. Variations on these two types of pessaries have been developed and include solid-ring pessaries of different sizes and blow-up bulb pessaries, also in a variety of sizes. Each seeks to distend the vaginal wall, hold the bladder and rectum in their normal positions, and maintain the uterus high in the pelvis. The Smith-Hodge pessary is one of a family of lever pessaries that holds the bladder neck behind the pubic symphysis and therefore may alleviate genuine urinary stress incontinence. The doughnut and blow-up pessaries work best by holding the cervix and uterus higher in the pelvis and usually do not have a positive effect on continence. In fact, many women with large cystoceles who have their pelvic relaxation treated with a doughnut pessary often become incontinent because the kinking of the urethra caused by the large cystocele is alleviated by the pessary therapy.

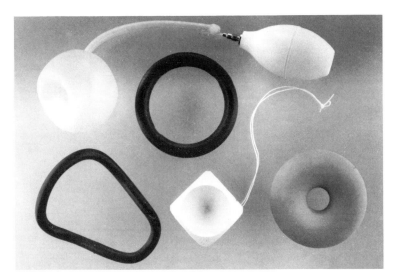

FIGURE 19-7. Various pessaries available commercially. *Top (left to right):* Milex inflatable ball; ring. *Bottom:* Smith-Hodge; Milex cube; doughnut.

Recently, the Milex cube has been developed in multiple sizes, and it is easy for the patient to remove, clean, and reinsert. It too holds the bladder and rectum in their proper position and tends to elevate the vaginal vault. This type of pessary has an advantage in women with weak or absent perineal bodies (Fig. 19-7).

The physician and patient should patiently seek the pessary that works best for the patient's individual needs and should not be discouraged by failure of a specific pessary. In general, the largest pessary that the patient can tolerate should be used. The patient should be advised that if the pessary falls out she should reinsert it. The most likely time to have the pessary fall out is during a bowel movement or with some other straining exercise. To prevent this from happening, the patient should be instructed to hold the pessary in place with a finger while she moves her bowels. Often reassurance that pessaries may fall out and can be replaced will be helpful for patients in attempting to maintain their use. Pessaries should be removed at least once a week and washed before replacement. Patients or their caregivers can often be trained to do this, but from time to time the patient should be seen by the physician and the vaginal vault inspected. It is wise to use estrogen cream or estrogen replacement therapy to ensure a greater health of vaginal epithelium during pessary use. Neglected pessaries can lead to vaginal ulceration and to partial embedding in the vaginal wall. Epithelial atypia may occur, as may hemorrhage and infection. Patients using pessaries should be followed closely.

No nonsurgical therapy will correct a cystocele, rectocele, enterocele, or prolapse, and a truly symptomatic patient should be offered surgical intervention appropriate for her particular circumstances. However, in many cases, nonsurgical therapy can be useful in the patient who is minimally symptomatic or a poor surgical risk or a patient who wishes to put off an operation for a period of time.

BIBLIOGRAPHY

Droegemueller W: Anatomy. In Droegemueller W, Herbst AL, Mishell DR, et al, editors: *Comprehensive gynecology,* St Louis, 1987, Mosby.

Henalla SM, Hutchins CJ, Robinson P, MacVicar J: Non-operative methods of treatment of female genuine stress incontinence of urine, *Br J Obstet Gynaecol* 9:222, 1989.

Henalla SM, Kerrwan P, Castleden CM, et al: The effect of pelvic floor exercises in the treatment of genuine urinary stress incontinence in women at two hospitals, *Br J Obstet Gynaecol* 95:602, 1988.

Kegel AH: Stress incontinence of urine in women. Physiologic treatment, *J Int Coll Surg* 25:487, 1956.

Miller DS: Contemporary use of pessary. In Sciarra J, editor: *Gynecology and obstetrics,* vol 1, Philadelphia, 1992, Lippincott.

Sulak PJ, Kuehl TJ, Shull BL: Vaginal pessaries and their use in pelvic relaxation, *J Reprod Med* 38:919, 1993.

Stenchever MA: Disorders of abdominal wall and pelvic support. In Droegemueller W, Herbst AL, Mishell DR, et al, editors: *Comprehensive gynecology,* St Louis, 1987, Mosby.

Zeitlin MP, Lebtherz TB: Pessaries in the geriatric patient, *J Am Geriatr Soc* 40:635, 1992.

CHAPTER 20

Office Urogynecology

GRETCHEN M. LENTZ

The primary care physician frequently is asked to evaluate and treat patients for lower urinary tract disorders ranging from infections to incontinence. Approximately 5% of medical care rendered in a gynecologic practice is related to the lower urinary tract.

Urinary incontinence is a common problem. It occurs in 8% to 10% of the population aged 15 to 64 years. Yarnell and St. Leger found that 5% to 15% of community-dwelling elderly women have incontinence. Other reports have found that 15% to 30% of women over age 60 have incontinence. About 40% to 50% of institutionalized elderly women have urinary incontinence. As the population ages and public awareness of incontinence continues to increase, physicians will need to understand the current testing and treatment options. Particularly important is the emphasis being placed on the conservative treatment of incontinence evidenced by the U.S. Department of Health and Human Services 1992 clinical practice guidelines on urinary incontinence.

Urinary incontinence has considerable social consequences in addition to the medical aspects, including social isolation, embarrassment, depression, and shame.

This chapter will review the anatomy and physiology of micturition, pertinent history, diagnostic tests, and therapy for many common lower urinary tract disorders. This information will be synthesized to help differentiate various types of urinary incontinence and provide treatment options. Many of the urinary tests may be done with simple office equipment and provide the clinician with useful information. However, more precise measurements require electronic urodynamic equipment. Identifying patients who require more sophisticated tests will be addressed.

FUNCTIONAL ANATOMY AND PHYSIOLOGY OF CONTINENCE

Although the bladder and urethra are described separately, it is important to remember that the bladder and urethra work together as one functional unit, both being derived embryologically from the urogenital sinus. Unlike the bladder and urethra, which are of endodermal origin, the trigone of the bladder is derived from mesodermal origin. Iosif, Batra, Ek, and others found that the trigone is responsive to sex steroid hormones.

The physiology of micturition depends on the two basic processes of urine storage and bladder emptying. For the bladder to be able to store urine effectively, it must have compliance, a physiologic property whereby the bladder pressure remains low with increasing volume of urine. The patient must have appropriate sensation of bladder filling without involuntary contractions. Continence is a function of both the bladder's ability to store urine and the urethra's ability to prevent flow of urine. The urethra must remain closed at rest and with increased intraabdominal pressure. Micturition relies on the ability of the bladder's detrusor muscle to contract and the urethra to relax in a coordinated fashion.

The lower urinary tract is controlled by the autonomic nervous system. The bladder is predominantly made up of β-adrenergic receptors (Fig. 20-1). Sympathetic stimulation relaxes the bladder and allows filling. The preganglionic sympathetic fibers to the bladder originate from the thoracolumbar segments of T10 to L2 and synapse in the ganglia of the superior hypogastric. The postganglionic sympathetic nerves continue in the hypogastric nerves and terminate in the ganglia of the vesical plexus.

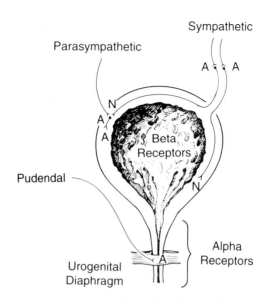

FIGURE 20-1. Nervous innervations of the bladder and urethra. *A*, Acetylcholine; *N*, norepinephrine.

The postganglionic adrenergic fibers innervate the blood vessels and smooth muscles of the bladder and urethra. Some adrenergic fibers terminate in the parasympathetic ganglion.

The bladder neck and urethra have predominately α-adrenergic receptors that cause contraction of the urethra when stimulated. In summary, sympathetic stimulation causes relaxation of the bladder and contraction of the urethra, and this results in continence.

The bladder is also innervated by the parasympathetic nervous system. The preganglionic parasympathetic nerves originate from S2 through S4 of the spinal cord and synapse in the ganglia of the bladder. Parasympathetic stimulation causes contraction of the bladder but has no effect on the bladder neck or urethra. Because atropine has only a partial response at the cholinergic nerve endings of the bladder, the experiments of Eaton, Birmingham, and Bates seem to indicate that there is a second neurotransmitter, possibly purinergic. The interganglionic connections between the sympathetic and parasympathetic systems suggest a regulatory mechanism on the bladder function at the ganglionic level.

The smooth muscle of the urethra is mainly composed of longitudinal and oblique muscle fibers that are under α-adrenergic control. The smooth muscle tension is distributed uniformly along the urethra and contributes approximately one third of the intraurethral pressure. The other two thirds of the intraurethral pressure are contributed by the vascular supply and the striated muscles. Studies have demonstrated that intraurethral pressure is reduced by 41% when patients receive curare and by 31% when there is obstruction of both common iliac arteries.

DeLancey demonstrated that women have two distinct groups of striated muscle that contribute to urethral pressure and support. The two groups are the striated urethral sphincter with the vaginal levator muscle attachments and the striated muscles of the urogenital diaphragm.

The urethra must be pliable so that the external forces may press against it. A rigid urethra, possibly resulting from multiple surgeries, radiation, or atrophy, may not close.

During increased intraabdominal pressures caused by coughing, the urethra maintains continence by two mechanisms: pressure transmission and striated muscle reflex contraction. A woman remains continent with coughing or sneezing if the intraabdominal pressure on the bladder is transmitted to the urethra in an equal manner, thus keeping the urethral closure pressure higher than that of the bladder pressure. This pressure transmission will not produce incontinence if the bladder neck is well supported.

Reflex pelvic floor contraction increases urethral pressure during coughing or any increase in intraabdominal pressure. Studies in urethral closure pressure profiles have demonstrated that increased urethral pressure precedes increased intravesical pressure during coughing.

PHYSIOLOGY OF MICTURITION

The urge to void becomes greater with increasing volume in the bladder even when the bladder pressure remains low. Voiding occurs whenever there is conscious or uncontrolled detrusor contraction.

Micturition is mediated under the cerebrocortical tracts. There are four main autonomic and somatic nervous system feedback loops. Loop I involves the frontal cortex and the brainstem, loop II involves the brain stem and the sacral micturition center (S2 through S4), loop III involves the sensory afferents in the detrusor muscle and the sacral micturition center, and loop IV involves the frontal lobe of the cerebral cortex to the urethral striated muscles via the sacral micturition center. Loop I inhibits micturition according to sensory information obtained from loop II. If no inhibitory information is sensed from loop I, activation of loop III occurs, allowing voluntary relaxation of the urethral sphincter in synchrony with detrusor contraction (loop II). Loop IV allows voluntary control of the striated external urethral sphincter.

The process of bladder control and micturition is a complex interplay of the nervous system, bladder muscle, and anatomy of the bladder neck and the urethra. An injury to any one part will cause bladder dysfunction. Neurologic diseases (such as multiple sclerosis, Parkinson's disease, cerebrovascular accidents, spinal cord injuries, diabetic neuropathy, and radical pelvic surgery) are examples of conditions that can greatly alter normal bladder function.

PATIENT EVALUATION
History

Taking a thorough urologic, gynecologic, neurologic, and general medical history is important in formulating a plan to care for patients with lower urinary tract complaints but it is often inaccurate for making a specific diagnosis. A detailed questionnaire can be completed by the patient and used to complement a physician-patient interview to determine the exact nature of the lower urinary tract complaint.

Specific urologic questions include determining the onset of the symptoms and frequency, the degree of disability, daytime and nighttime voiding patterns, urgency, frequency or dysuria complaints, voiding problems (such as hesitancy or straining to void), incomplete bladder emptying sensation, hematuria, and postvoid dribbling. It is also important to understand the impact the symptoms have on the patient's life.

If incontinence is the primary complaint, it is important to ask questions that distinguish stress incontinence from urge incontinence. Involuntary loss of urine with exertion (coughing, laughing, exercising, lifting) is often reported with stress incontinence. Urge incontinence is the involuntary loss of urine associated with a strong desire to void. Overflow incontinence may result in suprapubic pressure symptoms and constant dribbling. Continuous urine leakage even at night may be secondary to a genitourinary fistula, ectopic ureter, or a severe form of stress incontinence called intrinsic sphincter deficiency (discussed later). The latter condition often occurs after prior pelvic or incontinence surgery.

The frequency and volume of urine leakage can be difficult to assess; asking about the use of absorbant pads (type, number used per day) can help gauge the severity of the problem. Nocturnal enuresis as a child makes a diagnosis of detrusor instability more likely.

Other relevant urologic questions include a history of urinary tract infection, kidney stones, renal disease, or surgery. Prior pelvic surgery, particularly radical hysterectomy or radical vulvectomy history, should be carefully obtained. Radical vulvectomy with dissection around the urethra has been associated with stress incontinence. Symptoms of genital prolapse, menopausal status, hormone replacement use, prior obstetric history, history of neurologic disease, trauma, diabetes, and bowel habits may be pertinent and should be documented. Prescription and nonprescription drug use may aid in making a diagnosis because many classes of drugs have effects on the lower urinary tract (Table 20-1).

TABLE 20-1. Drugs with possible effects on the lower urinary tract

Class	Possible effects	Drug and usual indication	Action
Antihypertensives	Incontinence	Reserpine— hypertension Methyldopa— hypertension	Pharmacologic sympathectomy by depleting cate-cholamines
Dopaminergic agents	Bladder neck obstruction	Bromocriptine— galactorrhea Levodopa— Parkinson's disease	Increased urethral resistance and decreased detru-sor contractions
Cholinergic agonists	Decreased bladder ca-pacity and increased intravesical pressure	Digitalis— cardiotropic	Increased bladder wall tension
Neuroleptics	Incontinence	Major tranquilizers: prochlorperazine, promethazine, trifluoperazine, chlorpromazine, haloperidol	Dopamine receptor blockade, with internal sphincter relaxation
β-Adrenergic agents	Urinary reten-tion	Isoxsuprine— vasodilator Terbutaline— bronchodilator	Inhibited bladder muscle contrac-tility
Xanthines	Incontinence	Caffeine	Decreased urethral closure pressure

From Corlett RC: *Female Patient* 10:20, 1985.

Pelvic Examination

Inspection of the vulva, urethral meatus, and vagina is performed with a bimanual pelvic examination. A Sims' speculum or the posterior blade of a bivalve speculum should be used to visualize the anterior vaginal wall at rest and during straining. Descent of the urethra, bladder, and vagina can be noted. Assessment for vaginal atrophy is made visually. Urine in the vagina, particularly after pelvic surgery, may indicate a genitourinary fistula. The urethra is palpated for tenderness, purulent discharge, and masses to determine the presence of urethritis or diver-ticula.

A stress test can be performed to directly confirm urinary leakage. With the sensation of a moderately full bladder, the supine patient is asked to cough. If immediate urine leakage is noted, it is suggestive of stress incontinence. If a delay in leakage is noted after a cough or a large volume leaks, a cough-induced detrusor contraction may be present, suggesting detrusor instability. If there is no leakage seen, the patient should stand and the cough test should be repeated.

The Q-Tip test was first described by Crystal. This test evaluates the urethral axial positions at rest and at maximal cough or Valsalva maneuver. With the patient in the dorsal lithotomy position, a sterile cotton-tipped applicator lubricated with 2% lidocaine is gently introduced into the proximal portion of the urethra. By using a goniometer (Fig. 20-2), the resting angle and maximal coughing and straining angles are measured. The goniometer is positioned with zero degrees parallel with the longitudinal axis of the body. Therefore the normal resting angle of the Q-Tip may be plus or minus 10° with a deflection of 30° during straining. A Q-Tip straining angle of greater than 30° was previously thought to indicate urethral hypermobility. Caputo and Benson compared Q-Tip testing to perineal ultrasound and found that the Q-Tip test is not accurate in measuring urethrovesical junction mobility.

It is important to note that the Q-Tip test alone is not predictive of genuine stress incontinence (GSI). Normal continent women may have an abnormal Q-Tip test result. Montz and Stanton showed that 32% of patients with symptoms of stress incontinence with a positive Q-Tip test

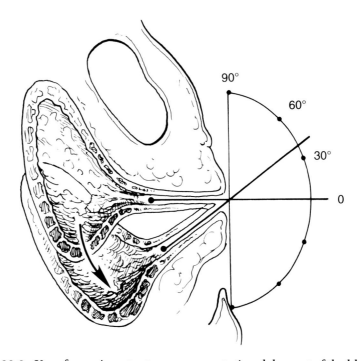

FIGURE 20-2. Use of a goniometer to measure rotational descent of the bladder and urethra.

had either detrusor instability or sensory urgency. Almost one third of patients in their study that had GSI had a negative Q-Tip test. Overall, the Q-Tip test is not diagnostic of GSI, nor is it an accurate measure of urethral mobility.

The elevation of the proximal portion of the urethra by placing fingers or instruments in the vagina (Bonney or Marshall test) is no longer used as a test to demonstrate the presumed effectiveness of surgery by elevating the urethrovesical angle. Bhatia and Bergman have demonstrated by urodynamic testing that elevation of the urethra by fingers or instruments causes urethral obstruction.

Neurologic Examination

Neurologic examination can be helpful in the workup, particularly if the history indicates possible neurologic disease. The evaluation includes assessment of T10 to S4 sensation, motor strength, tone, and reflexes. The sacral cord reflex arc (S1 through S4) is tested by a gentle stroking of the clitoris, labia minora, or anal skin. An intact sacral arc is indicated by a reflex contraction of the bulbocavernosus and anal sphincter. Rectal sphincter tone and strength are checked with digital rectal examination. A lack of reflex contraction or reduced rectal sphincter tone should be evaluated by a thorough neurologic examination. However, the clinical usefulness of this test appears to be limited because neurologically normal patients may not always have these reflexes.

URODYNAMIC TESTING PROCEDURE

The following tests are steps that may be taken in sequence for patients with urinary incontinence. Some tests may be eliminated depending on the clinical situation.

Uroflow

The urinary flow rate is measured mainly to screen women for voiding disorders. The patient who has a full bladder is asked to urinate into a container so that the volume may be measured. This gives an estimate of functional bladder capacity. A stopwatch can be used to time the complete voiding process, and the urine flow rate (milliliters per second) is calculated. The normal maximum flow rate is 25 ml per second, and the voiding time is 15 to 20 seconds. Abnormal uroflometry may show prolonged or interrupted flow patterns with reduced flow rate.

Electronic uroflometers are available, and a urinary flow pattern may be obtained. A special commode allows urine to be passed into a container where the amount of urine voided is measured over time and is traced on a single-channel recorder.

Figures 20-3 and 20-4 illustrate a normal uroflow pattern with a smooth curve and an abnormal uroflow pattern, respectively. Abnormal uroflow patterns may indicate a urethral outlet obstruction or a lack of detrusor contraction. Uroflometry has a wide variability in a normal woman, and it varies significantly with the volume voided. An exact diagnosis may not be made on the basis of this test.

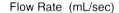
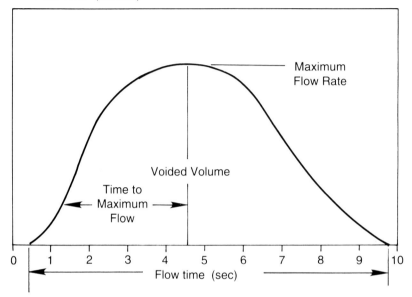

FIGURE 20-3. Diagram of uroflow.

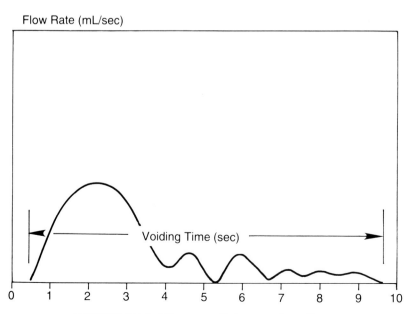

FIGURE 20-4. Diagram of abnormal uroflow.

Residual Urine

Residual urine measurement is indicated in all patients with incontinence to rule out overflow incontinence. It is also useful in patients with cystocele or voiding dysfunction. After micturition, a catheter is inserted into the bladder to measure the residual urine. A normal residual amount is less than 50 ml if the patient voided at least 100 to 150 ml. The residual urine may be sent for urinalysis and culture. A large residual (greater than 200 ml) indicates inadequate bladder emptying from either poor detrusor contraction, a large cystocele, or some other type of obstruction. Residual urine volume can also be accurately determined by ultrasound and avoids the discomfort of catheterization and risk of infection.

Urethrocystometrogram

Cystometry is used to assess bladder sensation, capacity, and compliance and identifies normal from overactive detrusor activity. The patient is placed in the dorsal lithotomy position, and the bladder is filled with room-temperature sterile water or saline solution through a Foley catheter. The volume of the patient's first sensation (first urge to void), normal desire to void (volume that the patient would usually go to the bathroom), and the bladder capacity (uncomfortable with a strong urge to void) are recorded. The normal range for the first sensation, normal desire to void, and bladder capacity are 100 to 150 cc, 200 to 350 cc, and 350 to 600 cc, respectively. Patients with denervation of the bladder do not have any filling sensation and have a large bladder capacity.

During the bladder fill, the bladder pressure may be measured in several different ways. The simplest office cystometry test is a single-channel system. A 50-cc syringe without the plunger is connected to the catheter and held above the level of the bladder. The sterile infusion media is added in 50-ml increments. The water level is closely monitored during filling. Any rise in the water column may indicate an uninhibited detrusor contraction. However, any increases in intraabdominal pressure or movement may cause the water level to rise and introduce artifacts.

Another way to perform office cystometry uses a double-lumen catheter. The bladder is filled through one port, and a bladder pressure measurement is accomplished through the other port with either a water column manometer or an electronic pressure transducer. The bladder pressure (cm H_2O) is a reflection of intraluminal pressure (P1) and intraabdominal pressure (P2). Thus it is necessary to subtract intraabdominal pressure from the measured bladder pressure to give the true bladder pressure (P3). The intraabdominal pressure may be measured indirectly by placing a pressure transducer inside either the rectum or the vagina. With a three-channel electronic recorder, P1 and P2 are recorded with an electronically subtracted P3. This allows more accurate measurements of bladder pressure because it avoids the artifacts mentioned previously.

TABLE 20-2. Indications for multichannel urodynamic studies for incontinence

Diagnosis is uncertain after basic evaluation
Voiding dysfunction is suspected
Prior incontinence surgery failed
High postvoid residual urine is found
Neurologic impairment
Leakage without warning or continuous incontinence
Prior gynecologic cancer treated with radiation
Prior radical pelvic surgery
Failed medical treatment for frequency and urge incontinence

Patients with normal bladder compliance have bladder pressures from 0 to 10 cm H_2O. Patients with poor compliance from either an unstable bladder or a contracted bladder have readings greater than 15 cm H_2O.

With a full bladder a cough stress test can be performed. The test is positive if water escapes from the urethral meatus. Occasionally, a patient with a history of GSI will not lose urine in an artificial office setting.

Specialized testing using multichannel urodynamics may be useful for patients with the indications listed in Table 20-2.

The urethral pressure profile gives a pressure reading throughout the urethra's length. Continence depends on the urethral pressure remaining above the bladder pressure; therefore it seems logical to quantify this difference. This test is accomplished with either a double-lumen catheter or a dual-sensor microtip transducer catheter. One lumen or sensor measures the bladder pressure, and the other (6-cm separation between the lumen or sensors) measures the urethral pressure. The urethral transducer is withdrawn from the bladder to the external urethral meatus, giving the urethral profile. Best results may be obtained by a mechanical puller at a speed of 0.5 to 1 mm per second. The bladder pressure, urethral pressure, and electronically subtracted urethral closure pressure are recorded. The maximum urethral closure pressure (MUCP) is determined by subtracting the bladder pressure (distal sensor) from the urethral pressure (proximal sensor). The profile also gives the functional urethral length and maximum urethral pressure.

The urethral closure pressure profile is the intraluminal pressure along the length of the urethra with the bladder at rest (Fig. 20-5). Normal urethral closing pressure is greater than 70 cm H_2O. Urinary incontinence may be found in women with low urethral pressure. Maximum urethral closure pressure has mainly been used to identify women with low urethral pressures (less than 20 cm H_2O), who may be at increased risk of surgical failure with standard incontinence procedures.

The effect of coughing on the urethral closure pressure may be obtained by having the patient cough while the urethral pressure is being measured.

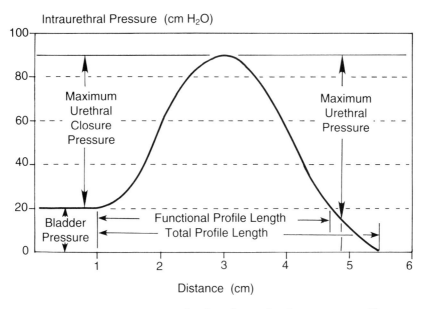

FIGURE 20-5. Diagram of a female urethral pressure profile.

A positive coughing test occurs when the urethral closure pressure is zero throughout the length of the urethra. A negative coughing test occurs when the closing urethral pressure is above zero throughout the length of the urethra. A pressure transmission ratio can be calculated, allowing quantification of the differences in urethral and bladder pressures with stress. The clinical usefulness of these profiles remains controversial because of the overlap between normal continent women and incontinent women.

Urethrocystoscopy

Endoscopy is frequently used to evaluate complaints related to the lower urinary tract. Endoscopy is easily performed in the office under local anesthetic such as 2% Xylocaine jelly. The entire length of the urethra may be visualized with a zero-degree Robertson urethroscope using a carbon dioxide (CO_2) gas medium. As proposed by Robertson, a single-channel gas cystometer with an electronic recorder can be used in many small offices to perform urethrocystometry. Normal values for CO_2 cystometry are about two thirds that of water.

With the gas flowing between 60 and 200 ml per minute, the urethroscope is advanced from the distal portion of the urethra to the bladder neck. The urethra is observed for infection (hyperemia with purulent discharge), condylomas, atrophy, and the presence of diverticula. Fibrosis with poor urethral mucosal coaptation, known as a drainpipe urethra, may indicate a more severe form of stress incontinence requiring additional evaluation.

DAY 1

Time	Fluid Intake (oz.)	Amount Voided (cc)	Activity or Symptoms	Leakage volume

DAY 2

Time	Fluid Intake (oz.)	Amount Voided (cc)	Activity or Symptoms	Leakage volume

FIGURE 20-6. Urinary diary.

With the urethroscope positioned at the proximal portion of the urethra (0.5 to 1 cm from the bladder neck), the urethrovesical junction may be seen to close with bladder filling. With the bladder filled with gas, the closed bladder neck can be evaluated by having the patient cough. If the patient has GSI, the proximal part of the urethra may be seen to open (funnel) during maximal coughing. The usefulness of this finding has been questioned because Versi and Cardozo found an open bladder neck in 50% of asymptomatic postmenopausal women on urodynamic testing with fluoroscopy. The urethra may also be seen to have rotational descent. Patients with bladder instability may have a bladder neck that does not close or one that alternatively opens and closes.

The entire bladder mucosa and trigone are evaluated by using a 60- or 70-degree urethroscope or cystoscope. Bladder tumor, stones, foreign objects such as suture material, inflammation, and infection may be visualized. Many physicians now use sterile water or saline for cystoscopy, and the role of gas urethrocystometry is limited.

Urolog

A diary of urinary habits monitors the amount and type of fluid intake, urine output volumes and time of void, number of incontinence episodes, and activity or symptoms when incontinent. This can be helpful in evaluating the patient's complaints of frequency, urgency, incontinence, and the severity of the problem. Lentz and Stanton showed a 3-day urinary diary to be as accurate as a weeklong diary for assessing women with frequency and urgency. An example of a urinary diary form is shown in Fig. 20-6.

GENUINE STRESS INCONTINENCE

Genuine stress incontinence, as defined by the International Continence Society, is the involuntary loss of urine that occurs when, in the absence of a detrusor contraction, the intravesical pressure exceeds the maximum urethral pressure. The definition implies that some form of cystometry has been performed to make this diagnosis.

History

In the medical history, a description of the patient's chief complaint and degree of disability is important. The patient with GSI complains of a leakage of urine whenever she coughs, sneezes, runs, or jumps. The amount of leakage may vary, but it usually consists of a small amount during a sudden increase in intraabdominal pressure. The increase in intraabdominal pressure during a cough is transmitted to the bladder, and during the short time that intravesical pressure exceeds MUCP, a small volume of urine is lost. However, large-volume leakage can occur, particularly in women with prior incontinence repairs or with intrinsic sphincter deficiency (ISD). This is one subtype of GSI and tends to be a more severe form of incontinence. It is seen less commonly than GSI from poor urethral support. It tends to occur after prior incontinence surgeries, trauma, or radiation. Leakage may occur secondary to gravity alone. Generally, the urethral support is excellent, and the problem is that the urethra no longer has any sphincteric function.

It is important to distinguish the loss of urine as a result of an uninhibited bladder contraction, which may often be misdiagnosed as GSI. In one study patients with a sole complaint of urinary stress incontinence had a 35% incidence of detrusor instability when studied with urodynamic tests.

Interpretation of Bladder Tests

Patients with GSI usually have normal neurologic findings. The resting urethral angle (Q-Tip) is normal, with a sharp rotational posterior descent that exceeds 30° on Valsalva maneuver. The Q-Tip test by itself does not differentiate GSI from other types of incontinence and as mentioned previously is not highly accurate. However, it can give at least a general sense of the presence of hypermobility and may add to the total clinical picture.

The presence of a cystocele, uterine descent, enterocele, or rectocele is noted by visual and bimanual pelvic examination. It is not uncommon for patients with anterior vaginal wall relaxation to have an enterocele, rectocele, or uterine prolapse. However, the presence of a cystocele does not indicate that the patient has GSI. Many patients with only cystoceles are continent, in contrast to patients with urethrocystoceles, who are often incontinent. Continence in patients with large cystoceles may be due to kinking and obstruction of the bladder neck during increased intraabdominal pressure. Surgical correction of the cystocele without correction of the urethrovesical angle may unmask GSI.

A patient with GSI may have a normal residual urine. If there is a large cystocele or a neurogenic bladder, the residual urine may be greater than 100 ml.

The bladder pressure and bladder capacity are generally normal in patients with only GSI. The patient may have a positive cough stress test either supine or standing. It is possible that under stress in the examination or laboratory setting the patient may be unable to demonstrate leakage.

Patients with GSI often have low urethral closure pressure (60 cm H_2O), but as mentioned there is considerable overlap with normal continent women. Extremely low urethral pressure (20 cm H_2O) has been associated with high failure rate after urethropexy. Previous studies have indicated that funneling of the proximal portion of the urethra with cough is an important finding in GSI. Funneling or spontaneous opening of the proximal aspect of the urethra while coughing may be visualized by urethroscope, vaginal ultrasound, or bead-chain urethrocystography. Funneling is the condition in which the posterior urethrovesical (PUV) angle opens greater than 120° with stress. Normal women have a PUV angle of 90° to 100° at all times, even under stress. Studies have shown that PUV angle measurements are not sensitive enough to diagnose GSI. Probably the bladder neck position and mobility are more important than the PUV angle in GSI diagnosis.

The urogynecologic examination may also include visualization of the urethra and bladder to determine concomitant diseases such as urethritis or cystitis. Patients with pure GSI have normal cystoscopic findings. Patients with intrinsic sphincter deficiency may have a patulous, poorly coapting urethra.

The most reliable method of diagnosing GSI is some form of urodynamic testing, and in the office this is easily accomplished with simple cystometry. Involuntary leakage in the absence of an involuntary detrusor contraction diagnoses GSI. In conjunction with a suggestive history and physical examination, this is sufficient information to begin a nonsurgical treatment program. A treatment program can be started without performing cystometry, but at least a urinalysis and postvoid residual urine should be done.

Nonsurgical Treatment for Genuine Stress Incontinence

Nonsurgical therapy for GSI has been given greater emphasis recently since the Agency for Health Care Policy and Research published its urinary incontinence guidelines in 1993. Treatment techniques range from simple measures such as fluid management and prompted voiding to behavioral strategies. These therapies have virtually no side effects, but they do require patient motivation and support and encouragement from the health care provider.

Pelvic floor muscle strengthening exercises are the major technique in the nonsurgical management of GSI. As described by Kegel, isometric exercise of the pubococcygeal muscles is of benefit. The patient is taught to contract the pelvic muscles that stop her from voiding. She is asked to contract these muscles for a count of 10 several times throughout the day. Kegel suggested that the exercise be done for 20 minutes three times a day. The amount of exercise necessary for an effective treatment is unknown. The different regimens in the medical literature include 12 minutes daily, five times every hour, 50 exercises daily, 100 contractions daily, and up to 300 contractions daily. Patients who benefit from exercises must continue them throughout life.

A common error in the exercise is tightening of the gluteal muscle instead of the inner pelvic floor muscles. Verbal directions are not sufficient instruction for learning pelvic floor muscle exercises. Probably the simplest way to ensure proper exercise technique is to perform a vaginal digital exam while the patient attempts to contract the pelvic floor muscles. More sophisticated intravaginal instruments such as balloons attached to a manometer or electronic devices have been used to teach patients to contract the right muscles. This is useful for patients who have difficulty localizing the levator ani muscles.

Drug therapy can be beneficial in the conservative treatment of incontinence. Postmenopausal women in the absence of estrogen frequently demonstrate lower maximum urethral closure pressure. The lower urethral pressure is believed to result from the lack of intrinsic muscular and vascular tone. Estrogen receptors have been demonstrated in the lower urinary tract, so estrogen replacement therapy has theoretically been thought to improve urethral function. However, studies found no direct estrogen effect on urethral function. To date there is no study confirming a beneficial response in stress incontinent women from estrogen, but most believe it is clinically useful and in some indirect way aids urethral pressure.

Estrogen replacement is also recommended when there is vaginal or urethral atrophy. The starting dosage of conjugated estrogen is 0.625 mg orally once a day. Progesterone may be prescribed for the last 10 to 14 days of the cycle or continuously in a lower dosage. Vaginal estrogen cream may also be of benefit even if the patient is on oral estrogen replacement.

Other medications for GSI treatment include the use of α-adrenergic stimulants such as phenylpropanolamine and ephedrine (Table 20-3). Phenylpropanolamine is an ingredient of over-the-counter diet pills and allergy pills. Imipramine, a tricyclic antidepressant, also has an α-adrenergic and detrusor-inhibiting effect.

Surgical Treatment

The surgical approach for urinary incontinence is to elevate the bladder neck back to its original anatomic location. There are many surgical procedures to accomplish this. One approach is the transvaginal approach as first described by Kelly and later modified by Kennedy. The paraurethral tissue is brought below the urethra so that the urethra is buttressed into a higher position. A cystocele may be corrected at the same time with this method.

Other surgical techniques are accomplished from the abdominal incision. The space of Retzius is opened, and sutures placed lateral to the urethra may be suspended from a number of anatomic sites. The periosteum of the pubic symphysis (Marshall-Marchetti-Krantz), central fibrocartilage of the pubic symphysis (Lee-Symmonds), Cooper's ligament (Burch), and the iliopectineal line (Richardson) are some of the sites used. Needle suspension operations are done primarily from a vaginal approach, and the sutures are suspended from the anterior abdominal fascia (Pereyra, Stamey). The different modifications include the use of either absorbable or permanent

TABLE 20-3. Drugs for genuine stress incontinence by increasing urethral resistance

Drugs	Dosage
α-Adrenergic drugs	
Ephedrine sulfate	50-100 mg PO* q12h
Phenylephrine	20 mg PO q12h
Phenylpropanolamine	25 mg PO q6h
Estrogen	
Conjugated estrogens	0.625 to 1.25 mg PO daily
Estradiol	2 mg PO daily
Imipramine	10-75 mg PO q12h

PO, Per os (orally).

sutures, and the number of sutures ranges from one to five sutures on each side of the urethra and bladder. All techniques described provide an 85% to 95% success rate at 1 to 2 years. Bergman and Elia published the only randomized surgical trial for the treatment of GSI. They allocated women to anterior colporrhaphy, Pereyra operation, or Burch colposuspension. At 5 years, the success rates were 37%, 43%, and 82%, respectively. This has brought into question the possible poor long-term success rates with anterior colporrhaphy and needle suspensions for GSI. The surgical technique of each procedure is beyond the scope of this chapter.

When these operations fail, it is important to determine if hypermobility is still present or if intrinsic sphincter deficiency is the cause of incontinence. If hypermobility exists in the absence of ISD, one of the suspension operations can be performed again or a urethral sling procedure done. If ISD is present, periurethral injection therapy is effective treatment. Previously polytetrafluoroethylene paste was used. Now, a biodegradable, bovine collagen substance has been approved by the Food and Drug Administration and can be injected in the office endoscopically. Success rates of 80% to 90% have been reported, although more than one injection session is often needed. Hypersensitivity to the bovine collagen occurs 2% to 3% of the time, so skin testing is required. A urethral sling or artificial sphincter operation can also be successful treatments for ISD.

TABLE 20-4. Outcomes of stress incontinence treatments*

	Treatment options				
	Behavioral technique			Surgical technique	
Outcome	Pelvic muscle exercise	Bladder training	Pharmacologic: alpha agonist	Retropubic suspension	Needle suspension
Percent cured	12	16	0-14	78	84
Percent improved	75	54	19-60	5	4
Total percent	87	70	19-74	83	88
Percent side effects	None		Minimal to 20	Unknown	
Percent complications	None		5-33	20	

From the Urinary Incontinence Guideline Panel: *Urinary incontinence in adults: clinical practice guideline,* AHCPR Pub No 92-0038, Rockville, Md, Agency for Health Care Policy and Research Public Health Service, and the US Dept of Health and Human Services, March, 1992.
*The figures used represent the average reported outcome within a given management option (e.g., behavioral, pharmacologic, or surgical) based on the literature review. The figures do not apply equally across specific treatments within a given management option (e.g., pelvic muscle exercise vs. oxybutynin vs. retropubic suspension) because the studies lack uniformity in many critical issues, including outcome criteria, types of subjects used, treatment protocol, follow-up period, and analytical method. The reader is referred to the guideline text for details.

A summary of GSI treatment results for nonsurgical and surgical therapy is presented in Table 20-4. This is taken from the Agency for Health Care Policy and Research (AHCPR) Urinary Incontinence Guidelines.

DETRUSOR INSTABILITY

As defined by the International Continence Society, *detrusor instability* is uninhibited detrusor contractions that occur spontaneously or on provocation, during the filling phase while the patient is attempting to inhibit micturition. The unstable detrusor may be asymptomatic, and its presence does not necessarily imply a neurologic disorder. Approximately 10% of patients with detrusor overactivity have a neurologic etiology (termed *detrusor hyperreflexia*), and 90% have an unknown etiology. The term *detrusor dyssynergia* is no longer used to avoid confusion with the International Continence Society voiding disorder termed *detrusor-sphincter dyssynergia*.

Detrusor instability may be associated with symptoms of urge incontinence, a condition in which involuntary loss of urine is associated with a strong desire to void (urgency). There are two types of urgency. Motor urgency is caused by an overactive detrusor, and sensory urgency is caused by increased sensation to void without any bladder contractions. Incontinence occurs commonly with motor urgency and less commonly with sensory urgency.

History

The patient is noted to have urge incontinence whenever there is an urge to void and there is an inability to inhibit the leakage long enough to reach the toilet. The urine loss is of moderate volume, with the patient losing most of the urine contained within the bladder at that time. Patients who complain of chronic "cystitis" without microbiologic evidence may have urge incontinence. Cantor and Bates found three symptoms to be most often correlated with urodynamic diagnosis of detrusor instability: nocturia, urge incontinence, and nocturnal enuresis.

Interpretation of Bladder Tests

Neurologic findings and the clitoral/anal reflex are normal with pure detrusor instability. The Q-Tip test is usually normal, and cystoceles or urethroceles are usually absent. Residual urine is normal (100 ml).

Supine and standing cystometrogram demonstrates spontaneous bladder contractions that cannot be inhibited. Detrusor-activating procedures such as coughing, heel bouncing, and hand washing are used to improve diagnostic sensitivity. The first sensation to void is at less than 100 cc, and the bladder capacity is small (200 cc). The MUCP is normal. The patient is unable to stop voiding once micturition has started.

With detrusor instability, it is important to look for infection or inflammation of the urethra or bladder. Urinalysis and culture are important. Outflow obstruction should be eliminated as a cause of the detrusor contractions. Also, detrusor instability can occur with severe genitourinary prolapse. One study found that 41% of women had uninhibited detrusor contractions on urodynamic testing when severe prolapse was present.

The bladder neck may be seen cystoscopically to "wink" or to open and close frequently during bladder filling with detrusor instability. The bladder neck may be seen to open shortly after a cough (but not immediately, as seen with GSI).

Again, the best method to reliably diagnose detrusor instability is urodynamic testing. However, a treatment trial can be started based on thorough history, physical examination, urinalysis, and postvoid residual urine.

Nonsurgical Treatment of Detrusor Instability

Nonsurgical therapy for patients with detrusor instability includes behavioral therapy and drug therapy. Patients who have detrusor instability with either motor or sensory incontinence are treated similarly (Table 20-5).

Behavioral therapy is best accomplished with bladder retraining. This is a program of progressively increasing the voiding interval to every 2 to 3 hours. The patient must suppress the urge to void, delay voiding, and urinate on a rigid time schedule. Strategies to resist the urge to void include sitting down if standing, crossing the legs, and performing a pelvic floor muscle

TABLE 20-5. Drugs for detrusor instability

Drugs	Dosage
ANTICHOLINERGICS	
Propantheline	15-30 mg PO* q4-6h
Methantheline bromide	50-100 mg PO q12-24h
ANTISPASMODICS	
Dicyclomine HCl	10-30 mg PO q6-12h
Oxybutynin chloride	2.5-10 mg PO q6h
Flavoxate HCl	100-400 mg PO q6-12h
Diazepam	5 mg PO q8h
TRICYCLIC ANTIDEPRESSANTS	
Imipramine HCl	25-75 mg PO q8-24h
SYMPATHOMIMETICS	
Terbutaline	2.5-5 mg PO q4h
CALCIUM CHANNEL BLOCKERS	
Nifedipine	10-20 mg PO q12-24h

*PO, Per os (orally).

contraction. She should resist the temptation to rush to the toilet and instead attempt to suppress the detrusor contraction. The ability to inhibit urination is under cortical (voluntary) control, and the bladder retraining program works to regain that voluntary control. Improvement rates of 74% have been reported by Millard. Less frequently used behavioral treatments include biofeedback, hypnosis, and psychotherapy.

Drug therapy includes anticholinergic and antispasmodic medications, tricyclic antidepressants, calcium channel blockers, and estrogen. Uninhibited detrusor contractions (motor incontinence) may be treated by anticholinergic agents, which increase bladder capacity by delaying and reducing the amplitude of involuntary contractions. Propantheline is one example and is a competitive inhibitor of acetylcholine at the postganglionic site. It is used in doses of 15 to 30 mg four times per day, and most anticholinergics are titrated up to a dosage of optimal benefit or when side effects become a problem. Side effects include dry mouth, constipation, dry eyes, blurred vision, tachycardia, urinary hesitancy or retention, confusion, and glaucoma. Anticholinergics are contraindicated in patients with narrow-angle glaucoma and should be used cautiously in women with cardiac arrhythmias.

Antispasmodic drugs have a relaxant effect on smooth muscle and most have anticholinergic effects. Oxybutynin (5 mg every 8 to 12 hours) is effective. Flavoxate is often used, but one study showed it to be no more effective than placebo. The side effects are similar to the anticholinergic medications.

Tricyclic antidepressants such as imipramine have efficacy with urge incontinence. These drugs have an unclear mechanism of action but seem to have anticholinergic and antispasmodic properties. They also have some α-adrenergic effect on the bladder outlet and urethra. Because of the sedative effect of imipramine, it is best used at night and for those patients who have frequent nocturia. The starting dose is much lower than that used for depression (10 to 50 mg once or twice per day) and can be titrated up as needed. Orthostatic hypotension, sedation, and the usual anticholinergic side effects can be problematic.

Calcium channel blockers have a depressant effect on the bladder muscle and anticholinergic properties. Their use in bladder problems has not been well studied but has been shown to cause urinary retention. Unfortunately, no bladder-specific calcium channel blockers are available in the United States. Terodiline hydrochloride was previously marketed in Europe and studied in the United States but was taken off the market because it induced serious cardiac arrhythmias.

The α-adrenergic agonists are useful in producing smooth muscle contraction at the bladder outlet and urethra. Phenylpropanolamine (75 mg twice daily) has been shown to be clinically useful by urodynamic studies. Its major side effects are dry mouth, anxiety, tachycardia, and hypertension. Ephedrine sulfate may also be used in doses of 25 to 50 mg four times daily.

Estrogen replacement in menopausal women has been shown to be effective in improving chronic irritative lower urinary tract symptoms. Estrogens stimulate the maturation of the urethral epithelium and increase blood flow through the urethra and the periurethral tissue. Nonetheless, studies have not shown improved detrusor function on objective testing, possibly because estrogen receptors are found much less frequently in the bladder and trigone than in the urethra. Estrogen may be helpful in women with frequency, urgency, and nocturia, but it does not appear to have a direct role in detrusor instability therapy. Studies have found that women with detrusor instability had less urine loss when on estrogen, although the result was not statistically significant.

Numerous studies have shown that electric stimulation delivered intravaginally or transrectally inhibits detrusor contraction. These battery-operated devices produce low frequency at moderate to high amperages and are of benefit to approximately 30% to 60% of patients with detrusor instability. Further research is needed to define electric stimulation's role for treating detrusor instability and the optimal stimulation protocol. Its use may be limited by patient acceptance because it can cause pain and discomfort.

Sensory urge incontinence may be caused by inflammation or infection producing an increased afferent sensation. The sensation leads to urinary loss in the absence of uninhibited bladder contractions. It is important that all patients with urge incontinence have a urinalysis and culture. The most common organism associated with acute uncomplicated cystitis is *Escherichia coli,* which accounts for approximately 80% of all acute infections. *Staphylococcus saprophyticus* accounts for 10% to 15%, and all other pathogens *(Klebsiella, Proteus)* are seen only 5% to 10% of the time. The pathogens are much different in complicated cases of cystitis (structural or functional urinary tract disorders or indwelling catheters). *Escherichia coli* accounts for only one third of these infections, with *Proteus, Klebsiella, Enterobacter, Streptococcus, Staphylococcus,* and *Pseudomonas* playing a much larger role. With the exception of urethritis, clinical infection is present when the bacteria colony count is greater than 100,000 organisms per ml. Appropriate treatment includes such agents as nitrofurantoin, trimethoprim/sulfamethoxazole, cephalexin, or a quinolone.

Patients with sensory urge incontinence may be treated with flavoxate or phenazopyridine hydrochloride. Oxybutynin is an effective antispasmodic with a mild anticholinergic effect.

Surgical Treatment

Urethral suspensions or plications are ineffective for urge incontinence. Denervations of the bladder may offer improvement, but further studies to prove their efficacy are necessary. Only patients with intractable symptoms should be considered for bladder augmentation cystoplasty or urinary diversion. Those are generally reserved for patients with neurologic disorders and detrusor hyperreflexia.

DETRUSOR HYPERREFLEXIA

Detrusor hyperreflexia is detrusor overactivity resulting from a relevant neurologic disorder. This term replaces undefined terms such as hypertonic, systolic, uninhibited, spastic, and automatic. This disorder is produced by a suprasacral lesion. It can be treated with the same therapy as indicated for detrusor instability, although care to watch for urinary retention is important.

MIXED INCONTINENCE

Approximately 15% to 35% of women with urinary incontinence have both detrusor instability and GSI. Treatment for these patients is more difficult. If standard surgery is performed for the mixed incontinence, the patient may persist with frequency, urgency, and urge incontinence, thereby producing an unfavorable surgical outcome. Behavioral and drug treatment for the bladder instability should be tried first. Imipramine is particularly useful in treating these conditions because of the combination of direct musculotropic relaxant effects and α-adrenergic agonist effectors. This leads to decreased detrusor activity and increased intraurethral pressure. If the bladder instability is adequately treated, conventional surgery may be performed for persistent GSI.

DETRUSOR AREFLEXIA

Detrusor areflexia, as defined by the International Continence Society, is caused by a lesion in the conus medullaris or by sacral nerve outflow. There is a complete absence of centrally coordinated bladder contraction. This term replaces words such as atonic, hypotonic, flaccid, and autonomic. This condition may be seen in patients after radical hysterectomies for cervical cancer. The treatment for this condition is

TABLE 20-6.   Drugs for treating detrusor areflexia

CHOLINERGIC AGONISTS	
Bethanechol	25-50 mg PO* tid
Carbachol	1-4 mg PO tid
ANTICHOLINESTERASE	
Distigmine bromide	2 mg PO daily

*PO, Per os (orally).

timed voiding by Valsalva maneuver, self-catheterization, or drug therapy (Table 20-6).

OVERFLOW INCONTINENCE

The International Continence Society defines *overflow incontinence* as the involuntary loss of urine associated with overdistention of the bladder. The patient urinates frequently in small amounts and has a sensation of continual bladder fullness but is unable to empty the bladder completely. Catheterization of the bladder is often productive of a large amount of urine in the range of 1000 to 1500 ml.

This condition may be caused by lesions in the central nervous system, multiple sclerosis, or diabetic neuropathy. It is treated by intermittent catheterization or continuous catheter bladder drainage. Pharmacologic therapy has not proved to be of benefit in treating this condition.

Overflow incontinence is more frequently found as a temporary condition associated with bladder trauma secondary to vaginal births or after radical pelvic surgery. The treatment is bladder drainage until the bladder is healed. Bladder drainage may be necessary in such cases for as short a time as 24 to 48 hours after vaginal delivery or for as long as 2 to 6 weeks after radical surgery.

VESICOVAGINAL FISTULA

Fistulas are a rare cause of incontinence in the United States. A fistula may occur after pelvic surgery, such as a simple or radical abdominal hysterectomy, cesarean section, or urethral diverticulum surgery, or after pelvic radiotherapy. Fistulas are a common problem in third-world countries because of complications of obstructed labor and delivery.

Patients with urinary fistulas have a true incontinence. Fistula sites include vesicovaginal (most common), urethrovaginal, and ureterovaginal fistulas. They may lose urine at all times. Frequently, the diagnosis may be made by observing urine drain from the vaginal cuff or from the base of the bladder. Instillation of methylene blue or indigo carmine dye into the bladder may allow the defect to be easily seen. If it is not visualized, a tampon can be placed in the vagina and inspected 30 minutes later for the presence of blue dye. Cystoscopy and intravenous pyelogram should be performed preoperatively to clearly identify the site and location in relation to the ureters.

Most fistulas can be repaired by the transvaginal route. The general principles of surgical repair of fistulas consist of either excising the fistula tract or freshing the fistula tract edge and a wide separation of the bladder from the vagina followed by a layered closure. The success rate for continence is 70% to 80%. A myocutaneous flap may be necessary, particularly with large fistulas or in patients with prior irradiation.

URETHRITIS

Patients with infection of the urethra may have various complaints, including frequency, urgency, and burning. They may complain of mild bladder discomfort, a sensation of incomplete emptying, incontinence, and painful intercourse.

Whereas cystitis by definition has a culture of a midstream specimen showing greater than 100,000 colonies per ml, lesser counts may be found with urethritis. In some patients who have been found to have pyuria and no organism, one must evaluate for *Chlamydia*, *Mycoplasma*, and acid-fast bacilli.

Mycoplasma does not grow well in culture, and it may be prudent to treat empirically with either tetracycline or erythromycin for 7 to 10 days.

If symptoms persist after treatment, urethroscopy and cystoscopy should be performed. Recurrent urinary discomfort, postvoid dribbling, and dyspareunia may indicate a urethral diverticulum. Digital massage of the anterior vaginal wall may reveal the presence of a tender mass and pus. A diverticulum may be seen with a urethroscope. The majority of the diverticula are found in the distal third of the urethra. Radiologic studies using a two-balloon catheter with dye may demonstrate a small, difficult-to-find diverticulum.

The treatment for diverticulitis includes antibiotics followed by surgery. If the diverticulum is located in the distal third of the urethra, it may be marsupialized (Spence procedure) or excised. If it is located in the proximal third of the urethra, the diverticulum is resected and the urethra repaired. This is a more difficult operation that may be complicated by urethrovaginal fistulas or strictures in approximately 1% to 4% of cases.

LOWER URINARY TRACT PAIN

Women frequently visit primary care providers with complaints of pain related to the bladder, urethra, or surrounding structures. Once acute cystitis has been ruled out, it is often difficult to evaluate the problem because pain sensations originating in the pelvis are poorly localized and much overlap exists in the multiple pelvic organ systems.

Lower urinary tract hypersensitivity is a generic term now often used to replace nonspecific diagnoses such as urethral syndrome, chronic trigonitis or urethritis, and chronic nonbacterial cystitis. Symptoms of frequency, urgency, and pain during any part of urination are common. The etiology is unknown, but symptoms may be triggered by many dietary factors, reduced fluid intake, prior episode of cystitis, trauma, menstrual cycle changes, or stress. Behavioral treatments can include gradually increasing water intake, working with a bladder retraining program to reduce urinary frequency, and avoiding foods and fluids that may be potential triggers (coffee, tea, carbonated beverages, alcohol, citrus fruits and juices such as cranberry juice, tomatoes, chocolate, and spicy foods). If pelvic floor muscle spasm occurs as a response to pain, learning pelvic floor muscle relaxation techniques may be important. Medications such as the tricyclic antidepressant amitriptyline, antispasmodics such as oxybutynin, phenazopyridine hydrochloride, or nonsteroidal antiinflammatory agents may be helpful.

Interstitial cystitis is a sensory bladder disorder of unknown etiology that causes pronounced urinary frequency, urgency, and pain. Patients may void up to every 15 minutes while awake and also have marked nocturia. The diagnosis is made according to symptoms and bladder studies (urodynamics and cystoscopy). Treatment strategies include behavioral techniques, oral medications, intravesical installations, and if necessary drastic surgical interventions.

When evaluating a patient with lower urinary tract pain, it is prudent to consider many other possible causes. Reproductive tract diseases such as vaginitis, sexually transmitted diseases, vulvar vestibulitis, and endometriosis should be considered. Musculoskeletal abnormalities can often involve the pelvic floor muscles, leading to pain and voiding difficulties. Bowel problems such as irritable bowel syndrome may play a factor. Also, other urinary tract problems previously discussed may be present (acute urethritis or urethral diverticulum).

BIBLIOGRAPHY

Abrams P, Blaivas JG, Stanton SL, et al: Standardization of terminology of lower urinary tract function, *Neurourol Urodyn* 7:403, 1988.

Anderson JT, Walter S, Vejlsgaard R: A clinical and bacteriological trial with dimethyl-sulfoxide (DMSO) in the treatment of severe detrusor hyperreflexia, *Scand J Urol Nephrol* 60:63, 1981.

Appell RA, Macaluso JN, Deutsch JS, et al: Endourologic control of incontinence with GAX collagen: the LSU experience, *J Endourol* 6:275, 1992.

Bates CP, Bradley W, Glen E, et al: First report of the standardization of terminology of lower urinary tract function. Procedures related to the evaluation of urine storage—cystometry, urethral closure pressure profile, units of measurement, *J Urol* 48:39, 1976.

Bates CP, Bradley W, Glen E, et al: The standardization of terminology of lower urinary tract function, *J Urol* 21:551, 1979.

Bates P, Bradley WE, Glen E, et al: Third report on the standardization of terminology of lower urinary tract function. Procedures related to the evaluation of micturition: pressure flow relationships, residual urine, *Br J Urol* 52:348, 1980.

Bates P, Bradley WE, Glen E, et al: Fourth report on the standardization of terminology of lower urinary tract function. Terminology related to neuromuscular dysfunction of lower urinary tract, *Br J Urol* 53:333, 1981.

Bates P, Glen E, Griffiths D, et al: Second report on the standardization of terminology of lower urinary tract function. Procedures related to the evaluation of micturition—flow rate, pressure measurement, symbols, *Br J Urol* 49:207, 1977.

Bates CP, Loose H, Stanton SLR: The objective study of incontinence after repair operations, *Surg Gynecol Obstet* 136:17, 1973.

Bent AE, Sand PK, Ostergard DR, Brubaker LT: Transvaginal electrical stimulation in the treatment of genuine stress incontinence and detrusor instability, *Int Urogynecol J* 4:9, 1993.

Bergman A, Elia G: Three surgical procedures for genuine stress incontinence: five-year follow-up of a prospective randomized study, *Am J Obstet Gynecol* 173:66, 1995.

Bhatia NN, Bergman A: Urodynamic appraisal of the Bonney test in women with stress urinary incontinence, *Obstet Gynecol* 62:696, 1983.

Bhatia NN, Bergman A: Use of preoperative uroflowmetry and simultaneous urethrocystometry for predicting risk of prolonged postoperative bladder drainage, *Urology* 28:440, 1986.

Bowen LW, Sand PK, Ostergard DR, et al: Unsuccessful Burch retropubic urethropexy: a case-controlled urodynamic study, *Am J Obstet Gynecol* 160:452, 1989.

Briggs RS, Castleden CM, Asher MJ: The effect of flavoxate on uninhibited detrusor contractions and urinary incontinence in elderly, *J Urol* 123:665, 1983.

Bump RC, Copeland WE, Hurt WG, et al: Dynamic urethral pressure/profilometry pressure transmission ratio determinations in stress-incontinent and stress-continent subjects, *Am J Obstet Gynecol* 159:749, 1988.

Bump RC, Fantl JA, Hurt WG: Dynamic urethral pressure profilometry pressure transmission ratio determinations after continent surgery: understanding the mechanism of success, failure, and complications, *Obstet Gynecol* 72:870, 1988.

Bump RC, Fantl JA, Hurt WG: The mechanism of urinary continence in women with severe uterovaginal prolapse: results of barrier studies, *Obstet Gynecol* 72:291, 1988.

Burch JC: Cooper's ligament urethrovesical suspension, *Am J Obstet Gynecol* 100:764, 1968.

Burgio K, Whitehead W, Engel B: Urinary incontinence in the elderly, *Ann Intern Med* 104:507, 1985.

Cantor TJ, Bates CP: A comparative study of symptoms and objective urody-namic findings in 214 incontinent women, *Br J Obstet Gynaecol* 87:889, 1980.

Caputo RM, Benson JT: The Q-tip test and urethrovesical junction mobility, *Obstet Gynecol* 82(6):892, 1993.

Cardozo LD: Genuine stress incontinence and detrusor instability—a review of 200 patients, *Br J Obstet Gynaecol* 87:184, 1980.

Corlett RC: Gynecologic urology. I. Urinary incontinence, *Female Patient* 10:20, 1985.

Crystle D, Charme L, Copeland W: Q-Tip test in stress urinary incontinence, *Obstet Gynecol* 38:313, 1971.

DeLancey JO: Correlative study of periurethral anatomy, *Obstet Gynecol* 68:91, 1986.

Dougherty M, Bishop K, Abrams R, et al: The effect of exercise in the circumvaginal muscles in postpartum women, *J Nurse Midwife* 34:8, 1989.

Eaton AC, Birmingham AT, Bates CP: Evidence for the existence of purinergic transmission in the human bladder and a possible new approach to the treatment of detrusor instability. Presented at the fifth annual meeting of the International Continence Society, Lund, Sweden, 1982.

Elkins TE, Drescher C, Martey JO, et al: Vesicovaginal fistula revisited, *Obstet Gynecol* 72:307, 1988.

Fall M: Electrical pelvic floor stimulation for the control of detrusor instability, *Neurourol Urodyn* 4:329, 1985.

Fall M, Erlandson BE, Sundin T, et al: Intravaginal electrical stimulation. Clinical experiments of bladder inhibition, *Scand J Urol Nephrol* 44(suppl):41, 1978.

Fantl JA, Smith PJ, Schneider V, et al: Fluid weight uroflowmetry in women, *Am J Obstet Gynecol* 145:1017, 1983.

Fantl JA, Wyman JF, Anderson RL, et al: Postmenopausal urinary incontinence: comparison between non–estrogen-supplemented and estrogen-supplemented women, *Obstet Gynecol* 71:823, 1988.

Fletcher TF, Bradley WE: Neuroanatomy of the bladder-urethra, *J Urol* 199:153, 1978.

Francis LN, Sand PK, Hamrang K, et al: A urodynamic appraisal of success and failure after retropubic urethropexy, *J Reprod Med* 32:693, 1987.

Gosling JA: The structure of the female lower urinary tract and pelvic floor, *Urol Clin North Am* 12:207, 1985.

Hadley EC: Bladder training and related therapies for urinary incontinence in older people, *JAMA* 256:372, 1986.

Haylen BT, Frazer MI: Measurement of residual urine volumes in women: urethral catheterization or transvaginal ultrasound, *Int Urogynecol J* 5:269, 1994.

Hendrickson L: The frequency of stress incontinence in women before and after the implementation of an exercise program, *Issues Health Care Women* 3:81, 1981.

Hilton P: The urethral pressure profile under stress: a comparison of profiles on coughing and straining, *Neurourol Urodyn* 2:55, 1983.

Hodgkinson CP: Stress urinary incontinence—1970, *Am J Obstet Gynecol* 108:1141, 1970.

Ingelman-Sundberg A: Partial bladder denervation for detrusor dyssynergia, *Clin Obstet Gynecol* 21:797, 1978.

Iosif CS, Batra S, Ek A, et al: Estrogen receptors in the human female lower urinary tract, *Am J Obstet Gynecol* 141:817, 1981.

Jorgensen L, Lose G, Andersen JT: Cystometry: H_2O or CO_2 as filling medium? A literature survey of the influence of the filling medium on the qualitative and the quantitative cystometric parameters, *Neurourol Urodyn* 7:343, 1988.

Kegel A: Progressive resistence exercise in the functional restoration of the perineal muscles, *Am J Obstet Gynecol* 56:238, 1948.

Kinn AC, Lindskog M: Estrogens and phenylpropanolamine in combination for stress urinary incontinence in post-menopausal women, *Urology* 32:273, 1988.

Krantz KE: Anatomy and embryological development of the urethra and bladder. In Slate WG, editor: *Disorders of the female urethra and urinary incontinence*, ed 2, Baltimore, 1982, Williams & Wilkins.

Latzko W: Postoperative vesicovaginal fistulas: genesis and therapy, *Am J Surg* 58:211, 1942.

Lee RB, Park RC: Bladder dysfunction following radical hysterectomy, *Gynecol Oncol* 11:304, 1981.

Lee RA, Symmonds RE, Williams TJ: Current status of genitourinary fistula, *Obstet Gynecol* 72:313, 1988.

Lee RB, Tamimi H: Urinary stress incontinence following radical vulvectomy, *Milit Med* 151:490, 1986.

Lentz GL, Stanton SL: Abstract, *AUGS*, Cambridge, Mass, 1992.

Lentz GL, Wiskind A, Stanton SL: Periurethral contigen *Bard* collagen injection for stress urinary incontinence: preliminary results, *Neurourol Urodyn* 10:451, 1991.

Lose G, Thuneborg P, Jorgensen L, et al: A comparison of spontaneous and intubated urinary flow in female patients. *Neurourol Urodyn* 5:1, 1986.

Marshall VF, Marchetti AA, Krantz KE: The correction of stress incontinence by simple vesicourethral suspension, *Surg Gynecol Obstet* 88:509, 1949.

Mattiason A, Ekstrom B, Andersson KE: Effects of intravesical instillation of verapamil in patients with detrusor hyperactivity, *J Urol* 141:174, 1989.

Meyhoff HH, Gerstenberg TC, Nordling J: Placebo: the drug of choice in female motor urge incontinence? *Br J Urol* 55:34, 1983.

Millard RJ, Oldenburg BF: The symptomatic, urodynamic, and psychodynamic results of bladder re-education programs, *J Urol* 130:715, 1983.

Mohide EA, Pringle DM, Robertson D, et al: Prevalence of urinary incontinence in patients receiving home care services, *Can Med Assoc J* 139:953, 1988.

Montz FJ, Stanton SL: Q-Tip test in female urinary incontinence, *Obstet Gynecol* 67:258, 1986.

Muller SC, Fronneberg D, Schwab R, et al: Selective sacral nerve blockade for the treatment of unstable bladders, *Eur Urol* 12:408, 1986.

Mundy AR: Long term results of bladder transection for urge incontinence, *Br J Urol* 545:642, 1983.

Norton P, MacDonald L, Stanton S: Distress associated with female urinary complaints and delay in seeking treatment, *Neurourol Urodyn* 6:170, 1987.

Ostergard DR: The effects of drugs on the lower urinary tract, *Obstet Gynecol Surv* 34:424, 1979.

Ostergard DR: The neurological control of micturition and integral voiding reflexes, *Obstet Gynecol Surv* 34:417, 1979.

Pereyra AJ, Lebherz TB: Combined urethro-vesical suspension and vagino-urethroplasty for correction of urinary stress incontinence, *Obstet Gynecol* 30:537, 1967.

Peters D: Terodiline in the treatment of urinary frequency and motor urge incontinence. A controlled multicentre trial, *Scand J Urol Nephrol Suppl* 87:21, 1984.

Richardson AC, Edmonds PB, Williams NL: Treatment of stress urinary incontinence due to paravaginal fascial defect, *Obstet Gynecol* 57:35, 1981.

Robertson JR: Ambulatory gynecologic urology, *Clin Obstet Gynecol* 44:72, 1974.

Robertson JR: Gas cystometrogram with urethral pressure profile, *Obstet Gynecol* 44:72, 1974.

Rosenzweig BA, Pushkin S, Blumenfeld D, Ghatia N: Prevalence of abnormal urodynamic test results in continent women with severe genitourinary prolapse, *Obstet Gynecol* 79:539, 1992.

Rud T, Andersson KE, Asmussen M: Factors maintaining the intraurethral pressure in women, *Invest Urol* 17:343, 1980.

Sand PK, Bowen LW, Ostergard DR: Uninhibited urethral relaxation: an unusual cause of incontinence, *Obstet Gynecol* 68:645, 1986.

Sand PK, Bowen LW, Ostergard DR, et al: The effect of retropubic urethropexy on detrusor stability, *Obstet Gynecol* 71:818, 1988.

Sand PK, Bowen LW, Panganiban R, et al: The low pressure urethra as a factor in failed retropubic urethropexy, *Obstet Gynecol* 69:399, 1987.

Sand PK, Brubaker LT, Novak T: Simple standing incremental cystome as a screening method for detrusor instability, *Obstet Gynecol* 77:453, 1991.

Sand PK, Hill RC, Ostergard DR: Supine urethroscopic and standing cystometry as screening methods for the detection of detrusor instability, *Obstet Gynecol* 70:57, 1987.

Sand PK, Hill RC, Ostergard DR: Incontinence history as a predictor of detrusor stability, *Obstet Gynecol* 71:257, 1988.

Sims JM: On the treatment of vesicovaginal fistula, *Am J Med Sci* 23:59, 1852.

Torring T, Pertersen T, Klemar B, et al: Selective sacral rootlet neurectomy in the treatment of strusor hyperreflexia. Technique and long-term results, *J Neurosurg* 68:241, 1988.

Ulmsten U, Andersson EK, Persson CGA: Diagnostic and therapeutic aspects of urge urinary incontinence in women, *Urol Int* 32:88, 1977.

Urinary Incontinence Guideline Panel: *Urinary incontinence in adults: clinical practice guideline*, AHCPR Pub. No. 92-0038, Rockville, Md, 1992, Agency for Health Care Policy and Research, Public Health Service, U.S. Department of Health and Human Services.

Vereecken RL, Das J, Grisar P: Electrical sphincter stimulation in the treatment of detrusor hyperreflexia of paraplegics, *Neurourol Urodyn* 3:145, 1984.

Versi E, Cardozo LD, Studd JW, et al: Internal urinary sphincter in maintenance of female continence, *Brit Med Jour Clin Res Ed* 292:166, 1986.

Walters MD, Shields LE: The diagnostic value of history, physical examination, and the Q-Tip cotton swab test in women with urinary incontinence, *Am J Obstet Gynecol* 159:145, 1988.

Wein AJ: Lower urinary tract function and pharmacologic management of lower urinary tract dysfunction, *Urol Clin North Am* 14:273, 1986.

Wein JA, Hanno PM, Dixon DO, et al: The reproducibility and interpretation of

carbon dioxide cystometry, *J Urol* 120: 205, 1978.

Yarnell JWG, St Leger AS: The prevalence, severity and factors associated with urinary incontinence in a random sample of elderly, *Age Ageing* 8:81, 1979.

Zeegers AGM, Kieswetter H, Kramer AEJL, et al: Conservative therapy of frequency, urgency and urge in continence: a double blind clinical trial of flavoxate hydrochloride, oxybutynin chloride, emepronium bromide and placebo, *World J Urol* 5:57, 1987.

CHAPTER 21

Outpatient Procedures in Gynecology

RICHARD M. SODERSTROM

Although the ability to perform surgical procedures in the office has been available for centuries, by the twentieth century, most minor gynecologic procedures had become hospital-based procedures. Incision and drainage of vulvar abscesses and minor skin biopsies were performed with regularity, but a procedure that invaded the uterus was reserved for the operating room. Near the end of the 1960s the advent of abortion reform introduced dilation and curettage (D & C) to the office setting out of a desire to make this procedure accessible at a low cost. Despite this change and experience, currently only 10% to 20% of gynecologists perform diagnostic or therapeutic D & C procedures in their office. As we move toward a managed health care environment, procedures that can be performed in an office setting will, by demand, find their place because of inherent costs in a hospital setting. This chapter will address those procedures that have been demonstrated as appropriate and safe when performed in the office.

ANESTHESIA

Some office procedures might be performed without anesthesia, but a thorough understanding of the principles of local anesthesia must be in place before attempting any of the following procedures. Once a gynecologist commands the knowledge and experience of outpatient anesthetic techniques, the opportunities to add more procedures become rapidly apparent. In some states, laws govern the use of any local anesthetic, requiring specific backup support should an untoward or idiosyncratic reaction occur. Prepared emergency kits have made it easy to fulfill these basic needs at a fair price (Fig. 21-1).

Complications

The complications that must be anticipated and treated fall into two groups: those caused by the untoward result of the normal pharmacologic actions of the local anesthetic and those resulting from trauma associated with the technique. The former are usually rapid and catastrophic but are readily reversible if immediate and correct therapy is instituted. If rapid diagnosis and treatment are not instituted, irreparable tissue damage may result.

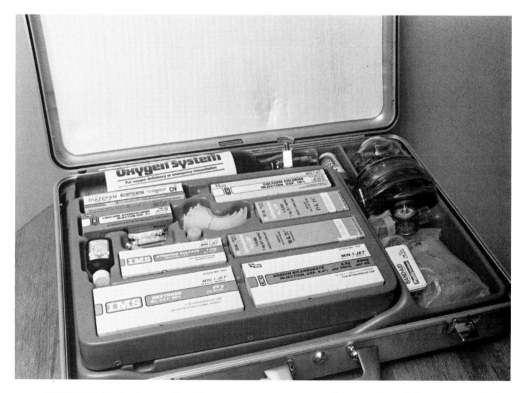

FIGURE 21-1. A cardiopulmonary resuscitation kit produced by Banyan (Abilene, Tex.).

Complications that fall in this group include systemic reactions to high blood levels of the local anesthetic or vasoconstrictor, systemic allergic reactions, and hypotension and hypoxia resulting from sympathetic blockade.

Complications resulting from trauma to the tissues usually produce gradual pathologic changes that do not immediately threaten the patient's life, although they may result in serious sequelae. These slowly developing sequelae should be treated correctly, but time alone will reveal the outcome. This group of complications includes hematomas, local tissue sloughs, neuritis, paresis, dermatitis, broken needles, and local reactions.

The keys to managing any of these untoward results are anticipation and preparedness. Complications will be rare if the physician observes the following prophylactic measures:

1. Carefully clean all reusable syringes with distilled water.
2. Autoclave by steam for 30 minutes at 255°F.
3. Use disposable local infiltration sets.
4. Do not exceed the concentration or toxic dose of the anesthetic.
5. Use as little premedication as possible.

Local Infiltration

There are several local infiltration kits available, consisting of the preparation solution, sterile towels, anesthetic agent, syringe, needles, and receptacles. For most local biopsies, a disposable tuberculin syringe with a 25-, 27-, or 30-gauge needle, an alcohol wipe, and a multidose anesthetic vial will suffice. One should use a sufficient amount of anesthetic, inject it slowly, and wait for it to take effect. An anesthetic (e.g., Nesacaine) may be rapid in its onset, but its duration of action may be short. Another anesthetic (e.g., Buffered Carbocaine) may be as quick in onset but lasts several times longer. Marcaine has the longest duration of action (without a vasoconstrictor additive), but it takes 5 to 10 minutes to set. For large lesions, insert the needle proximal to the nerve root distribution that supplies the area to be biopsied. For mucosal skin, such as vaginal and cervix, the local application of 20% benzocaine in polyethylene glycol is usually sufficient for small biopsies.

Paracervical Block

All gynecologists should become proficient in the administration of a paracervical block. It is useful both for surgical procedures and as a diagnostic tool. Its application for office D & C and hysteroscopy eliminates the need for these in-hospital procedures except in unusual circumstances. Unless the patient is in shock, an incomplete abortion can be quickly evacuated in the office using this local anesthetic technique. In patients with unexplained pelvic pain or dyspareunia, the use of a long-acting paracer-

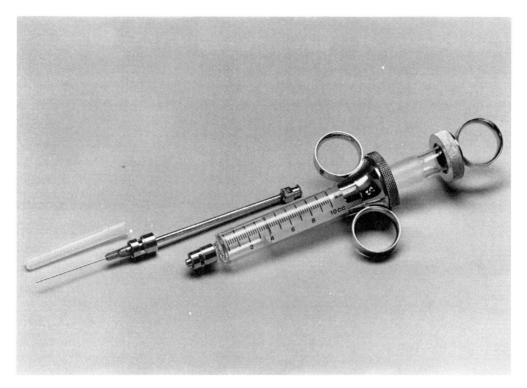

FIGURE 21-2. A reusable, three-ring syringe with a needle extender for paracervical block anesthesia.

vical block can assist the physician in determining whether the uterus or cervix is the site of discomfort. If a hysterectomy without adenectomy is considered for chronic pelvic pain, yet after a successful paracervical block the pain persists, the patient may be at increased risk for continued pain after the proposed hysterectomy.

In addition to the supplies needed for local infiltration anesthesia, a needle extender is frequently helpful because a long spinal needle may become unwieldy (Fig. 21-2). Some prefer a dental needle because of its rigid shaft. Buffered Carbocaine is an ideal agent because of its rapid onset, long duration of action, and low toxicity for the volume of fluid needed.

The application of Hurricaine ointment or gel before needle insertion helps eliminate the insertional pain. Some physicians inject in multiple places around the cervix into the paracervical fornix. Others choose the probable location of the uterosacral nerves and inject in that vicinity, usually described as the four o'clock and eight o'clock positions. A submucosal placement of the anesthetic agent is preferred. Because of the fanlike distribution of the uterosacral nerves, a large volume of anesthetic of low concentration gets better results than a small amount of higher concentration. Injecting 8 to 10 ml of anesthetic on each side of the cervix and waiting

5 to 10 minutes usually gives excellent results. Because the dome of the fundus of the uterus is supplied by the tenth thoracic nerve, that area of the uterus may perceive pain at the end of a D & C or when an instrument touches the fundus.

ENERGY SOURCES

There are two energy sources available for office procedures: the laser and the electrogenerator. Because of the keen interest in lasers for the operating room and office during the past two decades, the manufacturers of electrosurgical equipment have developed an array of instruments and generators that are more suitable for the gynecology office. Each has advantages, the laser being the most expensive. From the beginning, the laser was looked on as an instrument that deserved respect and basic understanding before the surgeon could use it. On the other hand, electrosurgery and its proper use was never taught with such caution; learning was usually left to hands-on experience at the operating table. Because of this new competition between these energy sources, they are now recognized as valuable tools that deserve equal respect and caution for them to be used properly. To use them in the office without a thorough understanding of the applied physics of each is not wise.

Lasers

Because of the cost and maintenance of all lasers used in gynecology, only a large clinic can afford to provide this method of energy to destroy or excise tissue. If one matches the power density (watts per square centimeter) between lasers and electrosurgery over the same amount of time and to the same tissue, the end result is the same. In other words, a watt is a watt. Many times the ease and simplicity of electrosurgery make it the tool of choice when the advantages of lasers are not required. For that reason, new electrosurgery systems that cost only one fifth of the average office-based laser are preferred in the average gynecologist's office.

Laser physics. Lasers produce waves of light energy within the electromagnetic spectrum and ultimately effect their work by producing heat. Laser is an acronym that stands for light amplification by stimulated emission of radiation. Here, radiation does not refer to ionizing-type radiation such as x-ray. It refers to a radiant body, one that emits light. Electricity is converted into light, which can be further intensified to cut, vaporize, or coagulate tissue. Through stimulated emission, atoms and molecules are energized and manipulated to produce this unique type of light.

Radiation heat transfer is important to both electrosurgical and laser modalities. This involves the transfer of thermal energy by electromagnetic waves (light and electricity). In this way, objects do not have to touch to transfer heat. Across a vacuum, heat may even be transmitted by radiation because it does not depend on the presence of matter. This is the essential mechanism of laser and electrosurgical devices. Lasers (any type of light) are of higher frequency than electrosurgical units, but both are forms of electromagnetic radiation. Radiation transfer means that laser beams contain no inherent heat. They transmit only radiant energy. Heat is created only when the tissue absorbs the transmitted radiation and converts it to motion in the tissue's atoms and molecules. This is the way a microwave oven works, only at lower frequencies than lasers. Highly vascular tissues have a high heat capacity and require higher powers to counteract the heat-sink effect of the blood flow.

Regular light sources such as light bulbs release this light energy in a random, chaotic emission of light. This results in incoherent white light with all colors combined, radiating in all directions. Laser light consists of the same photons of light as from ordinary light sources, but it is released in an organized fashion called stimulated emission. The light emitted is one energy (wavelength and color) and travels in one direction through space as a tight beam. The result is a coherent beam of bright light of one column, or at least pure colors. Thus laser light differs from regular light; it is coherent, monochromatic, and collimated.

Collimation allows the light waves to travel together as a tight, parallel beam. This allows the beam to be finely focused to intensify its effects and is the major characteristic allowing its surgical use. The superficial effects of the laser are due to localized heating when the light is absorbed by tissue. As tissue begins to heat, it blanches white as it coagulates, then shrivels as it desiccates, and finally turns to steam and vapor as it is vaporized above 100°C.

Several parameters control the delivery of laser energy to tissue. These include the power (watts, W), total energy delivered (watts and time), the color of the light, and the color and vascularity of the tissue. Power is simply a measure of the rate of energy delivered in joules per second and is expressed in watts. This applies equally to lasers or electrosurgery. Of greater importance is the amount of power that can be focused into a spot. This power density, or irradiance, of a laser is the number of watts per square centimeter of a spot and is the single most important factor in the effective application of a laser. The surface area of the spot size is controlled by the surgeon and the total power in watts set by the operator determines the power density, as follows:

$$\frac{W \times 100 \times .86}{\pi r^2} \text{ (expressed in W/cm}^2)$$

Therefore it is not the power that determines the surgeon's control of the beam's energy, but rather the power density or spot size. The larger the spot, the greater the power required to maintain the same power density. Thus a 0.6 mm spot set at 10 W delivers the same power density as a 2.0 mm spot set at 60 W. The total energy within any laser beam is expressed in joules (J). Power multiplied by delivery time equals the number of joules. One watt applied for 100 seconds equals 100 J, as does 100 W applied for one second.

It is important that the surgeon attend good hands-on training programs and work extensively with lasers in the operating room before attempting to learn to control these parameters in an office setting. When a laser is office based, it is usually a CO_2 laser because it provides a great deal of versatility in the "reach" it provides from the end of the colposcope. Its principal benefit is the precision and control it permits. The tissue effects of the laser occur at the surface, where it can be visually monitored via the colposcope; therefore this laser should not damage tissue beyond the view of the surgeon. Because the CO_2 laser beam is dispersed by water, injecting water under a lesion helps act as a backstop against undesirable deep penetration. A silver ENT mirror (without a glass face) can be used to deflect the beam into recesses too difficult to reach and control with standard electrodes. Each company supplies charts and calculations for its laser as to the proper settings recommended for various procedures.

Electrosurgery

Electrocautery is a term frequently used improperly when physicians mean electrosurgery. Electrocautery uses a direct electric current to heat a metal conductor with a high impedance so that the metal becomes physically hot. Tissue is then cauterized by touching the hot metal object to tissue. In contemporary surgery, few instruments employ the principles of electrocautery. Manipulating electrons through living tissue using an alternating current with enough current concentration (current density) to create heat within a tissue cell to tissue destruction is electrosurgery. Electrogenerators, or electrosurgical units, are machines that produce an alternating current of electricity at a frequency that will not stimulate muscle activity (500,000 to 3 million cycles per second). Whereas direct current flows in one direction only, alternating current flows to and fro, first increasing to a maximum in one direction and then increasing to a maximum in the other direction. This sinusoidal waveform can be interrupted or varied, creating different surgical effects.

The waveform of alternating current has a negative and a positive excursion, or peak. As it passes through each cell, the electrolytic polarity is agitated, creating cellular heat. The measurement from zero polarity to positive or negative polarity is called the peak voltage of the waveform. The measurement from plus peak to negative peak, which is twice peak voltage, is called peak-to-peak voltage. A pure cutting/desiccation (cut) waveform is a simple sinusoidal, undamped (nonmodulated) waveform and is generally produced by continuous energy (Fig. 21-3). An output waveform that is interrupted or varied (modulated or damped) is called a coagulating waveform.

When there is a continuous flow or waveform, the peak voltage need not be as high as with the damped waveform (coag) to create the same wattage. At the same level, however, when a coagulation effect must be enhanced, the damped waveform is preferable by pushing bursts of electrons through the tissue. The cooling effect of the off time between bursts allows for the coagulation effect. With the damped waveform a higher voltage than with an undamped waveform will briefly be present within the electric circuit. Most generators provide a blended current, which does not result from combined cutting and coagulating waveforms as is commonly thought. Instead, the blended waveform interrupts the current at variable intervals, delivering variable degrees of coagulating and cutting properties (Fig. 21-4). The degree to which the blended mode cuts or coagulates depends on the relative time interval that the current flow is on or off. Thus one of the tissue effects of electrosurgery depends on the various modes of delivering electric current.

Monopolar electrosurgery. As electrons, pushed with a given voltage, are concentrated in one specific location, heat within the tissue increases rapidly. This concentration phenomenon is defined as *current density*. The diathermy generator, an example of equipment using this principle, is familiar to most physicians. Here, electrons are passed through the body by applying two large metal conductors or plates on opposite sides of the body part to be heated. The electrons are pushed through the plate termed the *active electrode*. Electrons are received on the other plate, the *return (neutral) electrode*, or ground plate, after they leave the body. Once the

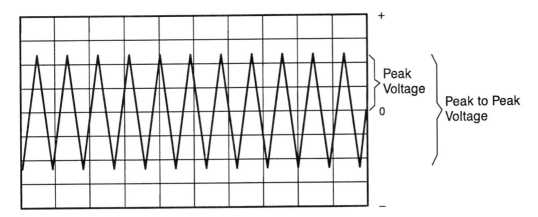

FIGURE 21-3. An undamped, or cut, waveform is a continuous delivery of energy.

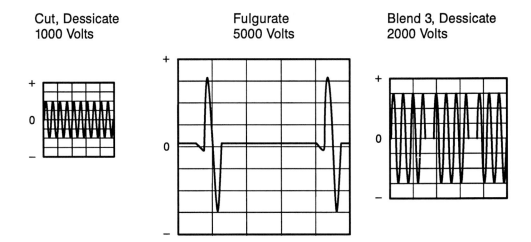

Cut, COAG, and Blend 3 set at 50 WATTS

FIGURE 21-4. As the generator is switched from one waveform to another, the voltage must change to match the designated power output. Note that the voltage increases as one selects a waveform from cut to blend to coag.

electrons enter the body (conductor) they are dispersed through the tissue toward the path of least resistance to the return electrode. Because current is dispersed over the entire surface area of both plates (low current density), the heat generated is of low intensity. If either plate or electrode is greatly reduced in size, however, current density (and thus heat) is increased accordingly (Fig. 21-5). Thus a small active electrode can create a burn (high current density) where the electrons enter the body. The electrons that leave the body through a small return electrode can produce another burn.

Like water, electrons flow through the path of least resistance. If tissue resistance is high but the corresponding voltage pressure is low, the current may cease to flow or may search out alternate pathways with lower resistance. When the voltage is increased, the electrons have more "push" to find an alternate path, which could be through a vital structure where the current might be condensed or where it might seek out an alternate return electrode (e.g., a cardiac monitor electrode). Therefore one should use the lowest voltage necessary to accomplish a given job and be sure that the dispersive electrode is in good contact with the patient and broad enough to reduce current density far below the level of tissue destruction. Isolated ground circuitry systems are desirable, as is a return electrode sentinel system, should an ineffective or incomplete return path be present.

Generators. There are significant differences among electrogenerators available for electrosurgical use. In general, generators that are set by a dial

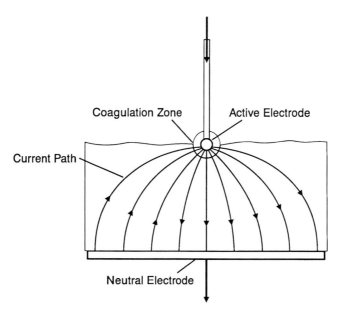

Coagulation Zone   Active Electrode

Current Path

Neutral Electrode

Distribution of current flow in the tissue
during monopolar HF surgical technique

FIGURE 21-5. When one electrode pole is reduced in size, the tissue in contact with
the smaller electrode is heated rapidly because of a higher current (power) density.

Copyright Reproductive Health Specialists, PS, Seattle, Wash.

of numbers are calibrated to the peak voltage output rather than the power
output, as is found in generators that have a digital liquid crystal display
window showing the output in watts. To determine the wattage output with
the "dial-a-number" generators, one must refer to an output graph found in
the manufacturer's manual; some generators have these output curves
printed on the top of the generator box. It should be understood that the
power output set by the company is the power available as one starts the
electrosurgical process but will fall off as the tissue impedance increases
during the heating of cellular fluids. Each generator is calibrated as to its
output measurements against a fixed resistance. For unipolar use, most
generators are calibrated against a 500-Ω load. Each generator has its own
power output characteristics, which are listed in the manual; with
experience, the proper settings can be found.

For general surgical use, most generators can produce a maximum of
8000 V in the coag mode. An 8000-V pressure can push electrons 5 mm
through room air under certain atmospheric conditions, which means that
arcing to distant tissue is improbable; most of the time generators are used
in the 1000- to 3000-V range. The waveform frequency is set above 350,000
cycles per second to prevent muscle stimulation. At frequencies below

100,000 cycles per second, undesirable muscle contraction (known as the faradic effect) can occur. The higher the frequency of a generator, the more leakage of current occurs, which can enhance a capacitance effect, especially worrisome in certain endoscopic procedures.

Most contemporary generators offer an isolated ground circuitry system to reduce the risk of monopolar energy seeking an alternative pathway to ground; older-model generators are known as ground referenced genera-tors. With an isolated, or "floating," ground system the electricity delivered to the patient and returned to the generator is created by an induction of current in transformers that are insulated from the frame of the generator. Should a break in the circuit occur, the electrons will not seek ground and thus no current will flow. This also reduces the risk of an aberrant burn to the surgeon unless he or she is leaning against the patient, thus becoming part of the isolated circuit.

Return electrode safety or sentinel systems are available that employ disposable return electrodes (called ground pads), which are usually two conductive pads side by side. Built-in monitors (called REM for return electrode monitor), through low-impedance feedback to the generators, measure pad-to-skin contact stability and power density contact by measuring the balance of contact between the two pads. If there is an imbalance or poor contact to the patient, an alarm sounds and the generator will not function. If the patient is awake, this system is not necessary because the patient will alert the surgeon of any heat created at the pad site. The return electrode should be orientated such that each pad is equally distant from and in close proximity to the operating site.

The basic principles of safety during electrosurgery are as follows:
- Place electrode pencils and electrodes in the safety holster when not in use.
- Use a monitored return electrode system.
- Select the lowest voltage that will create the desired effect.
- Use the manufacturer's recommended connection cables.
- Inspect instrument insulation before each use.
- Place the ground electrode near the site of surgery, usually the anterior thigh.

Biologic behavior of electrosurgery. Electrosurgery may be used to cut (*vaporize*) and coagulate deeply (*desiccate*) or superficially (*fulgurate*). These terms, frequently misused, stand for specific functions of electrosurgery and should be familiar to the surgeon. As mentioned, at the end of an electrode, the performance depends on the shape and size of the electrode, the frequency and wave modulation, the peak voltage, and the current coupled against output impedance. The tissue may be cut in a smooth, deliberate fashion without arcing, or it can be burned and charred. This great varia-tion of tissue effects is frequently ignored or misunderstood, which is

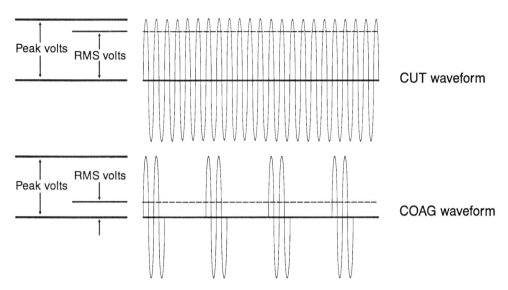

FIGURE 21-6. When the voltage is the same between cut and coag, the amount of power delivered in coag is only about one third that of cut.

why, in the past, some surgeons claimed that the laser provided better control of one's energy needs and promoted better wound healing.

Electrocoagulation may be carried out in many different forms, from slow, delicate contact coagulation (*desiccation*) to the charring effects of the spray coagulation mode (*fulguration*), at times leading to carbonization. The temperature differences may vary from 45°C to over 500°C.

The essential characteristic of cut waveforms is that they are continuous sine waves. That is, if the voltage output of the generator is plotted over time, a pure cut waveform is a continuous sine wave alternating from positive to negative at the operating frequency of the generator, 500 to 3000 kilohertz (kHz). The coag waveform consists of short bursts of radio frequency sine waves. With the sine wave frequency of 500 kHz, the coag bursts occur 31,250 times per second. The important feature of the coag waveform is the pause between each burst. If a coag waveform has the same peak voltage as a cut waveform the average power delivered (heat per second) will be less because the coag is turned off most of the time (Fig. 21-6).

Suppose that the coag waveform had the same average voltage (RMS voltage) as the cut waveform and thus could deliver the same heat per second. Because the coag is turned off most of the time, it can produce the same root mean square (RMS) voltage as the cut only by having large peak voltages and currents during the periods when the generator is on (Fig. 21-7).

A high-voltage coag waveform can spark to tissue without significant cutting effect because the heat is more widely dispersed by the long sparks

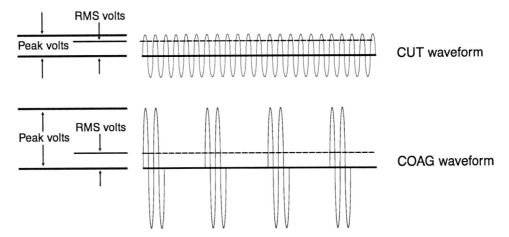

FIGURE 21-7. When the power settings are equal between cut and coag, the peak voltage of coag is about three times higher than cut.

and because the heating effect is intermittent. The temperature of the water in the cells does not get high enough to flash into steam. In this way the cells are dehydrated slowly but are not torn apart to form an incision. Because the high peak voltage is a quality of the coag waveform, it can drive a current through high resistances. In this way it is possible to fulgurate long after the water is driven out of the tissue and actually char it to carbon. *Coagulation* is a general term that includes both desiccation and fulguration.

Fulguration can be contrasted with desiccation in several ways. First, sparking to tissue with fulguration always produces necrosis anywhere the sparks land. This is not surprising when one considers that each cycle of voltage produces a new spark and each spark has an extremely high current density. In desiccation, the current is no more concentrated than the area of contact between the electrode and the tissue (Fig. 21-8). As a result, desiccation may or may not produce necrosis, depending on the current density. For an equal level of current flow, fulguration is always more efficient at producing surface necrosis; however, the depth of tissue injury is superficial compared with contact desiccation because with fulguration the sparks jump from one spot to another in a random fashion and thus the energy is "sprayed" rather than concentrated (Fig. 21-9). In general, fulguration requires only one fifth the average current flow of desiccation.

For example, if a ball electrode is pressed against moist tissue, the electrode will begin in the desiccation mode, regardless of the waveform. The initial tissue resistance is low and the resulting current is high. As the tissue dries out, its resistance rises until the electrical contact is broken.

DESICCATION

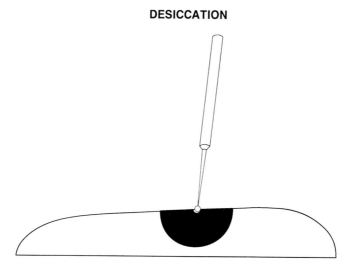

FIGURE 21-8. Desiccation occurs by touching the tissue before keying the generator, which creates deep penetration of heat and minimal charring of the surface tissue.

FULGURATION

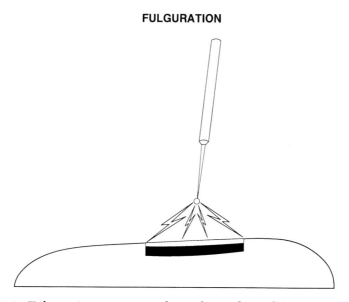

FIGURE 21-9. Fulguration sprays sparks to the surface of tissue, causing a rapid surface char with minimal heating of the deeper layers.

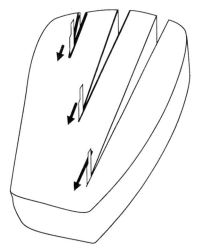

Influence of the speed of incision on the degree of coagulation

FIGURE 21-10. The tissue effect of increasing the speed of passage of a cutting electrode of the same size and at the same depth of cut.

Copyright Reproductive Health Specialists, PS, Seattle, Wash.

Because moist tissue is no longer touching the electrode, sparks jump to the nearest areas of moist tissue in the fulguration mode, as long as the voltage is high enough to make a spark. Eventually, the resistance of desiccated tissue stops the flow of electrons, limiting the depth of coagulation.

Electrosurgical electrodes can be sculptured to perform certain tasks. A microneedle, a knife, a wire loop, or even a scissor can be shaped and sized to a specific duty. When the waveform variables are added, cutters can be made to coagulate and coagulators can be made to cut. The faster an electrode passes over or through tissue, the less the coagulation effect, leading to more cutting. If the power setting and the electrode size remain constant, more desiccation of tissue of the adjacent tissue occurs the slower the electrode is passed through the tissue (Fig. 21-10). The more broad the electrode, the less cutting and more coagulation effect (Fig. 21-11). If one touches each electrode to the tissue before one keys the generator, desiccation occurs, but with more lateral charring in the coag than in the cut mode.

There is a point at which the desiccation effect is limited in depth by the impedance to flow at a fixed power setting. Interwoven into these acts are the output intensity and output impedance characteristics of the different electrosurgical generators. If a constant voltage can be maintained at a given power setting, which is variable as tissue resistance changes, lateral thermal damage is controlled, giving the surgeon a predetermined surgical

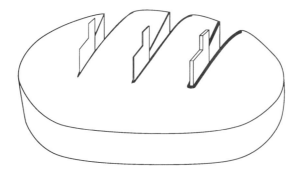

Influence of the shape of the electrode
on the degree of coagulation

FIGURE 21-11. The tissue effect of increasing the size of a cutting electrode if the speed and depth of cut is constant.

Copyright Reproductive Health Specialists, PS, Seattle, Wash.

effect. Using a constant-voltage generator controls the depth of coagulation independent of the cutting rate.

VULVAR PROCEDURES
Bartholin Duct Cysts or Abscesses

The Bartholin's duct abscess is an outpatient emergency that deserves prompt attention and a humane approach. Some might say that the insertion of the anesthetic needle may hurt more than the direct incision, but those words would probably come from a physician without personal experience. Often, after the incision is made, probing and separation of internal loculation demands anesthetic relief.

Because the disease is of the duct and not the gland, the incision should be made inside and behind the hymeneal ring at a convenient point, usually at 5 o'clock or 7 o'clock. Once the purulent material is release and cultured, a drain is usually placed into the dilated duct. In general, the Word catheter is chosen and left in place for several weeks (Fig. 21-12). The balloon should be large enough for retention purposes but not overdistended, otherwise the pain of the original distention may persist. On occasion, the patient may return in a few days with recurrent distention pain, and a small amount of fluid may need to be removed from the catheter bulb with a 25-gauge needle. By leaving this stent in place for several weeks, the epithelium of the duct will migrate out to the mucosa to establish a new, yet patent, foramen. Most would agree that this approach is applicable in 90% of acute and subacute Bartholin duct abscess, leaving removal or marsupialization to the minority of patients.

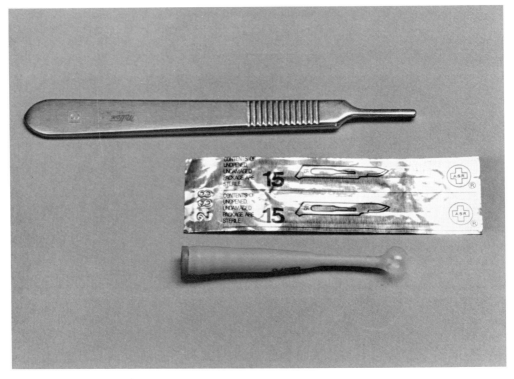

FIGURE 21-12. The Word catheter used to drain Bartholin's duct cysts and abscesses.

Warty Growths

Condyloma acuminatum can be excised or destroyed by chemical application, direct incision, or with a variety of energy sources. Local anesthesia is required for all but the chemical approaches. The recurrence rate is high, and frequent follow-up visits are common.

Of the chemical methods, podophyllin in 20% benzoin solution and trichloroacetic acid are the most popular. Each requires caution in application (apply only to the lesion), and strict instructions must be given to the patient to wash away the medication approximately 2 hours after application.

Lasers have been an effective treatment, especially when the lesions are many, confluent, and in recessed areas such as the rectum. Few clinics in private practice have a laser available, but some groups have shared or rented lasers for such purposes on specific days. Each laser has its own properties that dictate tissue destruction; each type of laser therefore must be understood by the surgeon before it is applied to skin lesions.

Although electrogenerators have been available in abundance since the 1930s, their use in condyloma eradication was not appreciated until the

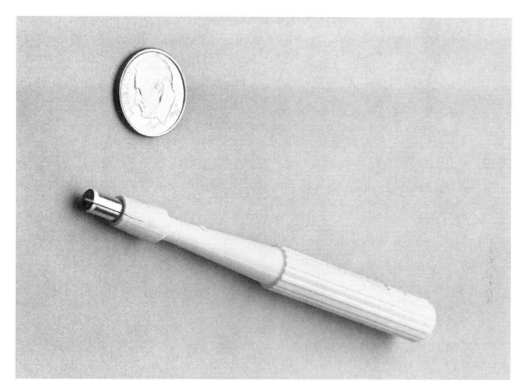

FIGURE 21-13. A Baker's punch for skin biopsy.

1990s. Using fine wire and needle electrodes to destroy or excise these lesions has been as effective as laser at a fraction of the cost. The important ingredient is understanding the comparison of spot size with lasers, or the area of electrode contact. When the two are equal in watts per square centimeter over time, the joules of energy cause the same effect.

OTHER VULVAR LESIONS

When in doubt, especially in asymmetric, pigmented lesions, excision is wise. For those under 7 mm in diameter a Baker's punch is swift and efficient (Fig. 21-13). After adequate local anesthesia is administered, the punch is rotated around the lesion 90° to the skin surface, drilling to a depth below the full dermis and then turning the punch parallel to the skin surface. The rotation of the punch will complete the biopsy. Some punches are disposable; as with disposable venipuncture needles, they are preferred. If a scalpel excision is necessary, elliptical incisions in the lines of Langer are best.

VAGINAL LESIONS

The need to remove a vaginal lesion is unusual, and should heavy bleeding occur it may be difficult to control. Fortunately, the paucity of nerve fiber in the vaginal canal allows the surgeon some leeway when a "quick" biopsy might be taken. The use of Hurricaine (benzocaine 20%) as a topical anesthetic that is rapidly absorbed by mucous membranes may be adequate by itself or as a prelude to the insertion of the anesthetic injection needle for the removal of large lesions. With the widespread use of loop electrosurgical excision procedure (LEEP) for cervical dysplasia biopsy and removal, small wire loops can make vaginal biopsies easy and swift.

CERVICAL PROCEDURES

The indications for cervical biopsy, cryosurgery, LEEP, and cervical cone biopsies are discussed in the chapter on colposcopy. All of these can be performed in the prepared office setting. For the cervical biopsy, Hurricaine ointment or spray is usually adequate anesthesia for direct biopsies. The colposcopic punch biopsy instruments need periodic maintenance because they dull easily with repeated use. After the biopsy is taken, silver nitrate or tannic acid solution, such as Monsel's solution or paste, is adequate in most cases. For persistent bleeding simple pressure packing may stop the bleeding, especially if the pack or pledget is soaked in a 1:1000 dilution of adrenalin, commonly used for bleeding nares. When all else fails, electro-surgical fulguration can be used.

If cryosurgery is chosen, the freezing procedure will create some of its own anesthetic effect, but cramping is common. With all cervical proce-dures, the preprocedural use of antiprostaglandin agents is helpful. The cryogenic application should establish an "ice ball" that extends about 5 mm beyond the edge of the cryogenic probe. Because of the radiator effect of the vascular bed in the cervix, the extent of the frozen tissue is limited. Cell death usually occurs 1 minute after the ice ball forms.

Loop Electrosurgical Excision Procedure

For use as biopsy tools in dermatology and gynecology, wire electrodes have been available for almost half a century. In gynecology, these loops have been used for cervical and "hot cone" biopsies. After such biopsies, anecdotal case histories of severe scarring, probably caused by high-voltage spark gap generators, led gynecologists to choose nonelectric methods of cervical biopsy by the 1950s. Although the rate was unclear, infertility after hot cone cervical biopsy occurred because of cervical stenosis. Today, a renewed interest in electrosurgical wire loop biopsy has surfaced in the form of loop electrosurgical excision process (LEEP) and large loop excision of transformation zone (LLETZ). As an outpatient procedure, LEEP or LLETZ surgery offers a one-time approach to a pesky problem plus an adequate and complete biopsy specimen. Made popular by British and French gynecologists, this excisional approach to cervical dysplasia gives a histologic confirmation of the entire lesion treated, unlike the random approach of colposcopic-directed biopsy followed by cryosurgery or laser ablation. To date, the long-term results after cervical healing are not available. No publication has evaluated different electrode loops matched with different electrogenerators or explored their thermal effect on the tissue left behind—the remaining, viable cervix.

Local infiltration of anesthesia is usually sufficient rather than a paracervical block. Using a 25-gauge needle a submucosal injection of 1 ml into the cervix at 2, 4, 8, and 10 o'clock for a total of 4 ml is enough. Some choose an agent with a vasoconstrictor, but with the proper electrosurgical settings it is not necessary.

Techniques for LEEP procedures. Performing LEEP procedures is a complete exercise in the applied principles of electrosurgery. The following features of LEEP procedures should be appreciated.

Electrode size. The thinner the wire, the higher the power density, giving a better cutting effect. Electrode wires thicker than 0.20 mm in diameter can cause deep coagulation up to a 10-mm depth depending on speed of excision and waveform.

Waveform. There is an increasing depth of coagulation as the waveform is blended from a pure, undamped waveform to a 50:50 ratio of undamped to damped waveform.

Power density. Besides the diameter or gauge of the wire used, the size and depth of the biopsy must be considered. As the electrode loop sinks deeper into the cervical tissue, the power density, as measured by the length and total surface area of wire loop penetrating the cervical tissue, decreases rapidly, losing the cutting effect created by a high-power density. To compensate for this change, one must increase the power output from the generator during the incision process or increase the speed of the electrode incision process. If the power output is adequate (usually at 60 W) but the loop is passed through the tissue at a slow pace, deep coagulation of the cervix may occur. When possible, it is preferable to use a generator with a low-output impedance because this keeps the energy fluctuations created by different tissue densities to a minimum.

Speed of incision. It is easier to increase the speed of incision than to manually adjust the generator with one hand as one presses the loop into, through, and then out of the area to be biopsied with the other hand. However, the loop wire should be rigid; a loop that bends or flexes reduces the speed of incision, leading to deep coagulation even when one uses a cut waveform. It appears that tungsten wire, because of its rigid characteristics (especially at higher temperatures), is preferred over stainless steel wire unless the yoke of the loop electrode handle can be shaped such that the stainless steel wire remains rigid (Fig. 21-14). Several new generators have been designed that are especially helpful in LEEP procedures. They control the flow of energy through a low-impedance feedback by controlling

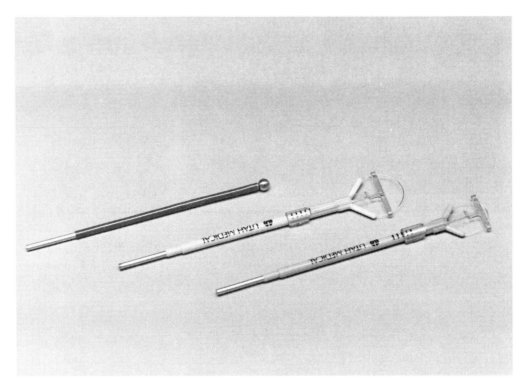

FIGURE 21-14. A fulgurating ball electrode and LEEP loops with depth gauge for the control of the depth of the biopsy. The gauge also makes the wire rigid for a better cutting effect.

voltage; the effect is similar to a speed-control device in an automobile. If a constant voltage can be maintained at a given power setting, which is variable as tissue resistance changes, lateral thermal damage is controlled, giving the surgeon a predetermined surgical effect. Using constant voltage controls the depth of coagulation independent of the cutting rate.

Other features. Because the vaginal fluids are rich in electrolytes, the vagina and cervix should be rinsed with a nonelectrolytic fluid before biopsy; the acetic acid solution used during colposcopy is adequate. The generator should be activated *before* the electrode touches the tissue, and the energy should be delivered in a continuous mode until the biopsy is complete. If, during the excisional biopsy, one turns the energy off, deep coagulation will occur during the restartup phase.

Care should be taken not to touch the metal speculum with the active electrode. Because the surface area of the metal speculum (in contact with the patient) is large, the current density is too low to cause a burn, but the effective frequency of the radio wave delivered through the speculum will be altered to a much lower frequency, which may stimulate involuntary muscle contractions of the patient. This will not be painful, but it will startle and be disconcerting to both patient and operator. The use of an insulated metal speculum is preferable.

It is better to cut and excise with minimal coagulation during the biopsy process and then use fulguration, not desiccation, to control spot bleeding. Because the power density of one spark is the same regardless of wattage used, using a high wattage, thus a big spark (at least 70 W in coag mode), makes it easier to keep from touching the tissue. Use a large ball electrode held close to yet off the bleeding site and switch to a damped (coag) waveform with high-voltage output. Should the operative field be obscured with electrolyte-rich blood, reduce the amount of blood with suction during the fulguration process. As an alternative, a slow irrigation with a nonelectrolytic solution (e.g., sterile or distilled water) will also allow effective spot fulguration with the ball electrode. Because water is a nonelectrolytic solution, the fulguration phenomenon is more precise if the oozing surface of the biopsy site is irrigated with water rather than a saline solution because the sparks will seek out the blood leaving the open blood vessel. Once fulguration is complete, the procedure is complete. Some physicians choose to apply Monsel's paste for extra security against postoperative bleeding.

Again, with LEEP or LLETZ procedures it is best to use a rigid loop electrode with a steady pace of transfer through the tissue to be biopsied. Choose an undamped waveform with minimal if any damped characteristics. A pure, undamped waveform delivered through an electrode transecting tissue at a slower rate will create some coagulation effect, which is a better choice than a partially damped waveform passed through a loop electrode that may stall because of inadequate power as it tries to pass through the cervical tissue.

When it is technically feasible, start the excisional sweep from bottom up rather than side to side. This allows the electrolyte-rich blood to flow away from the traveling electrode loop, and if the surgeon slips at the completed transection, the loop will hit the speculum rather than the vaginal wall. The same excisional maneuver should be used for the second excision of the endocervical canal (the LEEP cone biopsy), but because the size of the smaller loop increases the power density, the power should be reduced. For the large loop excisions, a setting of 60 W in pure cutting or blend gives the best results. For the endocervical biopsy loops, the power should be reduce to 30 to 40 W.

ENDOMETRIAL BIOPSY

Although there are many reusable metal curettes available for strip biopsy of the endometrial cavity, the use of suction cannulas or pipelles has a special benefit (Fig. 21-15). Besides being inexpensive and disposable, the suction offers a more complete sampling of the uterine cavity, provided the

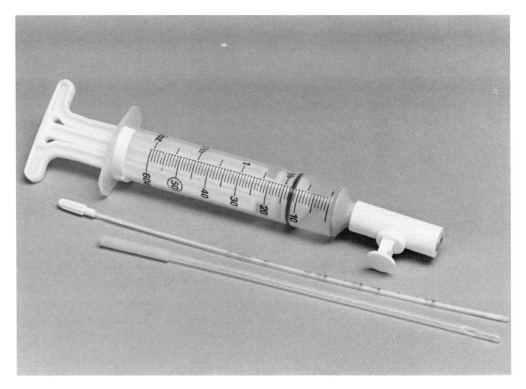

FIGURE 21-15. A suction syringe (IPAS, Caroboro, N.C.), a pipelle for endometrial suction biopsy, and a 4-mm suction cannula.

diameter of the suction cannula is not too small. In the postmenopausal patient in whom a relative cervical stenosis may be present, a 2- to 3-mm pipelle is preferred and may not require any local anesthesia. If the tissue received is only blood, it does not rule out an occult malignancy. If the tissue is scant or nonexistent and unexplained bleeding reoccurs, hysteroscopy should be performed. For those who are of menstrual age, a 4- or 5-mm cannula can be inserted without dilation, providing a generous biopsy of the endometrial tissue. The suction syringe is an excellent source of suction and is reusable for at least 20 to 30 procedures.

DILATION AND CURETTAGE

A paracervical-block anesthesia is necessary to perform a thorough curettage. The suction syringe can be used with suction cannulas up to 13 mm in size; it eliminates the need for an electric suction pump, is silent, and is easier to clean. Denniston dilators are nylon dilators that are reusable, autoclavable, inexpensive (about 50 dollars), and if needed allow one to dilate up to 12 mm (Fig. 21-16). The diameter is graduated or tapered along the shaft at a rate of 1 mm per 3 cm, which promotes efficiency in dilation yet prevents deep penetration unless excessive pressure is used.

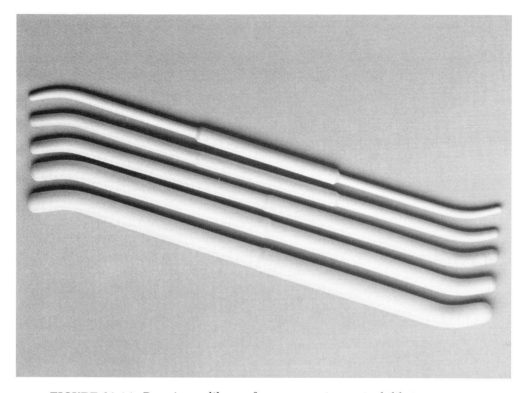

FIGURE 21-16. Denniston dilators for atraumatic cervical dilation.

There is little evidence that a therapeutic D & C is of any value. Except for the management of an incomplete or intentional abortion, the hysteroscope is preferable.

DIAGNOSTIC HYSTEROSCOPY

The deterrents to providing office hysteroscopy are the capital expense, lack of reimbursement for costs of materials by many third-party carriers, and a misconception that dilation of the cervix under paracervical block is difficult. Tables 21-1 and 21-2 list the equipment needed and the cost. If one realizes that the standard diagnostic hysteroscope and sheath has an outside diameter equal to that of the Progestasert intrauterine device, it becomes obvious that cervical dilation is not a problem. The Denniston dilator, 5 to 6 mm, is adequate if needed for dilation.

The indications for office hysteroscopy are listed in Table 21-3. It should be emphasized that for abnormal uterine bleeding, hysteroscopy should be reserved for patients for whom medical management has not been helpful. The ability to see and treat when medical therapy fails makes more sense than blindly curetting a cavity, usually in an incomplete fashion. It takes about 10 cases of diagnostic hysteroscopy to become proficient. Practicing

TABLE 21-1.   Office hysteroscopy instruments

Small, portable light source
Carbon dioxide insufflator, Hyskon, or continuous-flow office system
Video camera, tape recorder, and monitor (optional)
3-4 mm rigid hysteroscope (30-degree lens)
4-5 diagnostic sheath
Operating sheath
Deflecting bridge
Flexible biopsy forceps
Flexible scissors
Side-open speculum
Tenaculum
Paracervical block tray
Endometrial suction apparatus

TABLE 21-2.   Office hysteroscopy equipment—costs

Equipment	Cost
BASIC EQUIPMENT	
Telescope, 30-degree, wide-angle view	$2800
Hysteroscopy diagnostic sheath, 5 mm	$540
Hysteroinsufflator, CO_2	$1900
Light guide cable	$400
Light source	$700
Total	$6,340
Lease for 3 yr	$210/mo
OPERATING ACCESSORIES	
Operating sheath	$550
Deflecting bridge	$550
Flexible biopsy forceps	$350
Flexible scissors	$350
Total	$1,800
Lease for 3 yr	$55/mo
VIDEO EQUIPMENT	
Video camera	$3,700
Video coupler	$900
Video monitor	$1,200
Tape deck (8 mm)	$500
Total	$6,300
Lease for 3 yr	$210/mo
COMBINED COSTS	
Total cost	$14,400
Total lease package	$475/mo

TABLE 21-3. Indications for office hysteroscopy

Abnormal bleeding resistant to hormonal management
Directed biopsy rather than blind curettage
Removal of small, pedunculated intrauterine lesions (e.g., polyps)
Removal of foreign objects (e.g., intrauterine device, ossified products of conception, pieces of laminaria, suction catheter tips)
Infertility secondary to intrauterine pathology or congenital malformation

this skill in the operating room before a hysterectomy or laparoscopic sterilization procedure takes only a few extra minutes.

For diagnostic hysteroscopy, there are only two contraindications: the presence of active pelvic inflammatory disease and an intrauterine pregnancy. Operative procedures, such as the transection of uterine septae, resection of large myomas, endometrial ablations, and tubal canalization, are best reserved for the surgical theater. At present, all hysteroscopic sterilization techniques are considered investigational and fall under the scrutiny of the Food and Drug Administration.

For distention, CO_2, high-molecular-weight dextran (Hyskon), or continuous flow fluids is preferred. The initial expense of CO_2 equipment specifically designed for hysteroscopy and the messy characteristics of dextran have encouraged several instrument companies to develop continuous-flow diagnostic hysteroscopic systems (Fig. 21-17). With the aid of a self-contained, disposable inflow/outflow system, good visualization is easily accomplished without the frustration of bubbles so commonly confronted with CO_2, and the cost of the setup is half that of Hyskon.

Under direct vision, the hysteroscope is inserted into the cervical os; the distention medium acts as its own dilator to help lead the way. Most prefer a 30-degree lens so a more panoramic view can be obtain with the rigid lens system. By rotating the lens each cornu of the uterus is easily seen. Flexible hysteroscopes make cornual visualization even easier, but the ability to use accessory instruments is limited to small, flexible tools.

The use of the operating channel for office hysteroscopy increases the outside diameter of the hysteroscope sheath by several millimeters. Still, most patients under paracervical block anesthesia can be dilated beyond the largest office hysteroscope sheath. The larger the outside diameter of the operating sheath the larger the scissors, grasper, or biopsy forceps one can use, which is frequently desirable to receive adequate tissue. An even simpler approach is to see the lesion, remember its location, and blindly extract it with standard ovum or polyp forceps. Of course, the standard suction evacuation equipment can be used after one completes the diagnostic hysteroscopy. When excess blood obscures the view, irrigate

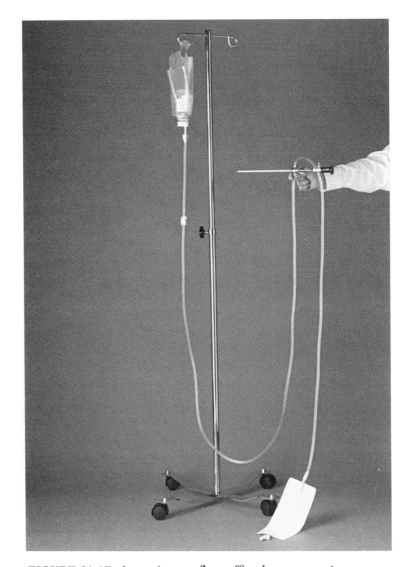

FIGURE 21-17. A continuous-flow office hysteroscopic system.

Courtesy CIRCON-ACMI, Stamford, Conn.

with saline, or aspirate with a 4-mm catheter when using CO_2 for distention.

Several suggestions for patient preparation should be considered. When possible, schedule during the proliferative phase. Administer a nonsteroidal antiinflamatory agent 1 hour before the procedure, or inject Toradol (30 mg) 30 minutes before the procedure. Inject 1% Carbocaine (plain) or 0.25% Marcaine (1 ml) in the anterior exocervix (tenaculum site) and 4 ml in each of four areas adjacent to the cervix, at 2, 4, 8, and 10 o'clock, approximately 3 to 5 mm deep. An alternative is to deposit 10 ml at 4 and 8 o'clock.

FUTURE OFFICE PROCEDURES

With LEEP cone procedures now possible in an office setting, for selected patients, shallow-cylinder cone biopsy using a Fleming cold cone knife is being evaluated. This will reduce the risk of excessive heat destruction of the endocervical canal caused by the smaller, endocervical LEEP loop. As new fiberoptic telescopes are perfected, the size of laparoscopes can be reduced without sacrificing light illumination. At present, researchers are evaluating the success of office laparoscopy for diagnosis and female sterilization. These scopes have an outside diameter between 2 and 3 mm, are semirigid, and can be used with state-of-the-art television cameras.

GLOSSARY

blend Term used when the electric current is interrupted between 20% and 50% of the time.

coag Term used to describe an interrupted electric current. In some generators, the period of interruption of current flow can be adjusted from 10% on to 50% on. At the same power settings, the voltage of the waveform is always higher than with cut.

collimation An organized emission of light energy waves, each synchronized and tightly grouped in the same direction and at the same amplitude.

cut Term used when referring to a continuous or undamped electric current. At the same power settings, the voltage of the waveform is always lower than with coag or blend.

desiccation The act of coagulating tissue *after* making contact with an active electrode. Either cut or coag may be used, but cut is preferable. Intracellular temperature stays below 100°C, which leads to cell shrinkage and dehydration.

electricity Movement of electrons between two oppositely charged poles, positive and negative.

electrocautery Transfer of energy by heat, such as a hot wire. Electrons do not move into the affected tissue; only heat is transferred.

electrosurgery The transfer of energy from an electrosurgical generator to tissue by means of energy packets (electrons).

energy (joules) Quantity of work produced over time. Energy (joules, J) = work (watts, W) × time (seconds).

faradic effect The electric stimulation of muscle responding to a frequency of electric current that is below 100,000 cycles per second.

fulguration The intentional application of sparks to tissue surface to coagulate surface bleeding. The coag waveform is preferable.

heat (thermal energy) Produced as electrons move from the low resistance of an electrosurgical probe to the high resistance of tissue. This energy may boil (vaporize) or denature (coagulate) tissue, depending on the extent and rapidity with which heat is generated.

impedance (ohms) Resistance to flow of electrons through a conductor. Although resistance refers to direct current through a uniform wire, such as copper, it is generally substituted for impedance. Impedance is correctly applied with changes in voltage (alternating or fluctuating), frequency (modulating, demodulating), or tissue type (lipid membranes, soft tissue, fibrous tissue, fat, muscle, bone, artificial appliances). It can measure the combination of tissue resistance and capacitance. Impedance in human tissue is generally 100 to 1000 Ω, and in the fallopian tube it is 400 to 500 Ω.

isolation ground circuity Safety feature using transformers that are not in contact with the parent generator such that the induced electrical flow "floats" in its own separate circuit. Should a break in the floating circuit occur, all energy within that circuit stops and does not seek ground.

laser Acronym that stands for light amplification by stimulated emission of radiation.

monopolar An electrode or electric system in which the active electrode is small (high current density) and the passive electrode is large (low current density). Most monopolar generators are calibrated against a 500-Ω load of resistance.

open circuit State in which a generator is activated before the active electrode touches tissue. This promotes higher voltage, especially in the coag mode, than activating the generator after touching the tissue. Open circuitry is used to start fulguration.

patient return electrode (grounding pad) A large pad (low current density) placed on the patient to complete an electrosurgical pathway.

power density The surface area of an electrode (or spot of a laser beam) in contact with tissue during energy flow. The *smaller* the spot of contact, the *greater* the heat effect for the same amount of time, increasing by the square root of the area of contact.

return electrode monitoring Dual-padded patient return electrode system designed to monitor irregular separation of the ground pad.

sparking (arcing, fulguration) The result of electric flow through gas (air, argon).

spot size The area of tissue affected by the delivery of either laser or electrosurgical energy.

vaporize To rapidly raise the cellular temperature above 100°C, which causes cell rupture and releases steam.

voltage (volts) The force (pressure) driving current.

watts (work) The amount of work produced by electron flow (current). Work (watts, W) = force (volts, V) × current rate (amperes, A).

waveform The oscillation characteristic of an alternating electric current from positive to negative.

waveform frequency The number of oscillations of an alternating electric current, usually between 350,000 and 4 million cycles per second in electrosurgery.

BIBLIOGRAPHY

Brooks PG: Hysteroscopic findings after unsuccessful D and C for abnormal uterine bleeding, *Am J Obstet Gynecol* 158:1354, 1988.

Daniel AG, Peters WA: Accuracy of office and operating room curettage in the grading of endometrial carcinoma, *Obstet Gynecol* 71:612, 1988.

Darney PD: *Handbook of office and ambulatory gynecologic surgery*, Oradell, NJ, 1987, Medical Economics Books.

Filmar S, Jetha N, McComb P, Gomel V: A comparative histologic study on the healing process after tissue transaction. I. Carbon dioxide laser and electromicrosurgery, *Am J Obstet Gynecol* 160:1062, 1989.

Gimpelson RJ: Comparison of accuracy of diagnostic D and C vs hysteroscopic biopsy, *Am J Obstet Gynecol* 158:489, 1988.

Gomel V, Taylor, PJ, Yuzpe AA, Rioux JE et al: *Laparoscopy and hysteroscopy in gynecologic practice*, Chicago, 1986, Year Book.

Grimes DA: Diagnostic dilation and curretage: a reappraisal, *Am J Obstet Gynecol* 142:1, 1982.

Larson DM, Johnson KK, Broste SK, et al: Comparison of D & C and office endometrial biopsy in predicting final histopathologic grade in endometrial cancer, *Obstet Gynecol* 86:38, 1995.

Luciano AA, Frishman GN, Kratka SA, Maier DB: A comparative analysis of adhesion reduction, tissue effects, and incising characteristics of electrosurgery, CO_2 laser, and Nd-Yag laser at operative laparoscopy, *J Laparoendoscopy* 2:305, 1993.

Luciano AA, Whitman GF, Maier DB, et al: A comparison of thermal injury, healing patterns and postoperative adhesion formation following CO_2 laser and electromicrosurgery, *Fertil Steril* 48:1025, 1987.

Odell RC: Biophysics of electrical energy. In Soderstrom RM, editor: *Operative laparoscopy: the master's techniques*, New York, 1993, Raven Press.

Pearce JA: *Electrosurgery*, London, 1986, Chapman and Hall.

Reich H, Vancaillie TG, Soderstrom RM: Electrical techniques. In Martin DC, editor: *Manual of endoscopy*, Baltimore, 1990, Port City Press.

Rodriguez GC, Yaqub N, King ME, A comparison of the Pipelle device and the Vabra aspirator as measured by endometrial denudation in hysterectomy specimens. *Am J Obstet Gynecol* 168:55, 1993.

Index

A

Abdomen, examination of, 32, 414, 415f
Abortion, 87-88, 191
    and abnormal bleeding, 436
    incomplete, 190, 568
    induced, 336, 338
    septic, Dalkon Shield and, 74
    spontaneous, 29, 77, 149, 470, 491
Abscess; *see also* Pelvic inflammatory disease
    Bartholin's and Skene's ducts, 279-281, 279f,
        280f, 581, 582f
    tuboovarian, 347, 349, 350t, 352
Accounting software, 9
Acetic acid, 337
Acne, 59, 72, 413
Actinomyces, 362t, 364, 365t
Acupressure/acupuncture, 202-203
Acute grief syndrome, 39-40
Acute salpingitis, 348
Acyclovir, 291
Adenocarcinoma of cervix, 381, 383-384
Adenomyosis, 200
Adhesions, 200, 204-205, 207
Adnexa
    in amenorrhea, 415-416
    pelvic masses, 479t
    in pelvic pain syndrome, 208
    twisted, 190
Adolescent patient
    mammography, 239
    with PID, 350
    sexual abuse, 97
    sexual activity and contraceptive use, 44-45, 46f
Adrenal androgens, 397t, 399
Adrenal hormones
    in amenorrhea, primary, 395t, 397t, 399
    fertility workup, female, 509
    oral contraceptives and, 58
Adrenarche, 390
α-Adrenergic agents, 552t, 553t, 556
Adrenocorticotropic hormone (ACTH), 154, 397t,
    398
Age
    and assisted reproductive technology outcomes,
        516, 517, 517f
    and breast cancer, 239, 255-256, 261, 264
    and infertility, 489, 490-491
    normal menstrual cycle, 386
    and oral contraceptive risk, 54, 55t, 56
    and urinary incontinence, 536-537
Agitated depression, 40-41
Alcohol-drug use, 41
    and bone density, 166
    and domestic violence, 105
    history taking, 29
    and infertility, 492
    and menopause, 153, 154

Alcohol-drug use—cont'd
    and PMS, 216
    and sexual response, 107, 108, 109
Alcohol injection, vulvar disorders, 303, 304f
Allen-Masters syndrome, 205
Alprazolam, 219
Ambiguous genitalia, 140-141
Amenorrhea, primary, 390-412
    breast development negative, 399-404, 400t,
        402f, 403f, 408-409, 410f
    breast development positive, 404-409, 405f,
        406t, 407f, 408f, 409f, 410-412, 411f, 412f,
        412t
    causes of, 390-393, 391f, 392f, 393f, 394-396t
    Depo-Provera, fetal masculinization with, 69
    diagnostic tests, 397-399, 397t
    evaluation, 393, 396-399
Amenorrhea, secondary, 413-426
    danazol and, 464
    definition, 387
    with Depo-Provera, 66-67, 67f
    history, 413-414
    hypothalamus/pituitary compartment, 416-420,
        417f, 418t, 419f, 421t
    normal menstrual function, 388, 389f, 390
    with Norplant, 71, 72f
    oral contraceptive side effects, 64
    ovarian compartment, 420-422, 423t
    physical examination, 414-416
    uterovaginal compartment, 423-426, 424, 425t,
        426t
E-Aminocaproic acid, 450
Amitriptyline, 210, 561
Amoxicillin, 337, 353
Ampicillin, 337, 353
Anabolic steroids, 171
Anatomy
    breast, 230-235, 231f, 232f
    pediatric patient, 119-123, 120f, 121f, 122f
    pelvic support, 523-525, 524f, 526f
Androgen insensitivity, 395t, 407
Androgenization
    hair growth patterns, 31, 32
    with norgestimate and desogestrel, 59, 60
Androgens, 154, 157; *see also* Testosterone
    in amenorrhea, primary, 395t, 397t, 399, 404
    labial agglutination, 140-142, 142f
    male fertility workup, 505
    menopause and, 149-150, 151f, 177-178
3α-Androstanediol glucuronide, 397t, 399
Androstenedione, 154
Anesthesia
    for hysteroscopy, 592
    outpatient, 567-570, 569f
Angiography, pelvic masses, 482
Annual checkup, 34-41
Anorchia, 395t, 403-404, 404t, 409